THE BIG PICTURE

MEDICAL MICROBIOLOGY

THE BIG PICTURE

MEDICAL MICROBIOLOGY

Neal R. Chamberlain, PhD

Associate Professor
Department of Microbiology and Immunology
A. T. Still University of Health Sciences
Kirksville, Missouri

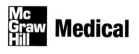 **Medical**

New York   Chicago   San Francisco   Lisbon   London   Madrid   Mexico City
Milan   New Delhi   San Juan   Seoul   Singapore   Sydney   Toronto

Big Picture Book: Medical Microbiology

Copyright © 2009 by The McGraw-Hill Companies, Inc. All rights reserved. Printed in China. Except as permitted under the United States copyright Act of 1976, no part of this publication may be reproduced or distributed in any form or by any means, or stored in a data base or retrieval system, without the prior written permission of the publisher.

1 2 3 4 5 6 7 8 9 0 CTPCTP 0 9 8

ISBN 978-0-07-147661-4
MHID 0-07-147661-X

This book was set in Minion by Aptara, Inc.   .
The editors were Susan Kelly, Michael Weitz and Karen Davis.
The production supervisor was Phil Galea.
Project management was provided by Sandhya Joshi, Aptara, Inc.
The text designer was Alan Barnett
The cover designer was Alan Barnett and Elizabeth Pisacreta .
Cover image caption: Macrophage engulfing tuberculosis vaccine. Colored scanning electron micrograph (SEM) of a macrophage white blood cell engulfing (red) *Mycobacterium bovis* bacteria (blue). This is the BCG (bacillus of Calmette-Guerin) strain of the bacteria, used in the vaccination for tuberculosis (TB). The bacteria is live but attenuated (weakened). The macrophage engulfs (phagocytoses) the bacteria and destroys them. The vaccine primes the immune system, without causing disease, so that it responds more rapidly if infected with TB bacteria. Magnification: ×3,500 when printed 10 centimeters tall.
Credit: SPL / Photo Researchers, Inc.
China Translation & Printing Service, Ltd., was the printer and binder.

This book is printed on acid-free paper.

Library of Congress Cataloging-in-Publication Data

Chamberlain, Neal R.
   Medical microbiology & immunology : the big picture / by Neal R.
Chamberlain.
         p. ; cm.
   Includes index.
   ISBN 978-0-07-147661-4 (soft cover : alk. paper) 1. Medical microbiology—Outlines, syllabi, etc. 2. Medical microbiology—Examinations, questions, etc. 3. Immunology—Outlines, syllabi, etc. 4. Immunology—Examinations, questions, etc. I. Title. II. Title: Medical microbiology and immunology.
   [DNLM: 1. Communicable Diseases—microbiology—Examination Questions. 2. Communicable Diseases—virology—Examination Questions. 3. Communicable Diseases—diagnosis—Examination Questions. 4. Immune System—Examination Questions. WC 18.2 C443m 2008]
   QR46 . C44 2008
   616 . 9'041—dc22
                                                                2008008352

International Edition:
ISBN 978-0-07-128728-9
MHID 0-07-128728-0
Copyright © 2009. Exclusive rights by The McGraw-Hill Companies, Inc., for manufacture and export. This book cannot be re-exported from the country to which it is consigned by McGraw-Hill. The International Edition is not available in North America.

DEDICATION

To my loving wife, wonderful children, and to the one who gave up everything
so that I might live this dream.

—*Neal Chamberlain*

CONTENTS

PREFACE

Patients don't walk into their physician's office and say, "I think I have typical pneumonia due to *Streptococcus pneumoniae*." Instead, patients describe their symptoms and how they feel. Physicians then complete a physical examination and draw upon their knowledge about pneumonia and the likely causes of the disease to develop a treatment plan. In other words, physicians must recognize disease and then determine causes.

Most microbiology professors don't live in a clinical world. Microbiologists know a lot about the microorganisms that cause human disease, and they go into great detail talking about them. They will then briefly tell you what diseases these pathogens cause. You then learn all these microbial characteristics and organize them by bacterial shape and Gram stain, viral family, fungal classification, or parasitic class, leaving the diseases to hang at the end of each microbial knowledge set.

This approach to teaching medical microbiology creates a dilemma when an attending physician says to his student physicians, "Dr. Chamberlain's chest radiograph indicates that he has pneumonia. Tell me the most common cause of typical pneumonia in this middle-aged male?" The way you learned microbiology requires that you recall a catalog of organism by organism to see which ones cause pneumonia. This takes several minutes and before you can answer, your attending says, "Don't you know that bacteria are the most likely cause of typical pneumonia and that the most common cause of this pneumonia is *Streptococcus pneumoniae*?" You walk away saying to yourself, "How did my attending get the answer so quick?" What the attending physician did was relearn medical microbiology. Instead of learning the microorganisms and recalling the diseases they cause, this physician learned how to identify a disease and then created lists of the microorganisms that caused that disease.

In the past, this reorienting of the students' medical microbiology knowledge was occurring while medical students were completing their clinical rotations. Unfortunately, case-based questions on USMLE and COMLEX, clinically oriented medical school course work, and recently revised medical school curricula require most medical students to reorient or organize their microbiology knowledge in a clinically relevant way even before they begin their clinical years. *The Big Picture Medical Microbiology* book was written to help you reorient or obtain medical microbiology knowledge in a clinically oriented way and to help you in your clinical rotations.

ORGANIZATION OF THE BOOK

- *The parade of microorganisms does not exist in this book.* This book is organized by organ systems and the infectious diseases caused by microorganisms in that particular system.

- The first chapter in each section presents a "Big Picture" overview that explains the organization of the organ system, some immunologic responses that the system uses to ward off infection, and the diseases as well as the common causes of the diseases that are discussed in chapters that follow within each section. Information in each chapter is discussed using similar headings of etiology, manifestations, epidemiology, pathogenesis, diagnosis, and therapy and prevention.

- About 280 color images are included to help you visualize many of the diseases; some of the images illustrate the results of laboratory tests that are used to identify certain pathogens.

- About 120 tables compare and contrast the various types of a particular disease, summarize the signs and symptoms of a disease, and quickly compare the causes of a disease.

- The last section of the book contains 100 case-based examination questions. Over 30 of the questions contain an image that is necessary for you to examine to correctly answer the question. The questions are in random order to better simulate actual board-type examinations.

- The Appendix contains 19 summary tables and 2 flow charts, which contain a variety of information about microorganisms that will help refresh your memory.

I hope you find this book helpful while studying for your medical school courses and examinations, when preparing to talk with attending physicians about patients in your clinics, and when preparing for USMLE and COMLEX.

—*Neal Chamberlain*

ACKNOWLEDGMENTS

I thank my father for advice he gave me when I was in college and was anxious about what I should do for a living. He said, "Son, do what you want to do, not what you have to do." Writing this book was something I have dreamed about for a long time. His words stayed with me and helped me through the times when I got stuck looking at a blank page.

I also thank Susan Kelly for all of her hard work as my editor. Her eye for detail, her expertise, and her problem-solving ability were essential to the successful completion of the book.

Thank you to Andi Lynch, a former graduate student and current medical student, class of 2008, who reviewed every chapter and provided invaluable comments while I continued to write and revise the manuscript.

My thanks go to Scott Anderson, DO, and my medical students for helping me reorient the ATSU infectious disease course to make it more useful in the clinics.

Lastly, I thank Gary Schilt, Robert Shaffer, and James Rider for many helpful discussions and suggestions while I was dreaming and thinking about how to write this book.

—*Neal Chamberlain*

SECTION 1

INTEGUMENT AND SOFT TISSUES

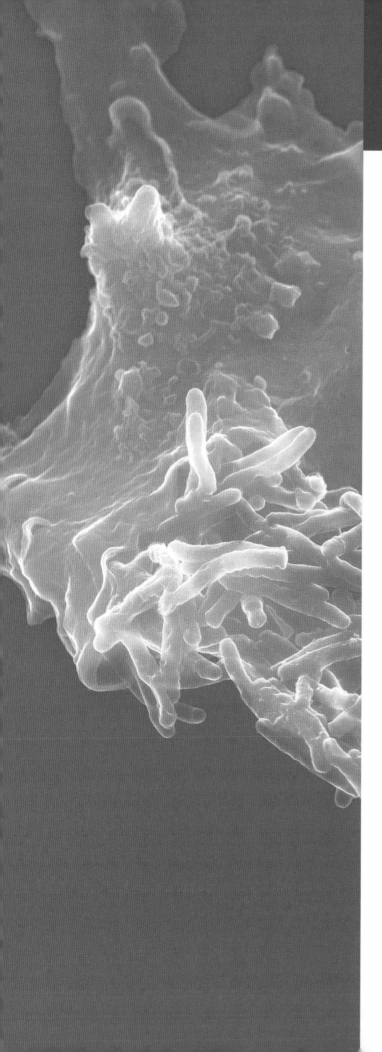

CHAPTER 1

THE BIG PICTURE: INFECTIONS OF THE INTEGUMENT AND SOFT TISSUES

OVERVIEW

The skin, the mucous membranes (e.g., gastrointestinal, respiratory, and urogenital tracts), and other membranous surfaces (e.g., eye) form a barrier that protects the body daily from microbial infections. The skin is the largest of these barriers and is the largest organ of the body. It provides a physical, chemical, and mechanical barrier that protects the body from dehydration, helps maintain proper body temperature, and protects the body from infectious agents.

The skin consists of two layers, the epidermis and the dermis. The epidermis consists of an outer layer of cornified keratinocytes called the stratum corneum. The most common fungal infections of the skin, the dermatophytic infections (e.g., tinea [ringworm]), are seen on and in this layer.

The dermis is composed of dense connective tissue with many white collagenous and elastic fibers. It is much thicker than the epidermis and contains many blood vessels, nerve endings, sebaceous glands, and hair follicles. Furuncles, carbuncles, and erysipelas are examples of diseases that can penetrate this region of the skin following a break in the protective epidermis.

HOW THE SKIN PREVENTS MICROBIAL INFECTIONS

The arid nature of skin prevents many microorganisms from colonizing on it (e.g., gram-negative bacteria). The continuous sloughing off of keratinocytes from the surface of the epidermis does not allow colonizers to overgrow and cause disease. The keratinocytes also provide a waterproof barrier that prevents entry of infectious agents into the body.

The sebaceous glands and the sweat glands secrete substances that inhibit the growth of many organisms. Sebaceous glands in the dermis secrete sebum, which contains a variety of fatty acids and lactic acid. Fatty acids kill most gram-positive bacteria and gram-negative cocci (e.g., *Neisseria* sp.). Lactic acid in the sebum reduces the pH of the skin surface and inhibits the growth of many microorganisms. The sweat glands secrete a

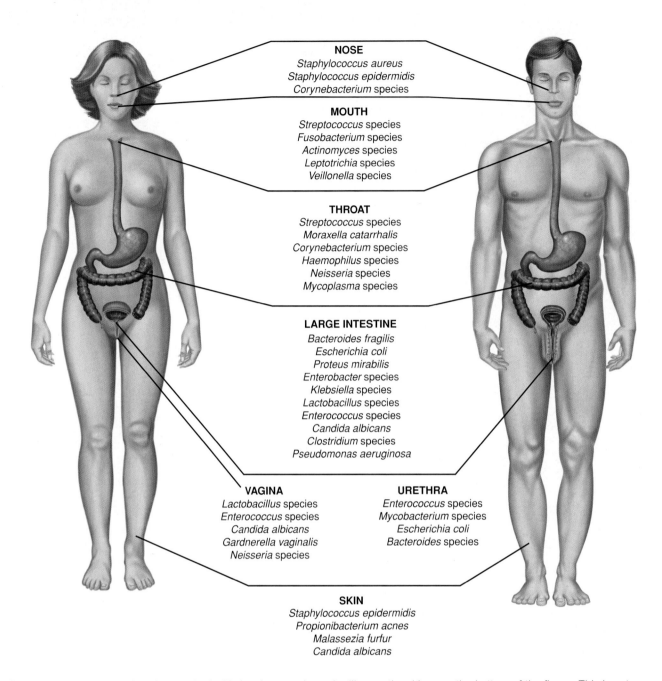

NOSE
Staphylococcus aureus
Staphylococcus epidermidis
Corynebacterium species

MOUTH
Streptococcus species
Fusobacterium species
Actinomyces species
Leptotrichia species
Veillonella species

THROAT
Streptococcus species
Moraxella catarrhalis
Corynebacterium species
Haemophilus species
Neisseria species
Mycoplasma species

LARGE INTESTINE
Bacteroides fragilis
Escherichia coli
Proteus mirabilis
Enterobacter species
Klebsiella species
Lactobacillus species
Enterococcus species
Candida albicans
Clostridium species
Pseudomonas aeruginosa

VAGINA
Lactobacillus species
Enterococcus species
Candida albicans
Gardnerella vaginalis
Neisseria species

URETHRA
Enterococcus species
Mycobacterium species
Escherichia coli
Bacteroides species

SKIN
Staphylococcus epidermidis
Propionibacterium acnes
Malassezia furfur
Candida albicans

Figure 1-1. Normal flora of the human body. Notice the organisms dwelling on the skin near the bottom of the figure. This is not a comprehensive list but rather the common normal flora organisms.

substance that contains lysozyme and high concentrations of sodium chloride. Lysozyme can catalyze the degradation of bacterial cell walls of certain bacteria, and the high content of sodium chloride in sweat can inhibit the growth of many bacteria. Skin secretions also contain microcidal peptides called beta defensins, which kill microorganisms by disrupting their membranes.

NORMAL FLORA OF THE SKIN

In spite of being a hostile residence for microorganisms, skin is still colonized by a number of microorganisms (Figure 1-1).

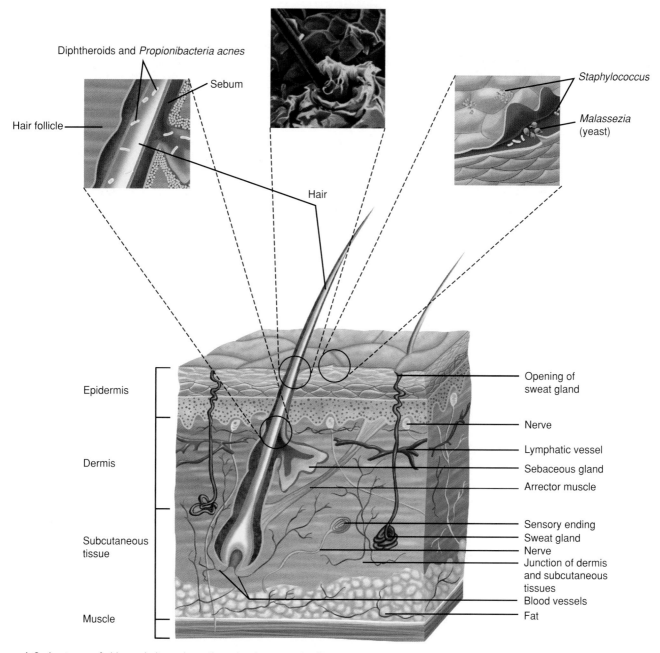

Figure 1-2. Anatomy of skin and sites where the microbes can dwell.

The normal flora (microbes) have the ability to prevent most pathogens from colonizing by preventing their attachment to the surface of the skin or by producing toxins that inhibit the growth of other microorganisms. Most microorganisms live in the superficial layers of the stratum corneum and in the upper parts of the hair follicles (Figure 1-2). Some areas of the skin are colonized more heavily than others (Figure 1-3). For example, moist areas such as the scalp, axilla, and perineum are more heavily colonized than drier areas such as the arms, legs, chest, and back.

Only a few microorganisms are capable of surviving in this hostile, moist environment. Gram-positive bacteria such as coagulase-negative *Staphylococcus*, *Corynebacterium*, and *Propionibacterium* are the most abundant colonizers of the skin.

Staphylococcus epidermidis is the most abundant inhabitant of the skin. *Candida* and *Malassezia* are the fungi that are commonly found colonizing the skin surface. Gram-negative bacilli such as *Enterobacter, Pseudomonas, Klebsiella, Escherichia coli,* and *Proteus* only inhabit the moister regions of the skin.

COMMON BACTERIAL CAUSES OF SKIN INFECTIONS

The most common bacterial causes of skin infection are *Staphylococcus aureus, Streptococcus pyogenes,* and *Propionibacterium acne. S aureus* can cause bullous impetigo, folliculitis, furuncles, carbuncles, cellulitis, myositis, scalded skin syndrome, and toxic shock syndrome (TSS). Most of these staphylococcal diseases result from invasion and destruction of the skin. Scalded skin syndrome and TSS are examples of bacterial diseases due primarily to toxins such as exfoliative or epidermolytic toxins and TSS toxin, respectively.

S pyogenes can cause impetigo, scarlet fever, erysipelas, necrotizing fasciitis, and streptococcal TSS. Impetigo, erysipelas, and necrotizing fasciitis are caused by invasion or colonization of the skin, whereas scarlet fever and streptococcal TSS are primarily the result of toxin (streptococcal pyogenic exotoxin [SPE] or erythrogenic toxin) production. *Propionibacterium acne* colonizes the hair follicles and is important in contributing to the formation of acne.

COMMON VIRAL INFECTIONS

Oral and genital herpes are caused by either herpes simplex virus type 1 (HSV-1) or HSV-2. Several types of wart-causing papillomaviruses (warts) infect millions of people each year worldwide. The common childhood exanthems are caused by viruses and are discussed in detail in Chapter 2 and are listed in Table 2-1.

COMMON FUNGAL INFECTIONS

Malassezia furfur, the dermatophytes *Microsporum, Trichophyton,* and *Epidermophyton,* and *Candida albicans* are the most common causes of skin infections, most of which are limited to the epidermis. *M furfur* and the dermatophytes are only able to infect the superficial keratinized layers of the epidermis. The dermatophytes can also infect the hair and nails. *C albicans* infections are usually restricted to the epidermis and cause intertrigo, folliculitis, paronychia, and onychomycosis.

HOW MICROORGANISMS INFECT THE SKIN

There are numerous infectious agents that cause skin lesions, which can occur via several modes: infection of the skin by the microbe, production of toxins by the microbe, or as an inflammatory response to a microbial infection. Most microorganisms infect the skin through breaks in the protective outer layers of the epidermidis or by infecting hair follicles. Breaks in the skin usually occur following trauma such as bites from insects, animals, or humans, needle sticks, scratches, or burns. If the hair follicles are clogged, they are more likely to become infected. These infections can penetrate deeper into the dermis and in some cases into the subcutaneous fat, fascia, and muscles under the skin causing severe disease (e.g., necrotizing fasciitis, myositis, and gas gangrene).

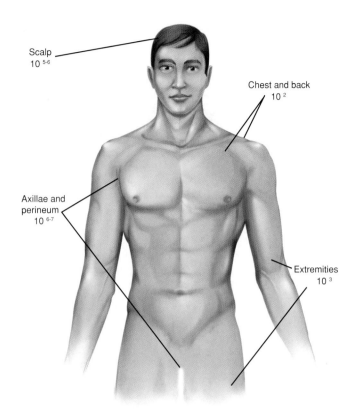

Scalp
10^{5-6}

Chest and back
10^2

Axillae and perineum
10^{6-7}

Extremities
10^3

Figure 1-3. Number of normal flora commensals per gram of skin.

TABLE 1-1. Types of Skin Lesions

Depressed Skin Lesions	Flat Skin Lesions	Elevated Skin Lesions	
Gangrene	Macule	Papule	Bulla(e)
Sinus	Patch	Plaque	Exudates (crusts)
Ulcer	Petechiae Purpura Ecchymosis Gangrene	Nodule Vesicle	Abscess Pustule Furuncle Carbuncle

Several different types of skin lesions can develop following a skin infection (Table 1-1). Macules are flat lesions that occur in the plane of the skin (Figure 1-4); ulcers are depressed lesions below the plane of the skin; and papules are elevated above the plane of the skin (Figure 1-5). Some skin lesions are characteristic of the infecting microorganism such as anthrax, which produces a black eschar, whereas other skin lesions such as childhood exanthems and erythematous rashes can be the result of several different organisms.

Not all skin lesions occur following infection of the skin. Some lesions occur following exposure to one or more toxins, and others occur as the result of damage to the capillaries. For example, leakage of small amounts of blood from the capillaries results in the formation of small nonblanching petechiae. If more capillary leakage occurs, purpura and ecchymosis can develop. Still other skin lesions, such as erythema nodosum, follow an inflammatory response to an infection occurring elsewhere in the body.

GROUPING INFECTIONS OF THE INTEGUMENT AND SOFT TISSUES

Infections of the integument and soft tissues can be grouped in several ways: by the microorganisms that cause the disease; by the depth of the infection or damage in the skin; or by the types of lesions produced by the microorganisms. Because most physicians must initially identify infections of the integument and soft tissues by lesions that are visible on a patient, these diseases will be presented based on the type of lesion produced. Chapters 2 through 5 will discuss infections of the integument and soft tissues; each of the chapters will discuss a different set of skin lesions and the microbes that cause them. Maculopapular rashes are discussed in Chapter 2. Chapter 3 discusses papules, plaques, and patches; Chapter 4 discusses vesicular, bullous, and purulent lesions; and Chapter 5 discusses petechial, hemorrhagic, ulcerative, and necrotic lesions.

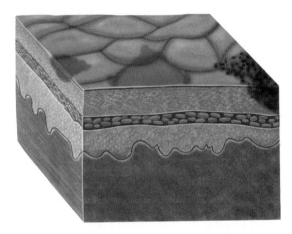

Figure 1-4. A schematic of a macule, which is a flat lesion usually less than 1 cm in diameter that can be brown, blue, red, or hypopigmented. Note the change in the color of the skin. The lesion cannot be felt but must be seen to be detected.

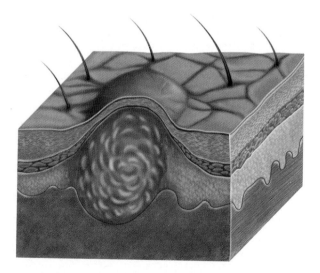

Figure 1-5. A schematic of a papule, a small (<0.5 cm in diameter) solid, elevated skin lesion. The top of a papule can be flat, pointed, or rounded.

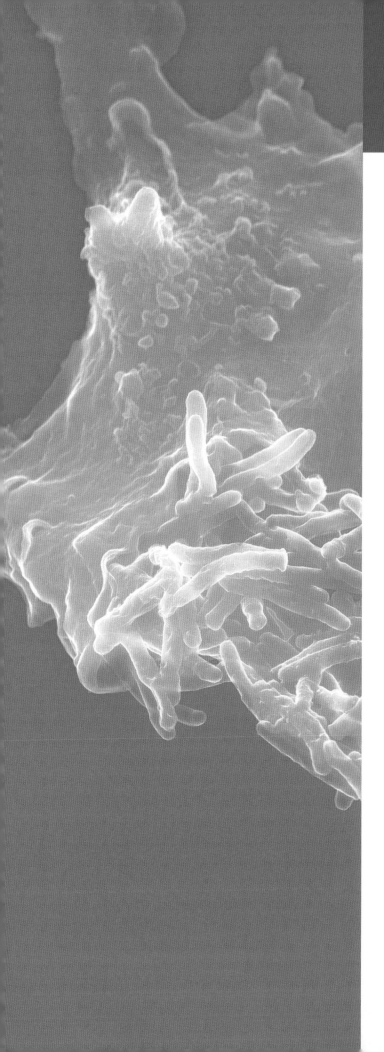

CHAPTER 2

MACULOPAPULAR RASHES

OVERVIEW

A macule is a flat lesion, usually less than 1 cm in diameter, and is a change in the color of the skin. Macules can be brown, blue, red, or hypopigmented; they cannot be felt but must be seen to be detected (Figure 2-1). A papule is a solid raised skin lesion that has distinct borders and is less than 1 cm in diameter (Figure 2-2). Maculopapular rashes are red or erythematous skin lesions with flat or slightly elevated areas in the rash lesion (Figure 2-3).

Table 2-1 lists several different diseases discussed in this chapter. Six of the diseases—erythema infectiosum, scarlet fever, exanthem subitum, rubeola, rubella, and enteroviral rashes—are frequently seen in children and have widespread lesions. Because the diseases are often difficult to distinguish from each other, they are discussed together in the following section. The other maculopapular diseases will be discussed separately, after the discussion of childhood exanthems.

CHILDHOOD EXANTHEMS

Exanthems are widespread rashes that are usually accompanied by systemic symptoms of fever, malaise, and headache. They can occur following a reaction to a microbial toxin, by microbial skin damage, or as an immune response to a microorganism. The common childhood exanthems are listed in Table 2-2.

ETIOLOGY

Viruses are the most common cause of exanthems. With the exception of scarlet fever, which is the only exanthem that is caused by a bacterium, all other childhood exanthems are caused by viruses (Table 2-3).

MANIFESTATIONS

Exanthems

The diseases classified as exanthems are quite similar in appearance and are easily misdiagnosed. Fortunately, most childhood exanthems have unique characteristics that aid in determining a diagnosis (Table 2-4).

Stages of erythema infectiosum

Erythema infectiosum skin lesions can appear in three stages. Immediately before the rash appears, there is a mild prodromal period that includes headache, coryza, low-grade fever, pharyngitis, and malaise.

- **Stage 1:** The exanthem begins with the classic slapped-cheek appearance when a bright red erythema appears abruptly over the cheeks (Figure 2-4A). Usually no erythema is seen on the nose or around the mouth or eyes. The exanthem usually has a sunburn-like appearance and fades within 2–4 days.

- **Stage 2:** Within 1–4 days after the appearance of the "slapped-cheek" rash, an erythematous macular-to-morbilliform eruption occurs primarily on the extremities. Morbilliform lesions are macules 2–20 mm in diameter, and can be confluent in certain regions (see Figure 2-4B). The rash is more commonly found on the extensor surfaces and can occasionally involve the palms and soles. Pruritus is rare.

- **Stage 3:** After several days, most of the eruptions that occurred in the second stage fade into a lacy pattern, which is most apparent on the proximal extremities. This reticulate (net-like) pattern is distinctly characteristic of erythema infectiosum and may be the only manifestation seen in some patients. The third stage lasts from 3 days to 3 weeks. Even after the rash begins to fade, it may recur intermittently over several weeks following exercise, sun exposure, friction, bathing in hot water, or a stressful event.

Roseola infantum

Roseola infantum is characterized by a history of high fever (40°C) followed by rapid defervescence. A rash appears after the patient no longer has a fever. This nonpruritic rash is an erythematous macular exanthem or a maculopapular exanthem beginning on the trunk and spreading to the extremities (Figure 2-5). The skin lesions are usually discrete and do not coalesce. The rash will blanch on pressure and will fade within a few hours to 2 days. A prodrome can occur and includes listlessness and irritability. Other symptoms include seizures, diarrhea, and cough.

Scarlet fever

Scarlet fever begins with a prodrome that includes pharyngitis, vomiting, fever, headache, and abdominal pain that precedes the rash from 1 to 2 days. The rash typically begins on the neck and extends to the trunk and extremities (Figure 2-6). This erythematous rash (scarlatiniform) is sandpaper-like in appearance (Figure 2-7) and blanches on pressure. The rash can be pruritic, but it is not painful. The patient's face is usually flushed with perioral pallor (Figure 2-8). After the rash has extended to the trunk and extremities, it becomes more intense along skin folds and produces lines of confluent petechiae, known as Pastia sign. During the first 2 days of the disease, the tongue has a

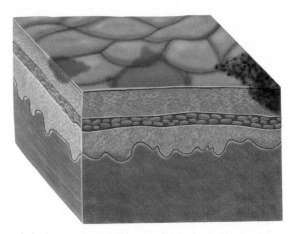

Figure 2-1. A macule showing the flat lesion with changes in the color of the skin. Macules can be brown, blue, red, or hypopigmented.

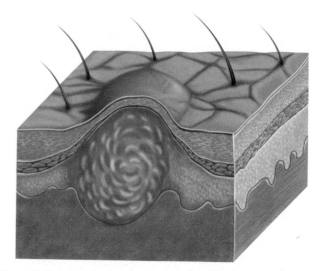

Figure 2-2. A papule showing the small, solid elevated skin lesion. The top of the papule can be flat, pointed, or rounded.

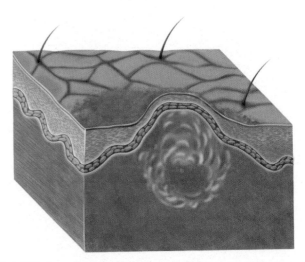

Figure 2-3. A maculopapular rash, an erythematous skin lesion with flat or slightly elevated areas in the rash lesion.

white coating through which the red and edematous papillae can be seen (white strawberry tongue).

The rash begins to fade 3–4 days after onset, and desquamation begins. This phase begins with flakes peeling from the face. Two days after the rash appears, the tongue also desquamates, causing a red tongue with prominent papillae (strawberry tongue) (Figure 2-9). Peeling from the palms and around the fingers occurs about 1 week later and can last up to 1 month.

Rubeola

Rubeola begins with a prodromal phase of coryza, conjunctivitis, nonproductive cough (known as the three Cs of rubeola), and fever. The prodrome is usually followed within 2–3 days by the pathognomonic Koplik spots—blue-gray macules 1–2 mm in diameter on an erythematous base that typically arises on the buccal, gingival, and labial mucosae (Figure 2-10). The maculopapular erythematous rash begins at the hairline and spreads to the trunk and extremities. The rash lesion concentration is highest above the shoulders and often coalesces (morbilliform rash) in this region of the body (Figure 2-11). The rash lasts about 4–6 days and then fades from the head downward. Patients usually recover fully within 7–10 days. Desquamation may occur, but it is usually not severe.

Rubella

Rubella begins with a prodrome, which includes fever, malaise, headache, coryza, and mild conjunctivitis (*patients do not have a cough*). The nonblanching rash appears 1–5 days after the beginning of the prodromal period (Figure 2-12). The faint pink maculopapular rash begins on the forehead and face and spreads caudally to the trunk and extremities. The rash may coalesce, resulting in a scarlatiniform (sandpaper-like) eruption (see Figure 2-7). Within 3 days, the rash fades, beginning at the forehead and face and fading caudally. Petechial lesions on the soft palate, called Forchheimer spots, may also be present. The patient usually has postauricular and suboccipital lymphadenopathy.

Enteroviral rashes

Enteroviral viruses can cause a large variety of rashes, and many patients will have fever, malaise, and headache. The rash may appear at the time the fever begins or it may appear near the end of the fever. The type of rash depends on the type of virus causing the exanthem. Echoviruses can cause a rubella-, measles-, or roseola-like rash. Roseola-like rashes typically appear after the temperature returns to normal, as is seen with roseola infantum. Echovirus 16 causes a roseola-type rash that has been named Boston exanthem. Coxsackie A viruses can cause pustular stomatitis and widespread vesicular lesions.

EPIDEMIOLOGY

All exanthems are found worldwide and are usually seen in children between the ages of 3 and 15 years.

TABLE 2-1. Maculopapular Rashes

Childhood exanthems	Infectious mononucleosis
• Enteroviral rashes	Secondary syphilis
• Erythema infectiosum (fifth disease, or slapped-cheek syndrome)	Rocky Mountain spotted fever
• Roseola infantum (exanthem subitum)	Toxic shock syndrome
• Scarlet fever	
• Rubeola (measles)	
• Rubella	

TABLE 2-2. Common Viral Childhood Exanthems

Virus	Disease
Coxsackie viruses	Enteroviral rash
Echoviruses	Enteroviral rash
Erythrovirus B19 (formerly called parvovirus B19)	Erythema infectiosum ("slapped-cheek syndrome," or fifth disease)
Human herpesvirus 6B (HHV-6B) and HHV-7	Roseola or exanthem subitum
Varicella-zoster virus (HHV-3)	Chickenpox and zoster (shingles)
Measles virus	Rubeola ("hard measles")
Rubella virus	Rubella (German measles)

TABLE 2-3. Causes of Childhood Exanthems

Causes of the Disease	Disease(s)
Erythrovirus B19	Erythema infectiosum, "slapped-cheek syndrome," or fifth disease
HHV-6 and occasionally HHV-7	Roseola infantum or exanthem subitum
Streptococcus pyogenes	Scarlet fever or scarlatina
Measles virus	Rubeola
Rubella virus	Rubella
Coxsackie A viruses and Echoviruses	Enteroviral rashes or viral rash

TABLE 2-4. Manifestations of the Childhood Exanthems

Disease and Cause	Prodrome	Disease Progression	Distribution of Rash	Unique Signs and Symptoms
Erythema infectiosum and Erythrovirus B19	Headache, coryza, low grade fever, pharyngitis, malaise	**Stage 1:** slapped-cheek appearance **Stage 2:** macular to morbilliform rash on extremities **Stage 3:** reticulate or lacy pattern of rash on extremities	Slapped cheek: sunburn-like rash on cheeks but usually not on nose or around mouth or eyes Rash on extremities: tends to be on extensor surfaces	Slapped cheek rash Reticular or lacy rash
Roseola infantum and human herpes virus 6 (HHV-6) or HHV-7	High fever with rapid defervescence	After fever recedes, rash appears	Rash begins on the trunk, spreads to extremities	High fever that occurs and goes away before the rash appears
Scarlet fever and *Streptococcus pyogenes*	Pharyngitis, vomiting, fever, headache, and abdominal pain precedes rash within 1–2 days	Rash (scarlatiniform) sandpaper-like in appearance and blanches on pressure Desquamation begins when rash starts to fade	Rash begins on neck, then extends to trunk and extremities	Perioral pallor, Pastia sign, White strawberry tongue (early), Strawberry tongue (during desquamation)
Rubeola and measles virus	Coryza, conjunctivitis, nonproductive cough (the 3 Cs), and fever	Maculopapular erythematous rash Lesions usually coalesce on trunk, forming a morbilliform rash	Rash begins at hairline, then spreads to trunk and extremities Rash concentration is highest above the shoulders	The three Cs of rubeola, Koplik spots
Rubella and rubella virus	Fever, malaise, headache, coryza, and mild conjunctivitis, without cough	Nonblanching rash: a faint pink, maculopapular rash, which may coalesce, resulting in a scarlatiniform eruption (sandpaper-like eruption)	Rash begins on forehead and face, spreading caudally to trunk and extremities	Forchheimer spots
Enteroviral rashes and coxsackieviruses or echoviruses	Fever, malaise, and headache	Large variety of rashes Rash may appear at the time fever begins or near the end of fever	Type of rash depends on type of virus causing the exanthem	

■ Erythema infectiosum is usually seen in patients in late winter to early spring.

■ Transmission is via aerosolized respiratory droplets.

Roseola infantum

Roseola infantum is most common during the spring and fall months. Infection with these viruses is common in children from 6 months to 3 years of age. About 80% of children in the United States are seropositive between the ages of 2 and 4 years. The viruses are shed in saliva and transmitted from latently infected adults to children.

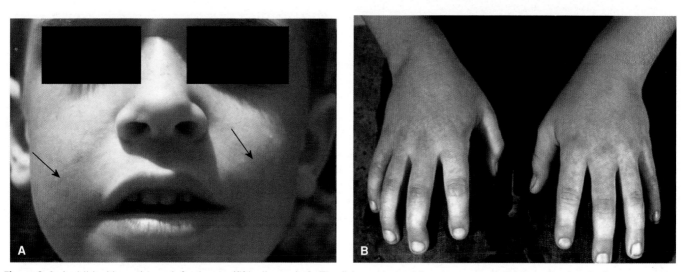

Figure 2-4. A child with erythema infectiosum (fifth disease). **A,** The "slapped-cheek" appearance. **B,** Rash on the hands. Images courtesy of the Centers for Disease Control and Prevention.

Scarlet fever

Scarlet fever is most common in children between the ages of 4 and 8 years of age, and usually occurs 12–24 hours after a pharyngeal infection caused by a pyogenic (erythrogenic) toxin-producing group A streptococcal infection. This bacterium is found in the oropharynx of 15–20% of healthy children and adults. The organism is transmitted by airborne respiratory particles from infected patients and asymptomatic carriers. Scarlet fever only occurs in 10% of patients with group A streptococcal pharyngitis.

Rubeola (Measles)

Rubeola, or measles, occurs only in humans and monkeys. The virus can be transmitted by direct contact, contaminated fomites, or droplet inhalation and is one of the most contagious exanthems, with a 90% attack rate. Due to universal vaccination, less than 100 cases of rubeola are reported in the United States annually (Figure 2-13).

Rubella

Rubella is found only in humans. Respiratory droplets transmit the virus, and it is most commonly seen in unimmunized children aged 5–9 years of age. Due to universal vaccination in the United States, less than 50 cases of rubella are reported annually (Figure 2-14).

Enteroviral rashes

Enteroviral rashes are transmitted person to person following contact with saliva or feces from infected patients. Most cases occur in infants during the summer months. About 10–15 million cases of this disease occur each year in the United States.

PATHOGENESIS

Erythema infectiosum

Erythema infectiosum is an immunologic response to infection of the virus. Acute infection leads to the production of specific

Day 1	Day 2	Day 3
Fever	Fever	Fever gone
40°C	38.9°C	Rash appears

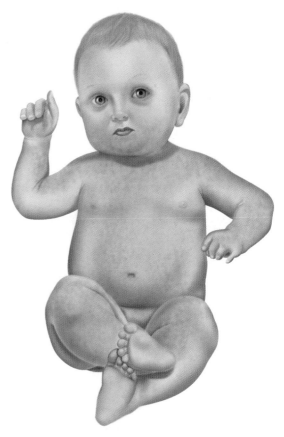

Figure 2-5. An infant with exanthem subitum (roseola) due to human herpes virus 6 (HHV-6) or HHV-7. The infant usually has a high fever for a few days, when the fever abruptly ends and the rash appears on the face, neck, and trunk.

IgM antibodies and subsequent formation of immune complexes. Clinical signs and symptoms result from the deposition of the immune complexes in the skin and joints of patients with this infection.

Roseola infantum

Roseola infantum is due to HHV-6 replication in the leukocytes and the salivary glands. Virus can be found in the saliva. There may be early invasion of the central nervous system (CNS), which may explain seizures and other CNS complications. Following the acute primary infection, HHV-6 remains latent in lymphocytes and monocytes.

Scarlet fever

Scarlet fever occurs 1–2 days after pharyngeal infections and following infection with *S pyogenes* of the skin and soft tissue, surgical wounds, or the uterus. Production of erythrogenic toxins (usually referred to as SPE A, B, C, and F) by *S pyogenes* causes the skin rash.

Measles virus

Measles virus causes rubeola and infects the upper respiratory tract or the conjunctival sac, leading to viral replication in the oral mucosa and regional lymph nodes. All lymph nodes and the major organs eventually are infected. Appearance of circulating antibodies causes viremia to cease and symptoms to disappear.

Rubella virus

Rubella virus initially replicates in the upper respiratory tract and in the cervical lymph nodes and is carried in the bloodstream to the skin, other lymph nodes, spleen, liver, joints, and CNS. Viremia can be detected up to 9 days before the rash develops. Neutralizing antibodies are detectable in the bloodstream, and the exanthem results from the antibody-virus complex.

Enteroviral rashes

Enteroviral rashes occur following ingestion of the virus. The virus attaches to epithelial cells in the gut and invades and replicates in the Peyer patches. A viremia occurs and seeds many organ systems, including the CNS, heart, lungs, heart, and skin.

DIAGNOSIS

Usually the diagnosis of exanthems is determined on clinical grounds. In several of these diseases, the distribution and the type of rash can be valuable in determining a diagnosis (Figure 2-15). Serologic tests or viral culture occasionally can also be helpful. Scarlet fever can be detected by culturing for *S pyogenes* or with a rapid strep test. *S pyogenes* produces beta hemolysis on sheep blood agar plates and is sensitive to bacitracin (Figure 2-16).

THERAPY AND PREVENTION

Supportive care is used in the treatment of viral exanthems. The mumps-measles-rubella vaccine is effective in preventing measles and rubella. Testing pregnant women for the presence

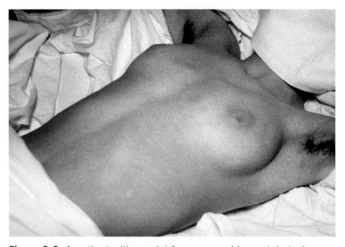

Figure 2-6. A patient with scarlet fever caused by certain toxin-producing strains of *Streptococcus pyogenes*. Note that the rash is darker in the axillae. Image courtesy of the Centers for Disease Control and Prevention.

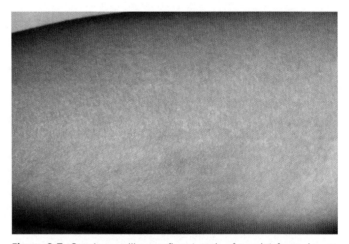

Figure 2-7. Sandpaper-like confluent rash of scarlet fever. Image courtesy of the Centers for Disease Control and Prevention.

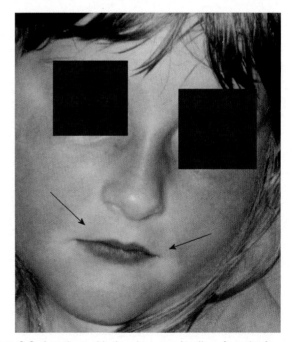

Figure 2-8. A patient with the circumoral pallor of scarlet fever.

of antibodies to rubella is valuable in determining if the fetus is at risk of infection following exposure to a person with rubella.

Patients with scarlet fever are usually treated with antibiotics. Treatment within 10 days of the appearance of symptoms can significantly reduce the chances of the patient developing rheumatic fever.

INFECTIOUS MONONUCLEOSIS

Infectious mononucleosis is a common cause of infection in adolescents. Most people have developed antibodies to the antigens of this virus by adulthood. Infectious mononucleosis can cause a rash in a certain subset of patients. Epstein-Barr virus (EBV) causes this disease and usually causes a regional lymphadenopathy due to its ability to infect B lymphocytes (see Chapter 24).

ETIOLOGY

EBV (also known as HHV-4) causes about 90% of cases of acute infectious mononucleosis in the United States.

MANIFESTATIONS

Patients with infectious mononucleosis usually have a **triad of symptoms,** including **fever** (38.3–38.9°C), **pharyngitis,** and **cervical lymphadenopathy** (Figure 2-17). The diffuse pharyngeal inflammation and tonsillar swelling can be severe and exudative or nonexudative. Nearly half of patients have splenomegaly. Petechiae on the hard and soft palates can be seen in 25–60% of patients. A maculopapular rash is usually faint, widely scattered, and erythematous, and occurs in 10–15% of patients. The rash is more common in young children.

Infectious mononucleosis is frequently misdiagnosed as a streptococcal pharyngitis, resulting in treatment with amoxicillin or ampicillin. About 80% of patients with EBV mononucleosis treated with these antibiotics develop a widely scattered maculopapular rash, which is often misdiagnosed as an allergic reaction to the antibiotic. To avoid treating viral infectious mononucleosis with an antibacterial antimicrobial agent, the pharynx should be swabbed and a rapid streptococcal antigen test performed or a throat culture for *Streptococcus pyogenes* should be performed to rule out streptococcal pharyngitis.

EPIDEMIOLOGY

- EBV is found worldwide and is common and relatively mild in children. The disease is usually more severe in young adults.

- Infection is most common in the 15- to 25-year-old age group.

- Approximately 90% of the population of the United States is seropositive for EBV by age 25.

- A skin rash develops in 10–15% of patients with infectious mononucleosis.

- Many individuals infected with EBV are asymptomatic and infectious. Children are more likely to be asymptomatic following infection.

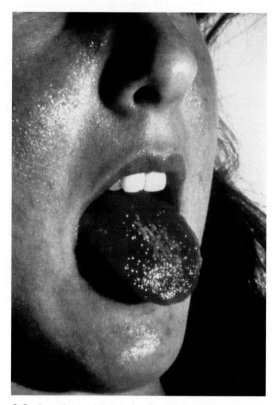

Figure 2-9. A patient with scarlet fever, showing the "strawberry tongue." Image courtesy of the Centers for Disease Control and Prevention.

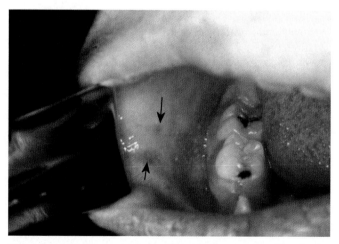

Figure 2-10. Pathognomonic Koplik spots in a patient with rubeola. Image courtesy of the Centers for Disease Control and Prevention.

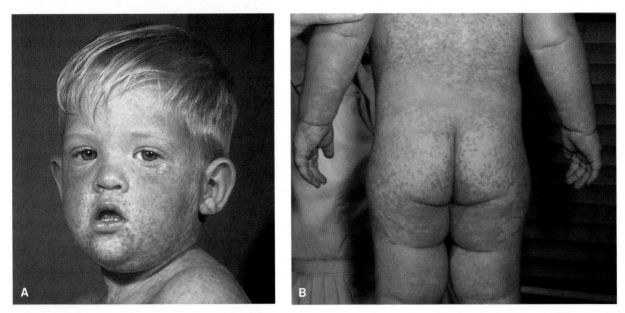

Figure 2-11. A, A child with rubeola. **B,** Rash on the trunk, which has coalesced in many places forming the typical morbilliform rash. Images courtesy of the Centers for Disease Control and Prevention, Barbara Rice.

■ EBV is transmitted via saliva or blood transfusions from infected or convalescent persons.

PATHOGENESIS

Disease is the result of viral replication and host immune responses to viral antigens.

1. EBV infects the B cells in the oropharyngeal epithelium.

2. The infected B cells spread the infection throughout the reticuloendothelial system (e.g., liver, spleen, and peripheral lymph nodes).

3. EBV infection of B cells results in a humoral (B-cell mitogen) and cellular response to the virus. EBV acts as a B-cell mitogen and causes multiplication of many different B cells, which are then activated to produce antibodies. Some of the B cells that are activated produce antibodies that react with EBV antigens; however, other activated B cells produce antibodies that do not react with EBV antigens but react with antigens from other mammals. The heterophil tests (Monospot and Paul-Bunnell tests) were developed because most patients with infectious mononucleosis due to EBV produce antibodies that will agglutinate other mammals' erythrocytes. The Monospot test uses horse erythrocytes, and the Paul-Bunnell test uses sheep erythrocytes.

4. The virus is usually not found free in the blood but is present in immune complexes. These complexes are believed to be responsible for the arthralgia and rash that occurs during the acute phase of the disease.

5. The T-cell response is essential in the control of EBV infection.

DIAGNOSIS

Laboratory studies used in the diagnosis of acute infectious mononucleosis

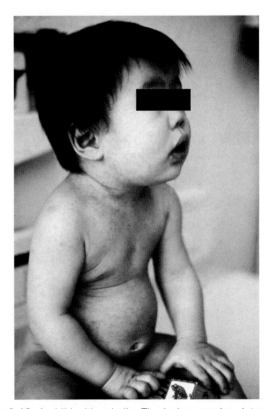

Figure 2-12. A child with rubella. The lesions are less intense and have not coalesced, as usually occurs in rubeola. Image courtesy of the Centers for Disease Control and Prevention.

1. A **complete blood cell count** (CBC) with differential. Leukocytosis with lymphocytosis is usually seen, and the presence of at least 10% atypical lymphocytes (Figure 2-18). Other etiologic agents can cause similar CBC results. To confirm a diagnosis of infectious mononucleosis, serologic testing must be performed.

2. A **positive serologic finding** for EBV includes heterophile antibody tests (**Monospot and Paul-Bunnell tests**) and **EBV-specific serology** (see Chapter 24). About 60–90% of adults are positive for EBV when tested during the first 2 weeks of the illness. Most children younger than age 2 are negative for the Monospot and Paul-Bunnell tests.

TREATMENT AND PREVENTION

Infectious mononucleosis is a self-limiting disease and usually only supportive treatment is needed. The virus is minimally contagious, and isolation is not necessary. Patients should avoid sharing items contaminated with saliva. Because splenomegaly can occur, patients should avoid heavy lifting and contact sports for at least 2–3 weeks during the acute stage of the illness.

SECONDARY SYPHILIS

Syphilis manifests in three stages—as primary, secondary, and tertiary syphilis. The stage with the most noticeable skin lesions is secondary syphilis. This stage of the disease produces many maculopapular lesions that cover most of the body. (Primary syphilis is discussed in Chapter 5.)

ETIOLOGY

Treponema pallidum is a spiral-shaped bacterium with a characteristic corkscrew motility. This bacterium is too narrow to stain and observe with conventional light microscopy. The most rapid method of visualizing *T pallidum* is darkfield microscopy.

MANIFESTATIONS

Neonatal syphilis
If skin lesions are present in neonates at birth, the lesions tend to be vesicular and bullous eruptions and are seen over most parts of the body, including the palms and soles. If skin lesions occur 1 week or later after birth, the skin lesions are widespread erythematous maculopapular lesions that resemble secondary syphilis in adults (Figure 2-19). Unlike the childhood exanthems and infectious mononucleosis, lesions in secondary syphilis can be seen on the **palms and soles.** Other symptoms include condyloma lata in the anogenital region, mucous patches on the oral, pharyngeal, and nasal mucosa, and snuffles (syphilitic rhinitis) (Figure 2-20).

Adults: secondary syphilis
In adults, secondary syphilis develops about 6–8 weeks after the appearance of the primary chancre and has a wide range of presentations. The most common systemic manifestations include

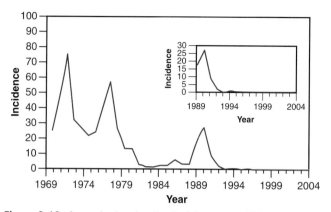

Figure 2-13. A graph showing the incidence per 100,000 population of rubeola from 1969 to 2004 in the United States. Image courtesy of the Centers for Disease Control and Prevention.

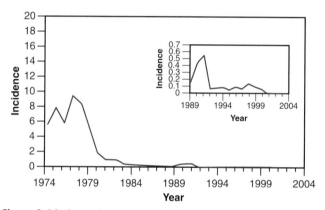

Figure 2-14. A graph showing the incidence per 100,000 population of rubella from 1974 to 2004 in the United States. Image courtesy of the Centers for Disease Control and Prevention.

malaise, fever, myalgias, and arthralgias, with a generalized body rash and lymphadenopathy. The rash is usually an erythematous maculopapular rash that can be seen over the entire body (Figure 2-21), including the palms and soles (Figures 2-22). The lesions will recede without treatment. Relapses of the rash may occur in about 20% of untreated patients. Other symptoms include condyloma lata in the anogenital region (Figure 2-23) and mucous patches on the oral, pharyngeal, and nasal mucosa (Figure 2-24).

EPIDEMIOLOGY

- The incidence of secondary syphilis is highest in sexually active men aged 25–45 years and in women aged 20–29 years (Figure 2-25).

- There are approximately 6000–7000 new cases of primary and secondary syphilis diagnosed each year (Figure 2-26), with incidence rates remaining highest in the southern part of the United States (Figure 2-27).

- About 300–500 cases of congenital syphilis are diagnosed each year in the United States.

- Syphilis infection rates are much higher in certain ethnic groups, such as blacks and Hispanics.

- Manifestations of secondary syphilis usually appear 6–8 weeks after the appearance of the primary chancre.

- Syphilis is a sexually transmitted disease.

PATHOGENESIS

Following intimate contact with a break in the skin, *T pallidum* penetrates the lower layers of the skin and multiplies at the site of penetration. The tissue destruction and lesions are thought to be primarily due to the patient's immune response to the infection. An inflammatory reaction occurs at the site of bacterial cell multiplication and causes a primary hard chancre (raised edematous ulcer), which is the lesion seen in primary syphilis. Histologic examination of the chancre demonstrates endarteritis and periarteritis and infiltration of the ulcer with macrophages and polymorphonuclear leukocytes.

Quite soon after penetrating the skin, some bacteria enter the bloodstream and are disseminated to almost every organ in the body, including the skin. In time, the organisms in the skin will multiply enough to cause an immune response. This immune response causes the lesions observed in secondary syphilis—mucocutaneous lesions with maculopapular lesions on the skin, and condyloma latum in moist intertriginous areas of the skin and in mucous patches associated with the mucous membranes. All of these lesions contain viable bacteria and are highly infectious. If the patient remains untreated, significant damage to the CNS, skin, and vasculature can occur, resulting in tertiary syphilis, which is extremely rare in the United States.

If a pregnant woman acquires syphilis, *T pallidum* can penetrate the placenta and infect the bloodstream of the fetus; about one fourth of fetuses die before birth, and one fourth die soon after birth. After in utero infection, the surviving patients can manifest signs early (before 2 years of age) or late (after 2 years of age), or both early and late. About 3 weeks after infection, the newborn usually develops skin lesions that are quite similar to

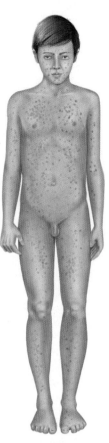
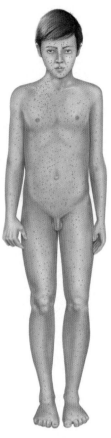

Measles   Rubella

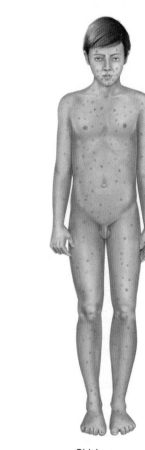

Scarlet fever   Chickenpox

Figure 2-15. The distribution and comparison of the rash of rubeola, rubella, scarlet fever, and chickenpox, which can be helpful in determining the diagnosis of these childhood exanthems.

those seen in adults who have secondary syphilis. The earlier the skin lesions appear following birth, the more severe the infection.

DIAGNOSIS

To obtain a diagnosis of secondary syphilis, it is important to complete a focused history and physical examination, perform serologic tests, determine sexual contacts, and, in some cases, perform darkfield microscopy of fluids from lesions (Figure 2-28). Two different serologic tests are used: screening tests and confirmatory tests. The screening test is a nontreponemal test that detects the presence of antibodies reactive with cardiolipin (reagin) in the patient's bloodstream. The nontreponemal serologic tests include the venereal diseases research laboratory (VDRL) and rapid plasma reagin (RPR) tests. False-positive results can occur; therefore a confirmatory test is required following a positive reagin test result. Confirmatory or treponemal tests include the *T pallidum* immobilization (TPI), fluorescent treponemal antibody absorption (FTA-ABS), and microhemagglutination assay for *T pallidum* (MHA-TP).

TREATMENT AND PREVENTION

Benzathine penicillin is the antibiotic of choice for treatment of primary and secondary syphilis. Over 50% of patients with secondary syphilis will have a Jarisch-Herxheimer reaction within 6–12 hours after initial antibiotic treatment. This reaction usually includes malaise, fever, headache, sweating, rigors, and temporary exacerbation of the skin lesions. The reaction usually subsides within 24 hours, but it may be severe, requiring hospitalization.

The nontreponemal serologic tests are helpful to determine the efficacy of the antibiotic treatment. Antibody levels to cardiolipin will decline after successful treatment. Antibody levels to treponemal antigens are detectable during the patient's lifetime, even following successful treatment.

Preventive measures include discouraging patients with syphilis from having sexual relations, identifying and treating their sexual contacts, and avoiding sexual contact with other syphilitic patients.

ROCKY MOUNTAIN SPOTTED FEVER

Rocky Mountain spotted fever (RMSF) is the most common rickettsial tick-borne infection in the United States. Contrary to what its name implies, very few cases of RMSF occur in the Rocky Mountain region of the United States.

ETIOLOGY

Rickettsia rickettsii is an obligate intracellular bacterium.

MANIFESTATIONS

About 5–10 days after a tick bite, a person diagnosed with RMSF may experience fever, nausea and vomiting, severe headache, myalgia, and anorexia. About 90% of patients present with a rash 3 days after the bite. ***A unique manifestation of this***

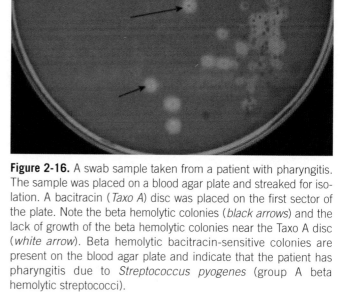

Figure 2-16. A swab sample taken from a patient with pharyngitis. The sample was placed on a blood agar plate and streaked for isolation. A bacitracin (*Taxo A*) disc was placed on the first sector of the plate. Note the beta hemolytic colonies (*black arrows*) and the lack of growth of the beta hemolytic colonies near the Taxo A disc (*white arrow*). Beta hemolytic bacitracin-sensitive colonies are present on the blood agar plate and indicate that the patient has pharyngitis due to *Streptococcus pyogenes* (group A beta hemolytic streptococci).

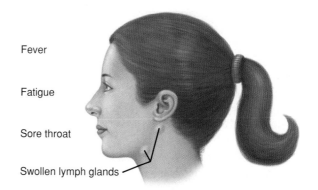

Fever

Fatigue

Sore throat

Swollen lymph glands

Figure 2-17. A schematic of a patient showing the manifestations of infectious mononucleosis.

disease is that the rash begins as erythematous macules on the wrists and ankles (Figure 2-29). The macules then become maculopapules and petechiae in about half of cases (Figure 2-30). The palms and soles usually are involved. Other manifestations include high fever that usually begins as the skin eruptions become evident. Most patients will also complain of a severe headache, nausea and vomiting, confusion, toxicity, stiff neck, and myalgia.

Damage to the circulatory system can cause severe disease in the lungs, kidneys, gastrointestinal system, and CNS. Damage to the blood vessels can also affect perfusion of various tissues resulting in partial paralysis of the lower extremities; gangrene requiring amputation of fingers, toes, arms, or legs; and conditions including hearing loss, loss of bowel or bladder control, movement disorders, or language disorders.

EPIDEMIOLOGY

▨ Approximately 250–1000 cases of RMSF are reported each year. More than half of cases of RMSF infections occur in the south central and southern Atlantic regions of the United States (Figure 2-31).

▨ The highest incidence of RMSF is in males, Caucasians, and children. Two thirds of cases occur in children younger than 15 years of age, and the peak age group is children aged 5–9 years.

▨ RMSF is the most severe and most common rickettsial disease in the United States. It is transmitted to humans during the late spring and summer months by the bite of an infected tick (ixodid [hard] tick) (Figure 2-32).

PATHOGENESIS

After the tick bite transmits the bacteria, the *Rickettsia* spread via lymphatics to the bloodstream and attach to vascular endothelial cells. The bacteria replicate in the endothelial cells, and after about 1 week clinical manifestations of infection are evident. Pathology in RMSF is due primarily to increased vascular permeability with a subsequent host mononuclear cell response. This systemic increase in vascular permeability can lead to edema, hypovolemia, and hypoalbuminemia. Vascular injury in the skin initially appears as blanchable erythematous macules. Eventually, the classic petechial rash of RMSF develops.

Vascular damage in the CNS can result in seizures, cranial nerve damage, and permanent blindness and deafness due to encephalitis and meningoencephalitis. Severe damage to the lungs can result in noncardiogenic pulmonary edema, interstitial pneumonia, and adult respiratory distress syndrome. Kidney damage results in decreased glomerular filtration rates and prerenal azotemia from hypovolemia. Focal hepatocellular necrosis occurs in 38% of patients and results in increased serum aminotransferase levels; hepatic failure does not occur.

Gastrointestinal endothelial cell injury leads to abdominal pain, nausea and vomiting, and diarrhea with many patients having guaiac-positive stools. About 30% of patients with RMSF are anemic; massive gastrointestinal bleeding can be fatal. Because RMSF is a multisystem disease, individuals can

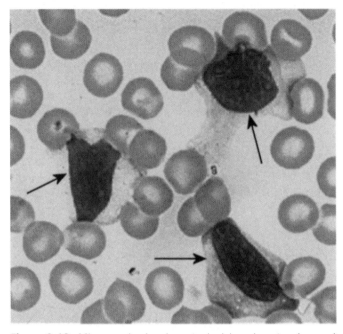

Figure 2-18. Micrograph showing atypical lymphocytes (*arrows*) representing several different viral diseases, including infectious mononucleosis, cytomegalovirus mononucleosis, viral hepatitis, and AIDS (acquired immunodeficiency disease syndrome).

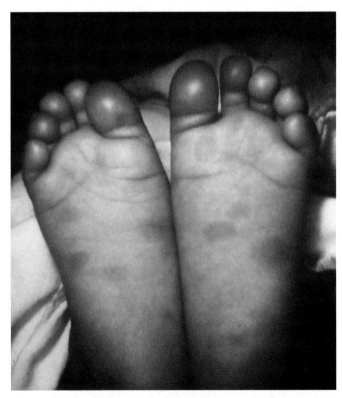

Figure 2-19. The feet of a neonate; note the syphilitic lesions on the soles of the feet. Image courtesy of the Centers for Disease Control and Prevention.

respond in different ways; in any particular patient, one organ system may be more affected than in other patients.

R rickettsii multiplies in the vascular endothelium and causes endothelial proliferation and perivascular infiltration, leading to hemorrhage and thrombosis. Hemorrhage of the capillaries causes the petechial skin lesions. Hemorrhage and thrombosis also appear to initiate the severe headache commonly seen in patients with RMSF. Muscle degeneration is characteristic, with muscle tenderness being a common complaint.

DIAGNOSIS

Several different tests are available to determine if a patient has RMSF. Culturing for the organism is rarely performed. An indirect immunofluorescence assay (IFA) can be performed on blood samples. Immunostaining of a biopsy of the rash can also be performed. Polymerase chain reaction (PCR) is now performed on blood and skin biopsies. Routine laboratory test results suggestive of RMSF include abnormal white blood cell count (leukocytosis: 11,000–30,000/mm^3 after the first week), thrombocytopenia, hyponatremia, or elevated liver enzyme levels.

THERAPY AND PREVENTION

Because of the severity of RMSF, treatment with doxycycline should be initiated *immediately* when there is a suspicion of the disease based on clinical and epidemiologic findings. Chloramphenicol is prescribed for patients who are pregnant. ***Treatment should not be delayed until laboratory confirmation is obtained.***

To avoid exposure to RMSF, limit exposure to ticks. An important method of preventing disease is for anyone exposed to tick-infested areas to promptly and carefully inspect and remove crawling or attached ticks. It usually takes several hours for an attached tick to transmit the RMSF bacterium; therefore prompt removal of attached ticks can prevent transmission of the disease.

TOXIC SHOCK SYNDROME

Toxic shock syndrome (TSS) is a relatively uncommon but severe systemic life-threatening disease that follows exposure to a bacterial superantigen produced by certain strains of *S aureus* and *S pyogenes*.

ETIOLOGY

The most common cause of TSS is *S pyogenes*, a gram-positive coccus, resulting in shock and multiorgan failure. Streptococcal strains producing either superantigen SPE A or C have been isolated in patients with TSS.

S aureus is a gram-positive coccus that also causes TSS. Staphylococcal TSS can occur during menstruation (known as menstrual TSS) or following a localized staphylococcal infection (nonmenstrual TSS). Menstrual TSS is nearly always caused by the superantigen exotoxin TSS toxin-1 (TSST-1).

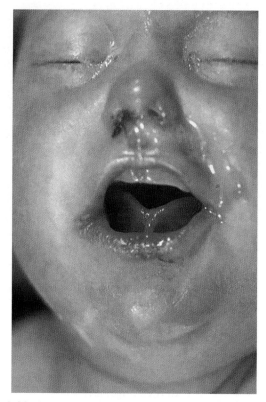

Figure 2-20. A neonate with syphilitic rhinitis (snuffles) due to *Treponema pallidum*. Image courtesy of the Centers for Disease Control and Prevention, Norman Cole.

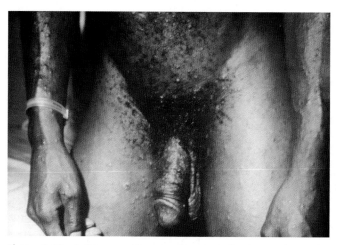

Figure 2-21. A 30-year-old man with generalized maculopapular eruptions of 1-week duration due to a secondary syphilitic infection. Image courtesy of the Centers for Disease Control and Prevention, VD, SCSD.

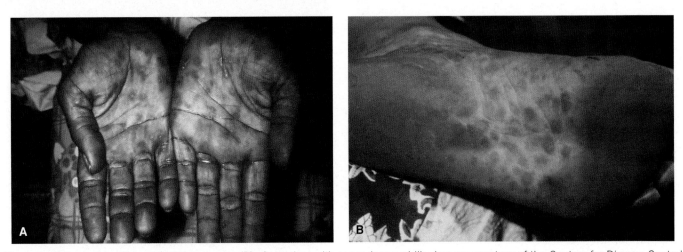

Figure 2-22. Lesions on the palms (**A**) and soles (**B**) of a patient with secondary syphilis. Images courtesy of the Centers for Disease Control and Prevention, Susan Lindsley.

About 50% of cases of nonmenstrual TSS are caused by strains of *S aureus* producing TSST-1. Other cases of nonmenstrual TSS are caused by strains of *S aureus*-producing enterotoxins.

MANIFESTATIONS

Streptococcal TSS is defined as any group A streptococcal (*S pyogenes*) infection associated with the early onset of shock and organ failure. A diffuse scarlatina-like erythema is seen in only about 10% of patients with streptococcal TSS.

Staphylococcal TSS is an acute-onset illness characterized by fever, hypotension, and rash and can lead to multiorgan failure and lethal shock. The rash appears later in the disease and has a sunburn-like appearance (Figure 2-33*A*). Desquamation frequently is seen in patients who survive (see Figure 2-33*B*). The desquamation is especially prominent on the palms and soles.

EPIDEMIOLOGY

- About 100 cases of **staphylococcal TSS** and 200–500 cases of **streptococcal TSS** are reported each year.

- People of any age can be affected, and many do not have any predisposing conditions. In some cases, however, viral infections such as chickenpox and influenza have provided a portal for infection. In other cases, the use of nonsteroidal anti-inflammatory agents may have masked the early symptoms or predisposed a patient to more severe streptococcal infection and shock. These infections have most often occurred sporadically.

- The mortality rate of streptococcal TSS is 30–70%.

- **Streptococcal TSS** occurs after an invasive infection (e.g., bacteremia, pneumonia) caused by a superantigen-producing strain of *S pyogenes*. Infection begins at a site of minor local trauma, which frequently does not result in a break in the skin. Many cases have developed within 24–72 hours of minor nonpenetrating trauma resulting in hematoma, deep bruise to the calf, or even muscle strain.

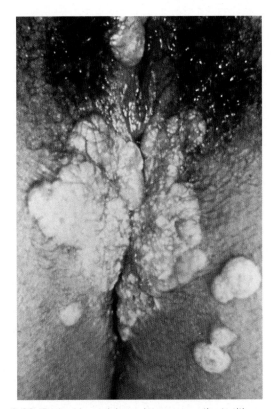

Figure 2-23. Perianal condyloma lata on a patient with secondary syphilis. Image courtesy of the Centers for Disease Control and Prevention.

- **Nonmenstrual staphylococcal TSS** can occur in healthy persons of any age, and commonly follows superinfection of an upper respiratory tract after viral infection. Other staphylococcal infections by superantigen-producing strains of *S aureus* can also cause nonmenstrual TSS (e.g., infected surgical wounds, abscesses, infected burns, and deep and superficial soft tissue infections). *S aureus* can be transmitted person to person and through contact with contaminated fomites.

- **Menstrual staphylococcal TSS** is defined as occurring during menstruation or within the 2 days preceding its onset or the 2 days following its cessation. This form of TSS is primarily but not exclusively associated with tampon use. The mortality rate is about 5% for both menstrual and nonmenstrual TSS.

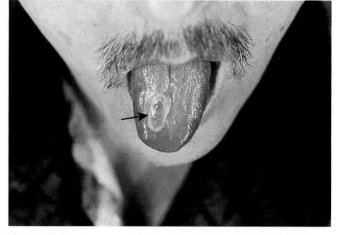

Figure 2-24. A mucous patch on the tongue of a patient with secondary syphilis. Image courtesy of the Centers for Disease Control and Prevention, Susan Lindsley.

PATHOGENESIS

Streptococcal TSS usually results following an invasive infection with *S pyogenes*. M protein on the surface of the bacteria contributes to invasiveness through its ability to impede phagocytosis of streptococci by human polymorphonuclear leukocytes. Production of streptococcal pyrogenic exotoxins A and C cause the signs and symptoms seen in streptococcal TSS.

Staphylococcal TSS can occur in menstruating women following overgrowth of *S aureus* in superabsorbent tampons or in tampons that remain in the vagina an excessive amount of time. *S aureus* is commonly found in the vaginal mucosa; however, only strains that produce TSST-1 are able to cause TSS. TSST-1 is the only superantigen in *S aureus* that can cross the mucosa and invade the bloodstream. The bacteria remain in the tampon and do not invade the surrounding tissues.

In nonmenstrual staphylococcal TSS, a localized infection with a TSS-associated superantigen-producing *S aureus* occurs before signs and symptoms of TSS are noticed. The localized lesion can be minute and escape notice. About one half of patients with nonmenstrual TSS have an *S aureus* isolate that produces TSST-1. Nearly all other patients have *S aureus* isolates that produce enterotoxin B, and a few patients with TSS have *S aureus* isolates that produce enterotoxin C.

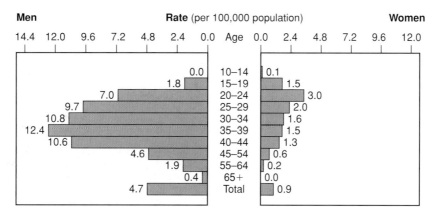

Figure 2-25. A graph showing age-specific and sex-specific rates for primary and secondary syphilis in the United States in 2004. Image courtesy of the Centers for Disease Control and Prevention.

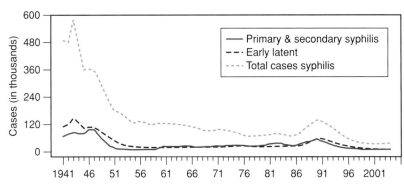

Figure 2-26. A graph showing reported cases of syphilis by stage of infection in the United States from 1941 to 2004. Image courtesy of the Centers for Disease Control and Prevention.

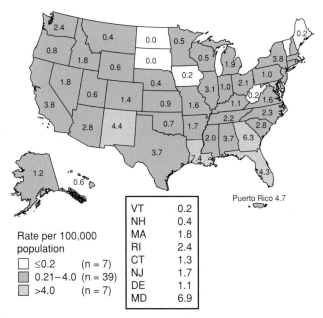

Figure 2-27. A map of the United States showing rates of primary and secondary syphilis by state in 2004. Image courtesy of the Centers for Disease Control and Prevention.

In both staphylococcal and streptococcal TSS, superantigens cause overactivation of the immune system, which activates immune cells to produce increased levels of cytokine.

1. Superantigens activate the immune system by simultaneously binding to major histocompatibility complex class II molecules and to the T-cell receptor molecules bearing a particular V-β region (Figure 2-34).

2. Superantigen binding results in the activation of numerous antigen-presenting cells and T cells, with subsequent systemic release of cytokines. Superantigens can stimulate over 20% of all T cells, whereas a conventional antigen stimulates only about 0.01% of the T cells.

3. The high levels of cytokine cause the clinical features of both staphylococcal and streptococcal TSS (i.e., fever, hypotension, rash).

4. The major cytokines released from antigen-presenting cells and T cells after activation by superantigens are tumor necrosis factor (TNF) α and β, interleukin-1 (IL-1), IL-2, and interferon-γ (IFN-γ).

   ○ TNF alpha and beta cause capillary leakage leading to peripheral pooling of blood and shock.

   ○ IL-1 causes fever.

   ○ IL-2 and IFN-γ cause a rash.

Production of antibodies to the M protein of *S pyogenes* will prevent invasive infections, and antibodies to its superantigens will prevent the symptoms associated with streptococcal TSS. Antibodies to *S aureus* superantigens, especially in the case of TSS induced by TSST-1, prevent the symptoms associated with staphylococcal TSS.

DIAGNOSIS

Streptococcal TSS can be difficult to diagnose and a set of clinical and laboratory criteria can aid in determining the diagnosis (Table 2-5). Because of the difficulty in diagnosing staphylococcal TSS, the Centers for Disease Control and Prevention has developed a case definition of five characteristic clinical criteria (Table 2-6).

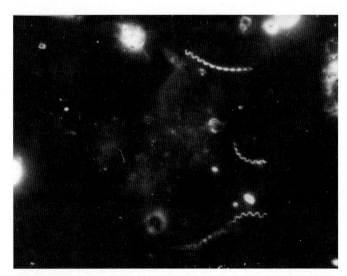

Figure 2-28. A darkfield micrograph of *Treponema pallidum*. Image courtesy of the Centers for Disease Control and Prevention, Susan Lindsley.

THERAPY AND PREVENTION

Treatment for **staphylococcal TSS** includes aggressive fluid replacement and intravenous treatment with antibiotics that are resistant to β-lactamase (e.g., oxacillin or nafcillin). In nonmenstrual TSS, searching for and removing the localized staphylococcal infection is essential.

Treatment of **streptococcal TSS** includes identification of the site of infection and surgical debridement, aggressive fluid replacement, intravenous immune globulin (IVIG), and intravenous antibiotics (e.g., penicillin G and clindamycin).

No vaccine is currently available for the treatment of TSS. Frequent handwashing and measures to prevent spread of these superantigen-producing bacteria can be helpful.

TABLE 2-5. Diagnostic Criteria for Streptococcal Toxic Shock Syndrome

1. Isolation of group A streptococcus (*Streptococcus pyogenes*) isolated from
   - Sterile site (blood, CSF)* *or*
   - Nonsterile site (skin lesion, pharynx)[§]

2. Clinical signs of severity[§]
   Hypotension (<90 mm Hg systolic pressure)
   Two or more clinical or laboratory abnormalities:
   - Renal impairment
   - Coagulopathy
   - Liver abnormalities
   - Acute respiratory distress syndrome
   - Extensive tissue necrosis
   - Erythematous rash (diffuse, scarlatina-like erythema)

*A definite case is made if *S pyogenes* has been isolated from a sterile site and the patient has hypotension and two or more clinical and laboratory abnormalities.

[§] A probable case is made if *S pyogenes* is isolated from a nonsterile site and the patient has hypotension and two or more clinical and laboratory abnormalities.

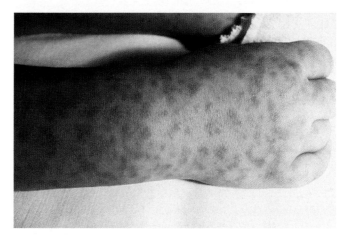

Figure 2-29. The right hand and wrist of a child showing the characteristic macules due to Rocky Mountain spotted fever. Image courtesy of the Centers for Disease Control and Prevention.

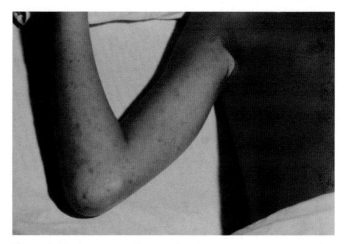

Figure 2-30. A patient with petechial lesions on the right arm following infection due to *Rickettsia rickettsii*. Image courtesy of the Centers for Disease Control and Prevention.

TABLE 2-6. Five Diagnostic Criteria for Diagnosis of Staphylococcal Toxic Shock Syndrome

1. Temperature >38.9°C

2. Systolic blood pressure <90 mm Hg

3. Widespread sunburn-like rash

4. Rash with subsequent desquamation (especially palms and soles)

5. More than three of the following manifestations:
   • Gastrointestinal: vomiting and diarrhea
   • Muscular: severe myalgias
   • Mucous membranes: hyperemia
   • Renal: high levels of BUN and creatinine; pyuria
   • Liver: hepatitis with serum bilirubin, AST, and ALT 2× normal
   • Blood: thrombocytopenia
   • CNS: disorientation without focal neurologic signs

A definite case fulfills all five clinical criteria, and a probable case fulfills four of the five criteria.
BUN, blood urea nitrogen; AST, aspartate transaminase; ALT, alanine transaminase; CNS, central nervous system.

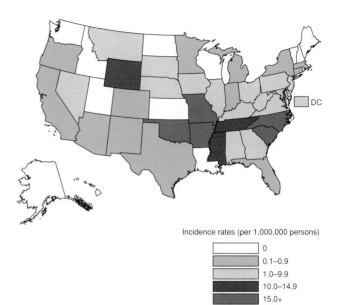

Incidence rates (per 1,000,000 persons)

	0
	0.1–0.9
	1.0–9.9
	10.0–14.9
	15.0+

Figure 2-31. A map of the United States showing the annual incidence of Rocky Mountain spotted fever (RMSF) in 2002. Although RMSF was first identified in the Rocky Mountain states, less than 1.5% of cases in the United States in 2002 were from that area. Image courtesy of the Centers for Disease Control and Prevention.

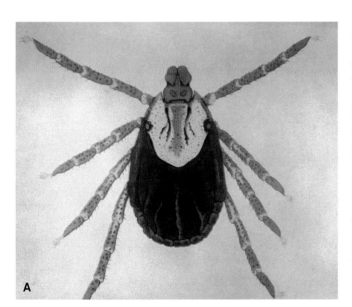

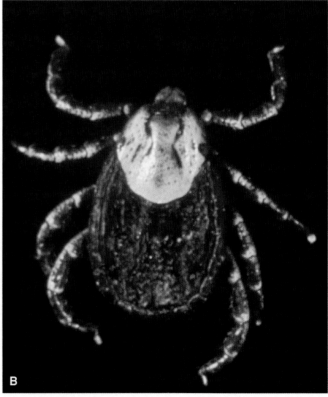

Figure 2-32. The American dog tick *Dermacentor variabilis* (**A**) and the Rocky Mountain wood tick *Dermacentor andersoni* (**B**), the two most common vectors of Rock Mountain spotted fever. Images courtesy of the Centers for Disease Control and Prevention, Andrew J Brooks.

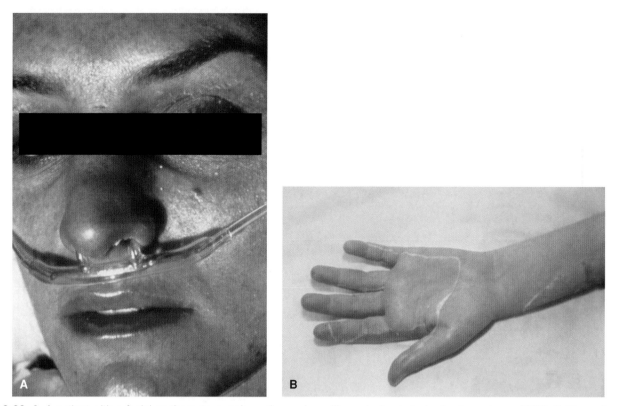

Figure 2-33. A, A patient with a facial erythematous rash, or the sunburn-like rash due to toxic shock syndrome (TSS). **B,** The patient's left palm shows desquamation, which develops late in the disease. Images courtesy of the Centers for Disease Control and Prevention.

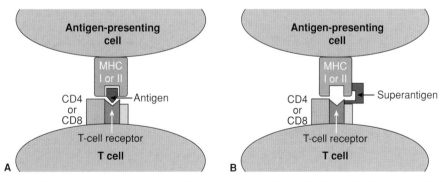

Figure 2-34. A diagram showing the interaction of an antigen (**A**) and a superantigen (**B**) with major histocompatability complex (MHC) and the T-cell receptor.

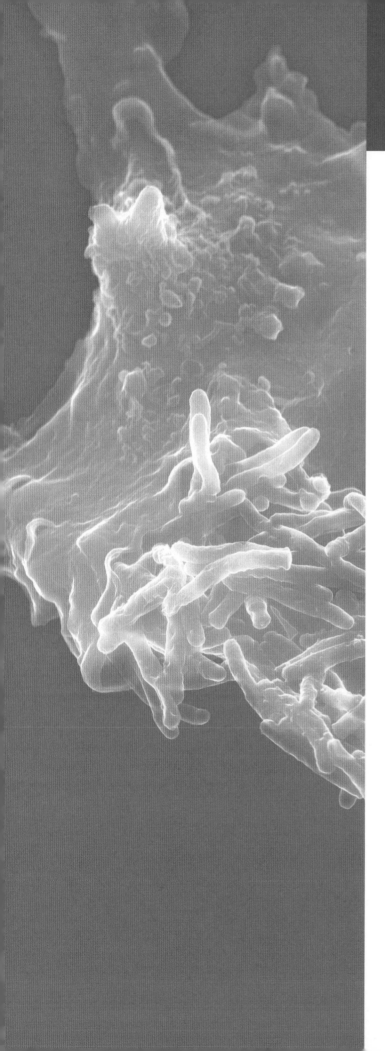

CHAPTER 3

PAPULES, PLAQUES, AND PATCHES

OVERVIEW

Plaques are elevated lesions larger than 1 cm in diameter, and are frequently formed by a confluence of many papules (Figure 3-1). Annular plaques are round lesions with a central area of clearing, and serpiginous plaques have a serpentine appearance. Patches are flat, nonpalpable lesions larger than 1 cm in diameter; in other words, patches are macules that are too large to be called macules. Papules are raised palpable lesions that are usually less than 1 cm in diameter (Figure 3-2).

This chapter is divided into discussions of hypopigmented and erythematous plaques, serpiginous and annular plaques, smooth papules, and verrucous (rough) papules (Figure 3-3; Table 3-1).

HYPOPIGMENTED PLAQUES: PITYRIASIS VERSICOLOR

Pityriasis versicolor (tinea versicolor) is an infection of the keratinized epithelial cells in the stratum corneum. The etiologic agent is considered a commensal and is present on the skin of most humans.

ETIOLOGY

Malassezia furfur is a dimorphic lipophilic fungus.

MANIFESTATIONS

Pityriasis versicolor is a common benign cutaneous fungal infection. Superficial hyper- or hypopigmented macules or patches appear on the chest or back (Figure 3-4).

EPIDEMIOLOGY

▪ *M furfur* is normal flora on the skin surface and can be isolated in 90–100% of adults.

▪ The prevalence of pityriasis versicolor is 2–8%. It is common in young adults.

▪ Some persons are genetically predisposed to pityriasis versicolor.

Patients with a deficiency in cell-mediated immunity are more likely to develop the infection (e.g., persons who are malnourished, infected with the human immunodeficiency virus [HIV], or are diabetic).

Pityriasis versicolor is usually found in warmer, more humid climates in the United States and in tropical areas worldwide. Fungal growth on skin is facilitated by higher temperatures and humidity.

PATHOGENESIS

M furfur infection remains in the stratum corneum. In patients with clinical disease, the organism is found in both the yeast (spore) stage and the filamentous (hyphal) form. Certain environmental and host factors can lead to the conversion of the saprophytic yeast to the parasitic mycelial morphologic form. *M furfur* produces dicarboxylic acids C9–C11, which inhibit tyrosinase. Tyrosinase is an enzyme involved in melanocyte pigment formation that causes hypopigmentation. In hyperpigmented macules, *M furfur* induces an enlargement of melanosomes, which are produced by melanocytes at the basal layer of the epidermis.

DIAGNOSIS

Diagnosis of pityriasis versicolor is usually determined following examination of the lesions. A Wood lamp can be used to demonstrate pale yellow to white fluorescence. Skin scrapings clarified with 10% KOH and stained with methylene blue may show round budding yeast cells and short fat hyphae described as **"spaghetti and meatballs"** (Figure 3-5).

THERAPY AND PREVENTION

Topical agents used to treat pityriasis versicolor include selenium sulfide, sodium sulfacetamide, and ciclopiroxolamine. Systemic treatment with ketoconazole, fluconazole, or itraconazole has also been shown to be effective. With either treatment, there is a high recurrence rate; therefore, prophylactic treatment with topical or oral therapy on an intermittent basis is usually necessary.

ERYTHEMATOUS PLAQUES: CUTANEOUS CANDIDIASIS

Candida albicans is a fungal commensal of the skin and can overgrow, causing infections of the skin and mucous membranes. Infections of the skin are common in immunocompetent persons and are becoming even more prevalent as the number of immunocompromised patients increases.

ETIOLOGY

The most common cause of cutaneous candidiasis is *C albicans*.

MANIFESTATIONS

Beefy-red, well-defined plaques with satellite plaques and pustules are usually found in moist intertriginous areas on patients

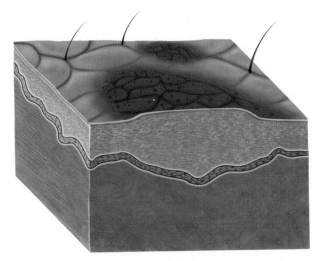

Figure 3-1. A plaque in the skin, depicted as a confluence of several papules.

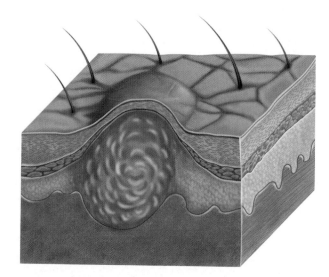

Figure 3-2. A papule in the skin.

with cutaneous candidiasis; areas include the groin, axillae, vagina, mouth, glans penis, angulus oris, and inframammary and obesity folds. Some of the more common manifestations are diaper rash (Figure 3-6), thrush (Figure 3-7), and perlèche (Figure 3-8). Thrush is an infection of the mucous membranes, which become fiery red and are covered partially or completely with a creamy-white, loosely adherent pseudomembrane. Perlèche fissures occur at angles of the mouth. Chronic mucocutaneous candidiasis is a form of widespread disease with chronic recalcitrant involvement of skin, mucous membranes, and nails (Figure 3-9).

EPIDEMIOLOGY

■ Immunodeficient or immunosuppressed patients—patients with diabetes mellitus, familial endocrinopathy syndrome, or macerated skin; diapered infants; and patients who are pregnant, obese, or immobile—are at increased risk of developing cutaneous candidiasis.

PATHOGENESIS

C albicans is normal flora of the skin in up to 50% of the general population. Predisposing factors can allow overgrowth of this organism, resulting in clinical manifestations. Cutaneous candidiasis infection is usually limited to the stratum corneum. Inflammation is augmented by the cell-mediated immune response.

DIAGNOSIS

Wet mounts of tissue samples in 10% KOH show spores, budding yeast, and pseudohyphae. Only *C albicans* and *C dubliniensis* produce germ tubes in medium containing horse serum and chlamydospores in cornmeal agar plates (Figure 3-10). The pustule or wet area of the lesion can be cultured on Sabouraud agar. Lesions do *NOT* fluoresce when exposed to a Wood lamp.

THERAPY AND PREVENTION

Topical treatment with antifungal creams containing nystatin or miconazole may be helpful. If topical treatment fails, treatment with systemic ketoconazole may eliminate the disease. It is important to prevent skin abrasions and to keep the area dry.

ERYTHEMATOUS PLAQUES: TINEA (DERMATOPHYTOSIS)

Dermatophytoses are superficial fungal skin infections that can occur on nearly every part of the body. Diagnosis often includes the location of the body affected by the organism—tinea capitis (head), tinea cruris (groin), tinea pedis (foot), tinea manus (hand), tinea barbae (beard), tinea faciei (face), and tinea unguium, or onychomycosis (nail).

ETIOLOGY

Microsporum, Trichophyton, and *Epidermophyton* (also called the dermatophytes) are the most common causes of

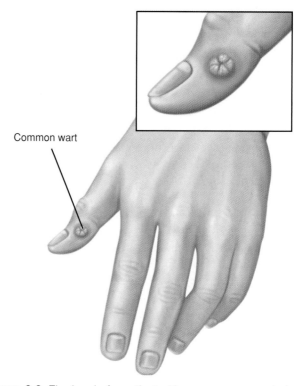

Common wart

Figure 3-3. The hand of a patient with a verrucous papule (common wart) due to the human papillomavirus.

TABLE 3-1. Papules, Plaques, and Patches

Hypopigmented plaques	Smooth papules
Tinea versicolor	Erythema nodosum
Erythematous plaques	Molluscum contagiosum
Candidiasis	Condyloma lata
Tinea	**Verrucous papules**
Erythrasma	Verrucae (warts, genital
Cellulitis	warts)
Erysipelas	Blastomycosis
Subcutaneous necrotizing	
infections	
Serpiginous or annular plaques	
Lyme disease	

dermatophytoses. Of the 40 different species that can cause tinea, only 6 cause 95% of all dermatophytoses. Onychomycosis is usually caused by *Trichophyton* but can also be due to infections with *Scopulariopsis, Fusarium,* and *C albicans.*

MANIFESTATIONS

Tinea lesions are usually pruritic erythematous macules that can become papular, annular, or confluent plaques with scaling or vesicles, or both. If the infection involves the scalp, hair loss is common (alopecia). This infection can involve any part of the skin or nails.

- **Tinea capitis:** Fungal infection of the scalp (Figure 3-11). The hair of the head, eyebrows, and eyelashes can also be involved, or the skin of the scalp alone can be infected. Nummular lesions to plaques and alopecia occur if the skin of the scalp is affected. Infections of the hair frequently result in broken hair (black-dot ringworm).

- **Tinea corporis:** Eczematous mildly erythematous plaques with central clearing and elevated borders on the trunk (Figure 3-12).

- **Tinea cruris:** Plaques present on the groin and perineum. There are usually no satellite lesions.

- **Tinea pedis:** Macerated scaling fissured toe webs; inflamed soles; thick friable toenails (Figure 3-13).

- **Tinea manuum:** Inflamed scaly palms.

- **Tinea unguium (onychomycosis):** Brown discoloration at the edge of the nails. Nails become soft, thick, and irregular and separate from the nail bed (Figure 3-14). Skin scales collect in the nail bed and lift the distal end of the nail. Tinea unguium usually results from untreated tinea pedis or tinea manuum.

EPIDEMIOLOGY

- Tinea accounts for 5% of all diseases that have a skin manifestation (~9 million cases per year in the United States).

- The incidence of dermatophyte infections varies with age, gender, ethnic group, and cultural and social habits.

- *The most common dermatophyte infection is tinea pedis.* Tinea capitis is common in children until they reach puberty, when it rapidly ceases to be a problem.

- Tinea capitis, tinea pedis, and tinea cruris are more common in men than in women. Tinea unguium on the fingernails is more common in women; however, the same infection on the toenails is more common in men.

- Several conditions predispose to chronic dermatophytosis, including moist environments (e.g., tropical climates, moist anatomic sites, and shower-room floors) and impaired cell-mediated immunity (e.g., immunodeficiency disorders, atopy, reticular malignancy, immunosuppressant drugs).

- Infections from zoophilic and geophilic dermatophytes tend to be more severe than infections from anthropophilic dermatophytes.

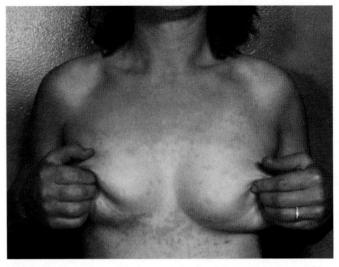

Figure 3-4. A patient with tinea versicolor due to *Malassezia furfur.* Image courtesy of the Centers for Disease Control and Prevention, Dr Lucille K Georg.

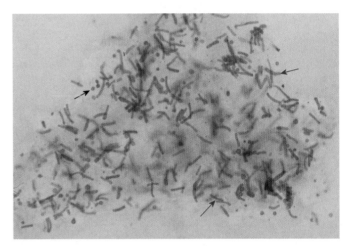

Figure 3-5. A micrograph showing the classic "spaghetti and meatball" appearance of *Malassezia furfur.* Black arrows point to the yeast cells ("meatballs"), and blue arrows point to the hyphal cells ("spaghetti") of this dimorphic fungus. Image courtesy of the Centers for Disease Control and Prevention, Dr Lucille K Georg.

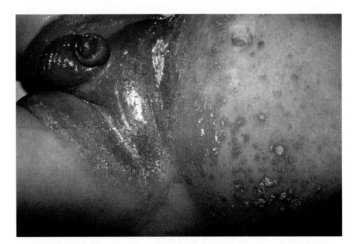

Figure 3-6. A photograph of the trunk of a young child with a severe case of diaper rash due to *Candida albicans.* Image courtesy of the Centers for Disease Control and Prevention.

■ Dermatophytes are transmitted from human to human (anthropophilic such as *T tonsurans* or *M audouinii)*, from nonhuman animals (zoophilic such as *M canis*), or from soil (geophilic such as *M gypseum*).

PATHOGENESIS

Fungi invade only the dead cornified layers of the skin, nails, and hair. Pathology results from the host's reaction to the fungus. The fundamental pathogenic mechanisms of dermatophytosis involve two distinct phases.

1. **Colonization:** Spores germinate on the skin, and the mycelium invades the stratum corneum. Deeper extension is restricted by the lack of iron, which is bound to the host's transferrin molecules and by the organism's growth requirement for keratin. Lateral extension continues for 1–5 weeks. After 2–3 weeks, the advancing border of the infection may become inflamed (ringworm lesions) due to a developing cell-mediated delayed-type hypersensitivity reaction.

2. **Host-parasite interaction:** Cell-mediated acute immune inflammation varies from erythema and edema of the dermis and epidermis to the formulation of vesicles and pustules. If epidermal integrity is breached, oozing and weeping of the tissue fluid occurs. Invasion of hair follicles results in inflamed nodules, deep-seated pustules, and abscesses. Inflammation tends to be most severe in geophilic species. Infections of the zoophilic species are intermediate in severity. Infections of anthropophilic species are milder than the two other species and may clear within 1–2 weeks.

Depending on the cell-mediated immune status of the patient, there are two basic results: (1) Normal cell-mediated immunity leads to an acute or inflammatory infection (which may heal spontaneously), or it will respond well to treatment. (2) Weak cell-mediated immunity results in chronic or noninflammatory infection with dryness, erythema, scaling, pruritus, and fissures. It relapses frequently and responds poorly to therapy.

DIAGNOSIS

Diagnosis of dermatophytoses is usually based on clinical appearance. Most lesions do not fluoresce when examined with a Wood lamp. A scraping of the lesions followed by 10% KOH treatment to eliminate the host cells is helpful. Occasionally, scrapings from the lesions are cultured on Sabouraud dextrose agar plates. Cultures are incubated at room temperature, with growth observed within 7–14 days.

THERAPY AND PREVENTION

Antifungal agents such as terbinafine, itraconazole, or fluconazole are helpful in treating onychomycosis. Tinea capitis can be treated with terbinafine. Tinea corporis, tinea cruris, and tinea pedis can be treated with over-the-counter clotrimazole or terbinafine. There is no vaccine or immunity following resolution of the infection; therefore, all patients with tinea infections should avoid environments where there is chronic moisture, areas with many spores (e.g., shower-room floors), and avoid wearing tight clothing.

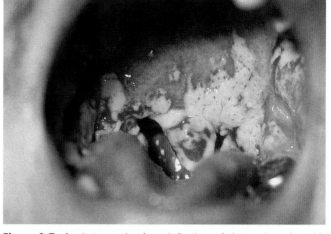

Figure 3-7. A photograph of an infection of the oral cavity with thrush caused by *Candida albicans*. Note the creamy appearance of the pseudomembrane and the erythematous appearance of the mucosa. Image courtesy of the Centers for Disease Control and Prevention.

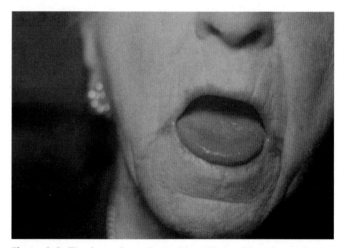

Figure 3-8. The face of a patient with perlèche. Note the erythema at the angles of the mouth, the site of perlèche. Image courtesy of the Centers for Disease Control and Prevention.

ERYTHEMATOUS PLAQUES: ERYTHRASMA

Erythrasma is a bacterial infection of the groin that is similar in appearance to tinea cruris and diaper rash. Differences in the fluorescence of the lesions following examination with a Wood lamp help in determining if the infection is erythrasma (coral-red fluorescence), tinea (usually does not fluoresce), or diaper rash (no fluorescence).

ETIOLOGY

Erythrasma is usually due to an organism in the normal flora called *Corynebacterium minutissimum* (gram-positive, rod-shaped bacteria).

MANIFESTATIONS

The lesions of erythrasma are brown to red-brown well-defined patches, which may have fine scale or epidermal wrinkling. They can be pruritic. Lesions are usually observed on the inner thighs, crural region, scrotum, and toe webs. The axillae, sub-mammary area, periumbilical region, and intergluteal fold can be affected but are less commonly reported.

EPIDEMIOLOGY

- Erythrasma occurs in about 4% of the population and is found worldwide.
- The infection is caused by a bacterium found in the normal flora and is facilitated by hot moist environments.
- Predisposing factors include excessive sweating, hyperhidrosis, obesity, diabetes mellitus, and other immunocompromised states.
- Obese middle-aged women or patients with diabetes mellitus are at increased risk.

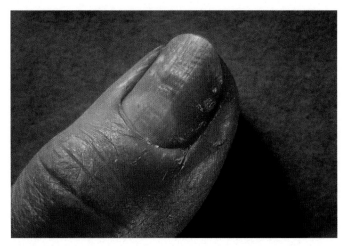

Figure 3-9. The fingernail of a patient with an infection due to *Candida*. Image courtesy of the Centers for Disease Control and Prevention, Sherry Brinkman.

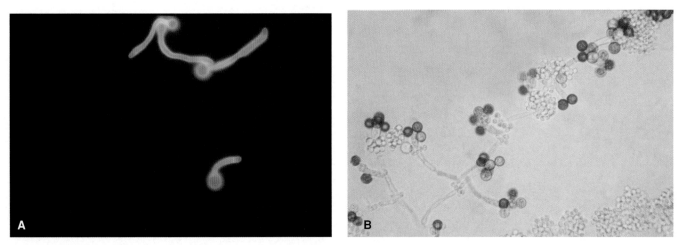

Figure 3-10. *Candida albicans* grown in special conditions to differentiate it from the other species in the genus. Only one other species of *Candida, C dubliniensis,* produces germ tubes and chlamydospores. **A,** Germ tubes of *C albicans* grown in media containing horse serum. A Calcofluor white stain was used to stain the organisms, which were visualized using a fluorescent microscope. **B,** Chlamydospores, the reproductive thick-walled structures of *C albicans* when grown in corn meal agar. Images courtesy of the Centers for Disease Control and Prevention, Mercy Hospital, Toledo, OH, Dr Brian Harrington, and the Centers for Disease Control and Prevention, Dr Godon Roberstad.

PATHOGENESIS

In patients with erythrasma, the bacteria invade the upper third of the stratum corneum and multiply in hot humid environments. The stratum corneum thickens, and the organisms can be seen in the intercellular spaces as well as within cells. *C minutissimum* can dissolve keratin fibrils.

DIAGNOSIS

The coral-red fluorescence seen when lesions are examined by Wood lamp is secondary to the production of porphyrin by bacteria. Skin scraping often reveals gram-positive rods after Gram staining. The skin scrapings also can be cultured to identify the organism.

THERAPY AND PREVENTION

Erythrasma can be treated with antiseptic or topical antibiotic such as fusidic acid cream and clindamycin solution. Extensive infections can be treated with oral erythromycin or tetracycline. To prevent recurrences, patients should be encouraged to improve hygiene, use antibacterial soaps to cleanse the area, and keep the area dry.

ERYTHEMATOUS PLAQUES: CELLULITIS

Cellulitis is an acute spreading infection of the dermis and subcutaneous tissues and results in pain, erythema, edema, and warmth.

ETIOLOGY

Many different bacteria can cause cellulitis; only a few are listed below.

- **Streptococcus pyogenes** (gram-positive coccus) is one of two common causes of superficial cellulitis. *Staphylococcus aureus* is the other common cause of a less extensive superficial cellulitis. It is commonly seen in association with wound or skin abscesses, and is a common cause of cellulitis that occurs in burn patients.
- **Gram-negative bacilli** (e.g., *Escherichia coli, Pseudomonas aeruginosa*) cause a superficial cellulitis resulting in granulocytopenia, foot ulcers in diabetic patients, or in severe tissue ischemia. *P aeruginosa* cellulitis and osteomyelitis often occur following trauma to the foot while inside an athletic shoe. It is also common in burn patients.
- **Streptococci groups B, C, D, and G** are less common causes of cellulitis.
- **Streptococcus pneumoniae** (gram-positive coccus) is characterized by a violaceous color and bullae.
- **Pasteurella multocida** (gram-negative rod) cellulitis is associated with dog or cat bites.

MANIFESTATIONS

Cellulitis infections are usually diffuse and can spread rapidly (Figure 3-15). Acute inflammation is seen within the subcutaneous solid tissues and is characterized by hyperemia and

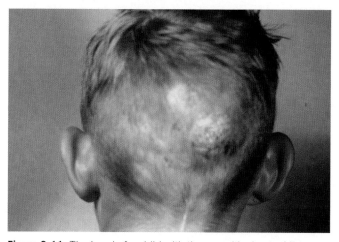

Figure 3-11. The head of a child with tinea capitis due to *Microsporum*. Image courtesy of the Centers for Disease Control and Prevention.

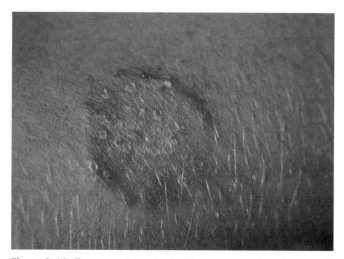

Figure 3-12. The arm of a patient with tinea corporis ("ringworm") lesions due to *Trichophyton mentagrophytes*. Image courtesy of the Centers for Disease Control and Prevention, Dr Lucille K Georg.

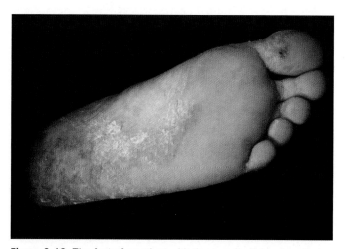

Figure 3-13. The foot of a patient with tinea pedis ("ringworm") due to *Trichophyton rubrum*. Image courtesy of the Centers for Disease Control and Prevention.

tenderness. The borders of the lesions are usually indistinct (Figure 3-16). Petechiae are common; however, large areas of ecchymoses are rare. Vesicles and bullae may develop and rupture, occasionally with necrosis of the involved skin. Histologic examination of a biopsy reveals leukocyte infiltration and edema without cellular necrosis or suppuration. Associated red streaking visible on skin proximal to the area of cellulitis is characteristic of ascending lymphangitis. Many patients do not appear ill; however, severe illness can occur. Manifestations include regional lymphadenopathy, fever, chills, malaise, tachycardia, headache, hypotension, and delirium. These symptoms may precede the cutaneous findings by just a few hours.

EPIDEMIOLOGY

- Facial cellulitis is more common in adults older than 50 years of age and in children 6 months to 3 years of age.

- Cellulitis is most common in the lower extremities.

- Conditions that predispose patients to increased risk of developing serious or rapidly spreading cellulitis include diabetes mellitus, immunodeficient status, varicella, impaired peripheral circulation (arterial insufficiency or venous stasis); lymphadenectomy following tumor excision such as mastectomy and postvenectomy status following stripping of the saphenous vein; and chronic steroid use.

- A cutaneous abnormality such as skin trauma, ulceration, tinea pedis, dermatitis, edematous tissue, and scars sustained from removal of the saphenous vein usually precedes cellulitis; there may be no predisposing condition or site of entry evident.

- Cellulitis following infection with gram-negative rods or fungi is more common in immunocompromised hosts.

PATHOGENESIS

A diffuse infection occurs in patients with cellulitis due to *S pyogenes* because streptokinase, DNase, and hyaluronidase break down cellular components that otherwise would contain and localize the inflammation. Spreading factors such as hyaluronidase, protease, and DNase are present in other bacteria and appear to be important in the pathogenesis of this disease. Cellulitis extends deeper into skin than does erysipelas (see below) and may result in osteomyelitis. Cellulitis results in serious systemic illness by uncontrolled spread to contiguous tissues, to the lymphatics, or to the bloodstream.

DIAGNOSIS

Diagnosis of cellulitis is usually based on clinical findings. Leukocytosis is commonly seen in the complete blood cell count (CBC). Unless there is pus or an open wound, the responsible organism is usually difficult to isolate, even on aspiration or skin biopsy. Results of blood cultures occasionally are positive. Serologic tests, especially a rising anti-DNase B titer, confirm a streptococcal cause.

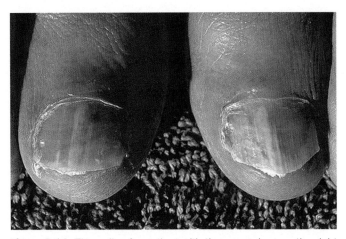

Figure 3-14. The nails of a patient with tinea unguium on the right and left great toes due to *Trichophyton rubrum*. Image courtesy of the Centers for Disease Control and Prevention, Dr Edwin P Ewing, Jr.

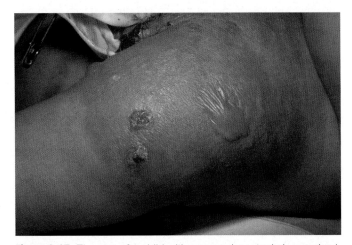

Figure 3-15. The arm of a child with a secondary staphylococcal cellulitis following vaccination for smallpox. Image courtesy of the Centers for Disease Control and Prevention, Allen W Mathies, MD, California Emergency Preparedness Office (Calif/EPO), Immunization Branch.

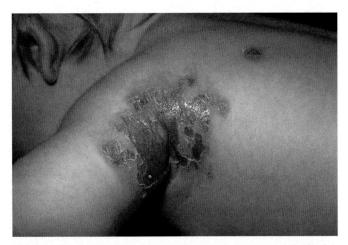

Figure 3-16. A child with a secondary staphylococcal cellulitis following vaccination for smallpox. The signs of cellulitis include the indistinct border, spreading erythema that surrounds the smallpox vaccination site, swelling, areas of purulence, and sloughing of necrotic skin. Image courtesy of the Centers for Disease Control and Prevention, Allen W Mathies, MD, California Emergency Preparedness Office (California EPO), Immunization Branch.

THERAPY AND PREVENTION

Oral or parenteral antibiotics are frequently used to treat patients with mild cellulitis. Patients with complicated cellulitis—cases where there is more extensive involvement, an underlying illness, or signs of systemic toxicity—usually must be admitted to the hospital and treated with antibiotics intravenously. Empiric antimicrobial agent coverage for *S pyogenes* and *S aureus* should be given. Outpatient regimens should include penicillinase-resistant synthetic penicillin (e.g., nafcillin), a first-generation cephalosporin (e.g., cephalexin), or a long-acting parenteral cephalosporin (e.g., ceftriaxone). Antibiotic prophylaxis can be given in cases of recurrent cellulitis.

ERYTHEMATOUS PLAQUES: ERYSIPELAS

Erysipelas is a superficial bacterial infection that extends into the cutaneous lymphatics.

ETIOLOGY

Over 80% of cases of erysipelas are due to infection with streptococci. *S pyogenes* (gram positive coccus) is present in over two thirds of cases, and group G streptococci (gram-positive cocci) are present in nearly a third of cases of erysipelas.

MANIFESTATIONS

Erysipelas is a superficial bacterial skin infection that extends into the cutaneous lymphatics. The lesions are raised and well demarcated with shiny bright red areas of dermal inflammation, which advance as the disease progresses (Figure 3-17). Edematous tender plaques are usually seen on the extremities or face. There is intense upper dermal edema, which tends to lift the epidermis except in areas where it is held down by hair follicles or sweat glands, resulting in the typical "**orange peel (peau d'orange) appearance**" (Figure 3-18). Extensions may have vesicles or bullae. The portal of entry may not be observed. Other symptoms include acute toxicity, fever, and pain.

EPIDEMIOLOGY

- The highest incidence of erysipelas occurs in patients aged 60 to 80 years.
- Erysipelas lesions are most commonly seen on the legs (in about 85% of cases), and the next most common location is the face.
- An interdigital fungal infection of the foot may provide a source for infection.
- Erysipelas is more commonly seen in patients who are immunocompromised and those with lymphedema.

PATHOGENESIS

In erysipelas, bacteria are usually initially inoculated into an area of skin trauma. Local factors such as venous insufficiency, stasis ulcerations, inflammatory dermatoses, dermatophyte infections, insect bites, and surgical incisions have all been

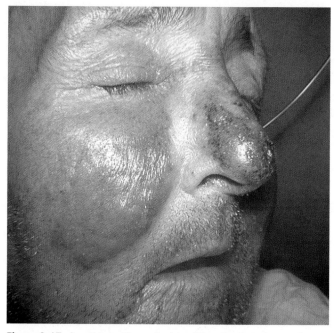

Figure 3-17. A patient with erysipelas of the cheek and nose. Image courtesy of the Centers for Disease Control and Prevention, Dr Thomas F Sellers, Emory University, Atlanta, GA.

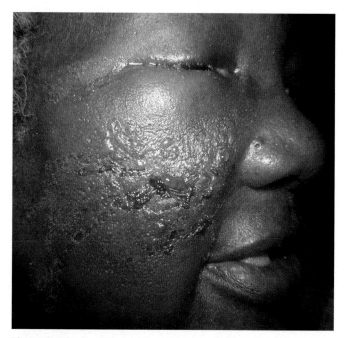

Figure 3-18. A patient with erysipelas. Notice the orange peel ("peau d'orange") appearance, the bullae, and the purulent material draining from the eye. Image courtesy of the Centers for Disease Control and Prevention, Dr Thomas F Sellers, Emory University, Atlanta, GA.

implicated as portals of entry. The source of the bacteria is usually from the host's nasopharynx. A history of recent streptococcal pharyngitis has been observed in up to 30% of patients. Other predisposing factors include diabetes mellitus, alcohol abuse, HIV infection, nephrotic syndrome, and other immunocompromising conditions. The infection rapidly invades and spreads via the lymphatic vessels, which can result in overlying skin "streaking" and regional lymphadenopathy.

DIAGNOSIS

Blood, wound, and nasopharyngeal samples should be obtained and cultured on blood agar plates; a CBC with differential should be ordered. Other laboratory tests may include erythrocyte sedimentation rate, urinalysis screening for hematuria and proteinuria, and antistreptolysin O and anti-DNase B titers. Neutrophilic leukocytosis is commonly seen in patients with erysipelas.

THERAPY AND PREVENTION

Elevation and rest of the affected limb are recommended to reduce local swelling and inflammation. Treatment includes oral or intramuscular injection of antibiotics such as penicillin, erythromycin, or azithromycin. Following treatment, the lesion usually desquamates but can resolve with pigmentary changes that may resolve over time. Predisposing skin lesions such as tinea pedis and stasis ulcers should be treated aggressively to prevent infections and superinfection.

ERYTHEMATOUS PLAQUES: SUBCUTANEOUS NECROTIZING INFECTIONS

The diseases in the category called subcutaneous necrotizing infections cause extensive destruction of the subcutaneous tissues and fascia, and some also cause extensive necrosis of the muscles (Figure 3-19). Diseases known as subcutaneous necrotizing infections include synergistic necrotizing cellulitis, necrotizing fasciitis, progressive bacterial synergistic gangrene, non-clostridial anaerobic cellulitis, clostridial cellulitis, and clostridial myonecrosis (gas gangrene).

ETIOLOGY

Table 3-2 is a summary of the etiologic agents that cause the various forms of subcutaneous necrotizing infections.

MANIFESTATIONS

Subcutaneous edema and necrosis are seen in the area of the subcutaneous necrotizing infection. The infected site is usually quite painful, and the overlying skin is hot and erythematous and edematous. With progression, violaceous discoloration and bullae, crepitus, palpable gas in tissues, and dermal gangrene may develop (see Table 3-2). When male genitalia are involved, the disease is called Fournier gangrene. Fever is nearly always present and accompanied by systemic toxicity, including

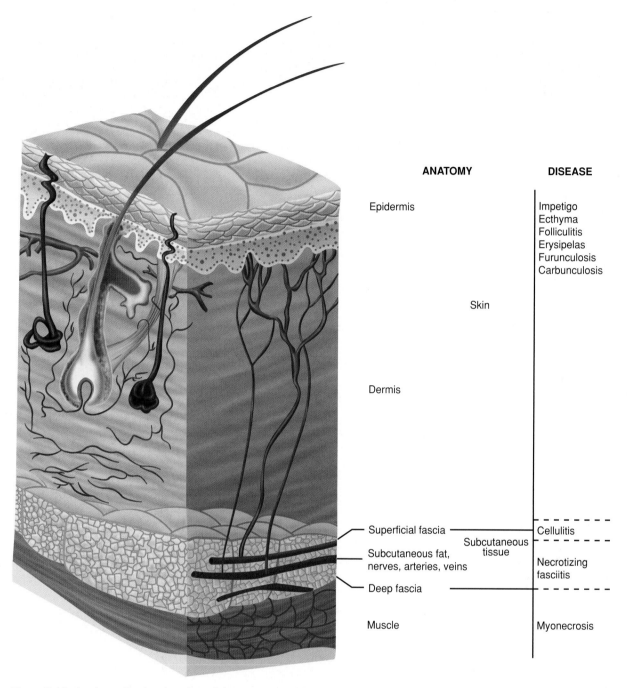

Figure 3-19. A schematic showing sites of damage caused by subcutaneous necrotizing infections compared to other infections of the skin.

tachycardia and altered mental status. Evidence of intravascular volume depletion, including hypotension, is common.

EPIDEMIOLOGY

About 1000 cases of clostridial myonecrosis occur each year in the United States. The mortality rate with treatment is 20–30%.

The most common site of involvement is an extremity, and may occur from infected cutaneous ulcers or infectious complications of previous injury.

The second most common site of involvement is the perineum, which is usually a complication of prior surgery,

TABLE 3-2. Subcutaneous Necrotizing Infections

Disease	Skin	Other Tissues Involved	Organisms	Predisposing Conditions	Systemic Toxicity	Progression of Infection in Tissue
Synergistic necrotizing cellulitis	Scattered areas of necrosis; usually involve perineum and legs; moderate gas production	Deeper compartments, including muscle	Anaerobes and aerobes	Diabetes mellitus, perirectal infections	Severe	Rapid
Necrotizing fasciitis	Erythematous cellulitis, usually at wounds moderate gas production	Fascia	*Streptococcus pyogenes* (most common); *Staphylococcus aureus*, anaerobes	Diabetes mellitus, abdominal surgery	Marked	Rapid, flesh eating; often fatal
Progressive bacterial synergistic gangrene	Central ulcer, surrounding purple hue, outer erythema usually at wounds; minimal gas production	Subcutaneous tissues	Microaerophilic streptococci, *S aureus*; enterobacteriaceae	Laparotomy with steel sutures	Minimal	Slowly progressive; often fatal
Nonclostridial anaerobic cellulitis	Minimal discoloration, usually at wounds; significant gas production	Subcutaneous tissues	Anaerobes or coliforms, or both	Diabetes mellitus	Moderate	Variable
Clostridial cellulitis	Minimal discoloration, usually at wounds; significant gas production	Subcutaneous tissues	*Clostridium* sp.	Local trauma or surgery	Severe	Rapid
Clostridial myonecrosis (gas gangrene)	Yellow-bronze, dark bullae, usually at wounds; moderate gas production	Muscle; little to no purulence in tissue	*Clostridium perfringens* iis the most common cause; other *Clostridium* species can cause the disease	Local trauma or surgery	Severe	Rapid

perirectal abscesses, periurethral gland infection, or retroperitoneal infections from perforated abdominal viscera.

■ Diabetes mellitus predisposes patients to subcutaneous necrotizing disease.

PATHOGENESIS

This bacterial infection extends into the subcutaneous tissue following trauma or due to an infection in an area contiguous to the subcutaneous necrotizing infection (see Figure 3-19). There is widespread undermining of surrounding tissue as well as the major findings of edema and necrosis of the subcutaneous tissues. Occlusion of small subcutaneous vessels leads to dermal gangrene. Muscle involvement is minimal or absent, except in cases of gas gangrene and synergistic necrotizing cellulitis.

Microscopic abnormalities may include intense white blood cell infiltration, microabscess formation, and necrosis in the subcutaneous tissue and adjacent fascia. An exception, however, is a patient with clostridial myonecrosis. Toxins produced by the bacteria in clostridial myonecrosis destroy the white blood cells, and very few are seen in the tissues of these patients. The subcutaneous arterioles and venules are often completely occluded. Ischemia, edema, and inflammation in the subcutaneous tissue decrease PO_2 and permit growth of obligate anaerobes (e.g., *Bacteroides*) while promoting anaerobic metabolism by facultative organisms (e.g., *Escherichia coli*). Anaerobic metabolism often produces hydrogen and nitrogen, which are relatively insoluble gases that may accumulate in subcutaneous tissues and cause crepitus or subcutaneous gas.

DIAGNOSIS

A CBC with differential usually reveals a polymorphonuclear leukocytosis. X-rays of the affected area often show soft tissue gas. The skin is red hot, tender, and markedly edematous and suggests an underlying necrotizing subcutaneous infection, which is a dermatologic emergency. Differentiation of cellulitis from clostridial gas gangrene, in which myositis and myonecrosis occur, is critical to proper management. Rapid progression of tissue damage or the development of bullae, ecchymoses, dermal gangrene, fluctuance, crepitus, or soft tissue gas requires surgical exploration. Blood cultures should be obtained. Pus aspirated into a syringe percutaneously or during surgery provides the most suitable material for Gram stain and aerobic and anaerobic cultures.

THERAPY AND PREVENTION

Gentamicin combined with clindamycin, or cefoxitin or imipenem alone is appropriate treatment of subcutaneous necrotizing infections pending results of cultures. Therapy involves incision and extensive debridement. Hyperbaric oxygen therapy is also used. Prevention involves proper care of wounds and trauma sites.

SERIPIGINOUS AND ANNUAL PLAQUES: LYME DISEASE

Lyme disease is the most common tick-borne illness in the United States.

ETIOLOGY

Lyme disease is caused by *Borrelia burgdorferi*, a bacterial spirochete.

MANIFESTATIONS

Within 3–32 days after a patient experiences a tick bite, a red macule will appear at the site. The macule expands radially with central clearing and swelling (e.g., erythema chronicum migrans, bull's eye, or annular erythema). This herald (bull's eye) lesion is seen in about 75% of all cases of Lyme disease and can become as large as 50 cm in diameter (Figure 3-20). In about 20% of patients, secondary skin lesions without the swollen center may occur elsewhere on the body. Other manifestations are variable and include a musculoskeletal flu-like syndrome consisting of malaise, fatigue, chills, fever, headache, stiff neck, myalgias, and arthralgias.

If Lyme disease is untreated, swelling, redness, and pain in one or a few large joints, usually the knees (e.g., arthritis), may develop in about 60% of patients. In about 15% of patients, neurologic abnormalities may occur and include headache, Bell palsy (Figure 3-21), bilateral facial palsy, paresthesias or pain due to peripheral neuropathy, and personality, cognitive, and sleep disturbances due to chronic encephalopathy. Myocardial abnormalities including palpitations, lightheadedness, and syncope, which may be a manifestation of varying degrees of heart block, are seen in about 8% of patients.

EPIDEMIOLOGY

- About 12,000 cases of Lyme disease occur in the United States each year, with the highest incidence in summer and early fall.

- The incidence is highest in children aged 5–10 years.

- The three regions in the United States with the highest number of cases are the Northeast (from Massachusetts to Maryland), the upper Midwest (especially Minnesota and Wisconsin), and the West Coast (especially northern California) (Figure 3-22).

- Deer, mice, sheep, and dogs serve as reservoirs for *B burgdorferi*.

- *B burgdorferi* is transmitted from animal reservoirs to humans via a bite from a hard-shelled tick (*Ixodes* sp.) (Figure 3-23).

PATHOGENESIS

The bacterium *B burgdorferi* causes many of the manifestations of Lyme disease, and some manifestations are probably due to the immune response to the bacterial infection. Although any body part can be infected, *B burgdorferi* shows a distinct tropism for the skin, central nervous system (CNS), heart, joints, and eyes. Once in the skin, the bacteria can either be eliminated by host defense mechanisms, remain viable and produce the pathognomonic skin lesion (erythema migrans), or disseminate via the lymphatics or blood. Hematogenous dissemination can occur within days to weeks following the initial infection. The bacterium then grows in the skin, heart, joints, CNS, and other parts of the body.

Stages of lyme disease

1. **Early stage localized disease** refers to isolated erythema migrans and an undifferentiated febrile illness. Most patients have erythema migrans.

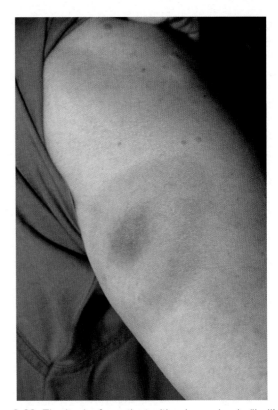

Figure 3-20. The back of a patient with a large classic "bull's eye" (erythema chronicum migrans) lesion on the posterior area of the right upper arm following a tick bite. Image courtesy of the Centers for Disease Control and Prevention, James Gathany.

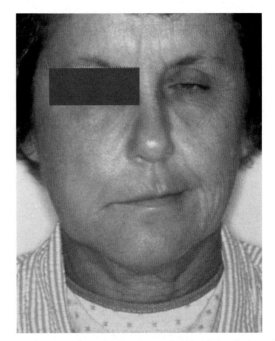

Figure 3-21. A patient with Bell palsy caused by *Borrelia burgdorferi*. Image courtesy of the Centers for Disease Control and Prevention.

2. **Early stage disseminated disease** refers to the extracutaneous manifestations and secondary skin lesions that occur during the first weeks to months after infection.

3. **Late stage disease** refers to later manifestations, usually in the CNS and joints, which occurs months to years later.

DIAGNOSIS

Presumptive diagnosis of Lyme disease is based on the typical erythema migrans rash and associated neurologic, cardiac, or rheumatic abnormalities. Definitive diagnosis requires a serologic test for the presence of antibodies to *B burgdorferi*. An ELISA that detects *B burgdorferi* IgM and IgG antibodies is usually performed.

THERAPY AND PREVENTION

Oral doxycycline, amoxicillin, or cefuroxime can be given to a patient bitten by a tick from an area that is endemic for Lyme disease. Patients with certain neurologic or cardiac forms of illness may require intravenous treatment with ceftriaxone or penicillin. To prevent tick bites, avoid tick habitats, wear appropriate clothing (long-sleeved garments and long pants) when outdoors, and use insect repellants. Because it can take several hours for the bacteria to infect a person, prompt removal of attached ticks can prevent infections.

SMOOTH PAPULAR LESIONS: ERYTHEMA NODOSUM

Erythema nodosum is an inflammatory disease of the deep dermis and subcutaneous fat.

ETIOLOGY

Table 3-3 lists the many different identified causes of erythema nodosum. Infectious causes are the most common and include bacteria and fungi.

MANIFESTATIONS

Erythema nodosum is characterized by discrete ill-defined nodules that are painful, hot, and tender (Figure 3-24). Lesions usually are seen on the anterior lower legs, but occasionally occur on the upper extremities and face. Lesions are usually symmetrical and change color over time. During the first week, lesions are bright red; by the second week, they become bluish to livid, and eventually the color fades to a yellowish hue resembling a bruise. The lesions disappear within 1–2 weeks as the overlying skin desquamates. Other manifestations include fever, malaise, and arthralgias, usually in the ankles, wrists, or knees. Other pathogen-specific manifestations may include pharyngitis, diarrhea, or chronic or atypical pneumonia.

EPIDEMIOLOGY

Erythema nodosum is most common in young adults aged 18–34 years.

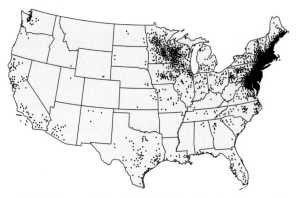

Figure 3-22. A map of the United States showing the number of reported cases of Lyme disease in 2005. One dot was placed randomly in each county for each case reported. Image courtesy of the Centers for Disease Control and Prevention.

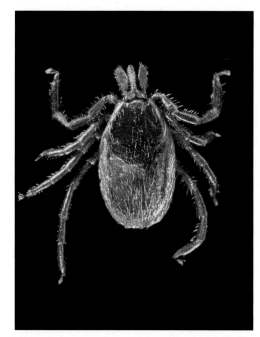

Figure 3-23. The dorsal view of an adult female western black-legged tick, *Ixodes pacificus*, which transmits *Borrelia burgdorferi*. Image courtesy of the Centers for Disease Control and Prevention, Dr Amanda Loftis, Dr William Nicholson, Dr Will Reeves, and Dr Chris Paddock.

TABLE 3-3. Causes of Erythema Nodosum

Cause(s)		Comment
Infections (most common cause)	Bacteria	*Streptococcus pyogenes* (most common cause of infections) *Salmonella* *Campylobacter* *Mycobacterium tuberculosis* *Mycoplasma pneumoniae* *Chlamydia trachomatis*
	Fungi	*Coccidioides immitis* *Histoplasma capsulatum* *Blastomyces dermatitidis*
Drug reactions	Sulfonamides Sulfonylureas Gold Oral contraceptives	
Other conditions	Ulcerative colitis Crohn disease Sarcoidosis Behçet disease	
Cancer	Hodgkin disease lymphoma	
Pregnancy		

▪ Women are affected more often than men, with a female-to-male ratio of 4:1.

▪ In children, erythema nodosum is usually caused by streptococcal upper respiratory tract infections.

▪ In adults, streptococcal infections and sarcoidosis are the most common causes of erythema nodosum.

▪ Less common causes of erythema nodosum (except in endemic areas) include coccidioidomycosis (southwestern United States), histoplasmosis (Ohio and Mississippi River valleys in the United States), primary tuberculosis, lymphogranuloma venereum, leprosy, ulcerative colitis, and drug reactions.

PATHOGENESIS

Erythema nodosum is a hypersensitivity reaction associated with the causes detailed in Table 3-3.

DIAGNOSIS

Deep-wedge biopsy in a patient with erythema nodosum will show septal panniculitis of subcutaneous tissue. A throat culture will exclude infection due to *S pyogenes*. Erythrocyte sedimentation rates are usually very high. Antistreptolysin O titer is elevated in some patients, but normal values do not exclude streptococcal infection. During the initial workup, antistreptolysin O titer levels should be obtained, since streptococcal disease is a common cause of erythema nodosum. An appropriate history of gastrointestinal complaints and a fecal examination

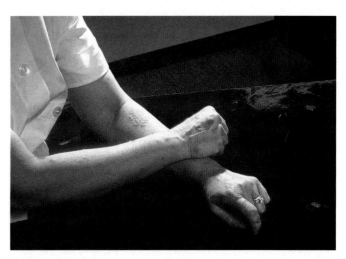

Figure 3-24. A patient with erythema nodosum on the arms and hands. Image courtesy of the Centers for Disease Control and Prevention, Margaret Renz.

can exclude infection due to *Salmonella* and *Campylobacter* organisms. Blood cultures should be obtained according to preliminary indications and findings.

THERAPY AND PREVENTION

Erythema nodosum usually regresses spontaneously; however, symptomatic relief can be obtained with nonsteroidal anti-inflammatory drugs (e.g., acetylsalicylic acid, ibuprofen, naproxen, indomethacin), and usually is all that is necessary. Recurrences following cessation of treatment are common. Prevention depends on the cause of erythema nodosum.

SMOOTH PAPULES: MOLLUSCUM CONTAGIOSUM

Molluscum contagiosum is a viral infection that produces papules with a central depression, and is most commonly seen in children younger than 5 years of age.

ETIOLOGY

Molluscum contagiosum virus is a large DNA poxvirus.

MANIFESTATIONS

Molluscum contagiosum lesions are translucent pink or flesh-colored, dome-shaped papules 2–10 mm in diameter. The center of the lesion is depressed (umbilicated) (Figure 3-25). Painless lesions occur in crops and may be pruritic and excoriated. Lesions can appear almost anywhere on the body, including the mucous membranes; they do not appear on the palms and soles.

EPIDEMIOLOGY

- Molluscum contagiosum is found worldwide.
- Prevalence of molluscum contagiosum in patients who are HIV positive may be as high as 5–18%.
- Lesions are usually observed on the chest, arms, legs, and face.
- Lesions are widespread and persistent in patients who are immunocompromised or have acquired immune deficiency syndrome (AIDS) and have low T-cell counts.
- The disease is self-limiting in patients with a normally functioning immune system; however, lesions can remain for years.
- Most infections occur in children and result from direct skin-to-skin contact or by contact with contaminated fomites (on bath towels, sponges, and gymnasium equipment).
- Molluscum contagiosum is usually a sexually transmitted infection in healthy adults. Few lesions are present and are usually limited to the genitalia, lower abdomen, or buttocks.

PATHOGENESIS

Molluscum contagiosum is a benign proliferation of epidermal cells that develops in response to poxvirus infection. The virus replicates in the cytoplasm of epithelial cells producing cytoplasmic inclusions; it may cause enlargement of infected cells.

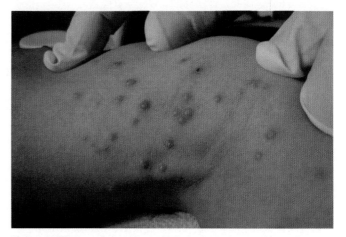

Figure 3-25. A patient with multiple lesions due to the molluscum contagiosum virus. Notice that several of the lesions are umbilicated in the center. Image courtesy of David Phillips, PhD, http://www.molluscum.com.

The severity of molluscum contagiosum is inversely related to the CD4 T-lymphocyte count. The infection usually resolves spontaneously without scarring over a period of weeks to years.

DIAGNOSIS

Diagnosis of molluscum contagiosum usually can be established based on the distinctive central umbilication of the dome-shaped lesions. If the diagnosis is uncertain, lesions can be biopsied. Characteristic intracytoplasmic inclusion bodies (molluscum bodies or Henderson-Patterson bodies) can be seen on histologic examination. Diagnosis of molluscum contagiosum can also be obtained by expressing the cheese-like substance from the center of the lesions, which contain molluscum bodies when Giemsa stained. Keratinocytes contain multiple intracytoplasmic inclusion bodies (Henderson-Patterson or molluscum bodies). Polymerase chain reaction (PCR) can be used to amplify viral DNA and detect the virus in material from the lesions.

THERAPY AND PREVENTION

Without treatment, molluscum contagiosum lesions will heal within several months or years. To prevent autoinoculation or transmission to close contacts, therapy may be beneficial and includes topical (e.g., podophyllin, trichloroacetic acid, cryotherapy with liquid nitrogen) and systemic agents (e.g., griseofulvin, methisazone, cimetidine). In immunocompromised patients, improvement of lesions can be observed following treatment with intravenous and topical ritonavir, cidofovir, zidovudine, or intralesional interferon alpha or topical injections of streptococcal antigen OK-432. To prevent spread, contact with infected persons should be avoided.

SMOOTH PAPULES: CONDYLOMA LATA

Condyloma lata are perimucosal skin papules that may be present in patients who have secondary syphilis. Refer to Chapter 2 for further discussion about condyloma lata.

ETIOLOGY

Condyloma lata are caused by *Treponema pallidum*, a thin bacterial spirochete (Figure 3-26).

MANIFESTATIONS

The lesions of condyloma lata are flattened, hypertrophic dull pink or gray papules that occur at the mucocutaneous junctions and in moist or intertriginous areas of the skin (Figure 3-27). Lesions are infectious.

EPIDEMIOLOGY

- Lesions of condyloma lata appear 6–8 weeks after the appearance of the primary chancre.
- The disease is usually acquired by unprotected sexual contact with an infected individual.

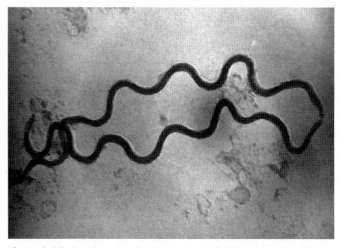

Figure 3-26. An electron photomicrograph of *Treponema pallidum*, which causes condyloma lata. Image courtesy of the Centers for Disease Control and Prevention, Joyce Ayers.

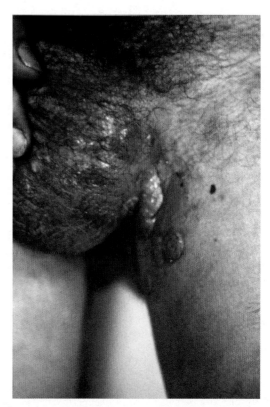

Figure 3-27. A patient with secondary syphilis and the lesions of condyloma latum. Image courtesy of the Centers for Disease Control and Prevention, Susan Lindsley.

PATHOGENESIS

See Chapter 2.

DIAGNOSIS

Lesions are similar to and frequently misdiagnosed as condyloma acuminatum (genital warts). As their name implies, condyloma lata are smoother and softer than the rough and hard condyloma acuminatum lesions.

THERAPY AND PREVENTION

Condyloma lata are treated with benzathine penicillin. Intimate contact with infected persons and with the lesions should be avoided.

VERRUCOUS LESIONS: VERRUCAE (WARTS)

Millions of people are infected each year by the human papillomavirus (HPV). Lesions can occur anywhere in the skin and on mucous membranes.

ETIOLOGY

Over 100 different types of HPV have been identified as agents of human infection.

MANIFESTATIONS

The most common clinical manifestations of HPV infection include common warts, flat warts, deep palmoplantar warts (myrmecia), and anogenital warts.

- **Common warts,** or **verruca vulgaris,** appear as hyperkeratotic papules with a rough irregular surface and range from less than 1 mm to larger than 1 cm. They can occur on any part of the body but usually are seen on the hands and knees. Lesions are usually caused by HPV type 2 and HPV-4 (most common), followed by types 1, 3, 27, 29, and 57.

- **Flat (plane) warts,** or **verruca plana,** are flat or slightly elevated flesh-colored papules that may be smooth or slightly hyperkeratotic and range in size from 1–5 mm. Patients may have only a few lesions or hundreds, which may become grouped or confluent. They may appear in a linear distribution as a result of trauma (Koebner phenomenon). Flat warts can occur anywhere; however, the face, hands, and shins are the most commonly affected areas. Regression of the lesions may occur, which usually is preceded by inflammation. HPV types 3, 10, and 28 usually cause these lesions.

- **Deep palmoplantar (myrmecia) warts** begin as small shiny papules and progress to deep endophytic, sharply defined round lesions with a rough keratotic surface that is surrounded by a smooth collar of calloused skin (Figure 3 28). Because this type of wart grows deep, it is likely to be more painful than common warts. Myrmecia warts that occur on the soles of the feet (plantar surface) are commonly found on weight-bearing areas (e.g., metatarsal head and heel). When warts occur on the hand, they tend to be subungual or periungual. Lesions are usually caused by HPV type 1 (most common), followed by types 2, 3, 4, 27, 29, and 57.

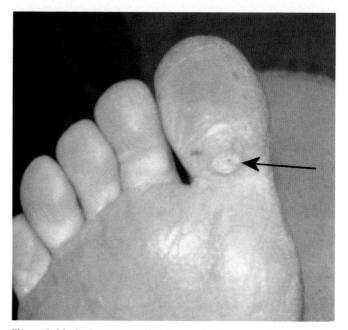

Figure 3-28. A plantar wart (*black arrow*) at the base of the patient's right great toe.

Anogenital (genital) warts, or condyloma acuminatum, are pink-to-brown papillomatous papules or nodules of the genitalia, perineum, crural folds, and anus (Figure 3-29). Warts vary in size and can form large exophytic cauliflower-like masses (Figure 3-30). Discrete papules 1–3 mm in diameter can be observed on the shaft of the penis. Lesions can extend into the vagina, urethra, cervix, perirectal epithelium, anus, and rectum. About 30 different HPV types are known to cause genital warts with types 6 and 11 being the most common.

EPIDEMIOLOGY

Warts are common worldwide and are estimated to affect about 7–12% of the population. In school-aged children, the prevalence is higher (10–20%). Increased frequency also is seen among immunosuppressed patients and meat handlers.

About 10% of the general population is infected by genital HPV at some point during their lifetime, with the highest incidence routinely observed in young adults aged 15–25 years.

The HPV viruses can resist desiccation, freezing, and prolonged storage outside host cells.

Predisposing factors include disruption to the normal epithelial barrier.

Most cases of HPV are transmitted by direct or indirect contact.

Anogenital warts are the most common sexually transmitted infection. Approximately 500,000–1,000,000 new cases of genital warts occur in the United States yearly.

PATHOGENESIS

The HPV virus infects the basal epidermal cells. As the cells differentiate and move to the surface, the virus becomes active and induces epidermal proliferation. Many warts resolve spontaneously within a few years. Cell-mediated immunity plays a significant role in wart regression. Patients with cell-mediated immune deficiencies are particularly susceptible to HPV infection, and lesions in these patients are very difficult to treat.

Many anogenital warts are benign. Patients with these infections receive intense clinical attention because of the increased risk of malignancy secondary to HPV infection. Some anogenital infections that are caused by HPV and are more likely to be malignant usually do not produce the wart-like lesion. HPV types 16, 18, 31, 33, and 51 (16 and 18 are most common) are commonly associated with anogenital malignancy (see Chapter 36).

DIAGNOSIS

The diagnosis of warts is usually based on clinical findings. Viral DNA identification using Southern blot hybridization is specific and quite sensitive and can be used to identify the specific HPV type present in tissue. PCR can be used to detect viral DNA; however, HPV DNA may not be present in older lesions.

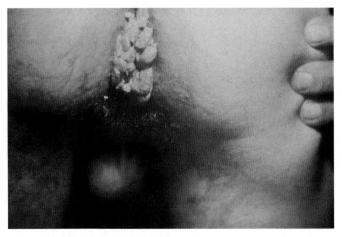

Figure 3-29. A patient with severe anogenital wart infection. Image courtesy of the Centers for Disease Control and Prevention, Dr Wiesner.

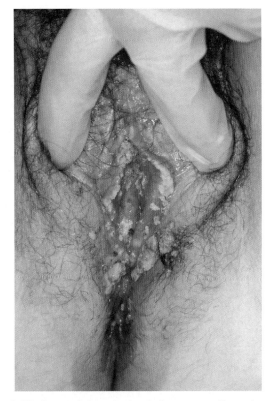

Figure 3-30. Anogenital warts due to human papillomavirus infection on and around the patient's labia. Image courtesy of the Centers for Disease Control and Prevention, Joe Miller.

In anogenital HPV infections that do not result in wart-like lesions, 5% acetic acid can be placed on the cervix of the patient. The areas of the cervix infected with HPV will produce an aceto-white reaction. PCR can be used to detect viral HPV DNA from cervical samples.

THERAPY AND PREVENTION

Treatment of warts can be difficult, with frequent failures and recurrences. Various procedures have been used and include application of topical agents such as salicylic acid and podophyllin; intralesional injections such as bleomycin and alpha interferon; systemic agents such as retinoids; and treatments with cryosurgery, lasers, plasters, curettage, electrodesiccation, and surgical excision. Most common warts usually disappear within 2 years without treatment. Contact with lesions should be avoided.

VERRUCOUS LESIONS: BLASTOMYCOSIS

Blastomycosis is a fungal infection that is also called North American blastomycosis or Gilchrist disease.

ETIOLOGY

Blastomyces dermatitidis is a thermally dimorphic fungus with a mold-to-yeast transition when infecting susceptible species. Organisms grown at 37°C and those obtained from a patient are in the yeast phase. When grown at room temperature, the organism becomes a mold.

MANIFESTATIONS

An infection of the lungs precedes the appearance of the skin lesions in patients diagnosed with blastomycosis, with skin lesions occurring in about 25% of patients. Slowly spreading papules (Figure 3-31) or papulopustules appear on skin with painless miliary abscesses less than 1 mm on the advancing border. As lesions enlarge, the centers heal with a scar. A fully developed lesion appears as an elevated verrucous patch, which is larger than 2 cm wide with an abruptly sloping purplish red abscess-studded border. Ulceration can occur after bacterial superinfection.

EPIDEMIOLOGY

■ Blastomycosis is endemic in the southeastern and south central states of North America, along the Mississippi and Ohio Rivers.

■ Outbreaks have been associated with occupational or recreational activities around streams or rivers with a high content of moist soil enriched with organic debris or rotting wood.

■ The incidence and severity of blastomycosis is increased in immunocompromised patients. One third of immunocompromised patients do not respond to therapy, and the mortality rate is 30–40%.

■ Untreated blastomycosis is slowly progressive and can be self-limited or fatal. If not treated, the mortality rate in patients

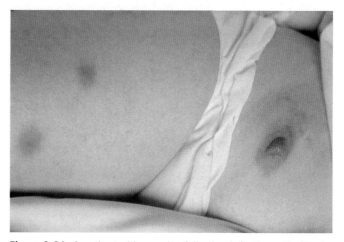

Figure 3-31. A patient with papules following infection with *Blastomyces dermatitidis*. Image courtesy of the Centers for Disease Control and Prevention.

with normal immune functioning can be as high as 60%; however, with appropriate treatment, the mortality rate can be reduced to about 10%.

PATHOGENESIS

Initially, *B dermatitidis* organisms are inhaled and infect the lungs. The conidia become yeast in the lung and are phagocytized by macrophages. The macrophages carry the organisms to other parts of the body (e.g., skin, bones, genitourinary tract, and other reticuloendothelial organs). The pulmonary infection can have three different outcomes:

- Resolution without involvement of other organs.
- Progressive pulmonary disease.
- Resolution of the pulmonary disease followed by infection of the skin, bones, genitourinary tract, and other reticuloendothelial organs.

At least 50% of primary infections are asymptomatic. Cell-mediated immunity plays a significant role in eliminating blastomycosis infection. Patients with cell-mediated immune deficiencies are particularly susceptible to this infection and can be difficult to treat. Resolution of the pulmonary disease does *not* result in calcifications in the lung.

DIAGNOSIS

Culture is definitive, but identification is aided by microscopy of sputum, pus, or urine specimens showing characteristic thick-walled unencapsulated yeasts (8–15 μm) with **broad-based buds** (Figure 3-32).

THERAPY AND PREVENTION

Amphotericin B is used to treat blastomycosis. Although immunocompromised patients living in or visiting areas that are endemic to blastomycosis cannot completely avoid exposure, they should be advised about reducing the risk of acquiring blastomycosis by avoiding certain occupational and recreational activities that would increase their risk of exposure (e.g., wooded areas along waterways).

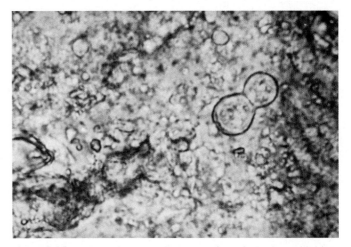

Figure 3-32. A smear from a lesion on the foot of a patient with blastomycosis. The yeast cell is undergoing broad-base budding. Image courtesy of the Centers for Disease Control and Prevention, ASCP, Atlas of Clinical Mycology II.

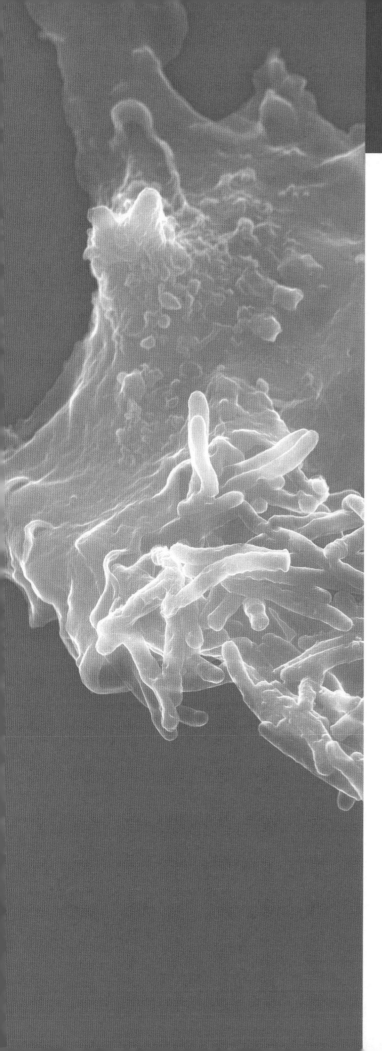

CHAPTER 4

VESICULAR, BULLOUS, AND PURULENT LESIONS

OVERVIEW

Vesicles and bullae are fluid-filled blisters (Figure 4-1). Vesicles are less than 1 cm in diameter, and bullae are larger than 1 cm in diameter. Purulent lesions are usually less than 1 cm in diameter (Figure 4-2). The diseases discussed in this chapter are listed in Table 4-1.

HERPES SIMPLEX VIRUS INFECTIONS

Herpes simplex viruses type 1 (HSV-1) and HSV-2 cause a variety of vesicular infections, including "cold sores," gingivostomatitis, vulvovaginitis, balanitis, and genital herpes.

ETIOLOGY

HSV-1 is also known as human herpes virus 1, or HHV-1, and causes most infections above the waist; 80% are due to HSV-1, and 20% are due to HSV-2. HSV-2 causes most infections below the waist; 80% are due to HSV-2, and 20% are due to HSV-1.

MANIFESTATIONS

Patients with HSV infections may feel a tingling over the area just before lesions appear. Other prodromal manifestations include a mild fever and occasional headache or malaise. HSV-1 and HSV-2 usually produce grouped vesicles on an erythematous plaque that later become pustules. Lesions rupture and produce shallow ulcers with an irregular edge covered by a yellow crust. Lesions can occur anywhere on the body; however, the usual sites are near the mouth (Figure 4-3) or on the genitalia (Figure 4-4). Sensory nerve involvement producing deep pain may occur as well as local lymphadenopathy. HSV-1 is the most common cause of cold sores and gingivostomatitis, whereas HSV-2 is the most common cause of vulvovaginitis, balanitis, and genital herpes. Over time, recurrences are usually less frequent and less severe.

EPIDEMIOLOGY

- HSV infections occur worldwide.

- Individuals of any age can be infected; however, primary infection with HSV-1 usually occurs in younger children and may cause severe gingivostomatitis.

- In the United States, about 70–90% of adults have been infected with HSV-1; about 22% of the entire population has been infected with HSV-2.

- HSV-2 infections are most common in sexually active young adults.

- HSV-2 seropositivity is about 40–50% in clinics that treat patients with sexually transmitted infections (STIs).

- Lesions can result from a primary infection or from reactivation of latent virus in the nerve ganglia.

- Recurrences may be precipitated by sun, trauma, fever, menses, or other stressful conditions.

- Asymptomatic individuals infected with HSV-1 and HSV-2 can shed the virus and infect others.

- HSV-1 infections are transmitted by respiratory droplets or direct exposure with infected saliva; HSV-2 infections are usually transmitted by genital contact.

PATHOGENESIS

HSV infections are the result of a cytotoxic infection with the formation of multinucleate giant cells. During primary infection, the virus invades sensory nerve endings and then migrates to the trigeminal ganglia (in HSV-1) or the sacral ganglia (in HSV-2) to establish a latent infection. Stress induces reactivation. HSV-1 and HSV-2 are lifelong infections.

DIAGNOSIS

The diagnosis of HSV is usually determined by clinical manifestations. A Tzanck test can be performed to reveal the presence of ballooned and multinucleated giant cells (Figure 4-5). Serology can be used to determine if the patient has been infected with HSV and the specific HSV virus that has infected the patient. Samples of the lesions can be obtained for polymerase chain reaction (PCR) analysis, or the viruses can be cultured in tissue culture.

TREATMENT AND PREVENTION

Without antiviral treatment, HSV lesions will usually resolve within 10 days; however, routine use of an antiviral agent is *not* suggested in patients with primary oral-labial herpes. Optimum therapeutic results usually occur when antiviral treatment is administered during the prodromal period. Antiviral agents can shorten the time to lesion healing and reduce the severity of the disease.

Acyclovir can be given to treat the primary infection and to suppress recurrences of genital herpes. Famciclovir and valacyclovir can also be given to treat recurrent episodes of genital herpes. Acyclovir is effective for mucocutaneous HSV in an immunocompromised patient and for suppressing oral herpes in immunocompromised patients who have frequent recurrences.

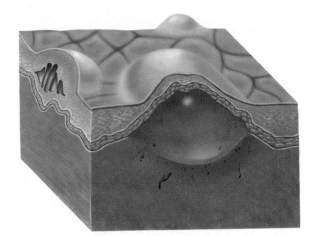

Figure 4-1. A vesicle (fluid-filled) skin lesion.

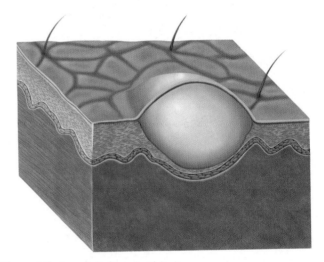

Figure 4-2. A pustule (purulent) lesion.

TABLE 4-1. Diseases that Result in Vesicular, Bullous, and Purulent Lesions

Vesicular and Bullous Lesions	Purulent Lesions
Herpes simplex skin lesions	Acne vulgaris
Varicella	Folliculitis, furunculosis, carbuncles
Herpes zoster	Herpetic whitlow
Hand, foot, and mouth disease	Gonococcemia
Herpangina	
Bullous impetigo (see Chapter 5)	
Vaccinia	

Herpes infections are lifelong and incurable. Treatment with antiviral agents does not cure herpetic infections, and patients should be encouraged to abstain from sexual contact when genital lesions are present and to use condoms when no lesions are present. Infections of neonates can be prevented by delivering the infant by Cesarean section if the mother is experiencing prodromal symptoms or if genital lesions are present at the time of delivery.

VARICELLA-ZOSTER VIRUS

Varicella (chickenpox) is a common childhood disease that results in widespread lesions over the entire body. Before universal vaccination, this viral infection was very common, with about 4 million cases reported each year. A varicella-zoster vaccine, approved in 1995, is an attenuated live virus used in the prevention of varicella. Similar to HSV infections, the varicella-zoster virus (VZV) establishes lifelong residence in the patient's nerves. *Zoster (shingles) is a localized recurrence of the VZV infection, and is a common disease of older adults.* Lesions in patients with zoster are usually restricted to one or two dermatomes and are not widespread.

ETIOLOGY

The etiologic agent of varicella and zoster is VZV (also known as HHV-3).

MANIFESTATIONS

Varicella

In varicella, crops of lesions 2–4 mm in diameter appear and progress from red macules to papules, to vesicles, to pustules, to crusts. The hallmark of varicella is the simultaneous presence of different stages of the rash (Figures 4-6). The vesicles are delicate and are often described as appearing as "dewdrops on rose petals." A centripetal pattern develops where there are more lesions on the trunk than on the extremities. Pruritus is variable. Young children infected with VZV usually have few signs of the illness and relatively few skin lesions. The disease is much more severe in older children and adults, and symptoms include a high fever, headache, malaise, myalgias, severe constitutional symptoms, and pulmonary involvement. Convalescence is usually much longer in these patients, and scarring following formation of skin lesions is more likely to occur.

Zoster

The lesions associated with zoster are more localized and follow activation of a latent infection with VZV. Groups of vesicles arise on red edematous tender plaques and are almost always unilateral and limited to one or two contiguous dermatomes (Figure 4-7). Lesions are usually seen on the costal region of the trunk. Vesicles become pustules that may coalesce to form larger bullae (Figure 4-8) and become hemorrhagic. Crusts form within 3–7 days and heal with or without scarring in about 2 weeks. The eruption is often very painful, and the pain can be disabling. Paresthesia and pain in the affected dermatomes may precede the eruption from 2 to 4 days and persist for weeks,

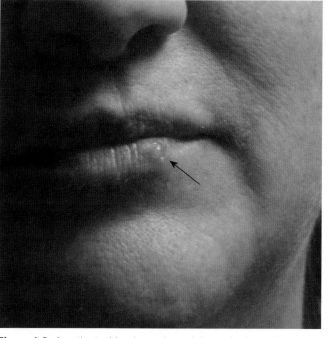

Figure 4-3. A patient with a herpetic vesicle on the lower lip.

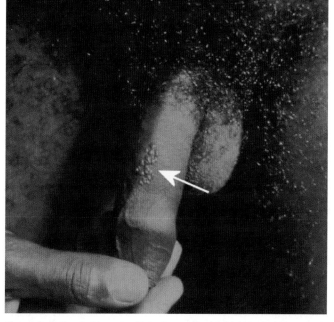

Figure 4-4. Genital herpes. Note the vesicular lesions (*white arrow*). Image courtesy of the Centers for Disease Control and Prevention, Dr M F Rein, Susan Lindsley.

months, or years after the eruption clears. The involved dermatome is usually hyperesthetic, and pain may be severe. Morbidity usually is confined to pain within the affected dermatome, and can be severe and persist well beyond the duration of active disease (postherpetic neuralgia). Sacral zoster may lead to acute urinary retention. Ophthalmic zoster (the ophthalmic branch of the trigeminal nerve) (Figure 4-9) may lead to conjunctivitis, keratitis, iridocyclitis, and paralysis of extraocular muscles. In immunosuppressed patients, VZV may disseminate to other regions of the skin and to visceral organs.

EPIDEMIOLOGY

Varicella

▨ About 25,000–30,000 cases of varicella are reported each year in the United States (Figure 4-10). Humans are the only known host.

▨ Varicella is an acute exanthematous disease that is most common in childhood (90% of cases are children). It affects susceptible children (those who are not vaccinated) before adolescence.

▨ About 95% of varicella cases occur in persons younger than 20 years of age.

▨ In children, the illness is usually self-limiting; however, at least 1% of children younger than 15 years of age experience a complication.

▨ In the United States, the mortality rate of varicella in children younger than age 14 is estimated at 2 per 100,000 cases.

▨ Only 5% of varicella cases occur in adults; however, adults experience more severe disease (hospitalizations are 18 per 1000 cases) and have a higher mortality rate (50 per 100,000 cases).

▨ The disease is highly contagious and is transmitted from person to person by droplet inhalation or direct contact. Household transmission rates are 80–90%.

Zoster

▨ Zoster is a reactivation of a previously latent VZV infection.

▨ Zoster affects 600,000–900,000 persons in the United States each year. Some patients will have several recurrences of zoster during a lifetime.

▨ The likelihood of developing zoster increases with age. The incidence is approximately 74 per 100,000 children younger than 10 years of age; 300 per 100,000 adults aged 35–44 years; and 1200 per 100,000 adults older than 75 years of age.

▨ Nearly 50% of individuals who are older than 80 years of age will develop zoster.

PATHOGENESIS

Varicella

VZV is acquired by inhalation of contaminated airborne droplets from an infected individual, and infects the conjunctivae or the mucosae of the upper respiratory tract. VZV then multiplies in regional lymph nodes of the upper respiratory tract, followed by a primary viremia. A second round of viral

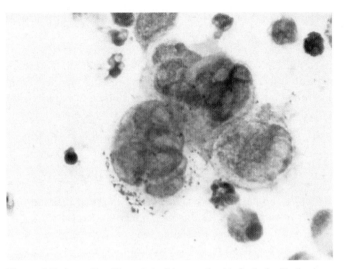

Figure 4-5. A positive Tzanck test in a patient infected with the herpes simplex virus. Image courtesy of the Centers for Disease Control and Prevention, Joe Miller.

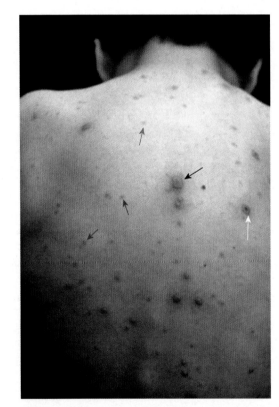

Figure 4-6. Varicella (chickenpox) lesions. Note the variety of lesions on the patient. The red arrow points to a macule; blue arrows point to a papule; the black arrow points to a pustule; and the white arrow points to crust. Image courtesy of the Centers for Disease Control and Prevention.

replication occurs in the internal organs and is followed by a secondary viremia, which results in viral invasion of capillary endothelial cells and the epidermis.

Early papular lesions of varicella are minute vacuoles surrounded by ballooning degeneration of epithelial cells within the prickle cell layer of the epidermis. Edema fluid accumulates within hours, elevating the stratum corneum to form a clear vesicle while multinucleated giant cells containing eosinophilic intranuclear inclusions form among the cells at the edges and base of the lesion. Vesicles begin to dry and fill with a cloudy fibrinous fluid containing leukocytes and desquamated epidermal cells. The lesions then crust and begin regeneration of the epithelial cells.

Meanwhile, the virus infects the sensory ganglia of the cranial nerves and the spinal dorsal root ganglia. The virus can remain latent in the nerves for decades. Suppression or waning immunity to VZV can result in reactivation and the signs and symptoms of zoster.

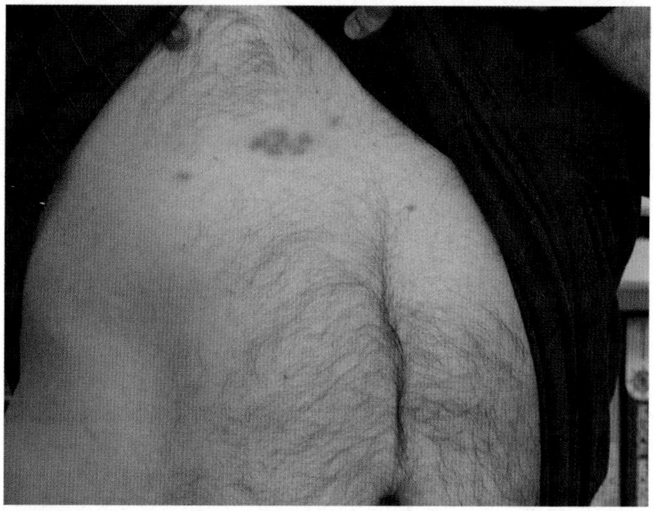

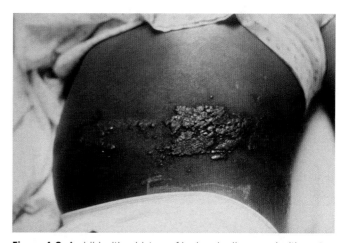

Figure 4-7. The upper body of a patient with zoster. Note the limited number of lesions compared to the patient with varicella.

Complications associated with varicella

- **Secondary bacterial infections** of skin lesions are the most common complication in children. The most common causes of these infections are *Staphylococcus aureus* and *Streptococcus pyogenes* and can result in septicemia, toxic shock syndrome, necrotizing fasciitis, osteomyelitis, bacterial pneumonia, and septic arthritis.

- **Pneumonia** is the leading cause of morbidity and mortality in adults, pregnant women, and in immunocompromised individuals.

- The second most common complication associated with varicella is involvement of the central nervous system. Complications can result in **acute cerebellar ataxia** or **encephalitis**.

- Inflammation of the liver can result in **hepatitis**. Reye syndrome can occur in a child with antecedent varicella who has been given salicylates. **Reye syndrome** begins with vomiting and a change in sensorium followed by signs of hepatic injury, hypoglycemia, and extensive fatty vacuolization of renal tubules and liver vessels.

Figure 4-8. A child with a history of leukemia diagnosed with zoster. Notice the extensive number of lesions that appeared to coalesce. Image courtesy of the Centers for Disease Control and Prevention.

Zoster

Individuals with no prior immunologic exposure to varicella virus (usually children) develop varicella, and those with circulating varicella antibodies develop zoster (older children and adults). Zoster most likely results from a failure of the immune system to contain latent VZV replication. It primarily involves the dorsal root ganglia and is characterized by vesicular eruption and neuralgic pain in the dermatome of the affected ganglia. Inflammatory changes occur in the sensory root ganglia and in the skin of the associated dermatome.

DIAGNOSIS

A diagnosis of varicella or zoster is usually determined based on clinical signs and symptoms. A Tzanck preparation, viral culture, direct fluorescence antibody (DFA) testing, and skin biopsy may be necessary to establish the diagnosis in atypical cases.

TREATMENT AND PREVENTION

Varicella is self-limiting in most patients, and supportive care is usually all that is needed. Treatment with acyclovir is recommended for adolescents and adults and children who are on corticosteroid or salicylate therapies and who are otherwise immunocompromised. The Varivax vaccine, approved in 1995, is an attenuated live virus that is given to children at 12 to 15 months of age.

In patients with zoster, acyclovir and its derivatives (i.e., famciclovir, penciclovir, and valacyclovir) have been shown to be effective in the treatment of active disease and the prevention of postherpetic neuralgia. Beginning therapy within 72 hours of onset of symptoms is more likely to result in shortening the duration of zoster and in preventing or decreasing the severity of postherpetic neuralgia. The varicella-zoster immune globulin can be given to prevent or modify clinical illness in individuals who are exposed to varicella or zoster or are susceptible or immunocompromised.

HAND, FOOT, AND MOUTH DISEASE

Hand, foot, and mouth disease is a childhood viral infection that results in vesicular lesions in the mouth and on the hands and feet. It is frequently confused with a foot and mouth disease that is also called hoof and mouth disease. Hoof and mouth disease is a disease of cloven-hooved animals and is caused by a virus of the picornavirus family. The virus that causes hand, foot, and mouth disease is a coxsackievirus that is very different from the virus that causes hoof and mouth or foot and mouth disease.

ETIOLOGY

The most common causes of hand, foot, and mouth disease are coxsackievirus A serotype 16 and enterovirus 71.

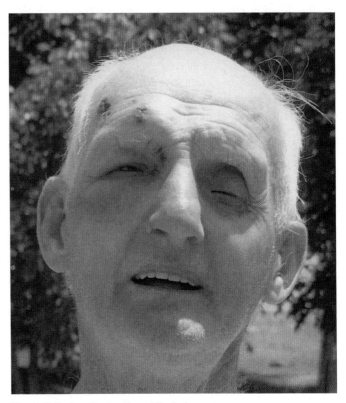

Figure 4-9. A patient with ophthalmic zoster.

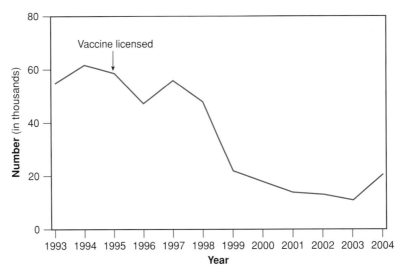

Figure 4-10. A graph showing the number of reported cases of varicella from 1993 to 2004 in Illinois, Michigan, Texas, and West Virginia. Note the decrease in the number of cases after introduction of the vaccine. Image courtesy of the Centers for Disease Control and Prevention.

MANIFESTATIONS

A brief prodrome precedes vesicle formation in hand, foot, and mouth disease and is characterized by low-grade fever (38.3°C), malaise, abdominal pain, and respiratory symptoms. The mouth is usually affected first with multiple small fragile vesicles, especially on the tongue, hard palate, buccal mucosa, lips, and pharynx. Rupture of the vesicles produces shallow ulcers. Multiple round or oval vesicles, 2–10 mm in diameter, are surrounded by red areolae and arise on the margins of palms and soles. *Other diseases that result in vesicular lesions do not cause skin lesions on the palms and soles.* Frequently, the lesions can be seen on the dorsa of the hands and feet, the buttocks, the lips, and the buccal mucosa. Vesicles occur along skin lines and become flaccid, or they rupture and crust and resolve within 7–10 days. The patient may also experience oral pain and sore throat. Complications include disseminated vesicles or maculopapules, aseptic meningitis, paralytic disease, or myocarditis.

EPIDEMIOLOGY

- Hand, foot, and mouth disease is more severe in infants and children than in adults. Usually the disease has a mild course.
- Coxsackieviruses are highly contagious and are a common cause of widespread outbreaks.
- Infection usually occurs in children and is often epidemic.
- Coxsackievirus A16 and enterovirus 71 may also cause myocarditis, pneumonia, meningoencephalitis, and death.
- Coxsackieviruses are transmitted from person to person by oral-oral and fecal-oral exposure.

PATHOGENESIS

After ingestion, the coxsackievirus adheres to and replicates in the nasopharynx and ileum. If local viral replication is limited, the disease remains asymptomatic. If the virus gains access to the regional lymphatic nodes and the reticuloendothelial system organs, minor or nonspecific disease may develop. The virus can spread via the bloodstream, causing a more severe and systemic illness.

DIAGNOSIS

Diagnosis is usually determined based on clinical signs and symptoms.

TREATMENT AND PREVENTION

Supportive care is usually needed. Contact should be avoided in epidemic situations.

HERPANGINA

Herpangina is an enteroviral infection that results in an acute febrile illness with small vesicular or ulcerative lesions on the posterior mucosal areas of the oropharynx.

ETIOLOGY

The most common cause of herpangina is coxsackievirus A (serotypes 2, 6, 7, 8, and 10). Occasionally, coxsackievirus B (serotypes 1, 2, 3, 4), echoviruses, adenoviruses, and other enteroviruses cause herpangina.

MANIFESTATIONS

Herpangina is an enanthem seen on the oral mucosal surfaces. The enanthem is characterized by the presence of gray-white minute papulovesicles about 1–2 mm in diameter. The lesions are surrounded by an erythematous halo, which then develops into a shallow ulcer. The lesions are self-limiting and disappear within 5–10 days. Lesions are most frequently found on the tonsils, uvula, soft palate, and anterior pillars of the tonsillar fauces. Other manifestations include a sudden onset of fever with sore throat, headache, anorexia, and frequently pain in the neck, abdomen, and extremities. Within 2 days after onset, the papulovesicular mucosal lesions appear and then ulcerate. Symptoms usually resolve by day 7. Vomiting and convulsions may occur in infants.

EPIDEMIOLOGY

- Herpangina tends to occur in epidemics, most commonly in infants and children.
- It is more common in summer and autumn in temperate climates and can occur anytime of the year in tropical climates.
- The viruses are highly contagious and are a common cause of widespread outbreaks.
- These enteroviruses are transmitted from person to person by oral-oral and fecal-oral exposure.

PATHOGENESIS

After ingestion, the coxsackieviruses adhere to and replicate in the nasopharynx and ileum. If local viral replication is limited, the disease remains asymptomatic. If the virus gains access to the regional lymphatic nodes and the organs of the reticuloendothelial system, minor or nonspecific disease may develop. Virus may be transmitted via the bloodstream, causing a more severe and systemic illness.

DIAGNOSIS

The diagnosis is determined based on the symptoms and characteristic oral lesions. Viral culture and serologic tests are definitive; however, these tests are not routinely performed.

TREATMENT AND PREVENTION

Mouth rinses with topical anesthetics (lidocaine 2%) or antihistamines (diphenhydramine hydrochloride) may lessen the oral pain. Good hygiene during epidemics can help to prevent infections.

VACCINIA

Vaccinia is a virus that was used to eradicate the world of smallpox and can cause significant pathology in some vaccine recipients. Because of these difficulties, universal vaccination with this organism is no longer recommended, following worldwide eradication of smallpox.

ETIOLOGY

Vaccinia virus is the virus present in the smallpox vaccine and is a hybrid relative of the smallpox and cowpox viruses.

MANIFESTATIONS

Primary vaccination to prevent smallpox results in a papule within 4–5 days. The papule then becomes a vesicle 2–3 days later, a scab within 14–21 days, and finally a permanent scar (Figure 4-11). When the normal vesicle forms, mild fever and regional lymphadenopathy may occur.

Vaccinia virus usually is administered by either intradermal scarification or injection. A bifurcated needle is used to apply the vaccine by inserting it in the skin of the upper deltoid region of the arm. Most adverse reactions involve the skin and central nervous system (Table 4-2). A progressive vaccinia infection can occur in patients who are immunosuppressed, particularly those with T-cell deficiencies. Erythema multiforme can also occur following vaccination with vaccinia.

EPIDEMIOLOGY

▪ Vaccinia infection typically occurs only after smallpox vaccination. Routine vaccination has *not* been performed in the United States since 1972.

▪ Persons who were at risk for the development of complications following vaccinia inoculation included young children, pregnant women, and persons with eczema or who were immunosuppressed.

PATHOGENESIS

Local ulceration and scar formation occur at the inoculation site.

DIAGNOSIS

Diagnosis of vaccinia is determined by a history of recent smallpox vaccination in patients with underlying conditions (e.g., B- and T-cell immune disorders, neoplasms of the reticuloendothelial system, immunosuppression by drugs, eczema, or pregnancy) and the presence of the typical lesions associated with the vaccinia virus. Samples are rarely sent for culture.

TREATMENT AND PREVENTION

Patients with smallpox who have serious complications (except those with postvaccinial encephalitis) are treated with immune globulin. Several hundred thousand doses of vaccinia vaccine

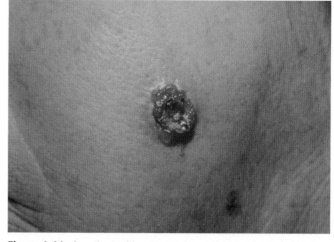

Figure 4-11. A patient with a secondary cutaneous vaccinia infection of the left cheek that developed following a smallpox vaccination. Image courtesy of the Centers for Disease Control and Prevention, Dr Robert Schecter.

TABLE 4-2. Frequency of Complications Related to Vaccinia Vaccination

Complication	Number of Cases
Death	First vaccination at 1 year of age: 5/1 million First vaccination at 1–4 years of age: 0.5/1 million First vaccination at 5–19 years of age: 0.5/1 million First vaccination at 20+ years of age: No data
Encephalitis	3/1 million primary vaccinees
Vaccinia necrosum	Approximately 1 patient per 1 million during primary or revaccination. Usually fatal over a period of several months
Eczema vaccinatum	1/100,000 primary vaccinees; 1/1 million revaccinees
Generalized vaccinia	Occasional occurrence in immunocompetent individuals 3/100,000 primary vaccinees; 1/1 million revaccinees
Accidental vaccinia	3/100,000–1 million vaccinees
Erythematous rash	Approximately 1/100,000 primary vaccinees*

*Incidence was somewhat higher when vaccination occurred in children younger than 1 year of age.

have recently been used to vaccinate the United States military; however, due to the increased concern surrounding the potential release of smallpox as a biologic weapon, the vaccine has also been made available to first-line health-care persons. **To prevent complications, persons with conditions that might predispose them to serious complications are not vaccinated**—this includes immunocompromised patients; persons with life-threatening allergies to polymyxin B, streptomycin, tetracycline, or neomycin; and persons with chronic skin conditions, especially atopic dermatitis.

ACNE VULGARIS

Acne vulgaris (acne) is a disease that significantly affects most teenagers worldwide; in some cases has caused lifelong physical and emotional scars.

ETIOLOGY

Propionibacterium acnes is a gram-positive bacteria that is a major inhabitant of skin. It and several other factors work together to cause these very common lesions.

MANIFESTATIONS

Several different types of acne lesions exist and include open or closed comedones, inflammatory papules, pustules, and nodules (Figure 4-12). Lesions are usually limited to the face, upper chest, and back. Inflammatory papules and nodules do not contain purulent material, but they are erythematous due to the inflammatory response. A comedo is a whitehead (closed comedo) or a blackhead (open comedo) without any clinical signs of inflammation. Pustules have the appearance of closed comedones but are surrounded by erythematous tissue. Scars from prior lesions may be present.

EPIDEMIOLOGY

▨ Acne usually appears during puberty and affects 85–100% of the population.

▨ During adolescence, acne vulgaris is more common in boys than in girls; however, in adulthood, it is more common in women than in men. About 10–20% of adults may continue to experience acne.

▨ Acne occurs on the areas of skin with the densest population of sebaceous glands, including the face, the upper part of the chest, and the back.

PATHOGENESIS

Four factors are responsible for the development of acne: (1) follicular epidermal hyperproliferation with subsequent plugging of the follicle; (2) excess sebum; (3) the presence and activity of *P acnes;* and (4) inflammation. Friction or trauma may rupture comedones and release inflammatory "foreign-body" material into the tissue. The comedo is a greasy plug consisting of keratin, sebum, and bacteria capped by a layer of melanin (to form the blackhead). The comedo of superficial acne may be closed or

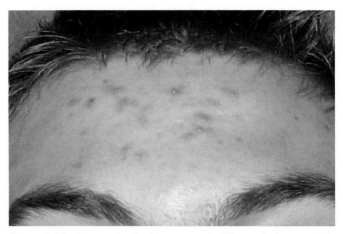

Figure 4-12. Acne vulgaris. Note several different lesions on this man's forehead.

open. The closed comedo is the precursor to the inflamed acne lesion (deep acne). Application of oils or other follicle-blocking substances or glucocorticoids can stimulate acne.

DIAGNOSIS

Diagnosis of acne vulgaris is usually determined based on clinical signs.

TREATMENT AND PREVENTION

Treatment of acne vulgaris includes the use of oral tetracycline or erythromycin, normal cleansing, and topical application of benzoyl peroxide, retinoic acid, or salicylic acid. Topical oils and excessive skin friction and facial scrubbing should be avoided.

FOLLICULITIS, FURUNCULOSIS, AND CARBUNCULOSIS

Folliculitis is a purulent bacterial infection of the hair follicle. Furuncles or boils are localized purulent inflammatory lesions of the skin and subcutaneous region. Carbuncles occur when several furuncles are connected subcutaneously by sinus tracts.

ETIOLOGY

Staphylococcus aureus is the most common cause of typical folliculitis, furunculosis, and carbunculosis. *Pseudomonas aeruginosa* is a common cause of folliculitis associated with a hot tub or whirlpool source ("hot-tub folliculitis"). Less common causes of these lesions are *Candida, Malassezia*, anaerobic bacteria, and diphtheroids.

MANIFESTATIONS

Folliculitis is a pinhead-sized erythematous papule topped by a superficial pustule located at the orifice of the hair follicle (Figure 4-13). Each pustule tends to be pierced by a hair. Lesions can be single or multiple and may occur at any hair-bearing site on the body. Lesions on the scalp may scar and cause permanent hair loss. Sycosis barbae is a deep folliculitis of bearded skin and is frequently a chronic condition.

Furunculosis is a focal purulent inflammation of the skin and subcutaneous tissue (Figure 4-14). **Carbunculosis** is a deeper infection producing multiple adjacent draining sinuses (Figure 4-15). Lesions begin as folliculitis and may be single (furuncle or boil), multiple and contiguous (carbuncle), or multiple and recurrent (furunculosis). Lesions initially are pruritic and mildly painful, followed by progressive local swelling and erythema. The overlying skin becomes very tender when pressure or motion is applied. The purulent lesions often rupture spontaneously and drain a purulent matter, bringing immediate relief of pain. Ruptured lesions then become violaceous and heal. Lesions can occur anywhere on hair-bearing skin and especially on buttocks, thighs, and abdomen. Carbuncles are usually found in the thick fibrous inelastic skin of the neck and upper back.

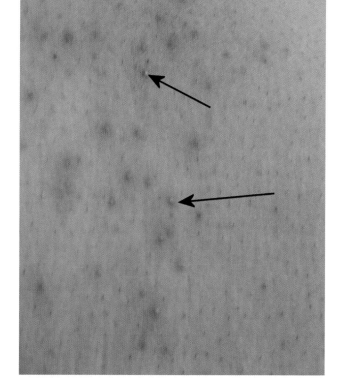

Figure 4-13. The inner thigh of a person with folliculitis caused by shaving the legs.

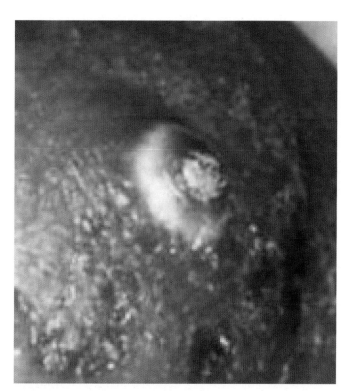

Figure 4-14. A furuncle. Image courtesy of the Centers for Disease Control and Prevention, Joe Miller.

EPIDEMIOLOGY

▨ Patients are usually in good health and most commonly 15–40 years of age.

▨ Predisposed individuals are usually obese, diabetic, or do not practice good hygiene.

PATHOGENESIS

Folliculitis occurs when hair follicles are blocked or damaged. If the lesion expands into the subcutaneous tissue, a furuncle forms. The impermeability of the skin of the upper back leads to lateral extension of the infection, producing a large indurated painful carbuncle with multiple ineffective drainage sites.

DIAGNOSIS

Diagnosis is usually determined based on clinical appearance of the skin lesions. Definitive diagnosis can be obtained by culturing the bacteria obtained from the purulent discharge or the erythematous base of the lesion.

TREATMENT AND PREVENTION

Over-the-counter antiseptics can be helpful in the treatment of folliculitis. Treatment of larger lesions may require warm wet compresses and incision and drainage. Systemic antibiotics may be required in severe cases. Lesions can be prevented by improving hygienic conditions.

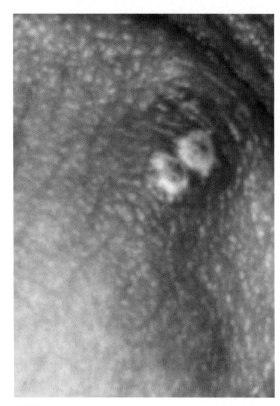

Figure 4-15. A carbuncle.

HERPETIC WHITLOW

Herpetic whitlow is a viral infection of the tissue around the fingernails. Many patients with this infection also have gingivostomatitis and have infected the digit by frequent sucking of the fingers.

ETIOLOGY

HSV 1 causes 60% of the infections, and HSV-2 causes the remaining 40%.

MANIFESTATIONS

Grouped vesicles that coalesce often can be seen on the fingers near the nails, usually on the dominant hand (Figure 4-16). Lesions can spread and become pustular. Symptoms include intense itching or pain at the lesion site, headache or malaise, and regional lymphadenopathy.

EPIDEMIOLOGY

▨ HSV is introduced by direct contact of skin with active herpes infection. In immunosuppressed persons, the virus may be autoinoculated from herpes labialis lesions.

▨ At-risk persons include nurses, dentists, and physicians who may have contact with oral or genital lesions on patients and children with herpetic gingivostomatitis who suck their thumbs.

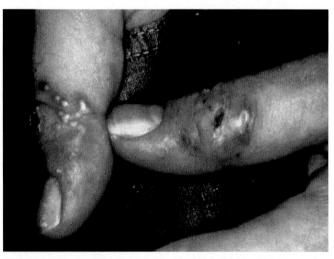

Figure 4-16. A patient with herpetic whitlow on both thumbs. Image courtesy of the Centers for Disease Control and Prevention.

In children, HSV-1 is the most common cause of herpetic whitlow. Infection involving the finger usually is due to autoinoculation from primary oropharyngeal lesions as a result of finger-sucking or thumb-sucking behavior in patients with herpes labialis or herpetic gingivostomatitis.

In health-care workers, infection with HSV-1 is more common than in the general population and usually occurs following unprotected exposure to infected oropharyngeal secretions of patients.

In the general adult population, herpetic whitlow is most often due to autoinoculation from genital herpes and is most frequently secondary to infection with HSV-2.

PATHOGENESIS

The virus enters via a break in the skin and causes edema, erythema, and local tenderness preceding the development of vesicular-pustular lesions.

DIAGNOSIS

Diagnosis of herpetic whitlow usually is based on clinical presentation; the patient has a history of oral herpes, genital herpes, or occupational risk factors. In children with herpetic whitlow, observation of gingivostomatitis is nearly pathognomonic. In adults, the presence of occupational risk factors or the presence of concurrent oral or genital herpes lesions strongly suggests the diagnosis of herpetic whitlow. Definitive diagnostic testing includes the Tzanck test, viral cultures, serology, fluorescent antibody testing, and DNA hybridization.

TREATMENT AND PREVENTION

Treatment is usually symptomatic and includes soaks and analgesics. Topical acyclovir reduces the severity and duration of the lesions following a primary infection. Oral acyclovir given during the prodromal period may prevent recurrences. Gloves should be worn to avoid infections.

GONOCOCCEMIA

Gonococcemia is defined as the presence of *Neisseria gonorrhoeae* in the bloodstream. Disseminated gonococcal infection occurs when organisms in the blood infect distant locations in the body. Disseminated gonococcal infection can result in a biphasic disease that initially manifests as polyarthritis, tenosynovitis, and dermatitis and is followed several days later by septic arthritis.

ETIOLOGY

N gonorrhoeae is a gram-negative diplococcus.

MANIFESTATIONS

The skin lesions in this dermatitis (gonococcemia) arise from disseminated gonococcal infection and begin as tiny red papules or petechiae, which may evolve into purpuric pustules, vesicles, or bullae (Figure 4-17). Widespread pustules 5–40 mm in diameter on an erythematous or hemorrhagic base are characteristic (Figure 4-18). Lesions are scattered over distal extremities, and one or two tender joints (purulent arthritis) are commonly seen (Figure 4-19). Other manifestations include fever, chills, polyarthralgia, tenosynovitis, and polyarthritis.

EPIDEMIOLOGY

▨ Gonococcemia is a disseminated STI, which in many cases occurs after asymptomatic *N gonorrhoeae* infection.

▨ It is most commonly seen in the adolescent and young adult population, with a peak incidence in males aged 20–24 years and females aged 15–19 years.

▨ Gonococcemia is more common in women and in patients with pharyngeal infections due to *N gonorrhoeae*.

▨ Women develop gonococcemia more frequently during menstruation and pregnancy.

▨ Gonorrhea is the second most often reported STI, with about 600,000 cases reported annually in the United States.

▨ Dissemination of gonorrhea to the bloodstream occurs in 0.5–3% of cases. Most individuals with gonococcemia do not exhibit any symptoms, except for septic arthritis.

PATHOGENESIS

N gonorrhoeae spreads from a primary infection site such as the endocervix, urethra, pharynx, or the rectum and disseminates to the bloodstream to infect other organs. Several different sites are infected, including the skin and joints. Factors that enable the organisms to enter the bloodstream include host physiologic changes, virulence factors of the organism, and defects in the host's immune response. Host factors include changes in the vaginal pH that occur during menses and pregnancy and the puerperium period, which causes the vaginal mucosa to become more suitable for the growth of the organism and provides increased access to the bloodstream.

Bacterial virulence factors involved in the disease process

▨ Pili help the bacteria adhere to the mucosal surface and prevent phagocytosis by macrophages.

▨ Lipo-oligosaccharides are a major component of the organism's outer membrane and cause excessive stimulation of cytokine release by the host's white blood cells, much like endotoxin does in gram-negative rod-shaped bacterial infections.

▨ Some strains of *N gonorrhoeae* that are quite pathogenic produce immunoglobulin A (IgA) proteases, which help the bacteria survive in the mucosa.

Patients with a deficiency in terminal complement components are less able to combat infection; about 13% of patients with disseminated gonococcal infection have a complement deficiency. Other causes of immunocompromise include HIV and systemic lupus erythematosus, which also predispose a patient to disseminated gonococcal infections.

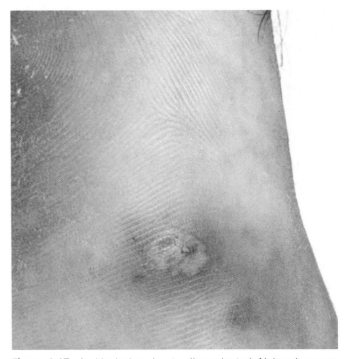

Figure 4-17. A skin lesion due to disseminated *Neisseria gonorrhoeae* infection. Image courtesy of the Centers for Disease Control and Prevention, Dr Wiesner.

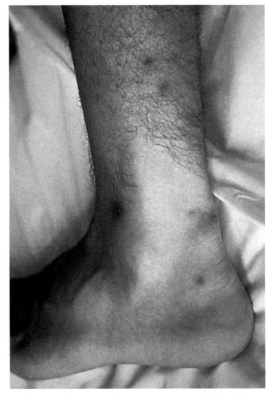

Figure 4-18. A patient with cutaneous lesions on the left ankle and calf due to disseminated *Neisseria gonorrhoeae* infection. Image courtesy of the Centers for Disease Control and Prevention, Dr S E Thompson, VDCD; J Pledger.

DIAGNOSIS

Patients with gonococcemia usually have an elevated white blood cell count. Samples of blood and synovial fluid should be obtained; blood samples will usually test positive at early stages. Rectal, genital, and pharyngeal samples should be collected for culture on Thayer-Martin agar. Results of Gram stain and culture of skin lesions may be positive. PCR and ligase chain reaction can be performed on urethral specimens and on first-void urine specimens to determine if a patient is infected with *N gonorrhoeae.*

TREATMENT AND PREVENTION

Treatment involves intravenous antibiotic therapy with ceftriaxone, cefotaxime, or ceftizoxime. Intimate contact with infected individuals should be avoided.

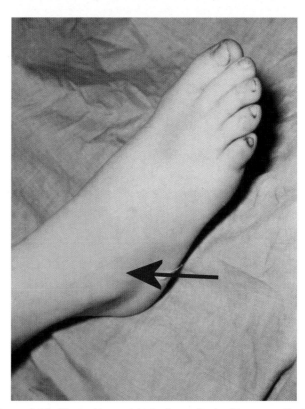

Figure 4-19. The ankle and foot of a patient with monoarticular arthritis due to *Neisseria gonorrhoeae.* Image courtesy of the Centers for Disease Control and Prevention.

CHAPTER 5

PETECHIAL, HEMORRHAGIC, ULCERATIVE, AND NECROTIC LESIONS

OVERVIEW

Petechiae are pinpoint, flat, round lesions caused by intradermal or submucosal hemorrhage (Figure 5-1). Hemorrhagic lesions are flat, irregularly shaped lesions larger than petechiae, and are also caused by intradermal or submucosal hemorrhage. Ulcers of the skin are a localized excavation of the skin surface and are produced by sloughing of inflammatory necrotic tissue (Figure 5-2). Necrotic lesions result when cells in the skin die and are destroyed by the progressive degradative action of various enzymes. Table 5-1 lists the diseases that result in petechia and hemorrhagic lesion formation, and Table 5-2 lists the diseases that result in ulcer and necrotic lesion formation. The diseases mentioned in these two tables will be discussed in this chapter.

ENDOCARDITIS

Endocarditis is an infection of the heart valves, and is characterized by vegetations that develop on the surface of the valves. The dislodged vegetations (septic emboli) are transported by the bloodstream and lodge in small vessels and cause petechial skin lesions associated with the disease. The disease will be briefly discussed here and more completely in Chapter 30.

ETIOLOGY

Several different organisms that cause endocarditis are listed in Table 5-3. The etiology depends on the condition of the valve, if the person is an intravenous (illicit) drug user or has a prosthetic heart valve, and the length of time the valve has been in place before an infection resulted in symptoms.

MANIFESTATIONS

Petechiae, splinter hemorrhages, Janeway lesions, and Osler nodes can occur following an infection of the heart valve. **Petechiae** are red nonblanching lesions that usually fade within

2–3 days. They usually appear in crops, especially in the conjunctivae (Figure 5-3), buccal mucosa or palate (Figure 5-4), upper chest, and extremities. **Splinter hemorrhages** are linear red-to-brown streaks that appear under the fingernails and toenails (Figure 5-5). **Janeway lesions** are small erythematous painless macules, plaques, or palpable purpura, and are usually observed on the palms and soles. **Osler nodes** are erythematous wheal-like tender nodules 2–15 mm in diameter, and are usually located on the pads of fingers and toes. They are frequently evanescent, lasting hours to days. Other manifestations of endocarditis include fever, fatigue, anorexia, weakness, myalgias, arthralgias, and malaise.

EPIDEMIOLOGY

- The incidence of endocarditis is 1.4–4.2 cases per 100,000 persons per year.

- Men are affected about twice as often as women.

- Over 50% of cases occur in patients older than 50 years of age.

- Skin lesions occur in 20–40% of patients.

- Endocarditis usually occurs in patients with prior damage to the surface of the heart valve; it is more common in intravenous (illicit) drug users and in patients who have a prosthetic heart valve.

- Infections of the native or prosthetic heart valves frequently occur following asymptomatic bacteremias from infected gingivaes, the genitourinary tract, or the gastrointestinal tract.

PATHOGENESIS

Infective endocarditis is usually preceded by the formation of a predisposing cardiac lesion. Damage to the endothelial cells that line the inside of the heart and the heart valve can result in the accumulation of platelets and fibrin, producing a nonbacterial thrombotic endocarditis. This sterile lesion serves as a site for bacteria to attach to in the bloodstream.

The microbial infection begins on the surface of the heart valves and forms vegetations containing bacteria, white blood cells, platelets, and fibrin. These vegetations can dislodge from the valves and settle in blood vessels, lowering perfusion of the tissues and resulting in skin lesions (e.g., petechiae, splinter hemorrhages, Janeway lesions). Immune complexes also occur, resulting in various immunologic phenomena (e.g., Osler nodes).

DIAGNOSIS

Diagnosis of endocarditis is difficult. Key signs include low-grade fever, fatigue, valvular insufficiency, a change in a preexisting murmur or a new cardiac valvular murmur, tachycardia, petechiae, Osler nodes, splinter hemorrhages, and hemorrhagic retinal lesions (Roth spots are round or oval lesions with small white centers). (For further discussion about diagnosis and the use of Duke criteria, see Chapter 30.)

TREATMENT AND PREVENTION

Treatment of endocarditis includes administration of antibiotics (see Chapter 30). In patients with prior heart valve

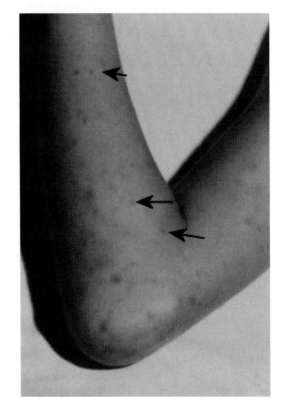

Figure 5-1. Petechiae on the arm of a patient. Arrows point to the lesions. Image courtesy of the Centers for Disease Control and Prevention.

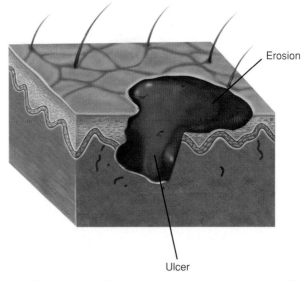

Figure 5-2. A schematic comparing a cutaneous erosion to an ulcer. Erosions are depressed areas of skin in which part or all of the epidermis has been lost. Ulcers occur when there is necrosis, and loss of the epidermis and dermis and can sometimes extend into the subcutaneous tissue.

damage, antibiotic prophylaxis prior to invasive dental procedures and genitourinary and gastrointestinal surgery is useful in preventing endocarditis.

MENINGOCOCCEMIA

Meningococcemia is a life-threatening infection of the bloodstream that causes inflammation and damage to the walls of the blood vessels (vasculitis). Damage to the blood vessels can cause hemorrhage into the skin and is a sign of this bacteremia.

ETIOLOGY

The cause of meningococcemia is *Neisseria meningitidis*, a gram-negative diplococcus. Thirteen capsular serogroups of the organism have been identified; however, only five serogroups (A, B, C, Y, W-135) cause most cases of meningococcemia.

MANIFESTATIONS

Acute meningococcemia produces erythematous macules, petechiae, purpura, and ecchymoses, with lesions commonly beginning on the trunk and legs in areas where pressure is applied by the patient's clothing (e.g., waistband, neck, ankles). A confluence of petechial and purpuric lesions results in hemorrhagic patches, often with central necrosis (Figure 5-6). Other manifestations include fever, weakness, headache, malaise, and hypotension; disseminated intravascular coagulation (DIC); Waterhouse-Friderichsen syndrome (fulminant meningococcemia) and meningeal irritation (i.e., rigidity, positive Kernig sign); and altered mental status.

EPIDEMIOLOGY

- About 2600 cases of meningococcemia occur in the United States yearly (Figure 5-7).
- Rates of meningococcal disease are highest among children younger than 4 years of age, with a second peak at 18 years of age.
- About 50–70% of patients with meningococcemia will also have signs and symptoms of meningitis (see Chapter 7).
- The case-fatality ratio is high (10–14%); 11–19% of survivors have serious health sequelae (e.g., hearing loss, amputation, cognitive impairment).
- Capsular serogroups B and C are associated with most cases of meningococcemia.
- Patients with complement deficiency (C5, C6, C7, or C8) are more likely to be diagnosed with meningococcemia.
- *N meningitidis* is a leading cause of bacterial meningitis and sepsis.
- *N meningitidis* is transmitted from person to person by respiratory secretions.

PATHOGENESIS

Humans are the only known reservoir of this bacterium (i.e., *N meningitidis*). About 2% of children younger than 2 years of age,

TABLE 5-1. Diseases that Cause Petechial and Hemorrhagic Lesions

Endocarditis
Meningococcemia
Gonococcemia (see Chapter 4)
Rocky Mountain spotted fever (see Chapter 2)

TABLE 5-2. Diseases that Cause Ulcerative and Necrotic Lesions

Impetigo	Ecthyma gangrenosum
Ecthyma	Gas gangrene (see Chapter 3)
Primary syphilis	Herpes simplex skin lesion (see Chapter 4)
Burn or wound infections	

TABLE 5-3. Conditions and Causes of Infectious Endocarditis

Condition of Valve or Patient	Causes*
Native heart valve	Viridans *Streptococcus* sp. *Staphylococcus aureus* Gram-negative bacilli HACEK group†
Prosthetic heart valve within 2 months post heart surgery	*Staphylococcus aureus* Coagulase negative *Staphylococcus* sp. Gram-negative aerobic bacilli Fungi
Prosthetic heart valve more than 2 months after heart surgery	Viridans *Streptococcus* species Coagulase negative *Staphylococcus* sp. *S aureus* Gram-negative bacilli Fungi
Intravenous (illicit) drug user	*S aureus* Gram-negative bacilli *Pseudomonas aeruginosa* (most common gram-negative bacilli) Viridans *Streptococcus* *Enterococcus* *Candida albicans*

*Causes are listed from most common to least common.
†HACEK group, *Haemophilus aphrophilus*, *H paraphrophilus*, *H parainfluenzae*, *Actinobacillus actinomycetemcomitans*, *Cardiobacterium hominis*, *Eikenella corrodens*, and *Kingella* sp.

5% of children up to 17 years of age, and 20–40% of young adults are asymptomatic carriers of *N meningitidis*. Overcrowded living conditions (e.g., college dormitories, schools, military camps) can significantly increase the carrier rate. Asymptomatic carriers are thought to be the major source of transmission of pathogenic strains.

N meningitidis uses pili to attach to mucosal epithelial cells, a concomitant viral infection allows *N meningitidis* to invade the bloodstream. Once in the bloodstream, *N meningitidis* damages the small blood vessels by direct invasion of endothelial cells and indirect damage following the release of endotoxin. The capsule on the surface of the bacteria prevents white blood cells from phagocytizing and killing the organisms. Meningococcal endotoxin causes the release of proinflammatory cytokines, which can result in severe hypotension, reduced cardiac output, and increased endothelial permeability (see Chapter 30).

Neonates are usually resistant to the disease because passively acquired maternal immunoglobulin G antibodies are present until approximately 6 months of age. As the child ages, asymptomatic exposure to a variety of strains of encapsulated and nonencapsulated *N meningitidis* increases protective bacterial immunity. Protective immunoglobulin M and immunoglobulin G are found in up to 95% of young adults.

DIAGNOSIS

Diagnosis of meningococcemia requires blood cultures. Gram stains revealing the gram-negative diplococci in samples from the skin lesions are usually diagnostic. If the patient is diagnosed with meningitis, cultures and Gram stains of the cerebrospinal fluid are also diagnostic.

TREATMENT AND PREVENTION

Treatment of meningococcemia requires administration of antibiotics (e.g., penicillin G) and supportive care. A tetravalent (A, C, Y, W-135) meningococcal conjugate vaccine licensed in 2005 is available for persons aged 11–55 years. Adolescents aged 11–12 years, students at high school entry, and college freshmen living in dormitories should be vaccinated. Unfortunately, no vaccine is currently available to prevent infection with *N meningitidis* serogroup B.

IMPETIGO AND ECTHYMA

Nonbullous impetigo is a superficial infection that causes shallow erosions in the skin that are covered by a honey-colored crust. Bullous impetigo occurs when the individual is infected with an epidermolytic toxin-producing strain of *Staphylococcus aureus*. Ecthyma infections extend deeper into the dermis, and when the crust is removed, a punched-out ulcer with a raised surrounding margin can be seen.

ETIOLOGY

S aureus and *Streptococcus pyogenes* cause nonbullous impetigo. Currently, *S aureus* is the most common cause of nonbullous impetigo, accounting for 50–60% of cases. About 20–45% of

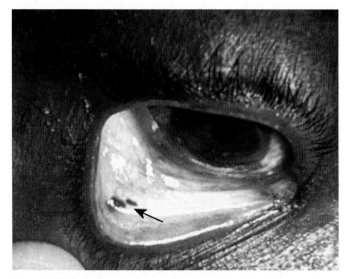

Figure 5-3. Petechiae in the conjunctiva of a patient. Image courtesy of the Centers for Disease Control and Prevention, Dr Thomas F Sellers, Emory University, Atlanta, GA.

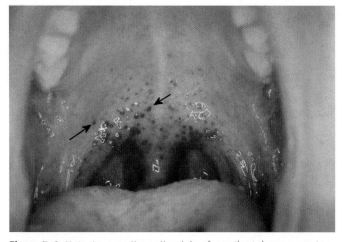

Figure 5-4. Petechiae on the soft palate of a patient. Image courtesy of the Centers for Disease Control and Prevention, Dr Heinz F Eichenwald.

cases are due to a combination of *S aureus* and *S pyogenes*. *S aureus* phage type 71 is associated with bullous impetigo. Ecthyma is caused by *S pyogenes*.

MANIFESTATIONS

Nonbullous impetigo begins as small vesicles that rupture quickly to form purulent erosions covered with **honey-colored, adherent thick crusts** (Figure 5-8). Lesions usually occur on the face or extremities. Lesions are superficial and limited to the epidermis, and are usually painless but may itch. Regional lymphadenopathy is common.

Bullous impetigo presents with **large superficial fragile bullae** on the trunk and the extremities (Figure 5-9). Only ruptured bullae usually are seen at the time of presentation, however. Lesions are painless, and are usually found on the face or extremities. Other manifestations frequently seen in patients with bullous impetigo are fever, diarrhea, and generalized weakness. These manifestations usually are not seen in patients with nonbullous impetigo. Regional lymphadenopathy is uncommon in this form of impetigo.

Ecthyma is an ulcerative form of impetigo that extends deeper into the dermis. It begins as a vesicle or pustule overlying an inflamed area of skin that deepens into a dermal ulceration with overlying crust. The **crust** is **gray-yellow** and is thicker and harder than the crust of impetigo. When the crust is removed, a shallow punched-out ulcer with a raised surrounding margin can be seen. Lesions are painful; the patient also may develop regional lymphadenopathy. Secondary lymphangitis and cellulitis can occur. Ecthyma heals slowly and, unlike impetigo, usually results in scarring.

EPIDEMIOLOGY

▨ *S aureus* colonizes the anterior nares of 30% of the general population.

▨ *S pyogenes* colonizes the oropharynx of 3–10% of the general population.

▨ Person-to-person spread of these bacterial pathogens is more likely in populations living in crowded conditions and with poor hygiene.

▨ Children are most at risk of developing **impetigo.** About 10% of children presenting to a clinic with skin infections have impetigo.

▨ About 90% of cases of **bullous impetigo** occur in children younger than 2 years of age.

▨ **Nonbullous impetigo** is much more common than bullous impetigo.

▨ Nonbullous impetigo, bullous impetigo, and ecthyma may occur at sites of eczema, arthropod bites, varicella, or traumatic erosions.

▨ **Ecthyma** usually occurs on the lower extremities of children, diabetic patients, and neglected elderly patients.

▨ Preexisting tissue damage (e.g., excoriations, insect bites, dermatitis) and immunocompromised states (e.g., diabetes

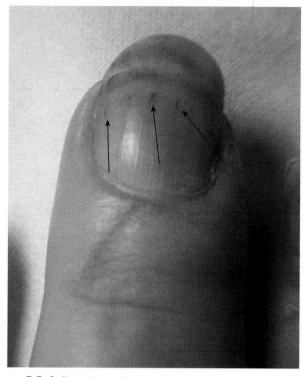

Figure 5-5. Splinter hemorrhages under the fingernail of a patient. Image courtesy of the Centers for Disease Control and Prevention, Dr Thomas F Sellers, Emory University, Atlanta, GA.

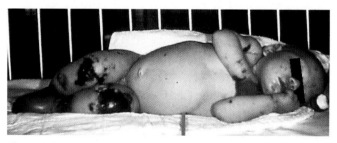

Figure 5-6. A 4-month-old infant with gangrene of the hands and lower extremities due to meningococcemia. Image courtesy of the Centers for Disease Control and Prevention, Mr Gust.

mellitus, neutropenia) predispose patients to the development of ecthyma.

- **Impetigo** and **ecthyma** are highly communicable to other sites (autoinoculation) or other persons (contagious).

PATHOGENESIS

S aureus and *S pyogenes* enter through damaged skin and are transmitted through direct contact. Although these diseases are caused by only two bacterial species, they can manifest in more than one form, including nonbullous impetigo, bullous impetigo, and ecthyma. The differences in manifestations are probably due to the bacterial strains involved and the relative activity of their exotoxins.

Bullous impetigo occurs when an individual is infected with a strain of *S aureus* that produces an exotoxin called epidermolytic toxin (formerly called exfoliative toxin). Epidermolytic toxin is a protease that degrades desmoglein-1, a glycoprotein that maintains cell-to-cell adhesion in the superficial epidermis. When desmoglein-1 is degraded, intercellular adhesion is disrupted and superficial blisters form. Nonbullous (impetigo contagiosa) and bullous impetigo lesions heal with no residual scarring. Scarring is common in ecthyma. Ecthyma infections extend deeper into the dermis than nonbullous and bullous impetigo and appear to be due to the particular strain of bacterium infecting the lesions.

Acute glomerulonephritis can occur as a complication of impetigo or ecthyma if the patient is infected with a nephritogenic strain of ***S pyogenes.*** The rate of cases of acute glomerulonephritis can be as high as 1% in patients with ecthyma.

DIAGNOSIS

Diagnosis of impetigo and ecthyma is usually based on the appearance of the lesions. Samples from the lesions can be Gram stained and cultured, but this is only rarely performed. A rising anti-DNase B titer indicates *S pyogenes* involvement and raises concern about acute glomerulonephritis. ASO titer usually does not rise following pyoderma.

TREATMENT AND PREVENTION

Bullous and nonbullous impetigo can be treated by cleaning the wound with gentle abrasion. Topical treatment with mupirocin is adequate for single lesions or small areas of involvement. Systemic antibiotics (e.g., cephalexin, erythromycin, dicloxacillin) are indicated for extensive involvement or for bullous impetigo.

Treatment of ecthyma depends on the progression of the lesions. Crusts can be removed by soaking or using wet compresses and by applying antibiotic ointment daily. Topical therapy with mupirocin ointment can be used for localized ecthyma. Patients with more extensive lesions usually require oral antibiotics (e.g., penicillin).

To prevent person-to-person spread of impetigo and ecthyma, avoid contact with the lesions. Good hygiene is important in preventing person-to-person spread and spread of the lesions on the patient. Using bactericidal soap and frequently

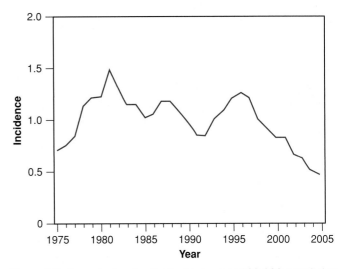

Figure 5-7. A graph showing the incidence per 100,000 population of invasive meningococcemia in the United States from 1975 to 2005. Image courtesy of the Centers for Disease Control and Prevention.

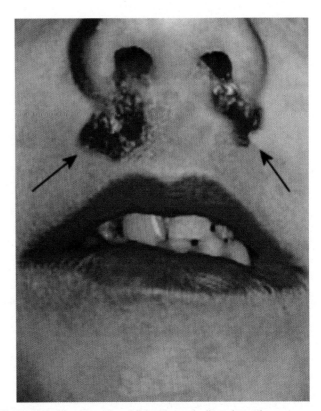

Figure 5-8. The face of a child with nonbullous impetigo.

changing bed linens, towels, and clothing can help in maintaining cleanliness.

PRIMARY SYPHILIS

Syphilis is a sexually transmitted infection that manifests in three stages as primary, secondary, and tertiary syphilis. The primary stage of syphilis results in an indurated chancre. For a more complete discussion of secondary syphilis, refer to Chapter 2.

ETIOLOGY

Treponema pallidum is a thin spirochete that presently has not been cultured in vitro.

MANIFESTATIONS

A painless papule progresses to a singular painless ulcer (chancre), which has a raised and indurated border (Figure 5-10). Chancres can occur on the penis, anus, and rectum in men, and on the vulva, cervix, and perineum in women. Chancres may also occur on the lips or the oropharyngeal or anogenital mucous membranes, and rarely on the hands or other parts of the body. Other manifestations include regional lymphadenopathy 3–4 days after the chancre appears.

EPIDEMIOLOGY

- In 2004, slightly less than 8000 cases of primary and secondary syphilis were reported in the United States.
- The South has the highest rates of primary and secondary syphilis, with 3.6 cases per 100,000 persons.
- Syphilis is a sexually transmitted infection.

PATHOGENESIS

T pallidum enters through the mucous membranes or skin. After 3–4 weeks, a red papule erodes to form a painless ulcer (chancre) with an indurated base, which, when abraded, exudes a serous fluid containing numerous spirochetes. In all stages of disease, perivascular infiltration of lymphocytes, plasma cells, and, later, fibroblasts causes swelling and proliferation of the endothelium of the smaller blood vessels, leading to endarteritis obliterans. Regional lymph nodes enlarge without tenderness.

DIAGNOSIS

Diagnosis of primary syphilis is based on physical examination, serologic tests, history of sexual contacts, and, if appropriate, darkfield examination of fluids from lesions for spirochetes.

TREATMENT AND PREVENTION

Benzathine penicillin is the antibiotic of choice in the treatment of primary and secondary syphilis. Over 50% of patients with early infectious syphilis, especially those with secondary syphilis, have a **Jarisch-Herxheimer reaction** (headache, fever, chills, myalgias, exacerbation of cutaneous lesions) within 6–12 hours of initial treatment.

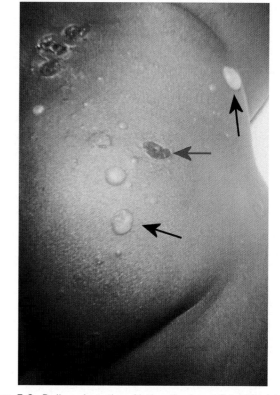

Figure 5-9. Bullous impetigo. Notice the large fluid filled bullae (*black arrows*) and the erythematous surface of a bullous lesion that ruptured and has lost the overlying epidermis (*blue arrow*). Image courtesy of the Centers for Disease Control and Prevention.

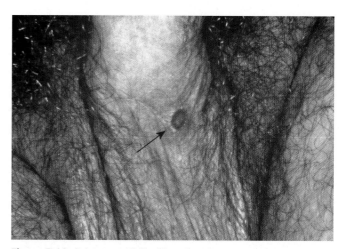

Figure 5-10. Primary syphilis. Note the chancre at the base of the penile shaft. Image courtesy of the Centers for Disease Control and Prevention, Dr NJ Fiumara, Dr Gavin Hart.

BURN OR WOUND INFECTIONS

Once the integrity of the skin is compromised, any number of organisms can cause damage. Protecting the wound or burn sites from contamination is vital in proper healing of the damaged sites.

ETIOLOGY

The common causes of burn or wound infections include *S aureus, Pseudomonas aeruginosa*, and *S pyogenes*.

MANIFESTATIONS

Infections of wounds and burns by *S aureus, P aeruginosa*, and *S pyogenes* results in tissue ulceration and degradation at the wound or trauma site. Other manifestations can include sepsis, septic shock, fever, and delayed wound healing.

EPIDEMIOLOGY

- *P aeruginosa* commonly contaminates water. *S aureus* is present in the anterior nares of 30% of the population and on the perineum of 10% of the population. *S pyogenes* is in the oropharynx of 3–10% of the population.

- Once the skin barrier is compromised, bacteria can contaminate the wound or burn and cause a destructive infection.

PATHOGENESIS

Burns or other wounds provide a highly nutritious medium for bacteria. Colonization may be limited to the eschar (nonviable skin debris on the surface), invade deeper tissues, or spread systemically through lymph and blood (septicemia). In burn patients, septicemia is often polymicrobic. Normal neutrophil function is a key determinant to limiting the severity of the infection.

DIAGNOSIS

The wound or burn site should be sampled and cultured to determine the specific organism that is the cause of the infection. In *P aeruginosa* infections, there may be a foul-smelling green-pigmented discharge, and necrosis may be evident. If skin lesions (ecthyma gangrenosum) distant from the burn or wound are present, the patient has developed sepsis. *S aureus* causes an insidious tissue-degrading infection that can eventually enter the bloodstream. *S pyogenes* infection can result in rapid tissue degradation with severe toxicity.

TREATMENT AND PREVENTION

Oral dicloxacillin is effective for treating both *S pyogenes* and *S aureus* infections. Imipenem-cilastatin or meropenem have been shown to be effective in treating *P aeruginosa* infections. Burn patients must have fluids and electrolytes restored intravenously as well as protection from infection of the burn sites.

ECTHYMA GANGRENOSUM

Ecthyma gangrenosum is a skin lesion that can occur following septic infections with *P aeruginosa*.

ETIOLOGY

P aeruginosa is the most common cause of ecthyma gangrenosum. Other bacteria and fungi occasionally have been associated with ecthyma gangrenosum.

MANIFESTATIONS

Lesions of ecthyma gangrenosum begin as red macules that enlarge and become slightly elevated papules, which become hemorrhagic and centrally necrotic with purple-to-black coloration (Figure 5-11). Previous (older) lesions are ulcers with a hemorrhagic crust or eschar. Lesions may be single, but are usually multiple with different stages of development. Lesions usually appear in the axillary or anogenital areas or the lower trunk and extremities.

EPIDEMIOLOGY

- Ecthyma gangrenosum occurs in 1.3–13% of patients with *P aeruginosa* sepsis, and is less common in patients who are not bacteremic.

- At-risk groups for ecthyma gangrenosum include immunocompromised neutropenic patients.

PATHOGENESIS

Impaired humoral or cellular immunity leads to increased susceptibility to infections with *P aeruginosa*. Breakdown of the skin allows the organism to disseminate. The lesions of ecthyma gangrenosum occur following perivascular bacterial invasion of arteries and veins in the dermis and subcutaneous tissues producing a necrotizing vasculitis. Perivascular involvement can occur by hematogenous seeding of the skin in bacteremic patients or by direct inoculation through the skin. Extravasation, edema, and necrosis around the vessel impede blood supply to the tissues, causing a secondary ischemic necrosis of the epidermis and dermis. Nodular lesions develop and proceed rapidly through the stages of central hemorrhage, ulceration, and necrosis.

DIAGNOSIS

Diagnosis of ecthyma gangrenosum can be obtained rapidly by Gram stain of fluid from the central hemorrhagic pustule or bulla. If no fluid is present, the eschar should be elevated and the underlying tissue swabbed for a Gram stain. Blood should be collected for culture to detect bacteremia.

THERAPY AND PREVENTION

Treatment of ecthyma gangrenosum usually requires the use of antipseudomonal penicillins, aminoglycosides, fluoroquinolones, third-generation cephalosporins, or aztreonam. Empiric therapy includes antipseudomonal penicillin (piperacillin) in combination with an aminoglycoside (gentamicin). Definitive therapy may be instituted after the organism has been identified and antibiotic sensitivity results are known.

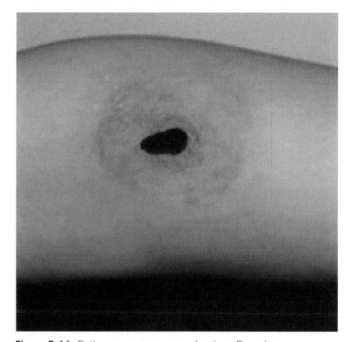

Figure 5-11. Ecthyma gangrenosum due to a *Pseudomonas aeruginosa* infection of the bloodstream.

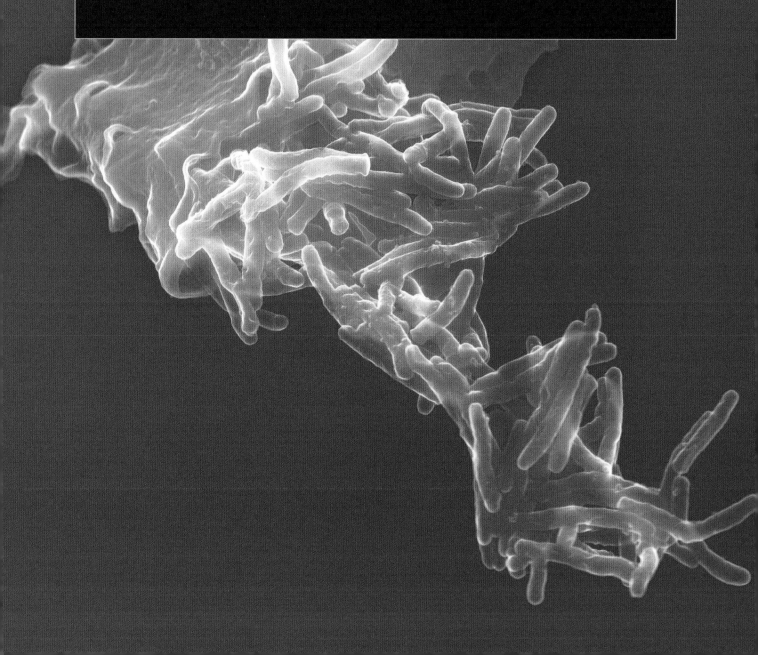

SECTION 2

CENTRAL NERVOUS SYSTEM

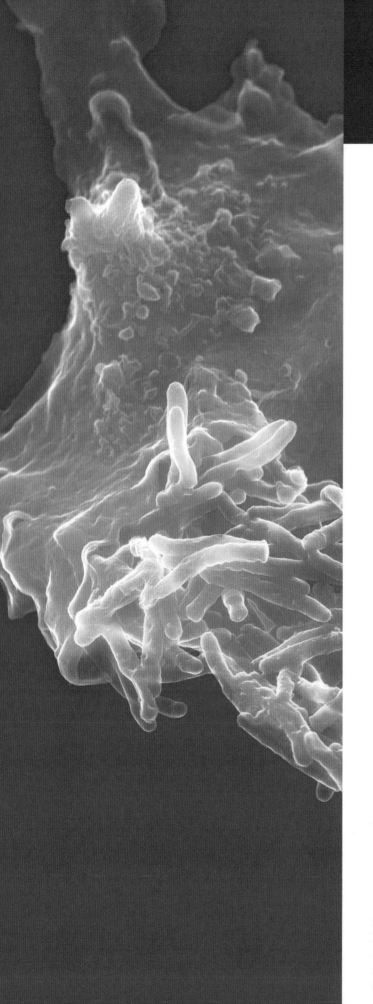

CHAPTER 6

THE BIG PICTURE: INFECTIONS OF THE CENTRAL NERVOUS SYSTEM

OVERVIEW

The central nervous system (CNS) consists of the cerebral cortex and the spinal cord. Infections of the CNS are rare; however when they do occur, they can rapidly become life threatening. Acute bacterial meningitis is a CNS infection, and it is one of the few infectious disease medical emergencies that requires rapid and aggressive therapy.

The cerebral cortex and the spinal cord are both located in confined spaces and have very limited ability to tolerate swelling associated with an inflammatory response to infection. Swelling of the CNS frequently results in tissue infarction and permanent neurologic sequelae or death.

The CNS is suspended in cerebrospinal fluid (CSF), which flows between the layers of the arachnoid and the pia mater, which are known as the leptomeninges (Figure 6-1). Most meningeal infections involve the leptomeninges.

The capillaries of the CNS differ significantly from capillaries in other parts of the body. The tight junctions of the endothelial cells lining the capillaries of the CNS are much less permeable and form the blood-brain barrier (BBB) (Figure 6-2). The BBB is difficult to cross and protects the CNS from pathogens and toxic substances. It also keeps certain serum components of the immune system (i.e., antibodies and complement) from getting into the CNS, delaying the immune response to an infection in the CNS. CNS infections are difficult to treat because the antibiotics used to treat them must be given at maximal (meningeal) doses to achieve therapeutic levels in the CNS, and they must be able to cross the BBB.

The impermeability of the BBB to immune system components, the difficulty of antibiotics reaching the CNS, and the nutrient-rich nature of the CSF allow pathogens that breach the BBB an excellent environment in which to multiply and cause significant pathology in a relatively short period of time. As a result, treatment of CNS infections, similar to the treatment of acute bacterial meningitis, must be rapid and aggressive.

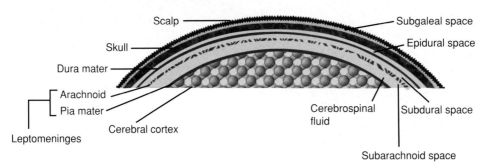

Figure 6-1. The relationship of the epidural, subdural, and subarachnoid spaces in the central nervous system. The cerebrospinal fluid is found within the leptomeninges, which are called the arachnoid and pia mater layers.

CNS infections are classified by the site of infection. **Meningitis** is an infection of the meninges, usually the leptomeninges. Viruses (e.g., enteroviruses) are the most common cause of meningitis in the United States. Enteroviruses cause a type of meningitis called **aseptic meningitis.** Bacterial causes of meningitis (e.g., *Streptococcus pneumoniae* and *Neisseria meningitidis*) are important to recognize because a patient with acute bacterial meningitis can die within a few hours. Bacterial causes of **neonatal meningitis** (e.g., *Streptococcus agalactiae* and *Escherichia coli*) are somewhat unique and physicians should become familiar with the infection and its manifestations in order to determine a correct diagnosis. Symptoms of **chronic meningitis** develop slowly and the causes (i.e., *Mycobacterium tuberculosis* and *Cryptococcus neoformans*) of this type of meningitis are important to recognize to determine the diagnosis.

Encephalitis is an infection of the cerebral cortex. Viruses are also the most common cause of encephalitis in the United States. Herpes simplex viruses, arboviruses, and rabies virus are important causes of encephalitis. Infections can occur in both the meninges and the cerebral cortex, resulting in a **meningoencephalitis.** Encephalitis and all the types of meningitis mentioned above will be discussed in Chapter 7.

Other CNS diseases include **poliomyelitis** and **tetanus,** topics that will be discussed in Chapter 8. Polioviruses replicate in the motor neurons of the anterior horns of the spinal cord, in the brain stem, and in the meninges, causing aseptic meningitis or an ascending paralysis called poliomyelitis. The toxin from *Clostridium tetani* blocks the release of the neurotransmitters in the spinal cord involved in inhibiting motor reflex responses to sensory stimulation. This causes a tetanic spasm of the muscles called tetanus (lockjaw).

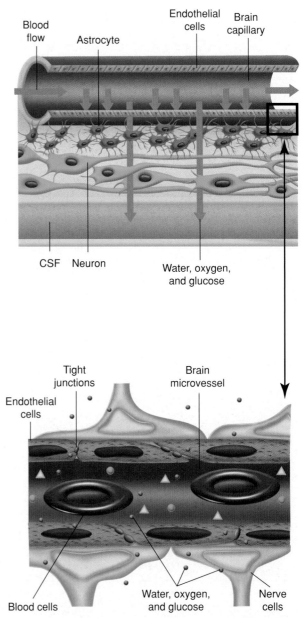

Figure 6-2. The blood-brain barrier (BBB). The BBB serves as a protective mechanism from harmful substances that may be in the bloodstream. The tight junctions between the endothelial cells that line the capillaries allow nutrients into the central nervous system but prevent blood cells and pathogens from entering when functioning normally. CSF, cerebrospinal fluid.

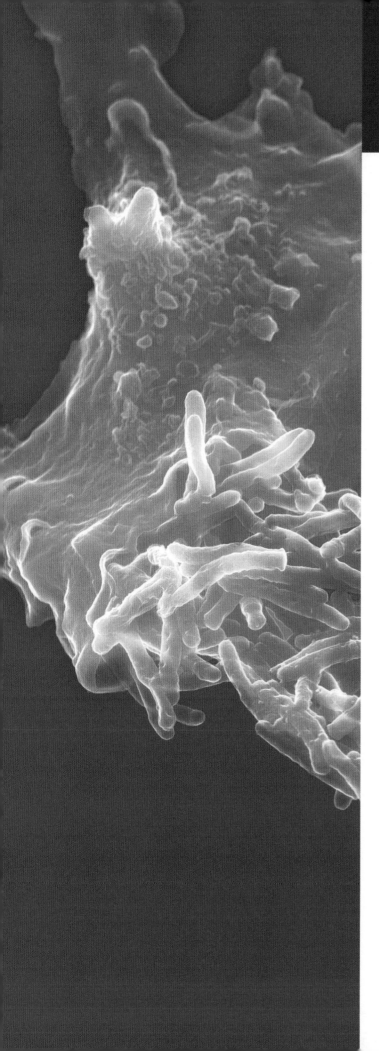

CHAPTER 7

MENINGITIS AND ENCEPHALITIS

MENINGITIS

OVERVIEW

Several different types of meningitis exist, and the differences are based on manifestations, etiology, and the age of the patient. The four types of meningitis discussed in this chapter include (1) aseptic (viral) meningitis, (2) infant meningitis, (3) acute bacterial meningitis, and (4) chronic meningitis. Aseptic, acute bacterial, and chronic meningitides can be differentiated based on manifestations and on laboratory tests. Infant meningitis is a type of meningitis with diagnosis based on the age of the infant and the specific manifestations and laboratory tests that indicate whether the infant has aseptic (viral) meningitis or acute bacterial meningitis.

ETIOLOGY

Aseptic meningitis
Aseptic meningitis is the most common type of meningitis and is usually the result of a viral infection; there are other common agents, however, that cause viral meningitis.

- **Echoviruses and coxsackieviruses A and B** are the most common causes of aseptic meningitis.
- Human simplex virus type 2 (HSV-2) aseptic meningitis can occur during primary genital infection. HSV-1 can also cause aseptic meningitis, but it is less common than HSV-2.
- Varicella-zoster virus (VZV), Epstein-Barr virus (EBV), and cytomegalovirus (CMV) can all cause aseptic meningitis.
- Human immunodeficiency virus (HIV) aseptic meningitis occurs during primary infection in 5–10% in patients who are HIV positive.

Infant meningitis
Causes of infant meningitis include viruses, bacteria, and parasites (Table 7-1). Diagnosing the specific cause of infant meningitis depends on which diseases (e.g., varicella) or organisms (e.g., *Streptococcus agalactiae*) the mother acquired during her pregnancy and the present age of the infant. Bacteria are

TABLE 7-1. Causes of Infant Meningitis

Viral	Comments	Bacterial	Comments	Parasitic
Enteroviruses	Most common cause in children <3 months of age	*Escherichia coli:* gram-negative rod	*E coli* and *S agalactiae*: most common causes in children <1 month of age	*Toxoplasma gondii*
Herpes simplex virus (HSV)	Vesicular skin lesions may be present in clusters	*Streptococcus agalactiae* (Group B streptococcus): gram-positive coccus		
Varicella-zoster virus (VZV)	Neonates with VZV infection present with a vesicular rash 9–15 days after appearance of mother's rash; vesicular skin lesions appear over entire body	*Listeria monocytogenes:* gram-positive rod	Occasional cause	
Cytomegalovirus (CMV)				

common causes of infant meningitis acquired within 1 month following birth; however, if an infant is diagnosed with meningitis after 1 month of age, viruses tend to be the more common cause of meningitis.

Acute bacterial meningitis

The common causes of acute bacterial meningitis depend on age, immune status, and whether the infection is community acquired or nosocomial. Table 7-2 lists information regarding causes of community-acquired acute bacterial meningitis and nosocomial acute bacterial meningitis.

Chronic meningitis

The most common cause of chronic meningitis in immunocompromised persons and persons with normal immune status is *Mycobacterium tuberculosis. Cryptococcus neoformans* is the most common cause of chronic meningitis in AIDS patients, and is the second most common infectious cause of chronic meningitis in all patients regardless of immune status. The HIV virus can also cause chronic meningitis in AIDS patients.

MANIFESTATIONS

Aseptic meningitis

The manifestations of aseptic meningitis are fever, headache, and nuchal rigidity, manifestations that are quite similar to those observed in acute bacterial meningitis (see below). Manifestations that may be more characteristic of a viral cause of meningitis include maculopapular rashes and conjunctivitis (commonly seen when caused by an echovirus) and lethargy but with **clear mentation** and **no focal neurologic findings.** Patients may occasionally experience tinnitus, vertigo, chest and abdominal pain, and paresthesia.

Acute bacterial meningitis

In patients with acute bacterial meningitis, an upper respiratory tract infection (e.g., sore throat, rhinorrhea, and nasal congestion) or ear infection may precede an abrupt onset of worsening fever and one or more meningeal symptoms (Table 7-3). The most common manifestations of acute bacterial meningitis include headache, fever, nuchal rigidity, and altered mental status (neurologic findings). Less than 50% of patients with acute bacterial meningitis have the classic triad of **fever, nuchal rigidity, and change in mental status;** however, nearly all patients have two of the four symptoms listed in Table 7-3.

Other signs and symptoms associated with acute bacterial meningitis

- Evidence of otitis media.
- Pharyngeal inflammation.
- Purulent nasal discharge is an indication that the patient may have a sinusitis infection that has resulted in meningitis. A clear nasal discharge may indicate a CSF leak and contamination of the meninges with normal flora from the nasal passages. In both cases, the common cause of acute bacterial meningitis is *Streptococcus pneumoniae.*
- If the patient has pneumonia, the acute bacterial meningitis that results is usually due to *S pneumoniae.*
- Diastolic heart murmur suggests endocarditis, and the acute bacterial meningitis that results is due to *Staphylococcus aureus.*
- Nonblanching petechiae or purpura are usually due to *Neisseria meningitidis* infection.
- Patients with severe *N meningitidis* infection may experience endotoxic shock with vascular collapse. Hemorrhage into the adrenals can result in Waterhouse-Friderichsen syndrome. Acute adrenal gland insufficiency and shock occur in 50% of patients with *N meningitidis* CNS infections.
- Ocular effects include lateral gaze palsy (abducens, or 6th, cranial nerve) and photophobia.
- **NOTE:** Papilledema, asymmetric response to light, and unilateral cranial deficits are rare in acute bacterial meningitis and are more common in space-occupying lesions in the brain.

Infant meningitis

When a neonate or infant presents with fever and lethargy or irritability, it is important to consider the diagnosis of meningitis even if the classic signs and symptoms are absent (i.e., fever, nuchal rigidity, and change in mental status). Other symptoms that may occur in a neonate or infant with meningitis include

- Poor feeding, vomiting, paradoxic irritability (i.e., quiet when stationary, cries when held), or high-pitched cry.
- Respiratory distress, apnea, and cyanosis.
- Bulging fontanelle.
- Hypotonia.
- Jaundice or rash (i.e., petechial, vesicular, macular, mucosal).
- Seizures or subdural effusions.

TABLE 7-2. Causes of Acute Bacterial Meningitis

Community-Acquired Acute Bacterial Meningitis

Neonates (Preterm to <1 month of age)
Escherichia coli: gram-negative rod
Streptococcus agalactiae (Group B streptococci): gram-positive coccus
Listeria monocytogenes: gram-positive rod

Persons 1 month to 50 years of age
Streptococcus pneumoniae, most common community-acquired cause of acute bacterial meningitis: gram-positive coccus
Neisseria meningitidis, common in crowded living environments (college dormitories, military training camps); more common in patients with complement deficiencies: gram-negative coccus

Persons older than 50 years of age, alcoholics, and impaired cell-mediated immunity
Streptococcus pneumoniae: gram-positive diplococcus
Listeria monocytogenes: gram-positive rod-shaped bacteria

Nosocomial Acute Bacterial Meningitis

Gram-negative rod-shaped bacteria (especially *Escherichia coli*)

Following endocarditis
Staphylococcus aureus usually: gram-positive coccus

Following ventricular shunt replacement
Staphylococcus epidermidis: gram-positive coccus
Staphylococcus aureus: gram-positive coccus
Enterococcus sp: gram-positive coccus
Bacillus subtilis: gram-positive rod
Corynebacterium sp: gram-positive rod

Syndrome of inappropriate antidiuretic hormone (SIADH) secretion (hyponatremia and hypovolemia of blood and inappropriately elevated urine osmolality). Symptoms can include nausea, vomiting, irritability, seizures, and stupor or coma.

CHRONIC MENINGITIS

Manifestations of chronic meningitis due to *M tuberculosis* include fever (38.3°C), unremitting headache, nausea, nuchal rigidity, and drowsiness, which can progress to stupor and coma. Symptoms usually progress slowly, but may suddenly increase in progression if damage from the infection causes thrombosis of a major cerebral vessel. The stages of tuberculous meningitis include (1) clear sensorium with abnormal CSF; (2) drowsiness or stupor with focal neurologic signs; and (3) coma.

Manifestations of chronic meningitis due to *Cryptococcus neoformans* progress slowly in immunocompetent patients with symptoms such as headache, nuchal rigidity, and a fever that tends to wax and wane. In AIDS patients, disease progression is rapid. Symptoms include severe intermittent headaches, confusion, personality changes that can progress to stupor, oculomotor palsies, decreased visual acuity, diplopia, hearing loss, hydrocephalus, and minimal nuchal rigidity.

EPIDEMIOLOGY

Aseptic meningitis

Aseptic meningitis is the most common form of meningitis, with about 10,000 cases reported each year in the United States. The incidence of this disease is 11 cases per 100,000 persons.

The incidence of aseptic meningitis decreases with age of the patient. Neonates are more likely to be diagnosed with aseptic meningitis and have the highest risk of morbidity and mortality.

The nonpolio enteroviruses (i.e., echovirus, coxsackieviruses A and B viruses) are the most common cause of aseptic meningitis and are spread via the fecal-oral route during the summer and early fall. Enteroviruses cause approximately 85% of all cases of meningitis. Coxsackievirus B causes over 60% of meningitis cases in children younger than 3 months of age.

HSV-1, HSV-2, CMV, and HIV-1 can be transmitted via sexual contact (heterosexual or homosexual). HIV-1 can also be transmitted percutaneously via intravenous substance use (e.g., illicit drugs).

VZV is transmitted by respiratory droplets.

EBV, HSV-1, and CMV are transmitted via infected saliva and other mucous secretions and are spread person to person.

Acute bacterial meningitis

Acute bacterial meningitis has become a disease of adults and is relatively uncommon, with an incidence of 3–4 cases per 100,000 in the United States.

TABLE 7-3. Signs and Symptoms of Acute Bacterial Meningitis

Sign and/or Symptom	Comments
Fever	Present in 95% of individuals; can last from 4 to 8 days after appropriate therapy has begun
Generalized severe, unremitting headache	May radiate down the neck Aspirin and over-the-counter pain relievers do not relieve pain
Neck stiffness (nuchal rigidity)	Occurs in around 90% of patients with acute bacterial meningitis Brudzinski or Kernig sign present
Altered mental status	Occurs in about 80% of patients Lethargic, stuporous, difficult to arouse, confused, disoriented, or in a coma More severe cases may result in loss of consciousness and grand mal or focal seizures Focal neurologic findings other than seizures can occur and include cranial nerve palsies, aphasia, and hemiparesis

- Bacterial meningitis occurs 20–100 times per 100,000 live births in the newborn period.

- *S pneumoniae* is spread person to person by respiratory droplets, and is the most common cause of acute bacterial meningitis.

- *Listeria monocytogenes* can be acquired following ingestion of commonly contaminated foods such as dairy products, hot dogs, and fish. *L monocytogenes* meningitis occurs more often in patients with depressed cellular-mediated immune responses (e.g., pregnant women, neonates, patients on immunosuppressive therapy, and patients with HIV and AIDS).

Infant meningitis

- Aseptic meningitis is the most common cause of infant meningitis.

- With the exception of HSV-2 meningitis, the clinical course of aseptic meningitis is usually self-limited, with complete recovery in 7–10 days.

- HSV infects 1500–2000 neonates each year. About 4% acquire HSV congenitally, with 86% during delivery and 10% postnatally. The highest risk of infant infection occurs when the onset of an outbreak of maternal primary herpes occurs near the time of labor and delivery.

- If a pregnant woman who is seronegative for VZV develops varicella skin lesions from a period of 7 days before giving birth until 2 days after giving birth, the neonate can acquire the virus from the mother and develop a severe multisystem disease that includes infection of the meninges. Seronegative mothers lack the maternal immunity needed to protect the infant from this severe VZV infection. The case fatality rate ranges from 25% to 40%.

- Neonates acquire *E coli* and *Streptococcus agalactiae* during passage down the birth canal. These organisms are the most common bacterial cause of meningitis in neonates younger than 1 month of age.

Chronic meningitis

- The risk of acquiring meningitis due to *M tuberculosis* increases with age across all racial and ethnic groups. The case rates are higher in minority racial and ethnic groups than in non-Hispanic whites; rates in Asians and Pacific Islanders are the highest, particularly in adults.

PATHOGENESIS

Aseptic meningitis

Echoviruses and coxsackieviruses gain access to the CNS hematogenously, the most common route. Penetration of the CNS via the neural route is from the nerve roots and usually is limited to HSV-1, HSV-2, VZV, and possibly some enteroviruses.

The viruses initially replicate in their target organ system (respiratory or gastrointestinal mucosa) and then gain access to the bloodstream. The primary viremia seeds the virus in the reticuloendothelial organs. If the replication continues and a secondary viremia occurs, the viruses then can infect the CNS. The viruses can cross the blood-brain barrier (BBB) directly at the capillary endothelial level or through natural defects (i.e., area postrema and other sites that lack a BBB). The inflammatory response is seen in the form of pleocytosis. Polymorphonuclear (PMNs) leukocytes are most abundant within the first 24–48 hours, followed later by increasing numbers of monocytes and lymphocytes. The CSF of a patient with viral meningitis will contain a high protein concentration, a normal glucose concentration, and a high leukocyte count of primarily lymphocytes (Table 7-4).

ACUTE BACTERIAL MENINGITIS

The most common means of transmission of bacteria to the meninges is through the bloodstream. Colonization and infections of the ears, sinuses, throat, lungs, heart, and gastrointestinal tract can all result in bacteremia. Once in the bloodstream,

TABLE 7-4. Important CSF Findings Used to Identify Aseptic, Acute Bacterial, and Chronic Meningitides

Test (adult values)	Aseptic Meningitis	Acute Bacterial Meningitis	Chronic (tuberculous and fungal) Meningitis
Opening pressure (60–180 mm H$_2$O)	Normal or slightly elevated	Elevated (>180 mm H$_2$O)	Normal or mildly increased for tuberculous Increased in fungal meningitis
Clarity (clear, colorless)	Clear or slightly turbid	Turbid; may clot	Clear to slightly turbid; if left to stand, a pellicle or faintly visible "spider's web clot" frequently forms
Protein (15–50 mg/dL)	Increased (50–100 mg/dL)	Increased (often >100 mg/dL)	Increased (average 224 mg/dL) for both
Glucose (45–85 mg/dL)	Normal or slightly decreased	Decreased (<45 mg/dL)	Decreased (<45 mg/dL) in tuberculous Sometimes decreased for fungal
CSF:serum glucose ratio (0.6)	>0.6	<0.3	≤0.4
White blood cells (<5/mL)	*Increased (≤500/mm^3); lymphocytes predominate	Increased (often >1000/mm^3), PMNs predominate	Increased (500/mm^3); initially PMNs then lymphocytes predominate in tuberculous; fungal lymphocytes predominate
Gram stain, acid-fast stain, India ink stain	No organisms	Shows organisms in ~75% of untreated cases	Acid-fast positive in about 25–40% of tuberculous meningitis 80–90% of fungal meningitis cases are positive for India ink staining (see Figure 7-3)
Culture	No organisms	Organisms grow in ~85% of untreated cases	Tuberculous meningitis cultures can take up to 4 weeks PCR amplification of bacterial DNA highly specific and much faster Fungal positive within 7 days for >90% of patients

CSF, cerebrospinal fluid; PMN, polymorphonuclear leukocyte; PCR, polymerase chain reaction.
*The CSF of early aseptic meningitis occasionally contains a predominance of PMNs; however, within 8–36 hours, lymphocytes predominate.

bacteria can settle in the large venous sinuses in the brain and then penetrate the dura and arachnoid and infect the CSF. Less common means of acquiring acute bacterial meningitis include breaks in the cribriform plate or defects in the base of the skull following basilar skull fractures. Head trauma can cause leakage of CSF into the middle ear or sinuses, and bacteria can then gain entrance into the subarachnoid space.

Once in the CSF, bacteria can grow rapidly, unimpeded by antibodies and complement. In time, the bacterial growth will attract PMNs to the infection site. The PMNs lyse, releasing toxic factors that result in necrosis and edema in the surrounding tissues. The inflammatory response causes the BBB to become more permeable to serum proteins. Glucose transport into the arachnoid and pia mater is reduced, causing a high protein concentration and a low glucose concentration in the CSF. The CSF of a patient with acute bacterial meningitis will contain a high protein concentration, a low glucose concentration, and a high leukocyte count of primarily neutrophils (see Table 7-4). Inflammation can also impede CSF flow resulting in cerebral edema. Intracranial pressure ultimately is increased and cerebral blood flow is decreased, resulting in hypoxia of the cerebral cortex and irreversible ischemic damage.

Chronic meningitis

Chronic meningitis due to *M tuberculosis* results from rupture of a tubercle into the adjacent subarachnoid space. *C neoformans* produces a capsule and melanin that protect the yeast cells from being phagocytized.

DIAGNOSIS

To obtain a definitive diagnosis of meningitis, it is necessary to perform a **lumbar puncture.** After lumbar puncture, empiric antimicrobial therapy can be initiated in most cases. The highest survival rates in cases of acute bacterial meningitis are obtained when antibiotics are administered to the patient within 30 minutes of arrival in the emergency department. In certain cases, a CT scan should be performed before lumbar puncture to ensure that no intracerebral masses are present in patients with focal neurologic deficits (i.e., dilated fixed pupils, Cheyne-Stokes respiration, decerebrate posturing, hemiplegia); patients with an abnormal level of consciousness (i.e., coma); patients with a history of CNS disease (e.g., mass lesion, stroke, or focal infection); patients with papilledema; patients who have had seizures within 1 week before presentation; or immunocompromised patients.

The following tests on the CSF will help in determining a diagnosis: CSF clarity, protein concentration, glucose concentration (compare with blood glucose), and white blood cell count (see Table 7-4). The CSF should also be smeared on a glass slide and Gram stained (Figures 7-1 and 7-2) and cultured. If certain bacterial pathogens are suspected (e.g., *S pneumoniae, S agalactiae, N meningitidis, E coli* K1), the CSF can be tested for bacterial capsular antigens by latex agglutination. CSF can be analyzed for *M tuberculosis* by acid-fast staining. *Cryptococcus* is the only encapsulated yeast that causes human infection and can be identified by an India ink stain of the CSF (Figure 7-3).

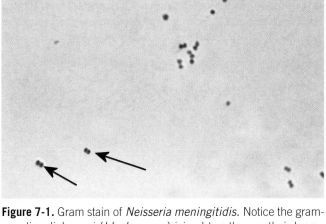

Figure 7-1. Gram stain of *Neisseria meningitidis.* Notice the gram-negative diplococci (*black arrows*) joined together on their longer side. Image courtesy of the Centers for Disease Control and Prevention, Dr Brodsky.

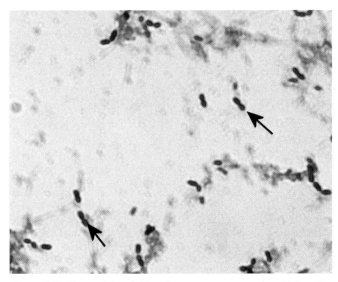

Figure 7-2. Gram stain of *Streptococcus pneumoniae.* Notice the gram-positive diplococci (*black arrows*) joined together on their shorter side. Image courtesy of the Centers for Disease Control and Prevention, Dr Mike Miller.

Other tests used to determine the cause of chronic meningitis include a chest radiograph and a tuberculin skin test, which may aid in the diagnosis of meningitis due to *M tuberculosis.* CT scan of the brain, with and without contrast, or MRI may show calcifications if the cause is CMV, toxoplasmosis, rubella, or HSV, whereas *Staphylococcus aureus, Citrobacter diversus, Proteus mirabilis,* and other bacteria can cause abscesses, which will have a well-defined border with a less opaque center.

THERAPY AND PREVENTION

If possible, antibiotic therapy should be delayed until blood and CSF samples have been collected. If not possible, performing the lumbar tap within 30 minutes after beginning antibiotic therapy increases the likelihood of culturing the CSF for bacterial causes of meningitis.

Aseptic meningitis

In the early stages of aseptic meningitis, CSF glucose concentration may be reduced and PMNs may predominate, mimicking bacterial meningitis. Patients should be given empiric antibiotics pending results of CSF culture, blood cultures, and follow-up lumbar puncture. In most cases, if the results of a repeat lumbar puncture 6–24 hours later show a predominance of lymphocytes, antibiotic therapy then may be discontinued. A negative CSF culture after 48 hours greatly reduces the probability of bacterial meningitis.

Acute bacterial meningitis

Once samples of blood and CSF are obtained, intravenous empiric therapy based on the most likely cause of the patient's meningitis should begin immediately (Table 7-5). If the cause of acute bacterial meningitis is known, specific therapy can then be initiated (Table 7-6).

Universal administration of *S pneumoniae* and *H influenzae* type b vaccines to infants has been shown to dramatically reduce the number of cases of acute bacterial meningitis in children. Administering the *N meningitidis* vaccine to college students who plan to stay in dormitories and to military recruits also has been shown to reduce the number of these infections.

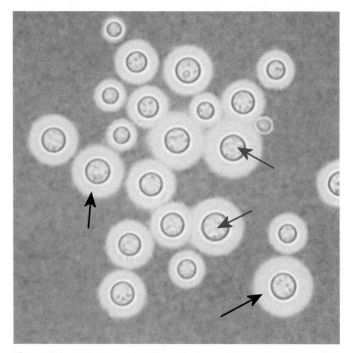

Figure 7-3. India ink stain of the capsule of *Cryptococcus neoformans.* This fungus is the *ONLY* encapsulated yeast that causes human infection. Notice the capsule (*black arrows*) not stained by the India ink and the yeast cells (*blue arrows*) surrounded by the capsule. Image courtesy of the Centers for Disease Control and Prevention, Dr Leanor Haley.

TABLE 7-5. Empiric Antimicrobial Therapy for Acute Bacterial Meningitis

Patient Profile	Etiology	Empiric Treatment
Preterm to <1 month	*Streptococcus agalactiae* (group B streptococcus), *Escherichia coli, Listeria*	Ampicillin + cefotaxime or ampicillin + gentamicin
1 month to 50 years	*Streptococcus pneumoniae, Neisseria meningitidis*	Cefotaxime or ceftriaxone + vancomycin + dexamethasone*
Age >50 years, alcoholism, impaired cell-mediated immunity	*S pneumoniae, Listeria,* and gram-negative bacteria	Cefotaxime or ceftriaxone + ampicillin + vancomycin + dexamethasone

*Dexamethasone blocks tumor necrosis factor production and reduces inflammation.

TABLE 7-6. Specific Antimicrobial Therapy Used to Treat Acute Bacterial Meningitis

Organism	Treatment
Streptococcus pneumoniae	Penicillin G or vancomycin (for resistant strains)
Neisseria meningitidis	Penicillin G or chloramphenicol
Listeria monocytogenes	Ampicillin + gentamicin
Staphylococcus aureus Methicillin-sensitive *S aureus* (MSSA)	Nafcillin or oxacillin + rifampin
Methicillin-resistant *S aureus* (MRSA)	Vancomycin + rifampin (also used to treat *Staphylococcus epidermidis*)
Enterobacteriaceae	Ceftriaxone + gentamicin (intrathecal and systemic)

If a person is exposed to a patient with meningitis, administration of certain antibiotics can prevent acute bacterial meningitis. For *H influenzae* exposure, rifampin should be given; for exposure to *N meningitidis*, rifampin, ciprofloxacin, or ceftriaxone should be given. To protect neonates from meningitis caused by *S agalactiae* (group B streptococcus), vaginal and rectal swab samples should be obtained from the pregnant woman (at 35–37 weeks' gestation). If cultures are positive for *S agalactiae*, administration of penicillin intrapartum can significantly reduce neonatal infections.

Infant meningitis

Because the causative agent usually is not known at presentation, all newborns or infants with meningitis should be treated aggressively, and antibiotics should be given to protect against the most common bacterial causes of meningitis. Antibiotics should be administered until all bacterial cultures have been negative for at least 72 hours. Empiric therapy for infants who are preterm or younger than 1 month of age includes ampicillin plus cefotaxime or gentamicin. If HSV infection is likely, acyclovir should also be given.

Antibiotics specific for identified bacterial agents are the same as those administered to patients with acute bacterial meningitis. However, ***chloramphenicol should NOT be administered to infants or to women who are pregnant or breastfeeding because fetuses and neonates lack the liver enzymes necessary to metabolize this drug.*** Drug toxicity can cause gray baby syndrome (e.g., hypotension, cyanosis, and frequently death). Treatments of other important etiologies for this age group are listed in Table 7-7.

Pregnant women with a history of genital herpes should be assessed before delivery, and a cesarean section should be performed if herpetic lesions or prodromal symptoms are present during labor rather than delivering the fetus vaginally. Pregnant women with no history of VZV infection should avoid exposure to patients with clinically apparent signs of this viral infection (e.g., chickenpox, zoster). They should also avoid contact with cat litter boxes (*Toxoplasma gondii*) and uncooked or undercooked meats (*T gondii* and *Listeria*).

TABLE 7-7. Antimicrobial Agents Used to Treat Infant Meningitis

Etiology	Treatment
HSV, VZV	Acyclovir
CMV	Ganciclovir
Enteroviruses	Immune globulin
HIV	Multidrug antiretroviral regimens
Borrelia burgdorferi (Lyme disease)	Ceftriaxone
Treponema pallidum (syphilis)	High-dose penicillin
Toxoplasma gondii	Pyrimethamine and sulfadiazine
Mycobacterium tuberculosis	Multidrug antimycobacterial regimens

HSV, herpes simplex virus; VZV, varicella-zoster virus; CMV, cytomegalovirus; HIV, human immunodeficiency virus.

Chronic meningitis

Tubercular, or tuberculous, meningitis is a severe bacterial meningitis caused by *M tuberculosis;* it is fatal if not treated within 5–8 weeks of symptom onset. A regimen of isoniazid, rifampin, pyrazinamide, and ethambutol should be administered for 12 months. Patients who have **fungal meningitis** should be given amphotericin B plus flucytosine until they are afebrile and cultures are negative; then treatment with amphotericin B plus flucytosine should be stopped and treatment with fluconazole should be given for 8–10 weeks.

ENCEPHALITIS

OVERVIEW

Encephalitis is an infection of the cerebral cortex that is viewed as a separate disease entity from meningitis. However, since the meninges are usually involved, patients can present with meningeal irritation (i.e., headache and nuchal rigidity) and encephalitis (i.e., meningoencephalitis). Viruses are the most common cause of encephalitis in the United States.

TWO MAJOR CATEGORIES OF ENCEPHALITIDES

1. Human-to-human diseases (e.g., herpesvirus encephalitis).
2. Zoonotic diseases acquired by direct contact with an animal (e.g., rabies) or via an insect vector that transmits the causative agent from animals to humans (e.g., West Nile fever, Eastern equine encephalitis).

ETIOLOGY

Human-to-human encephalitis

HSV-1 is the most common cause of encephalitis that is transmitted from human to human in the United States. Other viruses that can cause encephalitis include VZV, HSV-2 (seen almost exclusively in neonates), CMV, influenza virus, and HIV (i.e., HIV encephalopathy or AIDS dementia).

Zoonotic encephalitis

Zoonotic encephalitis is caused by an arbovirus (arthropod-borne viruses) or the rabies virus.

MANIFESTATIONS

Encephalitis

With the exception of rabies, the signs and symptoms of the different categories of encephalitis are quite similar and cannot be clinically differentiated. Common manifestations include severe headache, meningeal irritation (headache and nuchal rigidity), sensory or motor deficits similar to ataxia, and grand mal or focal seizures. Patients with encephalitis may experience visual or auditory hallucinations. They may perform peculiar higher motor functions such as continuous buttoning and unbuttoning of a shirt or placing their underwear over their outerwear. Viral encephalitis can cause personality changes, confusion, and sleepiness and can progress to coma and death.

Rabies

Patients who develop manifestations of rabies virus encephalitis experience an abrupt onset of hydrophobia. When attempting to drink water, the pharynx spasms, spreading to the respiratory muscles and causing shallow quick respirations and possibly hyperactivity. Seizures with coma usually follow these manifestations. Patients often experience pituitary dysfunction resulting in diabetes insipidus or inappropriate antidiuretic hormone secretion. Cardiac arrhythmias and autonomic dysfunction are also common. Death usually occurs within 1–2 weeks.

The manifestations of rabies begin 10–240 days after exposure; however, the usual incubation period is 30–90 days. The three clinical phases of the disease are prodromal, excitation, and paralytic (Table 7-8).

EPIDEMIOLOGY

Human encephalitides

- **Acute viral encephalitis** is an uncommon manifestation of certain common viral infections. This uncommon complication occurs most frequently in children and young adults.

- HSV-1 is the most common cause of sporadic encephalitis in the United States.

- About 4–7 cases per 100,000 of acute viral encephalitis occur each year in the United States.

- Some viruses that cause encephalitis are transmitted from human to human (e.g., HSV, VZV, EBV, HIV, influenza). An immunocompromised patient is more likely to develop encephalitis due to VZV and CMV.

- **HSV encephalitis** is the most common form of viral encephalitis and accounts for 10% of all cases of encephalitis in the United States. Most cases of HSV encephalitis appear to be due to the reactivation of HSV from the trigeminal ganglia.

Zoonotic encephalitides

- The **rabies** virus is transmitted primarily to humans following infected animal bites (e.g., bats and other mammals). Five animal species are recognized as reservoir species for the rabies virus: raccoons (eastern United States); skunks (north and south central United States and California); bats (in all states of United States except Hawaii); fox (Alaska, Arizona, and Texas); and mongoose (Puerto Rico).

- The **arboviruses** are transmitted from animals (e.g., birds) via an insect or arthropod vector (e.g., mosquito or tick, depending on the virus) to humans. A tick transmits the Powassan encephalitis virus. All other arboviruses endemic in the United States are transmitted by mosquitoes (Figure 7-4).

- Arboviruses are the most common episodic cause of encephalitis, with most cases of arboviral encephalitis occurring in the summer months when the vectors are most active.

- **West Nile virus** is the most common cause of **arboviral episodic encephalitis** in the United States. Elderly persons are more likely to develop encephalitis following West Nile virus infection.

TABLE 7-8. Symptoms of Rabies Encephalitis

Phase of the Disease	Signs and Symptoms
Prodromal phase	• Fever, headache, anorexia, malaise, • Itching, burning or tingling at the location of the bite • Restlessness, nausea, sore throat, increased saliva production, muscle stiffness • Dilated pupils • Increased sensitivity to light, sound, or temperature changes
Excitation phase	• Abnormal behavior, anxiety with depression and feelings of impending doom, confusion, or disorientation • Convulsions, delirium, insomnia, hallucinations • Positive Babinski sign • Hoarseness, hydrophobia • Papilledema, absence of corneal reflexes, dilation or constriction of the pupils which may be asymmetric and associated with hippos, strabismus, nystagmus, and diplopia
Paralytic phase	• Disappearance of hydrophobia • Progressive general flaccid paralysis • Apathy that progresses to stupor and then coma • Urinary incontinence • Peripheral vascular collapse

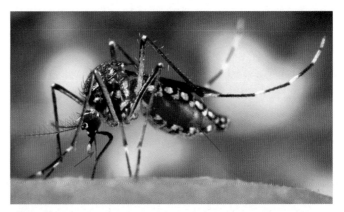

Figure 7-4. A mosquito obtaining a blood meal. Notice the blood-filled proboscis and the abdomen engorged with blood (*blue arrows*). Image courtesy of the Centers for Disease Control and Prevention, Frank Hadley Collins, Director, Center for Global Health and Infectious Diseases, University of Notre Dame, Notre Dame, IN.

Approximately 150 other arboviral encephalitis cases were reported yearly from 1995 to 2003 in the United States.

PATHOGENESIS

Encephalitis

The causative agent of encephalitis replicates outside the CNS and enters the CNS by a hematogenous route or by moving up neural (e.g., rabies, HSV, VZV) and olfactory (e.g., HSV) pathways. Some viruses (e.g., HSV) infect neurons causing damage. With other viral infections (e.g., CMV and EBV), most of the damage is due to the immune response to the viral infection.

After gaining access to the CNS, the virus can enter neural cells. Infections result in disruption of cell functioning, perivascular congestion, hemorrhage, and inflammatory response diffusely affecting gray matter more than white matter. Some viral receptors are only found in certain areas of the brain, which accounts for the localized damage associated with some of these viruses. For example, ***damage due to HSV is usually seen in the inferior and medial temporal lobes.***

Encephalitis following most viral infections results in non-specific histologic findings. However, the presence of ***Negri bodies in the hippocampus and cerebellum are pathognomonic of rabies virus infection*** (Figure 7-5). Cowdry type A inclusions with hemorrhagic necrosis in the temporal and orbitofrontal lobes are commonly associated with HSV infections.

DIAGNOSIS

Encephalitis

Laboratory tests helpful in the diagnosis of encephalitis include lumbar puncture to assess the CSF and CT scan or MRI with contrast to rule out brain abscess, stroke, or another structural disorder such as hematoma, aneurysm, or tumor. Viral culture can be performed on the CSF and on swab samples obtained from the throat. Even with these tests, a specific microorganism is identified less than 50% of the time. Tests for the detection of viral antigens in the CSF or identification of agents by reverse transcriptase polymerase chain reaction (RT-PCR) are available for some viruses, and the CSF profile is similar to that seen in aseptic meningitis. The CSF can also be assayed for virus-specific IgM and IgG using paired acute and convalescent samples.

Diagnosis of **West Nile virus encephalitis** is based on clinical suspicion and positive results of specific laboratory tests.

- West Nile virus or other arboviral diseases such as St. Louis encephalitis should be strongly considered in adults older than age 50 who develop unexplained encephalitis or meningitis in summer or early fall.

- The most efficient diagnostic method is detection of IgM antibody to West Nile virus in serum collected 8–14 days after onset of illness or CSF collected within 8 days of onset of illness.

- Identification of West Nile virus genome in CSF by RT-PCR.

Herpes encephalitis is clinically similar to other viral encephalitides but is strongly suggested by repeated seizures occurring early in the course of the disease and by signs indicating

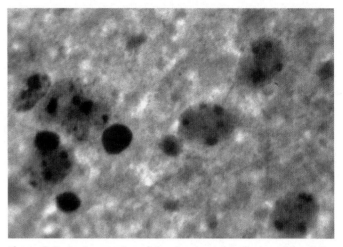

Figure 7-5. An impression slide of a dog brain that contained the intracellular Negri bodies due to rabies. Negri bodies are cellular inclusions found most frequently in the pyramidal cells of Ammon horn and the Purkinje cells of the cerebellum. Image courtesy of the Centers for Disease Control and Prevention, Mr G Heid.

temporal lobe involvement. An electroencephalogram usually demonstrates electrical spikes in the region of the infected temporal lobe. Erythrocytes in the CSF after an atraumatic lumbar tap also suggests HSV. PCR can detect HSV DNA in the CSF; however HSV is rarely isolated from the CSF.

Rabies

The animal vector should be euthanized and its brain examined for signs of rabies (see Figure 7-5). Pets (e.g., dogs, cats, ferrets) that do not appear sick may be confined and observed by a veterinarian for 10–14 days. If the pet remains healthy, it is considered to be free of rabies infection. Patients should not begin therapy unless the confined pet begins to show symptoms. If an animal shows signs of sickness, postexposure prophylaxis (see below) should begin immediately.

If the animal cannot be tested and if prodromal signs of rabies exist, tests can be performed on human patients. RT-PCR to detect rabies viral RNA can be performed on saliva or a skin biopsy can be taken from the posterior region of the neck at the hairline. Biopsies of the neck skin can be tested for viral antigen by immunofluorescent staining. Serum and CSF can be tested for antibodies to rabies by indirect immunofluorescence and virus neutralization tests. If no vaccine or rabies immune serum has been given, the presence of antibody to rabies virus in the serum is diagnostic and tests of CSF are unnecessary. Antibody to rabies virus in the CSF, regardless of immunization history, suggests a rabies virus infection.

THERAPY AND PREVENTION

Encephalitis

Treatment of encephalitis is supportive, usually resulting in hospitalization, intravenous fluids, respiratory support, and prevention of secondary infections for patients with severe disease. Ribavirin in high doses and interferon α-2b has some activity against West Nile virus in vitro, but no controlled studies have been completed on the use of these medications in treating West Nile virus encephalitis.

When HSV encephalitis cannot be ruled out, acyclovir must be started promptly, before the patient lapses into coma, and continued for at least 10 days to achieve maximal therapeutic benefit. Sometimes the initial lumbar puncture does not disclose a cellular pleocytosis, so treatment with acyclovir should not be delayed when the clinical picture is compatible with HSV encephalitis. The lumbar puncture should be repeated 24 hours later. Lymphocytosis is usually observed in the second CSF sample.

Mortality is directly related to mental status at the time treatment is initiated; therefore empiric treatment should be started as soon as HSV encephalitis is suspected. Permanent neurologic sequelae occur in 60% of patients even after treatment and can vary from mild deficits to severe disability. Up to 10% of patients will relapse.

Rabies

Only six patients in the United States have ever recovered following infection with the rabies virus. Of the six patients, five received rabies prophylaxis either before or after onset of illness.

Only one patient did not receive any rabies prophylaxis and survived. In 2004, a 15-year-old girl was bitten by a rabid bat about 1 month before symptoms began and was treated on day 6 of her illness with supportive care and neuroprotective measures. The neuroprotective measures included a drug-induced coma and ventilator support for 7 days. Intravenous ribavirin was also given. The exact reasons why this patient survived are not known, and the above treatment should be considered investigational. After symptoms appear, treatment is usually palliative (e.g., sedatives).

Following an animal bite, the wound should be cleaned by allowing it to bleed, and then it should be washed with soap and water. All pets should be immunized. Contact with bats and wild animals that are not behaving normally should be avoided.

Preexposure prophylaxis for rabies

Veterinarians and others who may be exposed to rabid animals should receive rabies vaccination. The most commonly used vaccine is produced in human diploid cell cultures and may be administered either intradermally or intramuscularly into the deltoid muscle. However, preexposure prophylaxis does not eliminate the need for additional therapy after a rabies exposure, but it simplifies therapy by eliminating the need for human rabies immunoglobulin and decreases the number of doses of vaccine needed. Furthermore, preexposure prophylaxis may protect patients whose postexposure therapy is delayed or those with inapparent exposures to rabies.

Postexposure prophylaxis for rabies

For patients who have not been immunized against rabies, the rabies vaccine should be given on days 0, 3, 7, 14, and 28. Rabies immunoglobulin should be administered into the tissues surrounding the wound. If more immunoglobulin remains, it can be infused into the wound area by injecting the remainder intramuscularly at a site distant from the vaccination site. Patients who have been immunized against rabies should receive two intramuscular doses of rabies vaccine on days 0 and 3, and rabies immunoglobulin should not be administered.

Prevention of arboviral encephalitis

- When outdoors, protective clothing should be worn and insect or tick repellent should be applied.
- Outdoor activity should be avoided at dusk and dawn when mosquitoes prefer to feed.
- Habitat for mosquitoes should be reduced by removing objects that collect water (e.g., old tires, garden containers).
- Habitat for ticks should be reduced by removing brush and weeds from around the home.
- Pets should be protected with repellent so that ticks are not brought into the home.
- Ticks should be removed as soon as possible after returning from the outdoors.

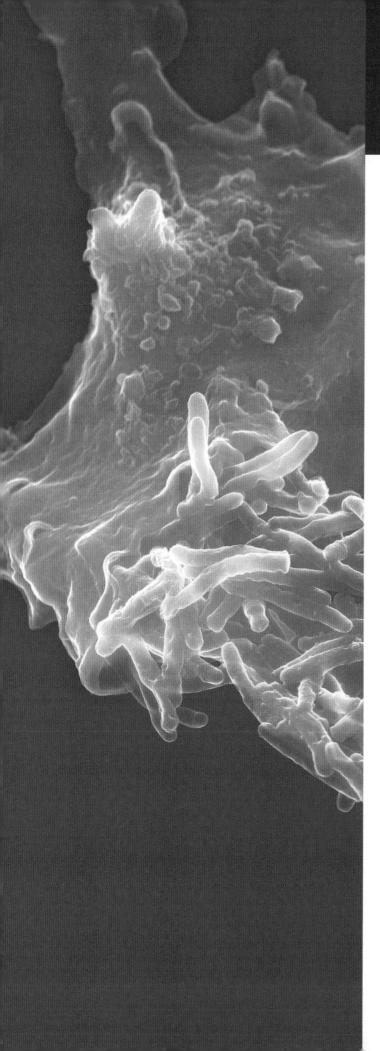

CHAPTER 8

POLIOMYELITIS AND TETANUS

OVERVIEW

There are two infectious diseases that will be discussed in this chapter, poliomyelitis and tetanus, and both of these diseases affect primarily the nerves of the spinal cord. Poliomyelitis is caused by an enterovirus. Tetanus is caused by a toxin produced by *Clostridium tetani*.

POLIOMYELITIS

Poliomyelitis (polio) is an acute viral infection of both the meninges and the motor neurons of the spinal cord and the brainstem.

ETIOLOGY

Poliomyelitis is caused by the poliovirus. There are three serotypes (1, 2, and 3) of this enterovirus that cause disease in humans.

MANIFESTATIONS

Most poliovirus infections are asymptomatic. However, symptomatic cases are characterized by two phases. The first phase is a nonspecific febrile illness, which is sometimes followed by aseptic meningitis or paralytic disease. Symptoms usually begin 6–20 days after exposure and include moderate fever, headache, vomiting, constipation, coryza, and sore throat.

The second phase begins 2–6 days after onset. The illness may subside entirely (abortive poliomyelitis), abate temporarily, or progress directly to involvement of the central nervous system (CNS). Early signs of paralytic polio include meningeal irritation (positive Kernig and Brudzinski signs), muscle weakness, hyperesthesia, severe muscle pain and spasms, and accentuated tendon reflexes. Babinski and Chaddock signs are present. The patient has **clear mentation.**

The second phase is followed rapidly by loss of motor function. One or both legs are involved in 60% of cases, and one or both arms are involved in 25% of cases. One in 200 cases of paralytic polio results in **irreversible paralysis** (Figure 8-1). If the diaphragm and intercostal muscles are involved, breathing capacity is reduced. There also may be respiratory obstruction, regurgitation, and aspiration of oropharyngeal secretions. Damage to the medullary respiratory center results in death in 2–5% of cases of children and in 15–30% of cases of adults. ***Sensory loss is rare in patients with polio.***

EPIDEMIOLOGY

▦ Poliomyelitis is a highly contagious infectious disease that is spread by the oral-fecal route or by contact with infectious saliva. After household exposure to wild poliovirus, more than 90% of susceptible contacts become infected.

▦ Humans are the only reservoir for poliovirus.

▦ Paralytic poliomyelitis is fatal in 2–5% of cases in children and in 15–30% of cases in adults.

▦ Polio is nearing worldwide eradication due to the efforts of the World Health Organization. In 2003, 784 confirmed cases of polio were reported globally, and polio was endemic in only six countries.

▦ The last cases of paralytic poliomyelitis caused by endemic transmission of wild virus in the United States were in 1979.

▦ From 1980 through 1999, 144 cases of polio were caused by the live oral polio vaccine. To eliminate vaccine-associated paralytic polio, only the killed polio vaccine has been used since 2000.

▦ Poliovirus infection results in lifelong immunity specific to the infecting viral serotype.

▦ Risk factors for paralytic disease include larger inocula of poliovirus, increasing age, pregnancy, strenuous exercise, tonsillectomy, and intramuscular injections administered while the patient is infected with poliovirus.

PATHOGENESIS

After ingestion of the poliovirus, the virus replicates in the oropharynx and the intestinal tract. Viremia follows, which can result in infection of the CNS. Replication of poliovirus in motor neurons of the anterior horn and brainstem results in cell destruction and causes the typical clinical manifestations of paralytic polio. Depending on the sites of paralysis, polio can be classified as **spinal** (weakness of legs), **bulbar** (weakness of muscles innervated by cranial nerves), or **spinobulbar** (combination of spinal and bulbar) disease. Progression to maximum paralysis is rapid (2–4 days), and is usually associated with fever and muscle pain and rarely continues after the patient's temperature has returned to normal. Spinal paralysis is typically asymmetric and more severe proximally than distally. Deep tendon reflexes are absent or diminished. Bulbar paralysis can compromise respiration and swallowing. After the acute episode, many patients recover some muscle function. Weakness or paralysis that remains after 12 months is usually permanent.

Post-polio syndrome

About 25–40% of patients who contracted paralytic polio during childhood may experience muscle pain and exacerbation of existing weakness or develop new weakness or paralysis after a

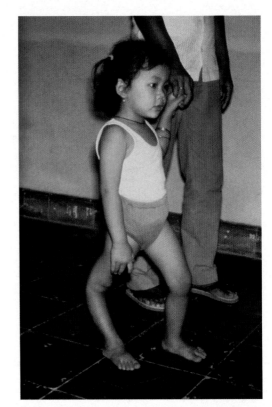

Figure 8-1. A child with a deformity of the right lower leg due to poliomyelitis. Image courtesy of the Centers for Disease Control and Prevention.

period of 30 to 40 years. Post-polio syndrome has been reported in people infected during the era of wild poliovirus circulation. Risk factors for post-polio syndrome include (1) the passage of more time since the acute poliovirus infection; (2) the presence of permanent residual impairment after recovery from the acute illness; and (3) female gender.

DIAGNOSIS

Specimens for virus isolation and serologic testing include **stool, throat swabs,** and **cerebrospinal fluid** (CSF). The greatest numbers of poliovirus can be obtained from stool specimens. In addition, an acute-phase serologic specimen should be obtained as early in the course of illness as possible, and a convalescent-phase specimen should be obtained at least 3 weeks later.

The following tests should be performed on stool specimens collected from persons who have suspected cases of polio.

- Isolation of poliovirus in tissue culture and serotyping of a poliovirus isolate as serotype 1, 2, or 3.

- Intratypic differentiation using DNA and RNA probe hybridization or polymerase chain reaction (PCR) to determine whether a poliovirus isolate is due to vaccination or is a wild virus.

- Acute-phase and convalescent-phase serum specimens should be tested for neutralizing antibody to each of the three poliovirus serotypes. A fourfold rise in antibody titer between acute-phase and convalescent-phase serum specimens is diagnostic for poliovirus infection.

THERAPY AND PREVENTION

There is no specific treatment for poliomyelitis. Supportive care includes monitoring of blood pressure; ability to handle secretions, to swallow, and to void; aid in respiratory ventilation; and examination for vocal cord weakness, breath sounds (e.g., signs of pulmonary edema, atelectasis, or pneumonitis), and evidence of thrombophlebitis).

Polio vaccines

In the United States, poliovirus vaccines have eliminated poliomyelitis caused by wild poliovirus. Until worldwide polio eradication is achieved, however, epidemics caused by importation of wild virus could occur if childhood vaccination were to cease. In 2000, the exclusive use of the inactivated (Salk) polio vaccine (IPV) was recommended because of the occurrence of vaccine-associated poliomyelitis. The vaccine consists of inactivated virus of serotypes 1, 2, and 3.

The oral (Sabin) polio vaccine (OPV) consists of serotypes 1, 2, and 3, but the virus is attenuated rather than inactivated. OPV remains the vaccine of choice for mass vaccination to control polio outbreaks. The use of OPV rather than the IPV in an outbreak setting is preferred due to the higher seroconversion rate after a single dose of OPV compared with a single dose of IPV and a greater degree of intestinal immunity induced by OPV. This increased intestinal immunity limits community spread of wild poliovirus.

TETANUS

Tetanus is caused by a toxin produced by *C tetani*. Following sensory stimulation, muscles will contract. To relax the muscles, inhibitory neurotransmitters must be released in the CNS. Tetanus toxin prevents release of these inhibitory neurotransmitters and causes the muscles to remain in spasm (Figure 8-2).

ETIOLOGY

Tetanus is caused by the anaerobic spore-forming, gram-positive, rod-shaped bacterium *C tetani*.

MANIFESTATIONS

The incubation period of tetanus varies from 3 to 21 days. The farther the injury site is from the CNS, the longer the incubation period. Three different forms of tetanus exist.

- **Local tetanus** is an uncommon form of the disease in which patients have persistent contraction of muscles in the same anatomic area as the injury. These contractions may persist for many weeks before gradually subsiding. Local tetanus may precede the onset of generalized tetanus, but it is generally milder.

- **Cephalic tetanus** is a rare form of the disease, occasionally occurring in conjunction with otitis media in which *C tetani* is present in the flora of the middle ear or following injuries to the head. There is involvement of the cranial nerves, especially in the facial area.

- **Generalized tetanus** is the most common type (about 80%) of tetanus. The spastic paralysis usually presents with a descending pattern. The first sign is **trismus** (lockjaw), followed by stiffness of the neck, difficulty in swallowing, and board-like rigidity of the abdominal muscles. Spasm of the facial muscles leads to a grotesque grinning expression termed **risus sardonicus** (Figure 8-3). Spasm of the somatic musculature may result in **opisthotonos,** a form of spasm in which the head and heels are bent backward and the body bowed forward (Figure 8-4). When spasms occur, they may be frequent and last for several minutes. Spasms continue for 3–4 weeks. Other symptoms include a temperature rise of 2–4°C above normal, sweating, elevated blood pressure, and episodic rapid heart rate. Complete recovery may take months.

Neonatal tetanus

Neonatal tetanus is a form of generalized tetanus that occurs in newborn infants (Figure 8-5). Symptoms usually appear 4–14 days after birth. Neonatal tetanus occurs in infants born without protective passive immunity because the mother is not immune. It usually occurs through infection of the unhealed umbilical stump, particularly when the stump is cut with contaminated instruments.

EPIDEMIOLOGY

- About 20–40 cases of tetanus are reported yearly.

- *C tetani* spores are found in soil and in animal and human feces. The spores enter the body through breaks in the skin and germinate under low oxygen conditions.

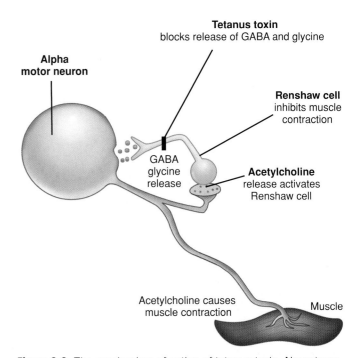

Figure 8-2. The mechanism of action of tetanus toxin. Neurotransmission is controlled by the balance between excitatory (acetylcholine) and inhibitory neurotransmitters. The inhibitory neurotransmitters (i.e., GABA [γ-aminobutyric acid], glycine) prevent depolarization of the postsynaptic membrane and conduction of the electrical signal. Tetanus toxin does not interfere with production or storage of GABA or glycine, but rather with their release. In the absence of inhibitory neurotransmitters, excitation of the nerves that stimulates muscle contraction is unrestrained, resulting in contraction of both extensor and flexor muscles and spastic paralysis.

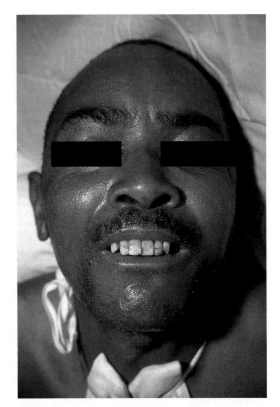

Figure 8-3. Risus sardonicus in a patient with tetanus. Image courtesy of the Centers for Disease Control and Prevention, AFIP, C Farmer.

- Puncture wounds and wounds with a significant amount of tissue injury are more likely to promote germination.
- Tetanus is *NOT* transmitted person to person.
- Tetanus occurs more commonly in intravenous substance abusers and following animal bites, deep wounds, and home births.

PATHOGENESIS

C tetani spores germinate and produce tetanospasmin (tetanus toxin) following injury and during anaerobic conditions in the tissue. Tetanospasmin initially binds to peripheral nerve terminals. The toxin is then transported within the axon and across synaptic junctions until it reaches the CNS. Once in the CNS, it binds to gangliosides at the presynaptic inhibitory motor nerve endings and is taken up into the axon. The toxin blocks the release of inhibitory neurotransmitters (i.e., glycine and gamma-aminobutyric acid [GABA]) into the synaptic cleft, which is required to inhibit the nerve impulses following sensory stimulation. Tetanospasmin cleaves a protein component of synaptic vesicles called synaptobrevin II, which aids in release of the inhibitory neurotransmitters into the synaptic cleft. Following sensory stimulation the muscles contract; if no inhibitory neurotransmitters can be released, the muscle will remain in spasm, causing the generalized muscular spasms characteristic of tetanus.

The shortest peripheral nerves are the first to deliver the toxin to the CNS, which leads to the early symptoms of facial distortion and back and neck stiffness. Seizures may occur, and the autonomic nervous system may also be affected.

DIAGNOSIS

There are no laboratory findings characteristic of tetanus. The diagnosis is determined based on clinical presentation of the disease. Early clues to the diagnosis of tetanus include a recent wound, no clear history of tetanus immunization, irritability, restlessness, headache, and low-grade fever.

THERAPY AND PREVENTION

All wounds should be cleansed, and necrotic tissue and foreign material should be removed. If tetanic spasms are occurring, supportive therapy and maintenance of an adequate airway are essential. Treatment should include muscle relaxants (e.g., curare, diazepam), assisted ventilation, and avoiding external stimuli that may trigger spasms (e.g., drafts of cold air, noise, turning on bright lights, attempting to drink).

Immunization is an essential component in treating tetanus. When the wound is dirty and likely to result in germination of *C tetani* spores and the patient has received fewer than three doses of tetanus vaccine, or it has been more than 5 years since the patient's last tetanus booster, the appropriate treatment includes diphtheria toxoid, tetanus toxoid, and acellular pertussis vaccine (DTaP) for a patient younger than age 7 or the Td booster in a patient older than age 7 and tetanus immune globulin (TIG) of human origin, administered distant to the vaccine administration site. A single intramuscular dose of TIG is recommended for children and adults. If the wound is not dirty or

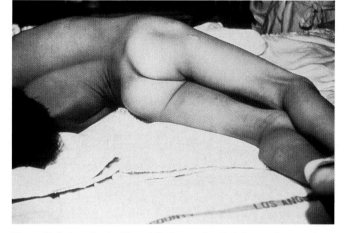

Figure 8-4. A patient with opisthotonos due to tetanus. Image courtesy of the Centers for Disease Control and Prevention.

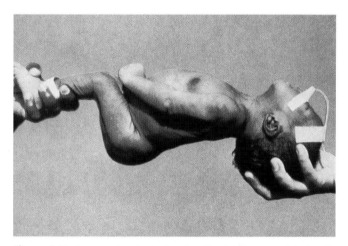

Figure 8-5. A neonate displaying bodily rigidity associated with neonatal tetanus. Image courtesy of the Centers for Disease Control and Prevention.

prone to tetanus but it has been more than 10 years since the patient's last booster, the vaccine without TIG should be administered.

Primary tetanus immunization, in which tetanus toxoid is combined with DTaP, is recommended for all children who are at least 6 weeks of age but younger than the age of 7. The recommended routine primary vaccination schedule is four doses given at 2, 4, 6, and 15–18 months of age.

Adult Td (tetanus and diphtheria toxoids) is the vaccine of choice for routine vaccination of children who are at least 7 years of age. Three doses constitute a primary series of Td. Due to waning antitoxin titers, most individuals have antitoxin levels below optimal levels 10 years after the last dose of tetanus vaccine. As a result, additional booster doses of tetanus and diphtheria toxoids (as Td) are required every 10 years to maintain protective antitoxin titers.

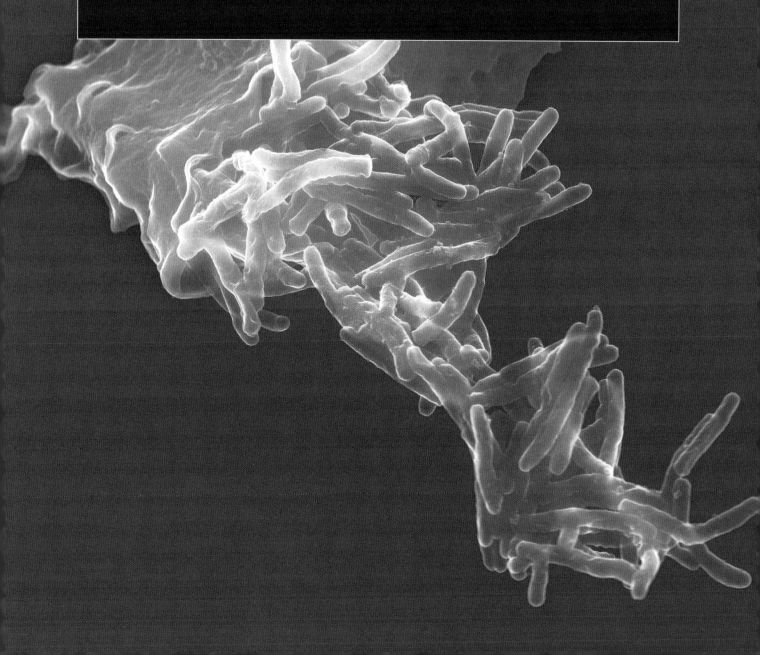

SECTION 3

EYES AND EARS

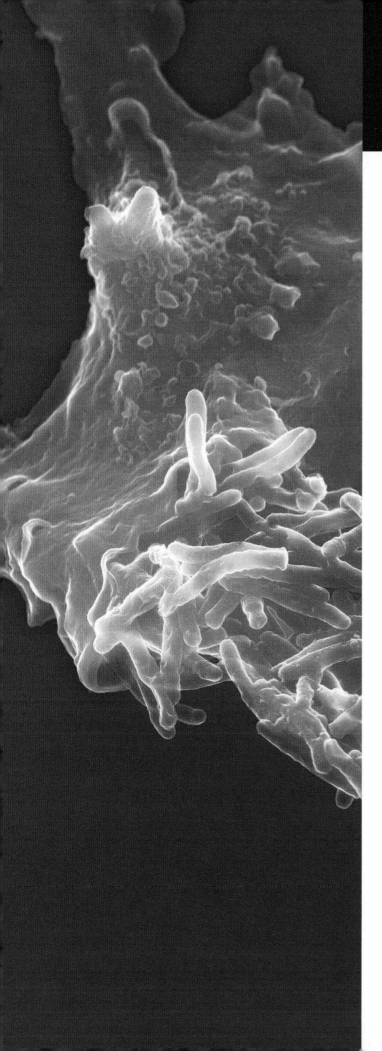

CHAPTER 9

THE BIG PICTURE: INFECTIONS OF THE EYES AND EARS

OVERVIEW OF EYE INFECTIONS

Chapter 10 will discuss common infections of the eyelids, the conjunctiva, and the cornea—specifically hordeola, conjunctivitis, and keratitis; these diseases along with other less common eye infections are also listed in Table 9-1. Figure 9-1 shows the eye and the surrounding structures where infections may occur. Because of highly specialized equipment necessary to diagnose these diseases, most patients with hordeola, conjunctivitis, or keratitis must be referred to an ophthalmologist.

Ocular infections can occur in the external and internal structures of the eye. The external structures of the eye include the eyelids, conjunctiva, sclera, and cornea, and infections of these structures can be quite common.

The major defense mechanisms that protect the external structures of the eye are the eyelids, eye blinking, tears, and the conjunctiva. The eyelids provide protection from trauma and close rapidly when the eye senses objects are nearing the surface of the eye. The eyelids maintain a moist surface of the eyes during sleep. Eye blinking helps to carry tears from the lacrimal gland to the lacrimal duct, and the flow of tears from the lacrimal gland constantly washes the eyes and helps to limit the growth of microorganisms and prevent infection. The tears contain secretory IgA and lysozyme; secretory IgA can bind to certain pathogens and prevent them from binding to the surface of the eye. Lysozyme is able to break down the cell walls of bacteria and kill bacteria that enter the surface of the eye. The conjunctiva contains many lymphocytes, plasma cells, neutrophils, and mast cells, which can respond to an infection of the conjunctiva by producing antibodies and phagocytizing the offending microorganisms. Cytokines are produced by some of these cells and cause inflammation, activate lymphocytes, and allow more white blood cells entry to the site of infection from the capillaries.

Trauma to the external structures of the eye is a common means of infection, and can be caused by organic material in the eye (which can cause fungal and protozoal infections of the cornea). Other sources of infection include improperly cleaned

TABLE 9-1. Diseases of the Eye and the Causative Agents

Area of Eye Affected	Disease	Most Common Infectious Cause(s)
Eyelids and surrounding tissues	Anterior blepharitis	*Staphylococcus aureus* or *S epidermidis*
Eyelids and surrounding tissues	Hordeola	*S aureus*
Eyelids and surrounding tissues	Periorbital cellulitis	Bacteremia: *Streptococcus pneumoniae* Trauma: *S aureus, Streptococcus pyogenes*
Eyelids and surrounding tissues	Orbital cellulitis	*S pneumoniae,* nontypeable *Haemophilus influenzae, Moraxella catarrhalis, S pyogenes, S aureus,* anaerobic bacteria
Lacrimal duct	Dacryocystitis	*S pneumoniae, S aureus, H influenzae, S pyogenes,* and *Pseudomonas aeruginosa*
Conjunctiva	Conjunctivitis	Viral: Adenoviruses Bacterial: *S aureus, S pneumoniae*
Conjunctiva	Ophthalmia neonatorum	*Chlamydia trachomatis,* most common *Neisseria gonorrhoeae,* Herpes simplex viruses
Cornea	Keratitis	Bacterial: *S aureus* Viral: herpes simplex virus 1 and 2

contact lenses, which can cause a serious infection of the cornea, known as keratitis. Eye infections can be caused by sources other than trauma; for example, microorganisms such as *Neisseria gonorrhoeae* cause infections to the external structures of the eye without being initiated by trauma. People who do not produce an adequate supply of tears are more likely to develop eye infections.

The internal structures of the eye include the iris, lens, vitreous humor, and retina. Infections of the internal structures of the eye usually require that the external structures be breached by trauma or an eye ulcer. Microorganisms can enter the bloodstream and carry infections to the internal structures of the eye causing chorioretinitis (e.g., cytomegalovirus). Infections of the internal structures of the eye are rare and are beyond the scope of discussion in this book.

OVERVIEW OF EAR INFECTIONS

Infections of the ear that will be discussed in Chapter 11 include otitis externa (also known as swimmer's ear) and malignant otitis externa, the invasive form of otitis externa, and otitis media. Otitis externa is an infection of the external auditory canal (Figure 9-2), and otitis media is an inflammatory disease of the mucosa of the inner ear (Figure 9-3).

The external auditory canal is protected from infections by the skin that lines the canal and by cerumen. The skin is a difficult environment for microorganisms to grow in because it is quite dry, contains certain antibacterial acids, produces antibacterial sebaceous secretions, and is constantly sloughing off (see

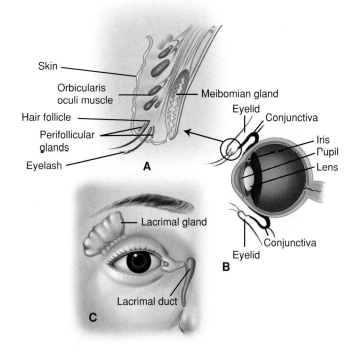

Figure 9-1. The eye and surrounding structures. **A,** Close-up of the meibomian gland, which is clogged in a patient with anterior blepharitis. **B,** Location of the conjunctiva, cornea, and anterior chamber of the eye. **C,** Positions of the lacrimal gland and duct.

Chapter 1). Cells formed in the center of the tympanic membrane migrate outwards from the umbo, a projection on the tympanic membrane where the malleus attaches to the eardrum, to the walls of the ear canal, and then toward the entrance of the ear canal. The cerumen in the canal is carried to the ear canal entrance taking with it microorganisms, dirt, dust, and particulate matter that may have entered the canal. Cerumen is produced in the ear canal and maintains a dry atmosphere that has some antibacterial and antifungal properties to protect the canal from infection.

Excessive amounts of moisture and trauma to the ear canal predispose an individual to otitis externa. People who swim frequently and those who are more likely to have impacted cerumen are more likely to develop otitis externa. Immunocompromised patients are more likely to develop infections of the ear canal that can spread rapidly to contiguous structures; these infections are diagnosed as malignant otitis externa.

Otitis media is an infection of the mucosa of the middle ear. The eustachian tube drains the middle ear and helps to prevent middle ear infections by providing ventilation, protection from infection, and clearance of fluid from the middle ear by mucociliary transport. If the eustachian tube remains open, proper drainage of fluid and ventilation occurs, and usually infections do not occur. However, if the tube is blocked, the middle ear is not ventilated and oxygen is absorbed from the middle ear cavity, producing a negative pressure that draws bacteria from the nasopharynx into the middle ear. If the eustachian tube does not drain fluid from the middle ear, bacteria can colonize, grow, and cause inflammation and more fluid accumulation.

Viral upper respiratory tract infections and allergies commonly cause inflammation and edema around the eustachian tube, causing it to close. Other factors that can affect drainage and ventilation of the middle ear by the eustachian tube include increased flexibility of the tube wall, muscular dysfunction associated with the cleft palate, scarring around the orifice of the tube, and anatomic abnormalities. Because of increased flexibility of the tube wall and the increased incidence of upper respiratory tract infections in children from 6 months to 18 months of age, otitis media is a very common infection in this age group.

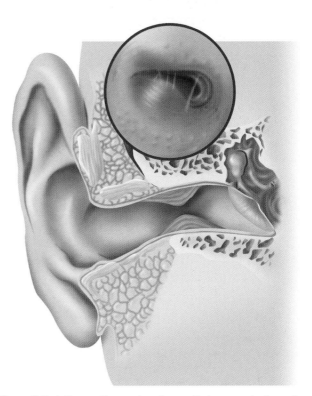

Figure 9-2. Inflammation and erythema that occurs in the external canal in otitis externa infection.

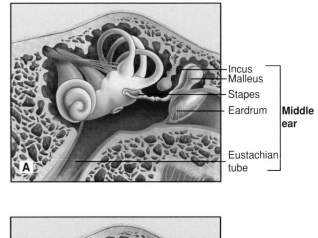

Incus
Malleus
Stapes
Eardrum   **Middle ear**

Eustachian tube

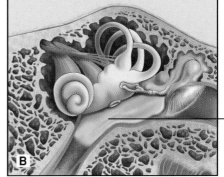

Otitis media

Inflammation and fluid

Figure 9-3. A, Anatomy of the middle ear. **B,** Inflammation and fluid accumulation that occurs in the middle ear in otitis media infection.

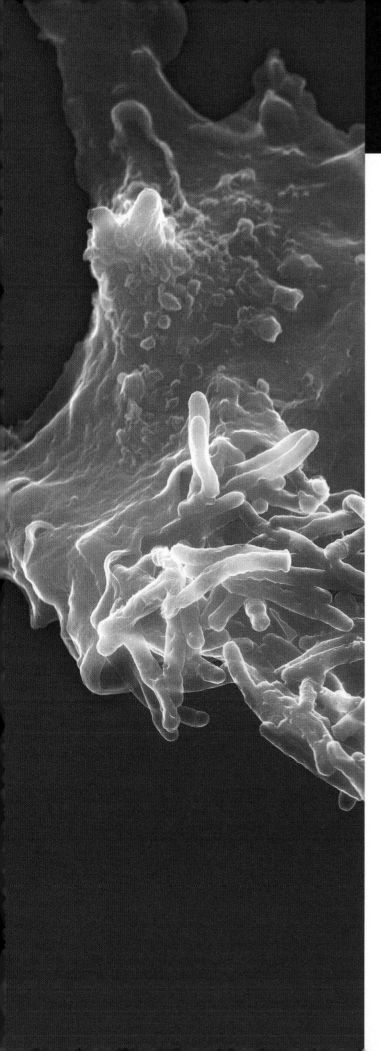

CHAPTER 10

INFECTIONS OF THE EYE

OVERVIEW

Several of the more common diseases of the external structures of the eyes that will be discussed in this chapter are hordeola (eyelid margin), conjunctivitis (conjunctiva), and keratitis (cornea).

HORDEOLA

Hordeola (styes) are relatively common and appear as acute purulent papules that occur at the lid margin.

ETIOLOGY

Staphylococcus aureus causes hordeola in 90–95% of the cases.

MANIFESTATIONS

Patients with hordeola present with an acutely swollen and edematous upper or lower eyelid with normal visual acuity and function. Conjunctivitis and a mucopurulent discharge may be present. The lids are sensitive to palpation, and there may be an associated pustular papule at the lid margin (Figure 10-1).

EPIDEMIOLOGY

- The number of cases of hordeola diagnosed each year is unknown; however, it is a relatively common disease.
- It is more commonly seen in patients in the third to fifth decades of life.

PATHOLOGY

An external hordeolum occurs following blockage and infection of the Zeiss or Moll sebaceous glands. An internal hordeolum occurs following a secondary infection of the meibomian glands in the tarsal plate. Both types of hordeola can occur as a complication of blepharitis (an inflammation of the eyelid margin due to blockage of the meibomian gland). Hordeola can spontaneously resolve, or it can result in a granulomatous inflammation known as a chalazion. Chalazia are more likely to form if the hordeola are not properly treated. If the infection in the hordeolum spreads to neighboring glands or other lid tissue anterior to the tarsal plate, it may lead to periorbital (preseptal) cellulitis.

DIAGNOSIS

Diagnosis of hordeola is usually determined after an examination of the lesion. Many chalazia are misdiagnosed as hordeola. Upon palpitation, hordeola usually are painful; chalazia are not painful.

THERAPY AND PREVENTION

Most hordeola drain spontaneously, especially if warm compresses are applied. If the hordeolum is external, the lesion can be drained by lancing it or by epilating nearby lashes. For internal hordeola, treatment includes application of warm compresses plus oral nafcillin and oxacillin. Good hygiene of the eyelid margin should be practiced to prevent hordeola formation.

CONJUNCTIVITIS

Conjunctivitis is an inflammation of the conjunctiva that results in dilatation of the blood vessels in the membrane. Dilatation then causes the white sclera of the eye to become red. A common name for this disease, pinkeye, is due to this inflammatory blood vessel dilatation.

ETIOLOGY

Many microorganisms and noninfectious entities can cause conjunctivitis. Of the infectious causes of conjunctivitis, bacteria and viruses cause about an equal number of cases of disease (Table 10-1). When conjunctivitis is associated with otitis media, the most common etiologies are bacterial, with 80% of cases caused by *Haemophilus influenzae* (nontypeable) and 20% of cases caused by *Streptococcus pneumoniae*. When a patient experiences conjunctivitis and pharyngitis, the most common etiology is adenovirus.

Viral conjunctivitis

Adenoviruses are the most common viral cause of conjunctivitis and can damage the cornea, resulting in a superficial keratitis. Herpes simplex virus type 1 (HSV-1) and HSV-2 are less common but are usually more serious in that they are more likely to cause keratitis (see below).

Bacterial conjunctivitis (pinkeye)

Staphylococcal and streptococcal species are the most common causes of purulent conjunctivitis. *S aureus, S pneumoniae, H influenzae,* and *Moraxella catarrhalis* all cause a purulent conjunctivitis. *Serratia marcescens, Pseudomonas aeruginosa,* and *Moraxella* species cause a purulent conjunctivitis that is more frequently seen in chronic care facilities (e.g., nursing homes). The bacteria *Neisseria gonorrhoeae* and *N meningitidis* can cause hyperpurulent conjunctivitis, which can infect the cornea causing significant damage. *N gonorrhoeae* is sexually transmitted. It can cause conjunctivitis in newborns (ophthalmia neonatorum), which can spread from the conjunctiva and rapidly infect the cornea. The corneal infection usually results in perforation of the cornea and vision loss (see Epidemiology).

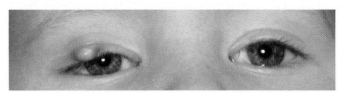

Figure 10-1. Hordeolum (stye) in the upper lid of the patient's right eyelid.

TABLE 10-1. Etiology of Conjunctivitis by Age Group

Etiology	Comment
Neonates (ophthalmia neonatorium)	
Chlamydia trachomatis	Neonate acquires infection following contact with an infected birth canal; **most common in neonates**; may also have pneumonia after conjunctivitis
Neisseria gonorrhoeae	Neonate acquires infection following contact with an infected birth canal; rapid loss of vision if not treated
Infants and children	
Haemophilus influenzae	Patient may also have otitis media
Streptococcus pneumoniae	Patient may also have otitis media
Adenovirus	Patient may also have pharyngitis
Enterovirus	Patient may also have pharyngitis
Adolescents and adults	
Adenovirus	Patient may also have pharyngitis
N gonorrhoeae	Patient may also have urethritis
C trachomatis	Patient may also have urethritis

Chlamydial conjunctivitis

Chlamydia trachomatis (serotypes D and K) causes inclusion conjunctivitis. It is common in sexually active teenagers and young adults, and is the most common cause of neonatal conjunctivitis (chlamydial ophthalmia neonatorum). It can also cause hot tub and swimming pool conjunctivitis (if pools are not chlorinated). *C trachomatis* (serotypes L1, L2, and L3) can cause ocular lymphogranuloma venereum.

MANIFESTATIONS

Inflammation in conjunctivitis causes the blood vessels in the conjunctiva to dilate and the underlying white sclera to appear red (Figure 10-2). The patient may have a sensation of fullness, burning, or of grit or a foreign body in the eye. (*Note:* **A patient with allergic conjunctivitis usually complains of itchy eyes but not burning, gritty, or foreign body sensation.**) Excessive tearing may also occur. A purulent discharge that is more abundant and common in bacterial causes of conjunctivitis may be seen. Dried exudate can "glue" the eyelid shut when the person wakes after an extended period of sleep, and there may be swelling of the eyelids. Vision usually is not impaired, and the cornea and pupil appear normal. Findings that are specific to the etiologic agent causing the conjunctivitis are listed in Table 10-2.

S pneumoniae and *H influenzae* can damage the blood vessels in the conjunctiva, which may result in petechial hemorrhages. Viruses and *Chlamydia* can cause the lymphatic tissue in the

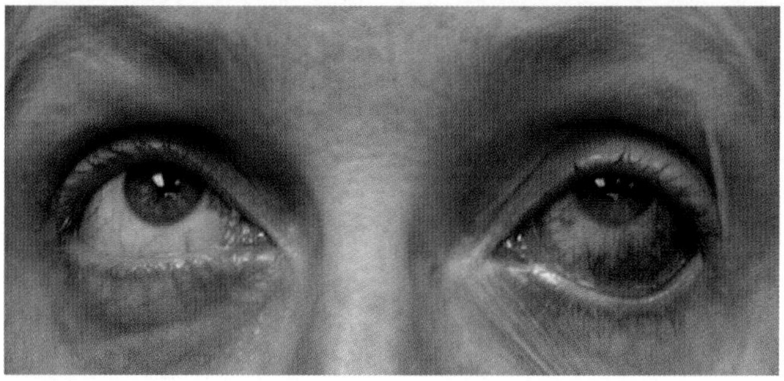

Figure 10-2. A patient with conjunctivitis in the left eye.

TABLE 10-2. Features that Distinguish Bacterial, Viral, and Chlamydial Forms of Conjunctivitis

Feature	Bacterial	Viral	Chlamydial
Conjunctival injection	Moderately severe	Minimal	Absent or minimal
Exudate	Moderate to profuse (polymorphonuclear)	Minimal (usually mononuclear)	Minimal in adults, copious in newborns
Sticking of lids upon awakening	Yes	No	Absent in adults, present in newborns
Papillae (palpebral conjunctiva)	Present	Usually absent	Present in adults, absent in newborns
Follicles (palpebral conjunctiva)	Usually absent	Present	Present in adults, absent in newborns
Preauricular lymphadenopathy	Absent	Present (common in epidemic Keratoconjunctivitis and herpes simplex virus infections)	Occasionally seen in adults, absent in newborns
Response to antibiotic therapy	Yes	No	Yes
Duration of untreated disease without treatment	Up to several weeks	Several weeks	Persistent

conjunctiva to hypertrophy, resulting in follicle formation (follicular conjunctivitis). Viruses and *Chlamydia* are also more likely to cause preauricular lymphadenopathy. Severe photophobia and foreign-body sensation occurs occasionally and is usually caused by an adenovirus (e.g., epidemic keratoconjunctivitis) when associated with keratitis.

Conjunctivitis of the newborn is any conjunctivitis with discharge occurring during the first 28 days of life. Ophthalmia neonatorum was the term used only to describe a hyperacute purulent conjunctivitis, caused by *N gonorrhoeae* in the first 10 days of life (Figure 10-3). Neonates with chlamydial or HSV conjunctivitis are presently also classified as having ophthalmia neonatorum. *C trachomatis* is the most common cause of ophthalmia neonatorum. The second most common is *N gonorrhoeae*, and HSV is a distant third.

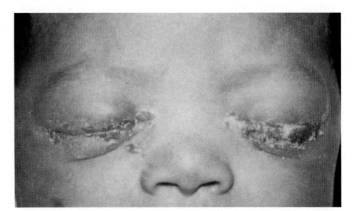

Figure 10-3. A neonate with hyperpurulent conjunctivitis (known as ophthalmia neonatorum) caused by *Neisseria gonorrhoeae*. Image courtesy of the Centers for Disease Control and Prevention, J Pledger.

EPIDEMIOLOGY

- Conjunctivitis is a very common infection and is responsible for approximately 30% of all eye complaints to family physicians. About 3% of all emergency department visits are due to ocular conditions.

- Conjunctivitis can occur at any age.

- The incidence of viral conjunctivitis increases in late fall and early spring.

- Viral conjunctivitis is usually associated with upper respiratory tract infections (e.g., coryza, pharyngitis). Patients usually have a history of a viral syndrome (upper respiratory tract infection), sexually transmitted infection, or fever blister, all of which can aid in diagnosis and in determining the likely cause of the conjunctivitis.

- Nearly all women with chlamydial eye infections have chlamydial infection of the genitalia, and slightly over half of men with chlamydial eye infection also have genitourinary symptoms.

- Conjunctivitis in patients with genitourinary tract infections typically occurs by autoinoculation.

- Three of the most common agents associated with follicular conjunctivitis, preauricular adenopathy, and superficial keratitis are adenovirus, *Chlamydia*, and HSV.

- ***Adenovirus is extremely contagious.*** If an adenovirus infection begins in one eye, it is common for it to rapidly affect the other eye. Sharing pillows, towels, computer keyboards, and anything in contact with infected eye secretions will transmit the infection.

- Transmission of ophthalmia neonatorum from the mother to the neonate occurs as the neonate passes down the infected birth canal.

PATHOGENESIS

Infectious agents adhere to the conjunctiva and overwhelm normal defense mechanisms (e.g., tearing, lysozyme) producing clinical symptoms of redness, discharge, and irritation. Conjunctivitis usually is a self-limited process; however, in immunocompromised patients and in patients with certain infectious agents, conjunctivitis can cause infections of the cornea that can be quite severe and threaten loss of sight.

Ophthalmia neonatorum in the neonate as a result of *N gonorrhoeae* can be invasive and can lead to rapid corneal perforation. **Chlamydial conjunctivitis** can lead to conjunctival scarring, which, if severe enough, may cause lid derangement and ingrown eyelashes. **Chlamydial pneumonia** can occur in infants up to 6 months after symptoms of conjunctivitis resolve.

DIAGNOSIS

Diagnosis of conjunctivitis is usually determined based on the clinical signs and symptoms. Examination of the exudates by Gram stain and culture and scrapings of the follicles are performed if patients do not improve within 48–72 hours despite treatment.

THERAPY AND PREVENTION

Treatment of viral conjunctivitis is usually supportive. Artificial tears help ease eye discomfort; cold compresses improve the swelling and discomfort of the lids; and antibiotic drops help prevent a secondary bacterial infection. Topical corticosteroids should only be prescribed by an ophthalmologist when substantial inflammation is present and HSV infection is excluded.

Treatment with antimicrobials and symptomatic therapy is recommended for patients presenting with simple bacterial conjunctivitis. Many topical antimicrobial agents may be used and include topical sulfacetamide, erythromycin, gentamicin, ciprofloxacin, or ofloxacin.

Gonococcal conjunctivitis may be part of a systemic disease that requires systemic treatment (e.g., norfloxacin, cefoxitin, ceftriaxone, cefotaxime, or spectinomycin). Patients who have chlamydial conjunctivitis should be treated with tetracycline, doxycycline, azithromycin, or erythromycin.

Prophylaxis for gonococcal and chlamydial forms of ophthalmia neonatorum consists of erythromycin or tetracycline ointment applied soon after birth.

INFECTION OF THE CORNEA: KERATITIS

Inflammation of the cornea is referred to as keratitis. Most cases of keratitis also involve the conjunctiva, leading to keratoconjunctivitis. Some of the agents that cause these infections can rapidly perforate the cornea, resulting in loss of sight.

ETIOLOGY

Bacteria are the most common cause of keratitis; however, many different microorganisms can infect the cornea, and clinical manifestations vary depending on the etiologic agent (Table 10-3).

MANIFESTATIONS

Because keratitis and conjunctivitis share several similar symptoms, keratitis can be difficult to correctly diagnose. The primary symptom of keratitis is eye pain. Each time the eyelid moves over the corneal ulcer, the patient experiences pain. Vision is impaired because of the haze in the cornea; photophobia and reflex tearing are also common. Severe inflammation may result in leukocytes collecting in the anterior chamber and settling, by gravity, to the bottom of the chamber, forming a

TABLE 10-3. Forms and Causes of Keratitis

Disease	Organism(s) Causing Disease	Comments
Bacterial keratitis	**Gram-positive cocci** *Staphylococcus aureus, Streptococcus pneumoniae, S epidermidis, S pyogenes, Streptococcus viridans*, enterococci, peptostreptococci	Most common cause of bacterial keratitis is *S aureus* *P aeruginosa* is a very destructive bacteria cause of keratitis, and is more common in hard contact lens wearers; exudate is often green, and the infiltrate is liquid like (e.g., "soupy")
	Gram-positive bacilli *Corynebacterium diphtheriae, Bacillus, Clostridium*	
	Gram-negative bacilli *Pseudomonas aeruginosa, Proteus mirabilis, Klebsiella pneumoniae, Serratia marcescens, Escherichia coli, Aeromonas hydrophila*	Liquid-like infiltrates can also occur in other gram-negative bacilli infections
	Gram-negative cocci or coccobacilli *Neisseria gonorrhoeae, N meningitidis, Moraxella, Pasteurella multocida, Acinetobacter*	*N gonorrhoeae* can also cause rapid destruction of the cornea in the newborn
	Other bacteria *Chlamydia trachomatis*	Ocular lymphogranuloma venereum is an uncommon cause of keratitis due to *C trachomatis* serotypes L1–L3
Viral keratitis	HSV-1, HSV-2, VZV, adenoviruses	HSV-1 and HSV-2 are the most common viral causes of keratitis Zoster (shingles) involving the ophthalmic branch of the trigeminal (CN III) nerve can result keratitis due to VZV Adenoviruses can cause epidemic keratoconjunctivitis which can cause damage to the conjunctiva and the cornea.
Fungal keratitis	Hyphal fungi (e.g., *Aspergillus, Fusarium*), *Candida albicans*	Rarely cause keratitis Fungal keratitis is usually seen following trauma to the cornea by organic material (e.g., tree branch)
Parasitic keratitis	*Acanthamoeba, Hartmannella*	Organisms are protozoan parasites; very rarely cause keratitis Infections occur in contact lens wearers and in persons who swim in stagnant ponds during warm summer months

HSV, herpes simplex virus; VZV, varicella-zoster virus; CN, cranial nerve.

hypopyon. Table 10-4 provides details that may help in differentiating keratitis from conjunctivitis.

Manifestations of bacterial causes of keratitis

▪ **S pneumoniae** produces a well-demarcated ulcer that has sharp margins and a gray base. The remainder of the cornea remains clear; a hypopyon occurs early in the infection.

- **N gonorrhoeae** can rapidly cause perforation of the cornea and is seen in the newborn of a mother infected with this bacterium.

- **P aeruginosa is one of the most destructive of the bacterial causes of keratitis.** Pain is severe, and the corneal ulcer spreads rapidly due to bacterial proteases. A large hypopyon usually forms, and perforation of the cornea is rapid. The exudate is often green, and the infiltrate is liquid ("soupy").

Manifestations of viral causes of keratitis

- **HSV-1 and HSV-2** may reactivate in the ophthalmic division of the trigeminal ganglia, causing a pathognomonic branching dendritic ulcer that stains with fluorescein (Figure 10-4).

- Reactivation of **varicella-zoster virus** from the ophthalmic branch of the trigeminal nerve (cranial nerve V) can result in shingles of the face and can infect the cornea. The clinical picture includes nondescript facial pain, fever, and general malaise. About 4 days after onset, a vesicular skin rash appears along the distribution of the trigeminal nerve. The vesicles will discharge fluid and begin to scab over within 1 week. Ocular involvement may include follicular conjunctivitis, epithelial and interstitial keratitis, uveitis, optic neuropathy, and even neurogenic motility disorders, especially fourth cranial nerve palsy (trochlear nerve palsy), which can cause vertical diplopia and the inability to look downward and inward. Vesicles at the tip of the nose (known as the Hutchinson sign) indicate a 75% likelihood of ocular sequelae. Corneal involvement may occur in varicella (chickenpox), but it is uncommon and usually benign.

- Epidemic keratoconjunctivitis due to adenoviruses is a form of viral conjunctivitis that presents as a bilateral, palpebral, follicular conjunctivitis with keratitis. Subepithelial corneal infiltrates are common and are typically concentrated in the central cornea.

Manifestations of fungal causes of keratitis

- Precipitating events of fungal keratitis are trauma with contamination by organic matter and the chronic use of glucocorticosteroid eye drops.

- Hypopyon is common. Ulcers are superficial and raised above the corneal surface.

- Slit-lamp examination reveals that the infiltrate tends to be irregular with an immune ring. Smaller satellite lesions may surround the main infiltrate.

EPIDEMIOLOGY

- Infection of the cornea is usually a bacterial infection; however, infection with HSV is quite common.

- Keratitis is much less common than conjunctivitis; without adequate treatment, however, it can cause significant damage to the cornea and loss of sight in the affected eye.

- Usually there is a small break in the corneal epithelium that allows entry of the microorganisms. Predisposition to keratitis may be due to trauma to the eye, abrasions from contact lenses, ocular surgery, and defective tear production.

TABLE 10-4. Features that Differentiate Conjunctivitis from Keratitis

Clinical Signs and Symptoms	Conjunctivitis	Keratitis
Vision	Normal	May be reduced
Pain	Gritty irritation	True pain
Conjunctiva	Diffuse injection	Ciliary flush
Exudate	Minimal to profuse	Usually none
Dried matter on lids	May be present	Absent
Photophobia	Absent	Present
Lacrimation	Usually absent	Present
Pupillary diameter	Normal	Usually small

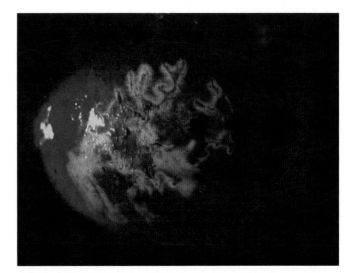

Figure 10-4. The eye of a patient with keratitis caused by a herpes simplex virus (HSV). Fluorescein dye has been placed on the affected eye. Notice the pathognomonic dendritic pattern of the ulcer caused by HSV. Image courtesy of the Edward S Harkness Eye Institute, College of Physicians and Surgeons, Columbia University, New York, NY.

- Immunosuppressed and diabetic patients are at increased risk of keratitis.

- Contact lens wearers who use tap water to clean their lenses are more likely to be diagnosed with parasitic and *P aeruginosa* keratitis. *P aeruginosa* keratitis is seen more commonly in hard contact lens wearers.

- Chronic use of glucocorticosteroid eye drops or eye injuries from organic material (e.g., a tree branch) are more likely to cause fungal keratitis.

PATHOGENESIS

Usually an injury to the corneal epithelium allows entry of a microorganism on the surface of the cornea and causes keratitis. When microorganisms gain access to the cornea, the rapidity and the extent of damage depends on the ability of the organism to produce various toxins and proteases. An inflammatory reaction to the infection results in leukocytes invading the anterior chamber of the eye, and in many cases a hypopyon will form. Some organisms, including *N gonorrhoeae*, *N meningitidis*, *Corynebacterium diphtheriae*, *Listeria*, and *Shigella* species, can gain entry to the cornea without prior trauma to the epithelium.

DIAGNOSIS

Oftentimes a patient who has conjunctivitis will also have keratitis. Keratitis can occur following conjunctivitis and, as a result, it is essential that the physician is able to recognize the differences in the symptoms associated with conjunctivitis and keratitis (see Table 10-4). Slit-lamp examination is useful in identifying potential causes of keratitis.

Bacterial keratitis without treatment can rapidly cause perforation of the cornea, causing loss of eyesight. Therefore, corneal scrapings should be sent for cultures as well as Gram stains. Corneal perforation can occur quickly in infections caused by *P aeruginosa*, and a green exudate may be present. A Wood lamp may be useful, since the ulcer associated with *P aeruginosa* fluoresces in ultraviolet light.

Viral keratitis can usually be diagnosed on clinical grounds and does not require culturing of corneal scrapings. A distinct dendritic lesion that fluoresces following topical administration of fluorescein is enough evidence to determine that HSV-1 or HSV-2 is the cause of the keratitis (Figure 10-4). Corneal scrapings from patients with **parasitic keratitis** when stained with calcofluor white will show cysts with fluorescent microscopy.

THERAPY AND PREVENTION

Treatment of bacterial keratitis must be rapid and aggressive.
Patients are usually hospitalized and watched closely for signs of further damage to the cornea (e.g., perforation, visual loss, and significant ulceration). Antibiotic therapy for most patients can be started based on the results of the Gram stain. Antibiotics are usually given topically; however if perforation is imminent, systemic therapy in addition to topical therapy should be instituted (Table 10-5). Prophylaxis against the gonococcal and chlamydial forms of ophthalmia neonatorum consists of erythromycin or tetracycline ointment, which should be applied shortly after birth.

TABLE 10-5. Antimicrobial Agents Used in the Treatment of Keratitis

Etiologic Agent	Antimicrobial Agent
Streptococcus pneumoniae	Bacitracin and gentamicin
Staphylococcus aureus (other gram-positive cocci)	Cephalosporin and bacitracin
Pseudomonas aeruginosa	Tobramycin or gentamicin
Other gram-negative bacilli *Escherichia coli*, *Klebsiella*, *Proteus*	Gentamicin
Chlamydia trachomatis	Doxycycline (erythromycin for neonates and infants)
Herpes simplex virus	Trifluridine or acyclovir (oral acyclovir given for several months after initial treatment can prevent recurrence)
Adenovirus	Cidofovir topical
Varicella-zoster virus	Famciclovir, valacyclovir, or acyclovir
Candida albicans	Amphotericin B and flucytosine
Hyphal fungi	Natamycin
Acanthamoeba	Neomycin and pentamidine isethionate

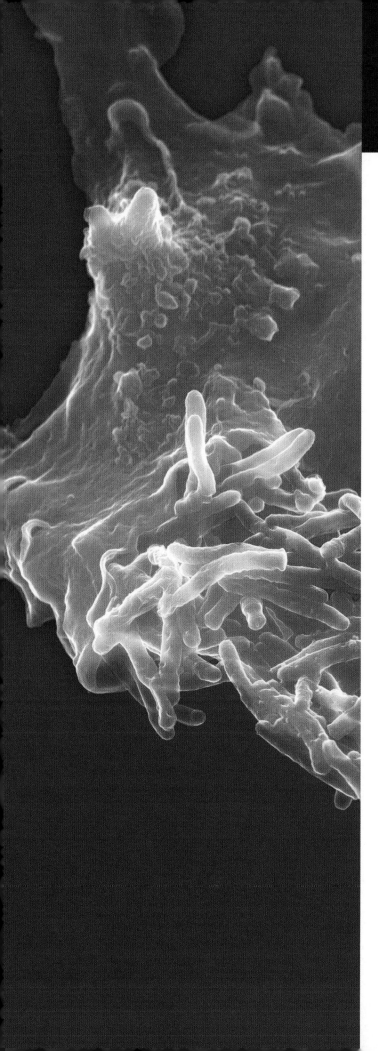

CHAPTER 11

INFECTIONS OF THE EAR

OVERVIEW

Two different ear infections that will be discussed in this chapter are otitis eternal and otitis media. Bacteria are the most common cause of infection in both of these diseases.

OTITIS EXTERNA

Otitis externa, or swimmer's ear, is an infection of the external auditory canal (Figure 11-1). Most cases occur because water is trapped in the external auditory canal, causing swimmer's ear. If the patient has diabetes mellitus or is immunocompromised in other ways, malignant otitis externa can occur.

ETIOLOGY

Gram-negative bacilli are the most common causes of otitis externa. *Pseudomonas aeruginosa* is the major pathogen associated with this disease and the most common cause of swimmer's ear and malignant otitis externa. Although *Staphylococcus aureus* is not as common a cause as gram-negative bacilli, it does cause otitis externa.

MANIFESTATIONS

A patient diagnosed with **otitis externa** may complain of ear pain, itching, and discharge. The pinna is usually tender, and the pain can be exacerbated by movement of the ear such as occurs when chewing. Other physical findings include redness and swelling of the external canal (see Figure 11-1). A fever may be present, but it is usually lower than 38.3°C.

In **malignant otitis externa,** a necrotizing infection can spread to the cartilage, blood vessels, and bone. The infection can involve the base of the skull, the meninges, or the brain, and can result in death. Cranial nerves VII, IX, X, and XII (i.e., facial, glossopharyngeal, vagus, and hypoglossal nerves, respectively) can also be involved. Malignant otitis externa should be suspected if the patient's temperature is higher than 38.3°C, if the initial pain is severe, or if regional lymphadenopathy of the preauricular, anterior, or posterior cervical chains is present.

EPIDEMIOLOGY

▨ Otitis externa occurs in 4 of every 1000 persons each year.

▨ It is most common in swimmers and divers who frequently get water trapped in the external canal.

▨ A combination of high humidity and perspiration can cause environmental moisture levels to increase, resulting in otitis externa.

▨ Other predisposing factors include high environmental temperatures, mechanical removal of cerumen, trauma following insertion of foreign objects (e.g., cotton swabs, fingernails, hearing aids, and ear plugs), and chronic dermatologic disease (e.g., eczema, psoriasis, seborrheic dermatitis, acne).

▨ Malignant otitis externa is more common in diabetic and immunocompromised patients.

PATHOGENESIS

The external auditory canal is the only skin-lined cul-de-sac in the human body. It is warm and dark and traps moisture readily, and is an excellent environment for the growth of bacteria and fungi. The skin in the canal is thin; the lateral third of the canal lies on top of cartilage, and the remainder of the canal has a base of bone. As a result, the skin lining the canal is easily traumatized. The elimination of debris, secretions, and foreign bodies is impeded by a curve at the junction of the cartilage and bone. The presence of hair, especially the thicker hair common in the ears of older men, can also prevent elimination of water and debris from the canal.

Cerumen (earwax produced in the ear canal) creates an acidic coat containing lysozymes and other substances that inhibit bacterial and fungal growth. The cerumen is also rich in lipids, which prevents water from penetrating to the skin and causing maceration. If too little cerumen is present, a person may be more susceptible to infections in the ear canal. Cerumen production that is excessive or overly viscous can lead to obstruction, retention of water and debris, and infection. The external ear canal is protected by epithelial migration that occurs from the tympanic membrane outward, carrying debris with it.

When the innate defenses in the canal fail or when the epithelium of the external auditory canal is damaged, otitis externa can occur. There are many factors that cause a person to be susceptible to development of otitis externa; however, the most common cause is **excessive moisture in the ear canal** that raises the pH and removes the cerumen. Once the protective cerumen is removed, keratin debris from sloughed off keratinized epithelial cells in the ear canal absorbs the water, creating a desirable medium for bacterial growth. Bacterial growth can cause inflammation, causing the infection to spread and damage the underlying cartilage or bone.

DIAGNOSIS

The diagnosis of otitis externa is usually determined based on clinical presentation and by direct inspection of the ear canal with an otoscope. Visualization and inspection of the tympanic membrane is essential to rule out otitis media. In some cases, the composition of the discharge can be helpful in determining

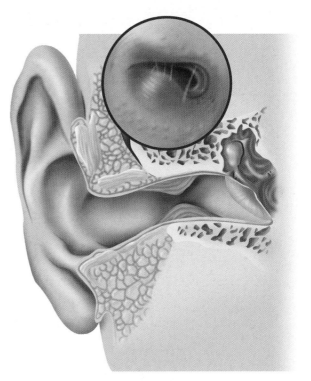

Figure 11-1. A schematic showing the inflammation and erythema that occurs in the external canal in otitis externa infection.

the etiologic agent involved. If the disease is an acute bacterial infection, the discharge may be thick white mucus. If the disease is a chronic bacterial infection, a bloody discharge containing granulation tissue is more common. Patients with malignant otitis externa frequently have a discharge (otorrhea) that contains foul-smelling yellow to yellow-green pus.

THERAPY AND PREVENTION

When treating patients with **bacterial otitis externa** (swimmer's ear), the ear canal should be cleansed and debris removed. Topical application of antimicrobial agents, including 2% acetic acid, ofloxacin, or neomycin with polymyxin B (or neomycin with hydrocortisone or with selenium sulfate) is usually effective in uncomplicated cases.

Systemic antibiotic therapy with imipenem is essential in the treatment of malignant otitis externa. Wound debridement is necessary. Swimmer's ear and malignant otitis externa can be prevented by avoiding behaviors that increase the moisture in the external auditory canal that result in trauma to the skin that lines the ear canal.

OTITIS MEDIA

Otitis media is an inflammatory disease of the mucosa of the inner ear with exudate production (Figure 11-2). Transient loss of hearing in children can result in delayed development of language and speech.

ETIOLOGY

Streptococcus pneumoniae, nontypeable *Haemophilus influenzae*, and *Moraxella catarrhalis* are the most common causes of otitis media. Other etiologic agents include *S aureus* and *Streptococcus pyogenes*. In children younger than 6 weeks of age, gram-negative bacilli (e.g., *Escherichia coli*, *Klebsiella*, *Pseudomonas*) commonly cause otitis media.

MANIFESTATIONS

The onset of acute bacterial otitis media is usually abrupt and produces pain in the ears and a feeling of fullness and fever. A patient also may experience vertigo, nystagmus, and tinnitus. There is no regional lymphadenopathy. Generally, there are no other symptoms except those of the viral respiratory infection or the allergic reaction that preceded the middle ear infection. In infants, the major manifestations of acute bacterial otitis media may be fever, ear pain, irritability, vomiting, and diarrhea.

EPIDEMIOLOGY

▪ Otitis media is common; 50% of children experience an episode before 12 months of age and 80% of children experience an episode by the age of 3.

▪ The infection can occur at any age, but it is most common in children aged 6 months to 3 years of age.

▪ Acute otitis media is the single most frequent diagnosis in febrile children. Boys are affected more often than girls.

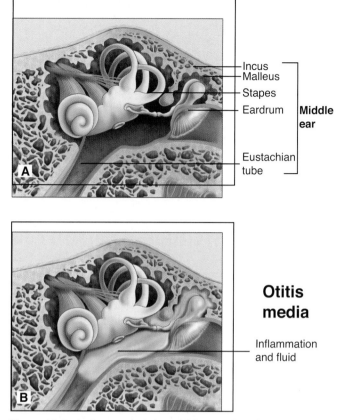

Figure 11-2. A, Anatomy of the middle ear. **B,** Inflammation and fluid accumulation that occurs in the middle ear during an episode of otitis media.

- Otitis media occurs more frequently in racial groups such as Inuits and Native Americans.

- Infants and children with purulent conjunctivitis, rhinitis, and sinusitis should be examined to determine if they have otitis media.

- Persons with antibody, complement, or phagocytic cell deficiencies are more likely to have recurrent otitis media.

- Cleft palate, attendance at a day-care facility, bottle-feeding, bottle-propping, secondhand smoke, and a family history of middle-ear disease all increase the likelihood of otitis media.

PATHOGENESIS

Children are more likely than adults to be diagnosed with otitis media because children have more flexible, shorter, and more horizontal eustachian tubes that are more susceptible to obstruction. Normally, the mucosa absorbs air in the middle ear. If the eustachian tube is partially or completely blocked, the continued mucosal absorption of air will cause negative pressure in the middle ear, which then produces a serous effusion that accumulates in the inner ear. If the obstruction of the eustachian tube resolves before the serous fluid becomes infected, fluid will drain from the inner ear without the need for treatment. However, if the serous effusion is infected by nasopharyngeal organisms carried into the inner ear by the negative pressure, an acute bacterial otitis media can develop. The neutrophils of the acute inflammatory response migrate into the cavity causing purulent serous fluid.

Children who develop otitis media usually have a preceding viral upper respiratory tract infection (e.g., respiratory syncytial virus or rhinovirus) followed within 5–10 days by abrupt onset of an acute bacterial middle ear infection. The acute inflammatory response to the initiating viral infection or to an allergic reaction causes the thin cuboidal lining of the middle ear cavity to swell, increasing the thickness of the lining to two to three times its normal size. When the orifice of the eustachian tube swells, the lumen becomes occluded and exudate accumulates. As more exudate accumulates, pressure in the inner ear increases causing the tympanic membrane to bulge outward. The pressure may also force purulent exudate into pneumatized portions of the petrous bone. The increased pressure can cause the tympanic membrane to rupture.

DIAGNOSIS

Distinguishing between acute otitis media and the more common otitis media with effusion is important, because the former may require antibiotic treatment and the latter does not. In both situations, fluid accumulates in the middle ear but *only in acute otitis media is the fluid infected.* Middle ear effusion is definitive for a diagnosis of otitis media when the patient also has ear pain, fever, vomiting, and diarrhea.

Bulging of the tympanic membrane is the highest predictive value when evaluating the presence of middle ear effusions (Figure 11-3). Other findings that indicate the presence of middle ear effusions include limited mobility of the tympanic membrane using pneumatic otoscopy and visualizing fluid behind the tympanic membrane or in the ear canal (with perforation).

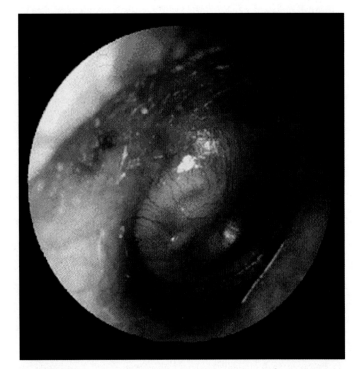

Figure 11-3. An image of the tympanic membrane of a patient with acute otitis media. Note the bulging tympanic membrane, the erythematous tympanic membrane, and the purulent effusion in the middle ear.

THERAPY AND PREVENTION

Most cases of otitis media resolve without antibiotic treatment. Afebrile patients older than 2 years of age who have no ear pain and no perforation of the tympanic membrane should be prescribed an analgesic (e.g., acetaminophen, ibuprofen) for symptomatic relief and should be observed. If the patient remains symptomatic by day 3, antibiotic therapy with amoxicillin should be started. If the patient does not meet the criteria for symptomatic treatment and observation, antibiotic treatment with amoxicillin should be given immediately.

Amoxicillin will not eliminate the infection when β-lactamase–producing organisms such as *H influenzae* and *M catarrhalis* are present. If the patient does not respond to amoxicillin treatment after 3 days, switch to amoxicillin-clavulanate or a third-generation cephalosporin (e.g., cefdinir). Patients allergic to β-lactam antibiotics such as amoxicillin can be treated with trimethoprim-sulfamethoxazole. Recurrences of episodes of otitis media can be reduced in patients with chronic or recurrent otitis media by the insertion of tympanostomy tubes.

Administering vaccines to children appears to prevent many episodes of otitis media. **Pneumovax** is used to vaccinate children older than 2 years of age. Each dose of the multivalent vaccine contains 23 types of capsular polysaccharide and immunizes the child against most strains of *S pneumoniae* that cause otitis media. However, Pneumovax is not effective in immunizing children younger than 2 years of age.

Prevnar is used to vaccinate children younger than 2 years of age. Each dose of Prevnar contains seven types of the *S pneumoniae* capsular polysaccharide conjugated to a nontoxic diphtheria toxoid. The *H influenzae* type b (Hib) vaccine is used to immunize children younger than 2 years of age and contains the capsule polysaccharide from serotype b organisms conjugated to a carrier protein.

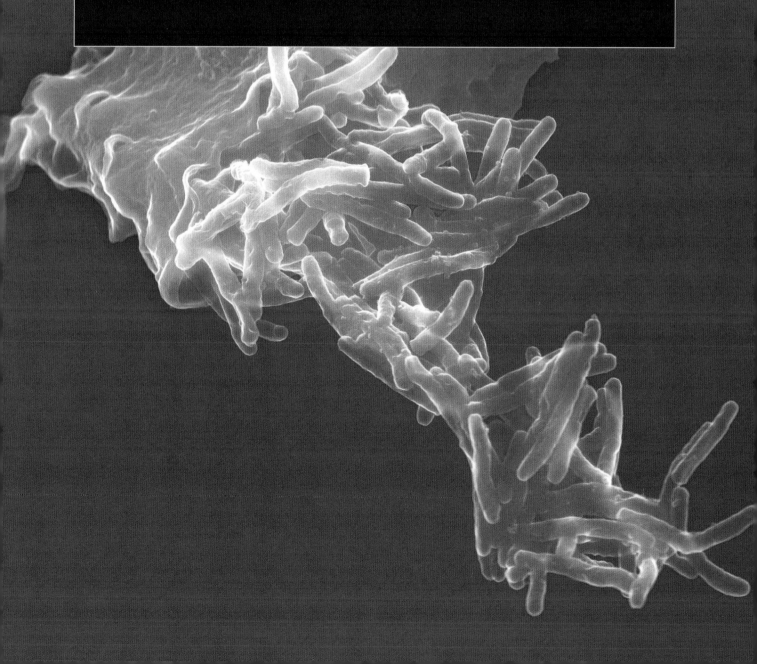

SECTION 4

RESPIRATORY TRACT

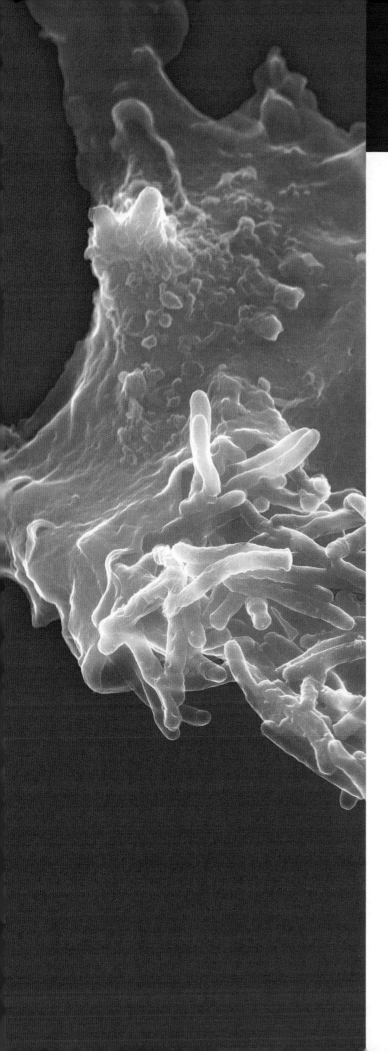

CHAPTER 12

THE BIG PICTURE: INFECTIONS OF THE RESPIRATORY TRACT

OVERVIEW

The discussion of the respiratory tract is divided into three different sections in this book: upper respiratory tract infections (Chapter 13), respiratory airway infections (Chapter 14), and lower respiratory tract infections (Chapter 15).

The respiratory tract is the most common site of infection by pathogens. Each year, children acquire between two and five upper respiratory tract infections and adults acquire one or two infections. The respiratory tract is a frequent site of infection because it comes in direct contact with the physical environment and is exposed to airborne microorganisms. A wide range of organisms can infect the respiratory tract, including viruses, bacteria, fungi, and parasites (Figure 12-1; Table 12-1).

The anatomy of the upper respiratory tract is composed of many features that help to rid the system of particles and pathogens. The nasal cavity has a mucociliary lining similar to that of the lower respiratory tract. The inside of the nose is lined with hairs, which act to filter larger particles that are inhaled. The turbinate bones ("baffle plates") are covered with mucus that collects particles not filtered by nasal hairs. Usually, particles 5–10 μm in diameter are either trapped by nasal hairs or impinge on the nasal mucosal surfaces.

After inhaled air moves through the nasal passages, the anatomy of the upper airway changes direction and causes many of the larger airborne particles to impinge on the back of the throat. The adenoids and tonsils are lymphoid organs in the upper respiratory tract that are important in developing an immune response to pathogens. Adenoids and tonsils are located in an area where many of these airborne particles are in contact with the mucosal surface.

A layer of mucus and ciliated cells covers the lower portion of the respiratory tract. Both single and subepithelial cells secrete mucus. Respiratory pathogens that reach the lower respiratory tract are trapped in the mucous layer and are driven upwards by ciliary action (the mucociliary elevator) to the back of the throat. The sneeze and cough reflexes are important

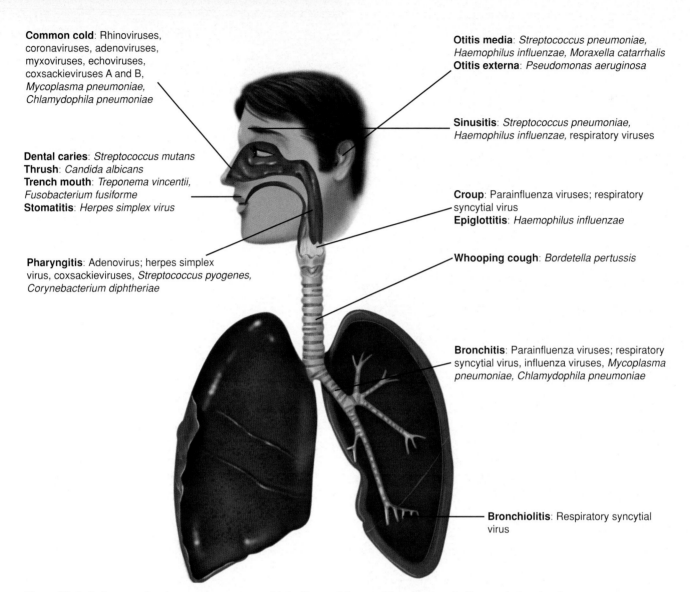

Common cold: Rhinoviruses, coronaviruses, adenoviruses, myxoviruses, echoviruses, coxsackieviruses A and B, *Mycoplasma pneumoniae*, *Chlamydophila pneumoniae*

Dental caries: *Streptococcus mutans*
Thrush: *Candida albicans*
Trench mouth: *Treponema vincentii*, *Fusobacterium fusiforme*
Stomatitis: *Herpes simplex virus*

Pharyngitis: Adenovirus; herpes simplex virus, coxsackieviruses, *Streptococcus pyogenes*, *Corynebacterium diphtheriae*

Otitis media: *Streptococcus pneumoniae*, *Haemophilus influenzae*, *Moraxella catarrhalis*
Otitis externa: *Pseudomonas aeruginosa*

Sinusitis: *Streptococcus pneumoniae*, *Haemophilus influenzae*, respiratory viruses

Croup: Parainfluenza viruses; respiratory syncytial virus
Epiglottitis: *Haemophilus influenzae*

Whooping cough: *Bordetella pertussis*

Bronchitis: Parainfluenza viruses; respiratory syncytial virus, influenza viruses, *Mycoplasma pneumoniae*, *Chlamydophila pneumoniae*

Bronchiolitis: Respiratory syncytial virus

Figure 12-1. A diagram showing common causes of infection and the resulting diseases in the respiratory tract.

mechanisms for clearing material that accumulates in or irritates the respiratory tract.

Most of the surfaces of the upper respiratory tract (including nasal and oral passages, nasopharynx, and oropharynx) are colonized by normal flora, which are regular inhabitants and rarely cause disease (Figure 12-2). The normal flora of the upper respiratory tract has two main functions that are important in maintaining the healthy state of the host: (1) These organisms compete with pathogenic organisms for potential attachment sites; and (2) they can produce substances that are bactericidal and prevent infection by pathogens.

There are no resident bacteria in the lower respiratory tract. Organisms that manage to enter the alveoli are usually eliminated by alveolar macrophages. **Alveolar macrophages are considered the most important means of eliminating the organisms when they enter the lungs.** Most bacteria (e.g., *Streptococcus pneumoniae*, *Klebsiella pneumoniae*, *Haemophilus influenzae*) that cause lung infections (e.g., pneumonia) produce a capsule that can prevent phagocytosis by the alveolar macrophage.

TABLE 12-1. Common Causes of Various Respiratory Diseases by Location

Disease Location	Disease	Group of Pathogen	Comments
Upper respiratory tract			
Nasal passages	Common cold	Viruses	Most common cause rhinovirus
Nasal sinuses	Rhinosinusitis	Viruses Bacteria	Viruses are most common cause of rhinosinusitis
Pharynx	Pharyngitis	Viruses, *Streptococcus pyogenes* and *Corynebacterium diphtheriae*	Viruses cause 90% of these infections
Respiratory airways			
Epiglottis	Epiglottitis	Bacteria	Usually *Haemophilus influenzae* type b
Trachea and bronchi	Bronchitis, tracheobronchitis, croup, laryngitis	Viruses	Usually caused by viruses
Bronchioles	Bronchiolitis	Viruses	Most common cause is respiratory syncytial virus
Lower respiratory tract			
Alveoli and alveolar sacs	Pneumonia	Bacteria	Most common cause in adults is *Streptococcus pneumoniae*

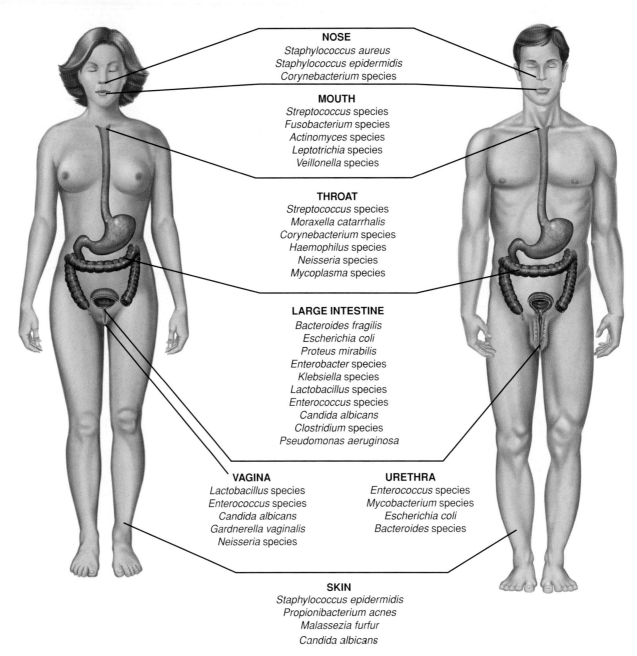

NOSE
Staphylococcus aureus
Staphylococcus epidermidis
Corynebacterium species

MOUTH
Streptococcus species
Fusobacterium species
Actinomyces species
Leptotrichia species
Veillonella species

THROAT
Streptococcus species
Moraxella catarrhalis
Corynebacterium species
Haemophilus species
Neisseria species
Mycoplasma species

LARGE INTESTINE
Bacteroides fragilis
Escherichia coli
Proteus mirabilis
Enterobacter species
Klebsiella species
Lactobacillus species
Enterococcus species
Candida albicans
Clostridium species
Pseudomonas aeruginosa

VAGINA
Lactobacillus species
Enterococcus species
Candida albicans
Gardnerella vaginalis
Neisseria species

URETHRA
Enterococcus species
Mycobacterium species
Escherichia coli
Bacteroides species

SKIN
Staphylococcus epidermidis
Propionibacterium acnes
Malassezia furfur
Candida albicans

Figure 12-2. Normal flora resident on the human body.

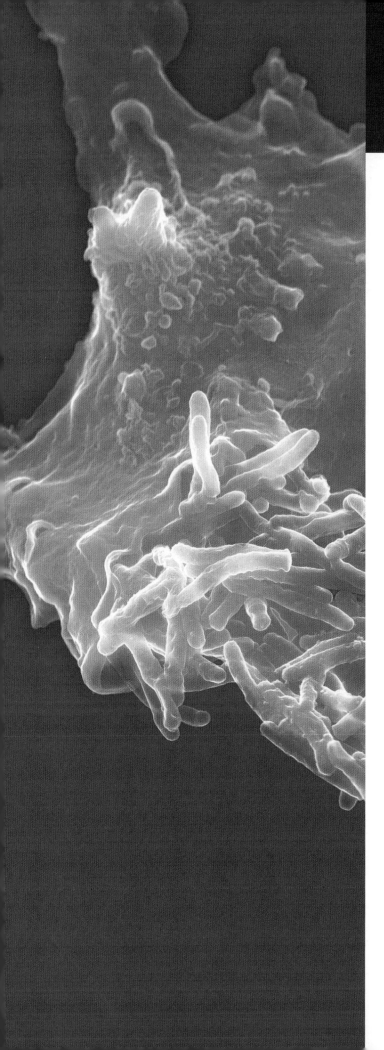

CHAPTER 13

INFECTIONS OF THE UPPER RESPIRATORY TRACT

OVERVIEW

This chapter will discuss infections of the upper respiratory tract, including infections of the nasal passages, paranasal sinuses, and the pharynx, and the organisms that cause these infections (Figure 13-1). The diseases that are discussed in this chapter are the common cold, rhinosinusitis, pharyngitis, and diphtheria. With the exception of diphtheria, viruses are the most common cause of all of these diseases.

COMMON COLD

The common cold is caused by a multitude of organisms; about 90% of cases are due to viruses.

ETIOLOGY

Most cases of the common cold are caused by rhinoviruses; there are at least 100 immunologically distinct rhinoviruses. Other causes of the common cold are listed in Table 13-1.

MANIFESTATIONS

Initially, the common cold begins with nasal stuffiness, sneezing, and headache. Rhinorrhea then occurs with increasing severity. General malaise, lacrimation, sore throat, slight fever, and anorexia are common in moderate to severe cases. If organisms enter the trachea and bronchi, a tracheobronchitis develops and there may be a cough and a feeling of substernal discomfort.

EPIDEMIOLOGY

- The common cold is worldwide in distribution.
- A child younger than 5 years of age will develop five to seven colds per year, and an adult will develop one or two.
- The common cold is seen mostly in winter months because more person-to-person contact occurs during this time of year.

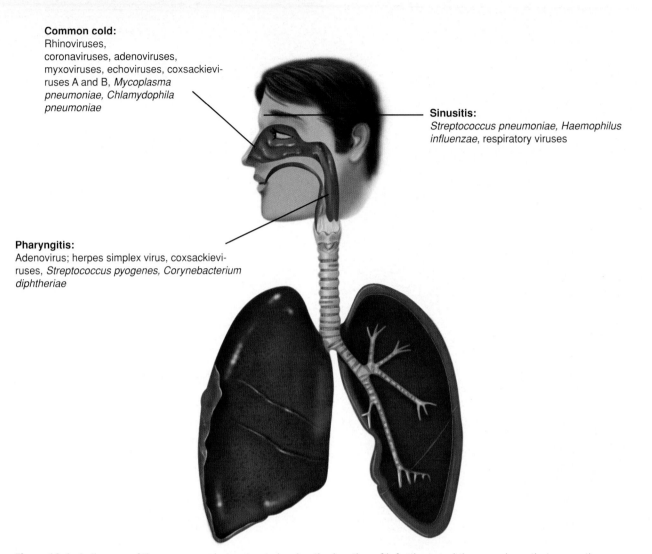

Common cold:
Rhinoviruses,
coronaviruses, adenoviruses,
myxoviruses, echoviruses, coxsackieviruses A and B, *Mycoplasma
pneumoniae, Chlamydophila
pneumoniae*

Sinusitis:
*Streptococcus pneumoniae, Haemophilus
influenzae,* respiratory viruses

Pharyngitis:
Adenovirus; herpes simplex virus, coxsackieviruses, *Streptococcus pyogenes, Corynebacterium
diphtheriae*

Figure 13-1. A diagram of the upper respiratory tract showing the location of infections and the organisms that cause them, as discussed in the chapter.

Viruses are spread person to person, usually during hand-to-hand contact (e.g., shaking hands).

PATHOGENESIS

The rhinovirus infects the nasal passages following direct contact of contaminated surfaces or via inhalation of infectious droplets. It then infects the cells lining the nasal passages and the pharynx following attachment to intercellular adhesion molecule-1 on the host cells. Inflammatory changes occur with hyperemia, edema, and leukocyte inflammation. The ciliated columnar epithelial cells are destroyed and slough off.

The pathology reaches its peak by days 2 to 5. Regeneration of the cells begins rapidly, with new cells formed by about day 14. The acute phase of the illness begins with a runny nose, when copious amounts of clear, mucoid nasal secretions are produced. After 1 to 2 days, a secondary bacterial infection by the normal flora causes the secretions to become mucopurulent. If severe, blockage of the sinus ostia or the eustachian tubes occurs, paranasal sinusitis or otitis media results. Complications are usually related to the infection extending to the lower respiratory tract and resulting in bronchitis.

DIAGNOSIS

Diagnosis of the common cold is dependent on the patient's symptoms, localization of the disease process, time of year, and afebrile course. Laboratory culture of the viruses and serologic testing is rarely performed.

THERAPY AND PREVENTION

Treatment of the common cold involves supportive therapy to ease the patient's discomfort, including zinc acetate lozenges and nasal gel containing zinc gluconate. Large doses of vitamin C may shorten the duration of the illness and decrease the severity of symptoms of the common cold. Handwashing and disinfecting contaminated objects can help to avoid acquiring the common cold as well as avoiding contact with others during the cold season.

ACUTE RHINOSINUSITIS

Acute rhinosinusitis is defined as inflammation or infection of the mucosa of the nasal passages and at least one of the paranasal sinuses and lasts no longer than 4 weeks. Rhinosinusitis occurs in about 32 million people each year in the United States. Rhinitis and sinusitis usually coexist and, therefore, the medical terminology has now changed from the term sinusitis to rhinosinusitis.

ETIOLOGY

Most cases of acute rhinosinusitis are due to respiratory viruses, which include rhinovirus, parainfluenza virus, respiratory syncytial virus, and adenovirus. However, acute rhinosinusitis can occasionally be complicated by a bacterial infection and is diagnosed as acute bacterial rhinosinusitis. The two most common causes of **community-acquired acute bacterial rhinosinusitis** are *Streptococcus pneumoniae* and nontypeable *Haemophilus influenzae*. The bacteria listed in Table 13-2 cause over 70% of the infections of the paranasal sinuses. Immunocompromised

TABLE 13-1. Some Infectious Agents that Cause the Common Cold

Agents*	Human Serotypes
Myxoviruses	
Influenza	A, B, C
Parainfluenza	1, 2, 3, 4
Respiratory syncytial virus	1 (possibly 2)
Human metapneumovirus	1 (possibly more)
Coronaviruses	1
Picornaviruses	
Rhinoviruses (*most common cause*)	>100 types
Coxsackievirus A	24
Coxsackievirus B	6
Echoviruses	31 (only types 11, 20, and 25 may cause respiratory illnesses)
Adenoviruses	34 (types 1, 2, 3, 5, 7, 14, and 21 are responsible for respiratory illnesses)
Mycoplasma pneumoniae	1

*Nonbacterial agents are responsible for >90% of upper respiratory infections in humans.

TABLE 13-2. Causes and Percentage of Cases of Community-Acquired Acute Bacterial Rhinosinusitis

Microorganism	Percentage of Cases	Comments
Haemophilus influenzae, nontypeable	35%	
Streptococcus pneumoniae	34%	
Anaerobic bacteria	6%	Anaerobic and polymicrobial infections are much more common in chronic rhinosinusitis
Gram-negative bacteria	4%	More common in hospital-acquired rhinosinusitis
Staphylococcus aureus	4%	
Moraxella catarrhalis	2%	More common in children
Streptococcus pyogenes	2%	

patients are also prone to fungal infections of the sinuses due to *Aspergillus* and *Mucor* species.

MANIFESTATIONS

Acute rhinosinusitis is characterized by mucosal inflammation of both the nose and the paranasal sinuses. Symptoms include sneezing, rhinorrhea, nasal congestion and postnasal drip, aural fullness, facial pressure and headache, sore throat, cough and fever, and myalgias. A viral upper respiratory tract infection usually precedes acute bacterial rhinosinusitis, and differentiating between a bacterial infection and a viral infection is difficult.

EPIDEMIOLOGY

- Respiratory viruses cause most cases of acute rhinosinusitis. Symptoms usually resolve within 5–7 days, and most people recover without medical treatment.

- Infection of the sinuses may follow the common cold, dental extractions, rhinitis due to allergies, and forcing water into the sinuses by jumping into water (e.g., diving).

- Infections of the sinuses develop most often during winter months when the common cold occurs more frequently.

- In approximately 2% of adults and 10% of children, acute bacterial rhinosinusitis can follow acute viral rhinosinusitis, allergic rhinitis, or other upper respiratory tract infections.

- Table 13-3 contains many of the predisposing factors that cause individuals to be more likely to develop acute bacterial rhinosinusitis.

- Patients with hospital-acquired infections are more likely to be infected with gram-negative organisms when they develop acute bacterial rhinosinusitis.

- Anaerobic acute bacterial rhinosinusitis infections are usually associated with dental infections or procedures.

TABLE 13-3. Acute Bacterial Rhinosinusitis: Predisposing Conditions

Viral infection
Allergic and nonallergic rhinitis
Anatomic variations
- Abnormality of the ostiomeatal complex
- Septal deviation
- Concha bullosa
- Hypertrophic middle turbinates
- Haller cells*
Topical nasal medications
Cigarette smoking
Diabetes mellitus
Swimming, diving, high-altitude climbing
Dental infections and procedures
Cocaine abuse

Rhinosinusitis is more common in patients with
- Cystic fibrosis
- Mechanical ventilation
- Head injuries
- Use of nasal tubes
- Samter triad[†]
- Sarcoidosis
- Wegener granulomatosis
- Immotile cilia syndrome
- Immune deficiency
  - Common variable
  - IgA
  - IgG subclass
  - Iatrogenic
  - AIDS (acquired immunodeficiency syndrome)

Note: Conditions are listed in order of relative frequency.
*Infraorbital ethmoid cells.
[†]Aspirin allergy, nasal polyps, and asthma.

PATHOGENESIS

The most common precursor to acute bacterial rhinosinusitis is a viral upper respiratory tract infection followed by sinus obstruction from the mucosal edema of inhalant allergies and by anatomic factors (e.g., nasal polyps). Obstruction of the paranasal sinusal ostia impedes drainage of mucus secretions. Bacteria then grow in these secretions, irritating the underlying mucosa and producing more secretions. Death and sloughing of the mucosal cells does occur, but cells will regenerate after the infection has cleared.

DIAGNOSIS

Diagnosis of **acute rhinosinusitis** is based on the patient's clinical signs and symptoms. Acute bacterial rhinosinusitis is correctly diagnosed about half the time based on clinical impressions. Acute bacterial rhinosinusitis and viral rhinosinusitis are difficult to differentiate because no single clinical finding can accurately distinguish between acute viral rhinosinusitis and acute bacterial rhinosinusitis. However, acute bacterial rhinosinusitis is more likely to become a chronic disease.

A diagnosis of **acute bacterial rhinosinusitis** is likely when a patient has symptoms of rhinosinusitis that include purulent nasal drainage that worsens after 5 days and persists beyond 10 days or is out of proportion to symptoms typically seen in viral upper respiratory disease. Signs and symptoms considered more likely to be due to a bacterial pathogen include high or persistent fever (>39°C), periorbital swelling, severe facial or dental pain, altered mental status, diplopia, and infraorbital hypesthesia.

Four signs and symptoms that appear to be most helpful in diagnosing a patient with acute bacterial rhinosinusitis are (1) purulent nasal discharge; (2) maxillary tooth or facial pain (especially unilateral); (3) unilateral maxillary sinus tenderness; and (4) worsening symptoms after initial improvement. Table 13-4 includes a criterion-based means of diagnosing acute bacterial rhinosinusitis.

THERAPY AND PREVENTION

Several different treatments can be employed to aid the patient in recovery. Symptomatic treatment is recommended for patients with acute viral rhinosinusitis; however, if a patient has acute bacterial rhinosinusitis, symptomatic and antibiotic treatment is recommended.

Symptomatic treatment
- Increase oral hydration with liberal use of nasal saline and steam to promote drainage.
- Antipyretics, analgesics (e.g., acetaminophen), and decongestants (e.g., oxymetazoline, phenylephrine, and naphazoline) may be needed for fever, headache, and facial pain.
- Mucolytics (e.g., guaifenesin) are helpful for thinning thick nasal secretions and especially for postnasal drip.

Antibiotic treatment
Recommendations for initial antibiotic therapy for patients with acute bacterial rhinosinusitis include amoxicillin or

TABLE 13-4. Signs and Symptoms Associated with the Diagnosis of Acute Bacterial Rhinosinusitis*

Major	Minor
Facial pain, pressure, fullness†	Headaches
Nasal obstruction and blockage	Fever (other than acute rhinosinusitis)
Nasal or postnasal discharge or purulence (by history or physical examination)	Halitosis
	Fatigue
	Dental pain
	Cough
Hyposmia, anosmia	Ear pain, pressure, fullness
Fever (in acute rhinosinusitis only††	

*The presence of two or more major signs and symptoms; OR one major and two or more minor signs or symptoms; OR nasal purulence on examination.

Acute bacterial rhinosinusitis is by definition an illness that lasts <4 weeks.

†Facial pain and pressure alone does *NOT* constitute a suggestive history in the absence of another finding listed in the major category.

††Fever alone in acute rhinosinusitis does *NOT* constitute a suggestive history in the absence of another finding listed in the major category.

cefdinir. If the patient is allergic to β-lactam antibiotics, trimethoprim-sulfamethoxazole or azithromycin can be prescribed.

No vaccines are available that prevent acute viral or bacterial rhinosinusitis; however, some patients can avoid future problems by

- Avoiding jumping in water without plugging the nose.
- Have septal deviations and polyps or foreign bodies surgically removed.
- Practice proper dental management.

PHARYNGITIS

Pharyngitis (sore throat) is a very common disease that results in over 15 million physician office visits each year in the United States. Most cases of pharyngitis are caused by viruses.

ETIOLOGY

Pharyngitis can be caused by many different microorganisms; however, 90% of sore throats in adults and 60–75% of sore throats in children are caused by viruses (Table 13-5). *S pyogenes* (beta-hemolytic group A *Streptococcus*) is the most common bacterial cause of acute pharyngitis.

TABLE 13-5. Some Viral Causes of Pharyngitis*

Virus	Associated Disorder or Symptom	Occurrence in Pharyngitis
Rhinovirus	Common cold	Common
Coronavirus	Common cold	Common
Adenovirus	Pharyngoconjunctival fever and acute respiratory disease	Common in military recruits and boarding schools
Herpes simplex virus types 1 and 2	Gingivostomatitis	Common
Parainfluenza virus	Cold and croup	Common in children
Coxsackievirus A	Herpangina (high fever, vomiting, diarrhea, abdominal pain) and hand-foot-and-mouth disease	Common
Influenza A and B viruses	Influenza	Common during flu season
Respiratory syncytial virus	Bronchiolitis and croup	Common in children
Epstein-Barr virus	Infectious mononucleosis	Common in adolescents during winter
Cytomegalovirus (CMV)	CMV mononucleosis	Less common
Human immunodeficiency virus (HIV)	Primary HIV infection	Infrequent (homosexual males and heterosexual females at highest risk)

*Viruses are the most common cause of pharyngitis.

MANIFESTATIONS

Fever, sore throat, edema, and hyperemia of the tonsils and pharyngeal walls are common findings in patients with viral and bacterial causes of pharyngitis (Figure 13-2). Other findings strongly suggest that a viral rather than a bacterial agent cause pharyngitis and include conjunctivitis, cough, coryza, hoarseness, and diarrhea; anterior stomatitis and discrete ulcerative lesions (see Chapter 4); and viral exanthem (see Chapter 2).

Patients with *S pyogenes* pharyngitis commonly present with fever and severe pain upon swallowing (generally of sudden onset). Headache, nausea and vomiting, and abdominal pain may also be present, especially in children. On examination, patients have tonsillopharyngeal erythema, with or without exudate, and tender, enlarged anterior cervical lymph nodes (lymphadenitis). They may also have a beefy red and swollen uvula; petechiae on the palate (Figure 13-3); excoriated nares (usually in children); and a scarlatiniform rash (see Chapter 2). However, none of these findings is specific for *S pyogenes* pharyngitis.

If untreated, a patient with *S pyogenes* pharyngitis can develop suppurative and nonsuppurative complications. Suppurative complications include peritonsillar abscess, cervical lymphadenitis, and mastoiditis. **The major nonsuppurative complication is rheumatic fever,** a complication that is more likely to occur in children with *S pyogenes* pharyngitis than in adults with this bacterial infection.

Rheumatic fever presents as a diverse set of clinical manifestations with onset of symptoms occurring within a few days to 5 weeks after a strep throat infection. A patient with rheumatic fever first presents with fever (38–40°C) and painful swelling of several joints such as the knees, elbows, or wrists. Severe rheumatic fever can result in damage to the valves of the heart.

EPIDEMIOLOGY

- Pharyngitis is common worldwide.
- Pharyngitis due to *S pyogenes* is usually a disorder of children aged 5–15 years.
- In temperate climates, it is most common during winter and early spring.
- Viruses are the most common cause of pharyngitis.
- With few exceptions (e.g., diphtheria), pharyngitis is benign and self-limiting.
- Viral pharyngitis is acquired by person-to-person contact and following contact with contaminated fomites.
- *S pyogenes* is transmitted by person-to-person contact.

PATHOGENESIS

In **viral pharyngitis,** viruses gain access to the mucosal cells lining the nasopharynx and replicate in these cells. Damage to the host is often caused by damage to the cells where the viruses are replicating.

In **bacterial pharyngitis,** *S pyogenes* attaches to the mucosal epithelial cells using M protein, lipoteichoic acid, and fibronectin-binding protein (protein F). It has a capsule composed of hyaluronic acid that prevents phagocytosis by host

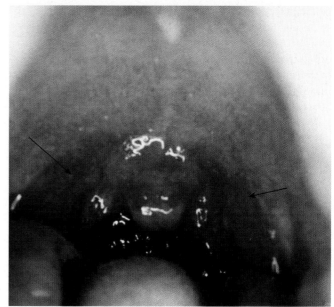

Figure 13-2. Inflammation of the oropharynx (soft palate) and tonsils in a patient with *Streptococcus pyogenes* pharyngitis. Notice the redness on the oropharynx and tonsils. (*Note:* Viral pharyngitis can appear similar to this image.) Image courtesy of the Centers for Disease Control and Prevention.

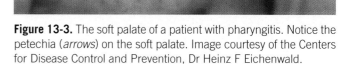

Figure 13-3. The soft palate of a patient with pharyngitis. Notice the petechia (*arrows*) on the soft palate. Image courtesy of the Centers for Disease Control and Prevention, Dr Heinz F Eichenwald.

macrophages. Because the hyaluronic acid in the bacterial capsule is identical to host hyaluronic acid, it facilitates bacterial survival by covering the bacterial antigens. Extracellular factors produced by *S pyogenes* during the infection include protease and hyaluronidase. These extracellular factors assist the bacteria in invading the mucosa. Direct extension to other sites can occur but due to the use of antibiotic therapy, this is now quite rare.

Nonsuppurative lesions resulting in rheumatic fever and glomerulonephritis still occur following throat infections caused by *S pyogenes*. It is believed that several bacterial antigens from *S pyogenes* share antigenic epitopes with the heart and renal tissues. An autoimmune reaction occurs in some patients following production of an immune response to these cross-reactive bacterial antigens and damages the patient's heart or kidneys. *Note: **Rheumatic fever and glomerulonephritis can occur after an episode of pharyngitis; only glomerulonephritis occurs after skin infections (e.g., impetigo).***

DIAGNOSIS

Viral infections of the throat are rarely cultured because of the mild self-limiting nature of the disease and the cost involved in culturing the pathogens. There are fewer cases of bacterial infections of the throat (compared to viral pharyngitis); however, delaying treatment of *S pyogenes* pharyngitis beyond 9 days after symptoms begin increases the patient's chances of developing rheumatic fever and suppurative complications (e.g., peritonsillar abscess, mastoiditis). Therefore, strategies for diagnosis of acute pharyngitis infections are primarily directed at identifying patients with *S pyogenes* pharyngitis who require antimicrobial therapy, as well as avoiding unnecessary treatment of patients diagnosed with acute viral pharyngitis.

The best means of determining which etiologic agent is causing the pharyngitis is to swab the patient's throat, culture the sample on blood agar plates, and demonstrate the growth of beta-hemolytic colonies that are catalase-negative, gram-positive cocci and are sensitive to bacitracin (Figure 13-4). *S pyogenes* rapid antigen detection tests are available and used clinically; however, these tests are not as sensitive as cultures.

Throat cultures are not necessary for proper diagnosis of all cases of pharyngitis, and this is especially true for adults. If a patient has clinical and epidemiologic features (e.g., cough, coryza, conjunctivitis, diarrhea) highly suggestive of a viral etiology, further testing is not needed (Table 13-6). However, if the patient has clinical and epidemiologic features highly suggestive of a bacterial etiology, further testing (e.g., cultures or rapid antigen tests) is needed.

Children younger than 18 years of age are more likely to develop *S pyogenes* pharyngitis, and are more likely to develop suppurative and nonsuppurative complications if not treated. Therefore, if a child is likely to have developed *S pyogenes* pharyngitis, as determined clinically and epidemiologically (see Table 13-6), further testing with rapid antigen detection tests and throat culture is indicated. If the result of the rapid antigen detection test is positive, a throat culture is *not* needed and the child should be treated with antibiotics. If the result of the rapid antigen detection test is negative, a throat culture should also be performed. A prescription for penicillin should be given if the result of either test is positive.

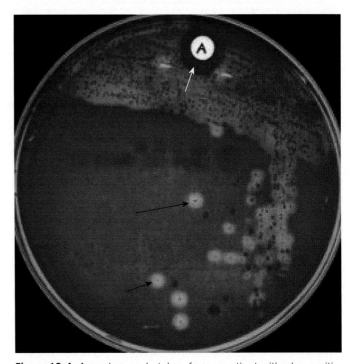

Figure 13-4. A swab sample taken from a patient with pharyngitis. The sample was placed on a blood agar plate and streaked for isolation. A bacitracin (Taxo A) disc was placed on the first sector of the plate. Note the beta-hemolytic colonies (*black arrows*) and the lack of growth of the beta-hemolytic colonies near the Taxo A disc (*white arrow*). Beta-hemolytic bacitracin-sensitive colonies are present on the blood agar plate and indicate that the patient has pharyngitis due to *Streptococcus pyogenes* (group A beta-hemolytic streptococci).

Rheumatic fever is a nonsuppurative complication of *S pyogenes* pharyngitis and resembles a number of other diseases that affect the joints (e.g., rheumatoid arthritis, systemic lupus erythematosus, serum sickness). Table 13-7 contains the Jones Criteria that is used in determining this diagnosis.

THERAPY AND PREVENTION

All patients with acute pharyngitis should be offered appropriate doses of antipyretics, analgesics, and supportive care.

Viral pharyngitis is treated with analgesics (e.g., acetaminophen); warm saline gargles will help lessen the pain. Fluids to avoid dehydration should be encouraged. Susceptible persons should be encouraged to limit contact with infected persons. An adenovirus vaccine is available for military personnel, but it is not warranted for use in the general population.

S pyogenes pharyngitis requires the use of an antimicrobial agent in addition to the treatment mentioned above for viral pharyngitis. Antimicrobial treatment has been shown to limit contiguous spread (e.g., peritonsillar abscess, cervical lymphadenitis, mastoiditis); prevent development of acute rheumatic fever (if given within 9 days of the appearance of symptoms); improve clinical signs and symptoms (if given within 2 days of the appearance of symptoms); rapidly decrease infectivity and thus reduce transmission of the bacterium to close-contacts (e.g., family, classmates); and allow for a rapid resumption to the patient's usual activities. Penicillin remains the drug of choice to treat *S pyogenes* pharyngitis; erythromycin is the drug of choice for patients allergic to penicillin. Patients should be encouraged to limit contact with uninfected persons.

Treatment of rheumatic fever includes antimicrobials to eliminate the *S pyogenes* resident in the pharynx and anti-inflammatory agents to suppress the clinical manifestations of the disease. Recurrence of rheumatic fever is more likely in patients who have had a previous episode of *S pyogenes* pharyngitis. Patients who have recovered from a bout of rheumatic fever should be protected from a second infection due to *S pyogenes* by chemoprophylaxis with a monthly dose of penicillin. This chemoprophylaxis should continue throughout the patient's childhood years. If permanent damage occurs to the heart, chemoprophylaxis should continue for the life of the patient.

DIPHTHERIA

Diphtheria is a bacterial disease that is now rarely seen in the United States because of successful universal vaccination (Figure 13-5). The vaccine does not affect the ability of the bacteria to colonize the oropharynx, however, but rather induces antibody production to inhibit diphtheria toxin. If vaccination were no longer available, diphtheria could once again become a common place disease.

ETIOLOGY

Corynebacterium diphtheriae is irregularly staining gram-positive, rod-shaped bacteria (Figure 13-6). Only strains of *C diphtheriae* that have toxin-producing lysogenic bacteriophage (β phage) can cause diphtheria.

TABLE 13-6. Clinical and Epidemiologic Findings Useful in the Diagnosis of Pharyngitis

Epidemiologic findings suggestive of *Streptococcus pyogenes* as the etiologic agent

Patient aged 5–15 years

Presentation in winter or early spring

History of exposure

Sudden onset of signs and symptoms

Clinical findings suggestive of *S pyogenes* as the etiologic agent

Sore throat

Fever

Headache

Nausea, vomiting, and abdominal pain

Inflammation of pharynx and tonsils

Patchy discrete exudates

Tender, enlarged anterior cervical nodes

Features suggestive of a virus as the etiologic agent

Conjunctivitis

Coryza

Cough

Diarrhea

Note: These findings, either individually or collectively, cannot definitively predict the presence of *S pyogenes* pharyngitis. They can identify persons with a high probability of being diagnosed with *S pyogenes* pharyngitis (and for whom throat culture or rapid antigen detection testing is indicated) or a low probability of *S pyogenes* pharyngitis (neither culture nor rapid antigen detection testing is necessary).

MANIFESTATIONS

Diphtheria results in pharyngeal pain, formation of a pseudomembrane seen on the tonsils and back of the oropharynx, regional lymphadenopathy ("bull neck" appearance as shown in Figure 13-7), edema of the surrounding tissues, fetid breath, low-grade fever, and cough. Airway obstruction can occur, and findings of tachypnea, stridor, and cyanosis are seen. The toxin can damage the cranial nerves and the heart, causing neurologic abnormalities (e.g., palatine palsy, difficulty swallowing, nasal regurgitation of liquids) and myocarditis.

EPIDEMIOLOGY

- The disease is worldwide in distribution. Only 1 or 2 cases of diphtheria are reported each year in the United States (see Figure 13-5).

- The largest outbreak in recent history occurred in the former Soviet Union in 1994, with nearly 48,000 cases of diphtheria and over 1700 deaths.

- *C diphtheriae* can colonize the oropharynx and the skin of persons immune to the disease without causing disease, which is how the organism remains in the population.

- Humans are the only known reservoir of *C diphtheriae*.

- The most common cause of death is due to diphtheria toxin damage to the heart.

- *C diphtheriae* is transmitted by respiratory droplets and by skin contact. Healthy carriers, convalescent patients, and patients incubating the disease are the optimum transmitters of infection.

PATHOGENESIS

C diphtheria colonizes the oropharynx and remains localized on the mucosal surfaces. Only *C diphtheriae* lysogenic for the bacteriophage (beta phage) carrying the toxin gene causes diphtheria. Damage to the pharynx is caused by the diphtheria toxin, which kills the mucosal cells by adenosine diphosphate ribosylation of elongation factor II and terminating protein synthesis. An inflammatory response to cell death and the dead cells form the pseudomembrane. The toxin can also bind to and damage the heart and nerve cells. The major complications of the disease are myocarditis and cranial nerve damage. Myocarditis is the more important of the two complications and causes the highest mortality. Cranial nerves are most sensitive to the toxin, resulting in difficulty swallowing and in nasal regurgitation of liquids.

DIAGNOSIS

Diagnosis of diphtheria includes observation of a pseudomembrane and bleeding upon removal of the membrane and severe cervical lymphadenopathy (see Figure 13-7). Neurologic abnormalities such as palatine palsy, difficulty swallowing, and nasal regurgitation of fluids are important clues in correctly diagnosing diphtheria. The oropharynx should be swabbed and samples cultured for *C diphtheriae*. The *C diphtheriae* strain isolated by culture should be assayed for diphtheria toxin production using the Elek test (immunodiffusion assay) or by polymerase chain reaction (PCR).

TABLE 13-7. Jones Criteria for Guidance in the Diagnosis of Rheumatic Fever*

Major Manifestations	Minor Manifestations
Carditis	**Clinical**
Polyarthritis	Previous rheumatic fever or rheumatic heart disease
Chorea	Arthralgia
Erythema marginatum	Fever
Subcutaneous nodules	**Laboratory**
	Increase in acute phase reactants: erythrocyte sedimentation rate, C-reactive protein, leukocytosis
	Prolonged P-R interval

*The presence of 2 major criteria **OR** 1 major and 2 minor criteria indicates a high probability of acute rheumatic fever, if supported by evidence of preceding group A streptococcal infection.
Supporting evidence of streptococcal infection: Increased titer of antistreptococcal antibodies, ASO (antistreptolysin O), other throat culture positive for group A Streptococcus, or recent case of scarlet fever.

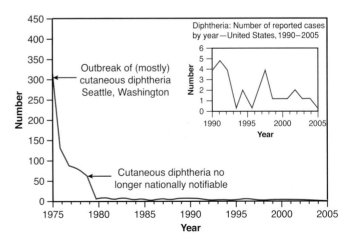

Figure 13-5. A graph showing the number of cases of diphtheria in the United States from 1975 to 2005. Image courtesy of the Centers for Disease Control and Prevention.

TREATMENT AND PREVENTION

A patient with diphtheria should be hospitalized, placed in isolation, and immediately treated with antiserum to the toxin. The most urgent task is giving the antiserum to neutralize the toxic affects of the diphtheria toxin. The second most urgent task is antimicrobial treatment with penicillin or erythromycin. The patient should also be given diphtheria vaccine to ensure immunity to the disease. Active immunization with the DTaP vaccine for children and the DT vaccine for adults will serve as protection from diphtheria.

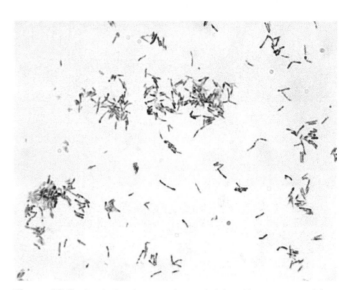

Figure 13-6. A photomicrograph containing the gram-positive, irregularly staining *Corynebacterium diphtheriae* bacteria. Image courtesy of the Centers for Disease Control and Prevention, Dr PB Smith.

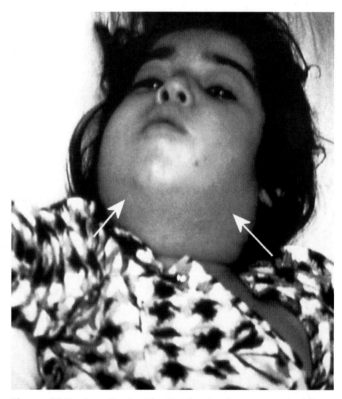

Figure 13-7. A patient with diphtheria. Severe cervical lymphadenopathy and edema cause the "bull neck" appearance characteristic of this disease. Image courtesy of the Centers for Disease Control and Prevention.

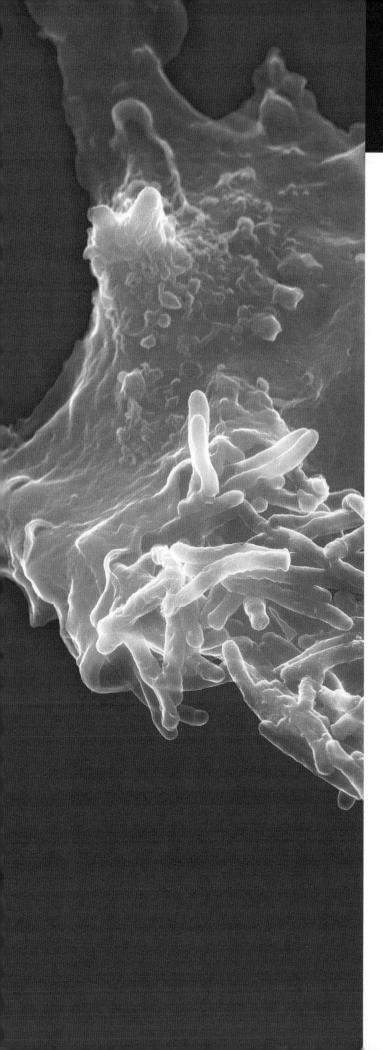

CHAPTER 14

INFECTIONS OF THE RESPIRATORY AIRWAYS

OVERVIEW

The respiratory airways discussed in this chapter include the airways from the epiglottis to the bronchioles. The infections discussed are croup (which includes acute laryngitis, laryngotracheobronchitis, and epiglottitis), acute bronchitis, bronchiolitis, influenza, and pertussis (Figure 14-1). All of the diseases discussed in this chapter, with the exception of epiglottitis and pertussis, are usually caused by viruses; epiglottitis and pertussis are caused by bacteria.

CROUP

Acute laryngitis, laryngotracheobronchitis (viral croup), and epiglottitis (bacterial croup) are acute inflammatory diseases, collectively called croup, and involve the upper airways (see Figure 14-1). *The most common and most serious risk of this group of diseases is obstruction of the airway.* This risk is particularly important to remember when treating very young children because the airways of young child are narrower than the airways of older children and adults.

ETIOLOGY

Parainfluenza virus type I is the most common cause of viral croup; other causes of viral croup and laryngitis are listed in Table 14-1. *Haemophilus influenzae* type b is the most common cause of epiglottitis (bacterial croup); Table 14-2 lists other causes of epiglottitis.

MANIFESTATIONS

Acute laryngitis

Acute laryngitis begins as an upper respiratory infection followed by dysphonia (hoarseness) (see Figure 14-1). Other symptoms may include odynophonia (pain when speaking), dysphagia (difficulty swallowing), odynophagia (pain when swallowing), sore throat, congestion, fatigue, and malaise.

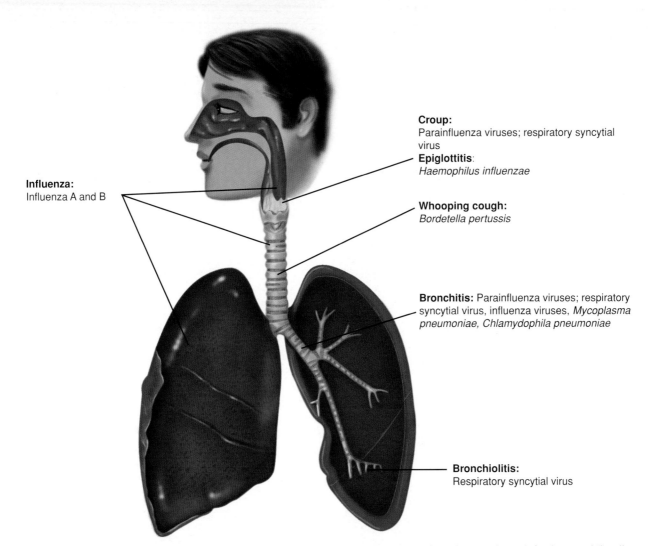

Influenza:
Influenza A and B

Croup:
Parainfluenza viruses; respiratory syncytial virus
Epiglottitis:
Haemophilus influenzae

Whooping cough:
Bordetella pertussis

Bronchitis: Parainfluenza viruses; respiratory syncytial virus, influenza viruses, *Mycoplasma pneumoniae, Chlamydophila pneumoniae*

Bronchiolitis:
Respiratory syncytial virus

Figure 14-1. A schematic of the respiratory airways showing the common causes of respiratory airway infections and the diseases they cause in the respiratory tract of humans.

Viral croup

Patients with viral croup or laryngotracheobronchitis have a fever (38–39°C), which is higher than occurs in laryngitis, and restlessness and air hunger, which is more severe than occurs in laryngitis. Croup begins with a prodromal mild upper respiratory infection with coryza, nasal congestion, sore throat, and cough that lasts 2–3 days; this is followed by hoarseness and a harsh, brassy, "bark-like" cough. Respiratory stridor usually occurs at night, often awakening the child from sleep.

Physical examination of the patient with croup may reveal minimal distress to severe respiratory failure due to airway obstruction. In mild cases, the results of the lung examination at rest usually are normal; however, mild expiratory wheezing may he heard during auscultation. Children with severe croup have primarily inspiratory stridor at rest with nasal flaring and suprasternal and intercostal retractions (Figure 14-2). Lethargy or agitation may be a result of hypoxemia. Other warning signs of severe respiratory disease are tachypnea, tachycardia out of proportion to the presence of fever, lethargy, pallor, and hypotonia (decreased muscle tone). The child may be unable to maintain adequate oral intake and may become dehydrated.

TABLE 14-1. Other Causes of Viral Croup

Viruses	Parainfluenza type II, influenza types A and B, adenovirus, respiratory syncytial virus, herpes simplex virus, rhinovirus, coxsackievirus A and B, echovirus

TABLE 14-2. Other Causes of Epiglottitis

Bacteria	Nontypeable *Haemophilus influenzae*, *Streptococcus* groups A, B, and C, *Streptococcus pneumoniae, Klebsiella pneumoniae, Staphylococcus aureus, Haemophilus parainfluenza, Neisseria meningitidis*
Viruses	Varicella zoster virus
Fungi	*Candida albicans*

Cyanosis is a late and ominous sign. Croup symptoms usually peak over 3–5 days and resolve within 4–7 days.

Epiglottitis

Epiglottitis is a medical emergency, and risk of mortality is extremely high. Signs and symptoms include acute onset and fever, sore throat, hoarseness, and a barking cough. There is retraction of the suprasternal notch (see Figure 14-2) and stridor with every breath. The throat is inflamed, and the epiglottis is swollen, stiff, and a beefy red color and can be seen by direct laryngoscopy. The disease can progress rapidly resulting in toxicity, prostration, severe dyspnea, and cyanosis. The physician should be watchful for *dysphagia, dysphonia, drooling, and distress—known as the four D's.*

EPIDEMIOLOGY

▫ Person-to-person contact is the usual means of spread of all types of croup.

Viral croup and acute laryngitis

▫ Young children are most susceptible to **viral croup,** which typically occurs in children 6 months to 3 years of age, with the mean age being 18 months. Boys are more likely than girls to develop croup.

▫ Viral croup has an annual peak incidence during the second year of life of 50 new cases per 1000 children.

▫ The incidence of viral croup decreases dramatically by 6 years of age.

▫ Viral croup occurs in late fall and early winter. The recurrence rate is 5%.

▫ Outcomes of viral croup depend of how ill the patient is, the age of the patient, and the adequacy of the treatment. Complications in severe cases include crusty exudates resulting in obstruction of the airways, segmental atelectasis, pneumothorax, obstructive mediastinal emphysema, and bronchopneumonia.

▫ Parainfluenza infections can cause viral croup anytime during the year. Influenza virus and respiratory syncytial virus infections tend to occur more frequently during the winter and early spring.

▫ **Acute laryngitis** usually occurs in persons aged 18–40 years of age. Although children are less likely to contract acute laryngitis, they can acquire the disease and are usually 3 years of age or older.

▫ Acute laryngitis is usually a mild self-limiting disease lasting 7–10 days.

Epiglottitis

▫ The *H influenzae* type b (Hib) vaccine has significantly reduced the incidence of epiglottitis from 10.9 per 10,000 to 0.63 cases per 100,000 persons.

▫ *H influenzae* type b is still the most common cause of epiglottitis.

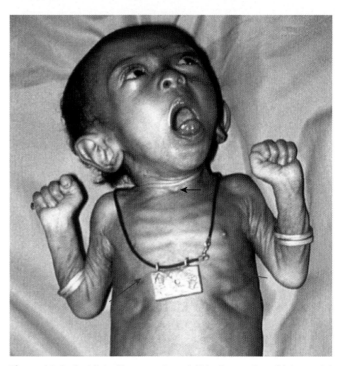

Figure 14-2. A child with suprasternal (*black arrow*) and intercostal (*blue arrows*) retractions. The child also has nasal flaring (*red arrow*). Image courtesy of the Centers for Disease Control and Prevention.

■ The median age of patients with epiglottitis has increased from 35 months of age to 80 months of age. Prior to 1994, the disease was usually seen in children 2–7 years of age.

■ The prevalence of epiglottitis in adults now surpasses the prevalence in children, which is due to the success of Hib vaccination of children.

■ The morbidity and mortality of epiglottitis can be very high, with bacteremia often resulting in meningitis, septic arthritis, or osteomyelitis.

PATHOGENESIS

Children have narrower airways than adults, which results in an increased number of complications associated with viral croup and epiglottitis.

Viral infection of the upper airways causes inflammation and edema of the larynx in **acute laryngitis;** viral infection in the larynx, trachea, and bronchi causes **viral croup**. Mucus is produced by the host and causes partial obstruction of the airway in both viral croup and acute laryngitis. Swelling of the vocal cords results in dysphonia. In viral croup, narrowing of the subglottic trachea in a child's airway results in audible inspiratory stridor. As viral croup progresses, the lumen of the trachea becomes obstructed further by fibrous exudates. The barking cough that occurs in patients with viral croup is caused by inflammation in the larynx and trachea.

Epiglottitis is a cellulitis of the epiglottis and the surrounding tissues. *H influenzae* type b colonizes the pharynx. The organisms colonize the epiglottitis and enter the tissues of the epiglottitis through minor breaks in the mucosal surface. The organisms then grow in the tissues and cause an inflammatory response that results in erythema and edema. A sore throat rapidly progresses to difficulty breathing, stridor, obstruction of the airways, and respiratory arrest. Local extension from the colonized nasopharynx through soft tissues is likely to be the cause of epiglottitis.

DIAGNOSIS

Diagnosis of **acute laryngitis** is based on the clinical signs and symptoms of the patient (see Manifestations). **Viral croup** is diagnosed by hoarseness, barking cough, and inspiratory stridor and retractions, which indicate airway obstruction (Table 14-3). A patient with viral croup will usually experience less restlessness and air hunger following treatment with racemic epinephrine or water-saturated air. These treatments do not have any affect on a patient with bacterial epiglottitis, however. *The steeple sign seen in an anteroposterior neck radiograph is characteristic of viral croup.* Viral cultures usually are not obtained.

The patient with **epiglottitis** should be handled with extreme care because airway closure can occur simply by placing a tongue depressor in the patient's mouth to examine the throat. Examination of the larynx can irritate the patient and cause airway closure and asphyxiation. Equipment for an emergency tracheostomy should be available during examination of a patient suspected of having epiglottitis. If the patient has bacterial epiglottitis, the etiologic agent should be determined. *H influenzae* type b, the most common cause of epiglottis, does

TABLE 14-3. Comparison of the Clinical Features of Viral Croup and Epiglottitis

Clinical Features	Viral Croup	Epiglottitis
Etiology	Parainfluenza virus	*Haemophilus influenzae* type b
Age of patient	6 month–3 years	2–7 years
Onset of disease	Gradual	Sudden
Fever	Mild	>38°C
Abnormal chest sounds	Bark-like cough, stridor	Muffled, guttural cough
Swallowing	Normal	Difficult, with drooling
Facies	Normal	Anxious, distressed, toxic

not grow on blood agar; therefore throat swabs and smears should be cultured on blood agar and chocolate agar plates. In epiglottitis, *H influenzae* is often in the bloodstream; therefore blood cultures are helpful. A leukocytosis can be seen in the complete blood count (CBC). *A positive thumb sign on lateral radiographs of the neck is diagnostic of epiglottitis.*

THERAPY AND PREVENTION

Acute laryngitis is a self-limiting infection, and symptomatic therapy usually is all that is necessary. *Treatment of viral croup requires maintenance of an adequate airway,* as follows.

- Humidification of air provides water droplets that penetrate the area of inflammation and add moisture to the mucosa. Methods used to deliver high humidity include croup tents, masks, and blow-by oxygen.

- Racemic epinephrine is effective in reducing stridor in children with stridor at rest or in children with more severe symptoms who are not responding to humidified oxygen.

- Dexamethasone, prednisone, or budesonide may help patients who have severe viral croup and are hospitalized or treated in the emergency department.

- Oxygen may be necessary if respiratory distress occurs.

- Patients should be kept in a quiet, calm environment; any treatment that separates the child from the parents should be avoided because separation can increase anxiety.

- If the patient is experiencing lack of air, tracheostomy should be considered.

Proper care and handling of the patient with epiglottitis can determine whether the patient lives or dies. *Treatment of epiglottitis involves securing the patient's airway by intubation and antibiotic therapy* with ceftriaxone or cefuroxime. Children should be sedated when being intubated to prevent them from pulling out the tube.

The Hib vaccine is the capsular type b polysaccharide conjugated to the diphtheria toxoid, and it has drastically reduced the incidence of epiglottitis in the United States. A child who has not received the Hib vaccine and who is exposed to a patient with epiglottitis should receive chemoprophylaxis with rifampin.

ACUTE BRONCHITIS

Acute bronchitis causes inflammation of the trachea and bronchi but does not involve the alveoli (see Figure 14-1); it is usually caused by viral agents (see below). Acute bronchitis occurs in patients of all ages but is most common in the young and in older persons. Chronic bronchitis, which is not discussed here, occurs in adulthood.

ETIOLOGY

Viruses are the most common cause of acute bronchitis. Acute bronchitis can be caused by the following agents.

- Respiratory viruses that infect the upper respiratory tract: Influenza viruses A and B, parainfluenza viruses, adenovirus, respiratory syncytial virus, herpes simplex virus, rhinovirus, coxsackievirus groups A and B, and echovirus.
- *Mycoplasma pneumoniae*
- *Chlamydophila pneumoniae*

MANIFESTATIONS

Manifestations of bronchitis include a cough (which is nonproductive at first but can become mucopurulent), substernal pain, and fever (38.3–38.9°C). Physical findings will reveal an infected pharynx; rhonchi and moist crackles can be heard upon auscultation. Several hours before symptoms of bronchitis develop, the patient will experience malaise, headache, coryza, and sore throat. Chest radiographs do not reveal consolidations or infiltrates, as seen in patients with pneumonia; therefore, a chest radiograph can be helpful in differentiating bronchitis from pneumonia.

EPIDEMIOLOGY

- Acute bronchitis usually occurs after a previous upper respiratory tract infection with extension of the infection to the bronchial tree.
- It is most common in the winter months, similar to most other respiratory diseases.
- Air pollution increases the number of cases of bronchitis.
- Acute bronchitis is a self-limiting disease in healthy adults and resolves within 7–10 days.
- Predisposing factors for the development of acute bronchitis in children include poor nutrition, allergy, deficiencies in IgG_2, IgG_3, and IgG_4 subclasses, and rickets.
- Older patients who have emphysema or chronic respiratory disease (e.g., tuberculosis) are more likely to develop acute bronchitis.

PATHOGENESIS

Acute bronchitis usually follows a viral upper respiratory tract infection that extends into the trachea, bronchi, and bronchioles and results in a hacking cough and sputum production.

The inflammation results in hypersecretion of mucus in the bronchial airways. The cough reflex aids in the elimination of mucus secretions from the airways. In time, bacteria can colonize the damaged airways causing the sputum to be purulent. If the patient is healthy, the viral infection is eliminated and the mucous membranes return to normal within 7–10 days. Mucociliary clearance of the airway may be delayed in patients who smoke or who are exposed to smoke because of excess mucus production and loss of ciliated cells, which lead to a productive cough. These patients are more likely to develop chronic bronchitis.

DIAGNOSIS

Diagnosis of acute bronchitis is based on clinical signs and symptoms. Differentiation between bronchitis and pneumonia is nearly impossible to determine based on clinical grounds unless chest radiographs demonstrate infiltrates or consolidation consistent with pneumonia. If the patient's temperature is elevated, a bacterial bronchitis may be present. Healthy persons usually improve with few complications.

THERAPY AND PREVENTION

Bronchitis in an otherwise healthy person is almost always self-limiting. Supportive therapy with analgesics (e.g., acetaminophen), antipyretics (e.g., ibuprofen), antitussives (e.g., dextromethorphan), and expectorants (e.g., guaifenesin) is recommended. If the patient has a fever and if the sputum becomes purulent, it may be necessary to identify the bacterial pathogen by culturing the sputum and treating the patient with erythromycin or azithromycin.

There are no preventative measures available to treat all of the possible agents that can cause bronchitis. The influenza virus vaccine is available to prevent bronchitis due to this agent.

BRONCHIOLITIS

Bronchiolitis causes inflammation of the bronchial tree as low as the bronchioles but does not involve the alveoli (see Figure 14-1). Because infants have narrower airways, bronchiolitis is usually a disease of infants younger than 1 year of age.

ETIOLOGY

The most common cause of bronchiolitis is respiratory syncytial virus; other causes include human metapneumovirus, parainfluenza viruses, and adenoviruses.

MANIFESTATIONS

Early symptoms of bronchiolitis are similar to symptoms of a viral upper respiratory tract infection and include mild rhinorrhea, cough, and sometimes a low-grade fever. In some infants and young children, the infection extends downward into the lower respiratory tract causing paroxysmal cough and dyspnea. Other common symptoms include tachypnea, tachycardia, fever (38.5–39°C), diffuse expiratory wheezing, respiratory crackles, nasal flaring, intercostal retractions (see Figure 14-2), grunting, vomiting (especially posttussive), cyanosis, and hyperinflation of the lungs and depression of the diaphragm.

EPIDEMIOLOGY

- The incidence of bronchiolitis parallels respiratory infections in older children and adults and is most common during fall and winter months.

- Although infection with respiratory syncytial virus may occur at any age, the clinical disease bronchiolitis develops only in infants and young children. About 75% of cases of bronchiolitis occur in children younger than 1 year of age and 95% occur in children younger than 2 years of age, with a peak incidence at 2–8 months of age. The infection is usually self-limiting.

- Bronchiolitis is an acute viral infection with a favorable outcome; fatalities rarely occur.

- About 95% of children aged 2 have serologic evidence of past infection with respiratory syncytial virus; the presence of antibodies to this virus does not confer immunity.

- Risk factors include age younger than 6 months, bottle feeding, prematurity (born before 37 weeks' gestation), exposure to cigarette smoke, and crowded living conditions.

- The virus is transmitted from person to person by direct contact with nasal secretions or by airborne droplets.

PATHOGENESIS

Bronchiolitis is usually a viral infection of the small airways (bronchioles). Infection of the bronchiolar respiratory and ciliated epithelial cells produces increased mucous secretion, cell death, and sloughing, followed by a peribronchiolar lymphocytic infiltrate and submucosal edema. Debris in the bronchioles and edema of the walls of the bronchioles results in critical narrowing and obstruction of these airways. Decreased ventilation of portions of the lung causes ventilation-perfusion mismatching resulting in hypoxia. The expiratory phase of respiration also causes dynamic narrowing of the airways resulting in decreased air flow from the lungs and air trapping. The patient must work harder to breathe, which is due to increased end-expiratory lung volume and decreased lung compliance. The debris present in the bronchioles is cleared by macrophages. The pulmonary epithelial cells regenerate within 3–4 days after the infection clears.

DIAGNOSIS

The diagnosis of bronchiolitis involves observation of the patient's signs and symptoms, chest radiographs, and antigen testing for respiratory syncytial virus in nasal washings. Chest radiographs should include anteroposterior and lateral views, which may show hyperinflation and patchy infiltrates, air trapping, focal atelectasis, flattened diaphragm, increased anteroposterior diameter, and peribronchial cuffing.

Antigen tests of nasal washings provide rapid and accurate detection of respiratory syncytial virus. A positive culture or direct fluorescent antibody test result can confirm the diagnosis of respiratory syncytial virus bronchiolitis. Nasal washings should be obtained from children who are hospitalized and children at risk for severe disease.

THERAPY AND PREVENTION

Patients with bronchiolitis may require supplemental oxygen and replacement of electrolytes and fluids. Empiric treatment with beta agonists (e.g., albuterol) may be helpful in some cases. Anticholinergics (e.g., ipratropium) inhibit smooth muscle contraction and are useful in patients with severe bronchospasm. Treatment of respiratory syncytial virus with ribavirin is usually used only in select patients with high risk of serious infection (e.g., patients with congenital heart disease or cystic fibrosis).

To prevent bronchiolitis, **RespiGam** (immunoglobulin reactive with respiratory syncytial virus) or **palivizumab** (humanized monoclonal antibody reactive with respiratory syncytial virus) can be given to high-risk patients, including infants born prematurely, patients with cystic fibrosis, patients who have hemodynamically significant acyanotic or cyanotic congenital heart disease, or patients who are immunodeficient.

INFLUENZA

To emphasize the importance of the disease, influenza is discussed as a separate topic in this chapter. Although it is a self-limiting disease, severe complications leading to fatalities are seen in the very young, the elderly, patients with underlying cardiovascular and pulmonary diseases, and women in the third trimester of pregnancy.

ETIOLOGY

The causative agent of influenza (or flu) is the influenza virus; the three different antigenic types of the virus are A, B, and C. Virus types A and B cause most epidemics and sporadic outbreaks of flu worldwide. Type C is usually seen as a mild disease of the very young, and rarely causes a flu epidemic. By age 15, nearly everyone has developed antibodies to the virus.

A distinctive terminology is used when discussing influenza A virus—the type of influenza virus, the geographic location where it was first isolated, the month it was first isolated, the year it was first isolated, and the H and N antigens expressed (e.g., A/Ann Arbor/1/86/H1N2—an influenza virus type A, first isolated in Ann Arbor, Michigan, in January of 1986, that is a H1N2 type). Influenza B viruses are identified by type, where it was first isolated, and the date first isolated but *NOT* by the H and N types.

MANIFESTATIONS

Symptoms of influenza include abrupt onset of fever (38.9–40°C), chills, rigors, headache, congested conjunctiva, extreme prostration with myalgia in the back and limbs, nonproductive cough, and injection of the pharynx and conjunctiva. Fever usually abates within 3–4 days, and recovery usually is complete within 1 week. Cough and malaise may persist for 2 weeks or longer.

In the very young, the elderly, patients with underlying cardiovascular and pulmonary diseases, and women in the third trimester of pregnancy, the condition may worsen with persistent fever, marked prostration, cough with rales, and pneumonia. The pneumonia usually is due to a secondary bacterial

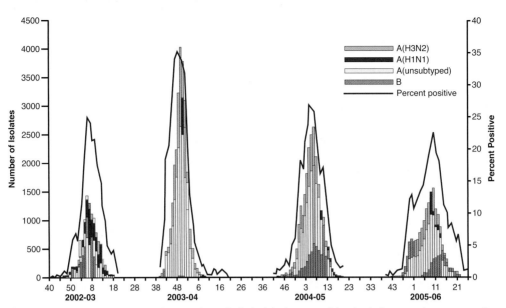

Figure 14-3. A graph showing the number of clinical isolates positive for influenza virus versus the week of the year the isolates were obtained from 2002 through 2006. Notice the seasonal nature of the influenza epidemics. Image courtesy of the Centers for Disease Control and Prevention.

infection, which can include *Staphylococcus aureus, H influenzae, Streptococcus pneumoniae,* or *Streptococcus pyogenes.*

EPIDEMIOLOGY

- Adults are infectious from 1 day before symptoms begin through approximately 5 days after onset of illness. Severely immunocompromised persons can shed the virus for weeks to months.

- Rates of influenza infection are highest among children, but rates of serious illness and death are highest among persons aged 65 or older and persons of any age who have medical conditions that place them at high risk for complications from influenza (e.g., pulmonary or cardiac disease).

- Epidemics of influenza usually occur every year during the winter months and are responsible for an average of approximately 36,000 deaths per year in the United States (Figure 14-3).

- Epidemic flu is cyclic and is usually caused by virus types A or B. Epidemics of type A occur every 2–3 years. Epidemics of type B occur every 4–6 years. Epidemics usually occur from late autumn to early spring.

- The most common complications associated with influenza infection are pneumonia and death. The overall mortality rate is about 1%. Influenza can exacerbate underlying medical conditions (Table 14-4) and lead to secondary bacterial pneumonia or primary influenza viral pneumonia.

- Young children with influenza infection can develop symptoms mimicking bacterial sepsis and have high fevers. Some children hospitalized with influenza may have febrile seizures.

- Influenza viruses are spread from person to person primarily by the coughing and sneezing of infected persons.

Avian influenza

- Avian influenza is caused by influenza A virus H5N1, which primarily infects birds.

TABLE 14-4. High-Risk Groups Likely to Develop Serious Complications Following Infection with the Influenza Virus

The following groups, listed from highest priority to lowest, should receive the influenza vaccine:

- Persons aged ≥ 65 years with comorbid conditions*
- Residents of long-term care facilities
- Persons aged 2–64 years with comorbid conditions*
- Persons aged ≥ 65 years *without* comorbid conditions*
- Children aged 6–23 months
- Pregnant women
- Health-care personnel who provide direct patient care
- Household contacts and out-of home caregivers of children <6 months

---

*Comorbid conditions include respiratory disease (e.g., asthma, emphysema), heart disease, metabolic disease (e.g., diabetes mellitus), kidney disease, and blood disorders (e.g., anemia).

- Outbreaks of H5N1 among poultry have occurred in Africa, East Asia, the Pacific, South Asia, the Near East, Eurasia, and Europe.

- More than 300 human cases of H5N1 were reported worldwide to the World Health Organization during the period of 2003 to 2007. The mortality rate is high, at about 60%. Most patients acquired the infection after direct close contact with infected poultry or contaminated surfaces.

- A few rare cases of human-to-human spread of H5N1 virus have occurred, although transmission did not continue beyond one person.

PATHOGENESIS

The influenza viruses are segmented single-strand RNA viruses. Influenza types A and B viruses have eight RNA segments, and influenza type C virus has seven RNA segments. The RNA codes for five structural proteins and three nonstructural proteins. Protein M and nucleoprotein NP are used to place the virus into types A, B, and C. The hemagglutinins (H antigen) and the neuraminidases (N antigen) are important in the pathogenesis of influenza—the H antigen is required for binding of the virus to the cell, and the N antigen helps the mature virus escape from the cell.

In addition to the major types of the influenza A virus, there are also subtypes of the virus that are determined by the H and N antigens. There are four antigenic types of H antigen (i.e., H1, H2, H3, and H5) and two antigenic types of N antigen (N1 and N2) that infect humans. Antibodies to one type of H or N antigen are not effective in protecting a person from being infected by another type of the H or N antigen.

Influenza viruses can infect other animal hosts (e.g., ducks, swine). Two different influenza A viruses can infect the same animal host cell, and as long as the viruses that result from this dual infection have the right number and kinds of RNA segments, they can cause infection in another host.

If two viruses are circulating in a population of swine (e.g., influenza A H5N2 virus and influenza A H1N1), the viruses can co-infect one animal. Suppose, for example, that one of these two viruses, the influenza A H1N1 virus, infected several persons the previous year. Because of their ability to produce antibodies that inactivate the influenza A H1N1 virus, those who survived the influenza A H1N1 infection would not acquire this viral infection again the following year. However, if influenza A H1N1 virus and influenza A H5N2 virus co-infected a pig and reassorted their viral RNA segments, an influenza A H5N1 virus could result. The influenza H5N1 virus could cause the next influenza epidemic in humans if they were exposed to the infected pig with the reassorted virus. These major changes in H or N types are called shifts (Figure 14-4).

Mutations can also occur in the H and N genes that result in slight changes in the H or N antigens. These slight changes are called antigenic drift (Figure 14-5). Influenza A viruses undergo both shift and drift, whereas influenza B viruses only undergo drift in their H and N antigens.

If a susceptible person inhales droplets containing the influenza virus, the virus attaches to the epithelial cells lining the respiratory airways as well as to the nasal turbinates. The

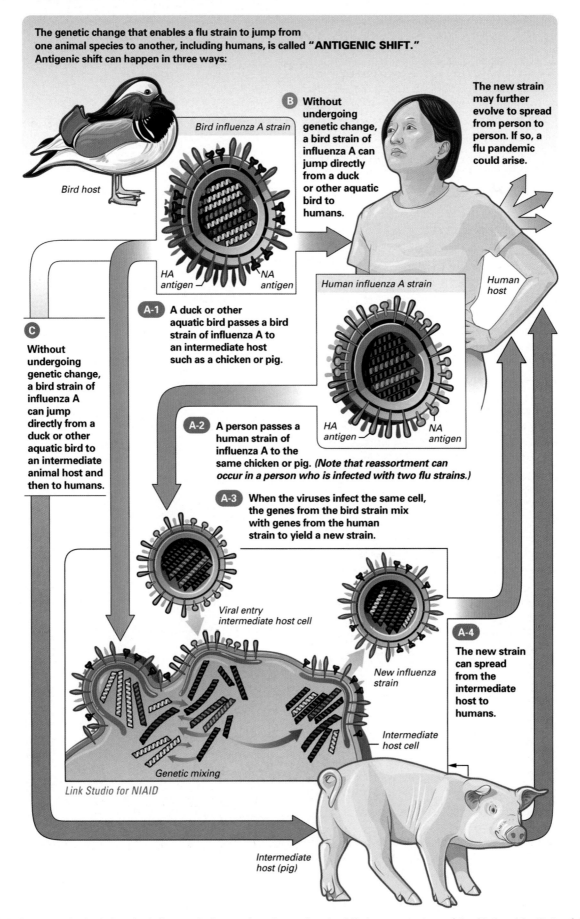

The genetic change that enables a flu strain to jump from one animal species to another, including humans, is called "ANTIGENIC SHIFT." Antigenic shift can happen in three ways:

Bird host

Bird influenza A strain

HA antigen *NA antigen*

B Without undergoing genetic change, a bird strain of influenza A can jump directly from a duck or other aquatic bird to humans.

The new strain may further evolve to spread from person to person. If so, a flu pandemic could arise.

A-1 A duck or other aquatic bird passes a bird strain of influenza A to an intermediate host such as a chicken or pig.

Human influenza A strain

Human host

C Without undergoing genetic change, a bird strain of influenza A can jump directly from a duck or other aquatic bird to an intermediate animal host and then to humans.

A-2 A person passes a human strain of influenza A to the same chicken or pig. *(Note that reassortment can occur in a person who is infected with two flu strains.)*

HA antigen *NA antigen*

A-3 When the viruses infect the same cell, the genes from the bird strain mix with genes from the human strain to yield a new strain.

Viral entry intermediate host cell

New influenza strain

A-4 The new strain can spread from the intermediate host to humans.

Intermediate host cell

Genetic mixing

Link Studio for NIAID

Intermediate host (pig)

Figure 14-4. A schematic depicting the influenza A virus undergoing antigenic shift. Image courtesy of the National Institute of Allergy and Infectious Diseases.

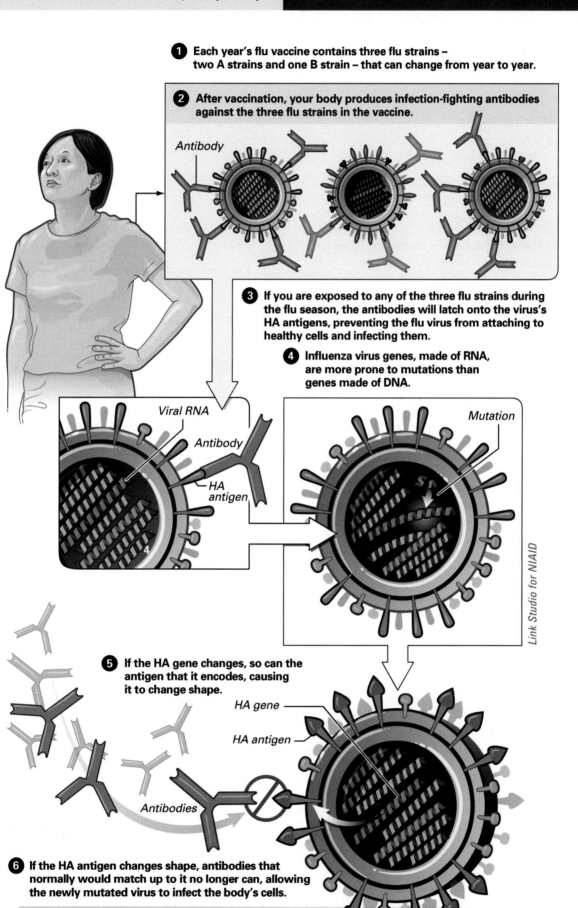

1 Each year's flu vaccine contains three flu strains – two A strains and one B strain – that can change from year to year.

2 After vaccination, your body produces infection-fighting antibodies against the three flu strains in the vaccine.

Antibody

3 If you are exposed to any of the three flu strains during the flu season, the antibodies will latch onto the virus's HA antigens, preventing the flu virus from attaching to healthy cells and infecting them.

4 Influenza virus genes, made of RNA, are more prone to mutations than genes made of DNA.

Viral RNA

Antibody

HA antigen

Mutation

Link Studio for NIAID

5 If the HA gene changes, so can the antigen that it encodes, causing it to change shape.

HA gene

HA antigen

Antibodies

6 If the HA antigen changes shape, antibodies that normally would match up to it no longer can, allowing the newly mutated virus to infect the body's cells.

This type of genetic mutation is called "**ANTIGENIC DRIFT.**"

Figure 14-5. A schematic depicting the influenza virus undergoing antigenic drift. Image courtesy of the National Institute of Allergy and Infectious Diseases.

virus replicates in the cells, causing desquamation of ciliated epithelium, hyperplasia of transitorial cells, edema, hyperemia, congestion, and increased secretions. Pneumonic complications without secondary bacterial infections can occur; however they usually are due to a secondary infection with bacteria (commonly *S aureus*).

DIAGNOSIS

Diagnosis of influenza is difficult in that there are no pathognomonic signs and the infection can be easily confused with other respiratory tract infections. Influenza can be differentiated from the common cold because the flu results in a high fever but the common cold is an afebrile disease. Differentiating influenza pneumonia from atypical pneumonia may be difficult however; the onset of atypical pneumonia is usually insidious whereas influenza is rapid in onset. Definitive diagnosis requires laboratory procedures such as isolation of the virus or serologic tests. A fluorescent antibody directed against the influenza virus is available to directly test nasal swabs collected from febrile acutely ill patients.

THERAPY AND PREVENTION

In uncomplicated cases of influenza, recovery is usually complete, with no residual effects. Supportive care is recommended for patients with healthy immune systems. Antipyretics and analgesics can provide relief for fever and muscle pain.

Antiviral drugs for influenza are an adjunct to influenza vaccine for controlling and preventing influenza. Four licensed influenza antiviral agents are available in the United States: amantadine, rimantadine, zanamivir, and oseltamivir. Amantadine and rimantadine are effective against influenza A viruses but not against influenza B viruses. Amantadine and rimantadine can be used in chemoprophylaxis and in the treatment of influenza A viral infections in adults. Only amantadine can be used in the treatment of influenza A viral infections and chemoprophylaxis in children aged 1 year or older. Rimantadine can only be used for chemoprophylaxis in children.

Zanamivir and oseltamivir are chemically related antiviral drugs known as neuraminidase inhibitors that have activity against both influenza A and B viruses. Both drugs are approved for treating uncomplicated influenza infections. Zanamivir is approved for treating persons aged 7 years or older, and oseltamivir is approved for treatment of persons aged 1 year or older and for chemoprophylaxis of influenza among persons aged 13 years or older.

Influenza vaccination contains three different influenza viruses (two As and one B). Vaccination and chemoprophylaxis with amantadine, rimantadine, or oseltamivir are useful for the prevention of disease in high-risk groups. Vaccination campaigns begin in mid-October and end in mid-November. Vaccination is recommended for the high-risk groups listed in Table 14-4.

PERTUSSIS

Pertussis (also known as whooping cough) was once a rare disease but is now becoming more common in the United States.

The word pertussis means cough, and the pathognomic whoop following a paroxysmal coughing episode aids greatly in determining the diagnosis. In the United States, *Bordetella pertussis* causes about 95% of cases of pertussis, and *B parapertussis* causes the other 5% of cases.

ETIOLOGY

B pertussis is a gram-negative coccobacillus.

MANIFESTATIONS

Pertussis is a coughing illness that lasts at least 2 weeks and has one of the following manifestations: paroxysms of coughing, inspiratory "whoop," or posttussis vomiting without other apparent cause. The incubation period for pertussis is 7–10 days, which is followed by the **catarrhal phase.** During the catarrhal phase, the disease is indistinguishable from an upper respiratory tract infection. The person is most infectious during this phase, which is characterized by the insidious onset of coryza, sneezing, low-grade fever, and a mild occasional cough similar to the cough of the common cold. The cough gradually becomes more severe and after 1–2 weeks, the second, or paroxysmal, stage begins.

The **paroxysmal phase** begins with episodic sudden coughing and generally lasts 2–4 weeks. The cough is so severe that patients are unable to sleep or eat. The whoop, if present, results from inspiratory stridor and is pathognomonic. The patient has paroxysms of numerous rapid coughs. ***When paroxysm ends, a long inspiratory effort is usually accompanied by a pathognomonic high-pitched whoop.*** During such an attack, the patient may become cyanotic. Vomiting and exhaustion commonly follow the episode. The patient usually appears normal between attacks. Paroxysmal coughing attacks occur more frequently at night, with an average of 15 attacks per 24 hours. Severe cases result in hemoptysis, subconjunctival hemorrhages, hernias, seizures, and death.

Adults with pertussis infection may complain of chronic cough. They may be asymptomatic or they may present with an illness that ranges from a mild cough to classic pertussis, with persistent cough lasting more than 7 days. Inspiratory whoop is uncommon.

PATHOGENESIS

B pertussis is inhaled on respiratory droplets and attaches to the ciliated epithelium in the trachea. The pertussis toxin causes almost all of the tissue damage in the trachea. The pertussis toxin adenosine diphosphate ribosylates guanine–nucleotide-binding protein, affecting regulatory mechanisms in the ciliated cells that line the host's trachea. This causes death and sloughing of the ciliated cells. Other products of importance are the tracheal cytotoxin and a filamentous hemagglutinin. The cytotoxin kills the cells that line the trachea, and the filamentous hemagglutinin is important in the attachment of *B pertussis* to the ciliated cells. Large amounts of mucus are produced in response to the infection and cause the patient to cough. The neurologic effects of infection are associated with hypoxia, lymphocyte plugging, and intracerebral hemorrhage.

EPIDEMIOLOGY

▪ Pertussis occurs worldwide and results in one million deaths a year, with most of the deaths occurring in underdeveloped countries.

▪ The number of cases of pertussis has rapidly increased in the past few years (Figure 14-6); adolescents and adults account for most reported cases (Figure 14-7).

▪ Older patients have better outcomes than younger patients.

▪ Up to 50% of cases of children with pertussis can be traced to adults with a chronic cough. A carrier state does not exist; however persons in close contact with symptomatic patients may transiently harbor the organism.

▪ The most severe cases of pertussis are in children younger than 12 months of age. Prognosis is dependent on the age of the patient, the state of health, and availability of supportive care.

▪ The risk of nonfatal neurologic damage due to infection is at least 6–10 times greater than the risk associated with immunization against pertussis.

▪ The disease is highly infectious. Infection does not ensure protection from a second infection with *B pertussis*.

▪ Humans are the only natural hosts; the disease is transmitted person to person via aerosolized droplets.

DIAGNOSIS

The presence of the whoop is pathognomonic for pertussis. Laboratory procedures necessary for diagnosis include nasopharyngeal aspirates plated on Bordet-Gengou medium, immunofluorescent staining of nasal secretions for *B pertussis*, and serologic testing (ELISA) with acute and convalescent sera. *An elevated white blood cell count with a lymphocytosis is usually present in children,* which is unusual for a bacterial infection. Most bacterial infections result in an increase in neutrophils rather than an increase in lymphocytes.

THERAPY AND PREVENTION

Antibiotics are ineffective in shortening the course of pertussis infection once the patient has entered the paroxysmal stage. If antibiotics are given, erythromycin is the drug of choice and will eradicate the organism from secretions and decrease spread of the infection to others and, if initiated early, may modify the course of the illness.

Supportive care is essential in the prevention of hypoxia and pulmonary complications. An antibiotic effective against pertussis (e.g., azithromycin, erythromycin, or trimethoprim-sulfamethoxazole) should be administered to all close contacts of persons with pertussis, regardless of age and vaccination status.

The best means of preventing pertussis is vaccination. The most commonly used vaccine is the acellular pertussis vaccine (DTaP), which is mixed with diphtheria and tetanus toxoids and is given to children 6 weeks to 6 years of age. Because of the waning immunity of adolescents and adults to pertussis and asymptomatic infections that spread to unprotected infants, vaccine recommendations have been expanded to give persons older than 10 years of age the tetanus-diphtheria-acellular pertussis vaccine rather than the tetanus-diphtheria vaccine for their scheduled booster shot.

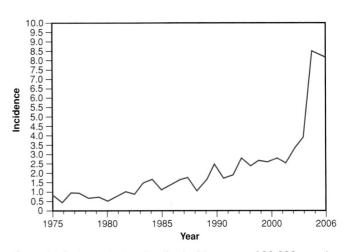

Figure 14-6. A graph showing the incidence per 100,000 population of pertussis in the United States from 1974 to 2005. Notice the rapid increase in the number of cases of the disease from 2002 to 2004. Image courtesy of the Centers for Disease Control and Prevention.

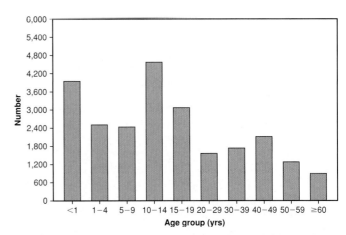

Figure 14-7. A graph showing the number of cases of pertussis, by age group, in the United States in 2005. Notice that about 60% of cases of pertussis occurred in patients aged 10 years and older. Vaccine recommendations encourage using the tetanus-diphtheria-acellular pertussis vaccine for these persons rather than the tetanus-diphtheria vaccine. Image courtesy of the Centers for Disease Control and Prevention.

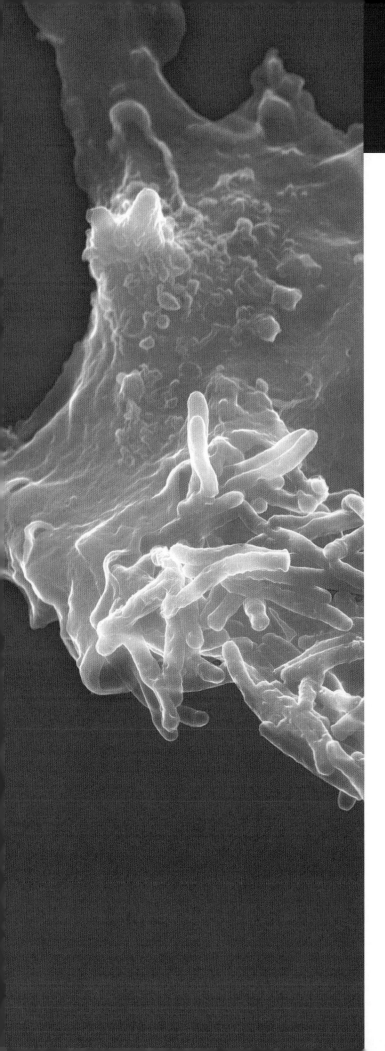

CHAPTER 15

INFECTIONS OF THE LOWER RESPIRATORY TRACT

OVERVIEW

Lower respiratory tract infections cause disease in the alveolar sacs, and the resulting infections are called pneumonia. This chapter will discuss the various types of pneumonia (i.e., typical, interstitial, chronic, and fungal pneumonia) and the agents that cause them.

PNEUMONIA

Pneumonia is an infection of the alveoli or the walls of the alveolar sacs. Diagnosis of pneumonia is relatively straightforward; however, since so many microorganisms can cause pneumonia, determining the cause of a particular patient's pneumonia can be very difficult.

ETIOLOGY

Numerous microorganisms can cause pneumonia, but most cases are caused by bacteria. The common causes of pneumonia are dependent on the immune status of the patient, the location where the patient acquired the pneumonia, the age of the patient, and the type of pneumonia the patient manifests (e.g., typical versus interstitial pneumonia). The clinical and epidemiologic factors are used to determine the most likely cause of each individual case of pneumonia. Table 15-1 lists causes of pneumonia by age of the patient; Table 15-2 lists causes of pneumonia according to the location where the disease was acquired and the immune status of the patient; Table 15-3 lists causes of pneumonia acquired from unusual exposure; Table 15-4 lists causes of pneumonia by time of onset and where acquired; and Table 15-5 lists the most common causes of various types of pneumonia diagnosed in the United States.

MANIFESTATIONS

Many patients who are diagnosed with pneumonia mention having previous flu-like symptoms or an upper respiratory tract infection. A patient with pneumonia will frequently continue to have symptoms of upper respiratory tract infection and develop respiratory symptoms that are indicative of a lower respiratory tract infection—cough, dyspnea, sputum production, and tachycardia. Pneumonia is even more likely to be the diagnosis if the patient also has a fever (**an exception is neonates who are diagnosed with afebrile Chlamydia trachomatis pneumonia**) and auscultatory findings that may include abnormal breath sounds, dullness to percussion, wheezes, and crackles (rales).

Pneumonias can be classified based on how rapid the pneumonia manifests. Acute onset pneumonias develop within 24–48 hours and are common in patients with typical pneumonia. The patient's only complaint may be an upper respiratory infection but manifestations of **typical pneumonia** rapidly develop—high fever, shaking chills, dyspnea, tachycardia, productive cough with purulent sputum production, toxic facies, and consolidations in the lungs as seen on chest radiographs (Figure 15-1; Table 15-6).

Interstitial pneumonia (atypical pneumonia) has a subacute onset; it may take several days to 1 week before the patient

TABLE 15-1. Common Causes of Pneumonia Listed by Patient Age

Age of Patient	Most Likely Organisms Causing the Pneumonia
Neonatal (0–1 month)	*Escherichia coli, Streptococcus agalactiae* (group B)
Infants (1–6 months)	*Chlamydia trachomatis,* respiratory syncytial virus
Children (6 months–5 years)	Respiratory syncytial virus, parainfluenza viruses
Children (5–15 years)	*Mycoplasma pneumoniae,* influenza virus type A
Young adults (16–30 years)	*M pneumoniae, Streptococcus pneumoniae*
Older adults	*Streptococcus pneumoniae, Haemophilus influenzae*

TABLE 15-2. Causes of Pneumonia Listed by Location Where Disease Was Acquired or by the Immune Status of the Patient

Location or Patient's Immune Status	Most Common Causes of Pneumonia	Infrequent Causes of Pneumonia
Community acquired typical pneumonia	*Streptococcus pneumoniae, Haemophilus influenzae, Klebsiella pneumoniae*	*Staphylococcus, Moraxella catarrhalis, Neisseria meningitidis*
Nosocomial pneumonia typical pneumonia	Gram-negative aerobic bacilli (*Enterobacter, Klebsiella, Acinetobacter, Pseudomonas*), *Staphylococcus aureus,* anaerobic bacteria, standard bacteria*	*Legionella, S pneumoniae*
Community acquired primary interstitial pneumonia	*Mycoplasma pneumoniae,* respiratory viruses,[†] influenza virus, *Chlamydophila pneumoniae, Legionella* sp.	Adenovirus, *Chlamydophila psittaci, Chlamydia trachomatis,* primary tuberculosis, acute fungal pneumonias
Hematogenous pneumonia	*Staphylococcus, Streptococcus*	Gram-negative aerobic bacilli
Opportunistic pneumonia occurring in immunocompromised host	Standard bacteria*, *Pneumocystis jirovecii,* cytomegalovirus, herpes simplex virus, *Nocardia,* opportunistic fungi (e.g., *Candida, Phycomycetes mucor, Aspergillus*)	*Legionella, Listeria, Histoplasma, Coccidioides*
Pneumonia acquired by environmental exposure	*Histoplasma capsulatum, Coccidioides immitis, Chlamydophila psittaci, Mycobacterium tuberculosis*	*Burkholderia mallei, Burkholderia pseudomallei Coxiella burnetii, Yersinia pestis, Pasteurella multocida, Paracoccidioides*
Aspiration pneumonia	*Prevotella melaninogenicus, Fusobacterium nucleatum, Peptostreptococcus, Peptococcus,* and other anaerobes, *Staphylococcus,* gram-negative aerobic bacilli	

*Standard bacteria refer to the bacteria that commonly cause community-acquired pneumonias.
[†]Respiratory viruses include influenza, parainfluenza, and respiratory syncytial virus.

TABLE 15-3. Disease, Causative Agent, and Environmental Source of the Patient's Disease

Disease	Causative Agent	Source
Psittacosis (parrot fever)	*Chlamydophila psittaci*	Infected birds
Q fever	*Coxiella burnetii*	Contact with placenta of cattle, sheep, and goats; consumption of unpasteurized milk
Histoplasmosis	*Histoplasma capsulatum*	Soil contaminated by starling, chicken, and bat excreta (Ohio and Mississippi river valleys)
Coccidioidomycosis	*Coccidioides immitis*	Soil in Southwestern United States
Cryptococcosis	*Cryptococcus neoformans*	Pigeon excreta and debris
Plague	*Yersinia pestis*	Contact with wild prairie dogs and infected pets; flea bites; person to person
Melioidosis	*Burkholderia pseudomallei*	Soil
Tularemia	*Francisella tularensis*	Ticks and deerflies; following aerosolization of dead infected animal carcasses by lawn mowers and string weed cutters

develops signs and symptoms of pneumonia—low-grade fever, chills, paroxysmal cough with mucoid sputum or no sputum production, well-appearing facies, and infiltrates in the lungs as seen on chest radiographs (Figure 15-2; see Table 15-6).

Chronic pneumonias can take several weeks to 1 month for symptoms to fully develop. Patients usually present with a history of night sweats, low-grade fever, significant weight loss, productive cough with purulent sputum production, and dyspnea; coin lesions (Ghon focus) in the lungs are seen on chest radiographs.

Symptoms of **aspiration pneumonia** are similar to other acute onset pneumonias, except patients experience recurrent chills rather than a shaking chill, and consolidations in the dependent lung segments are seen on chest radiographs. About one half of patients with aspiration pneumonia will produce foul-smelling sputum (Figure 15-3; Table 15-7).

Some causes of pneumonia that result in unique signs and symptoms

▪ **Legionnaire disease** caused by *Legionella* sp. can result in pneumonia with relative bradycardia, abdominal pain, vomiting, diarrhea, hematuria, mental confusion, abnormal results on liver and renal function tests, and increases in serum creatinine phosphokinase levels.

▪ **Psittacosis** due to *Chlamydophila psittaci* (formerly known as *Chlamydia psittaci*) can result in pneumonia with relative bradycardia, epistaxis, Horder spots, splenomegaly, and a normal or low leukocyte count. This disease is associated with caretakers of psittacine birds.

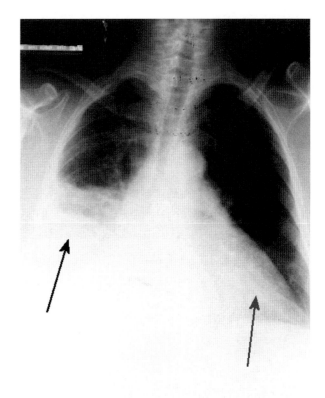

Figure 15-1. A chest radiograph of a patient with Q fever. Notice the consolidations in the right lower lung (*arrow*) and the thickened pericardium (*arrow*). Image courtesy of EM Scrimgeour et al. First report of Q fever in Oman. Emerging Infectious Diseases. Jan-Feb 2000. vol. 6, no. 1. Available at http://www.cdc.gov/ncidod/eid/vol6no1/scrimgeourG2.htm#Dispatches.

TABLE 15-4. Causes of Pneumonia by Time of Onset, Location Where Acquired, and Transmission

Time of Onset	Location Where Pneumonia was Acquired	Transmission	Causative Agents
Acute	Community acquired	Person to person	*Streptococcus pneumoniae, Mycoplasma pneumoniae, Haemophilus influenzae, Staphylococcus aureus, Klebsiella pneumoniae, Neisseria meningitidis, Moraxella catarrhalis*, influenza virus, *Streptococcus pyogenes*
Acute	Community acquired	Animal or environmental exposure	*Legionella, Francisella tularensis, Coxiella burnetii, Chlamydophila psittaci, Yersinia pestis* (plague), *Bacillus anthracis* (anthrax), *Burkholderia pseudomallei* (melioidosis), *Pasteurella multocida* (pasteurellosis)
Acute	Community acquired	Person to person in infants and young children	*Chlamydia trachomatis* (an afebrile pneumonia), respiratory syncytial virus and other respiratory viruses, *Streptococcus agalactiae* (Group B), *S aureus*, cytomegalovirus, *S pneumoniae, H influenza*
Acute	Nosocomial pneumonia	Person to person	Enterobacteriaceae, *Pseudomonas aeruginosa, Acinetobacter calcoaceticus, S aureus*
Subacute interstitial	Community acquired	Person to person	*M pneumoniae*, influenza virus
Subacute	Nosocomial or community acquired	Aspiration	Mixed anaerobic and aerobic gram-negative enteric bacteria, are usually polymicrobial
Subacute or chronic	Nosocomial or community acquired	Person to person or aspiration in the immunocompromised	*Pneumocystis jiroveci*, cytomegalovirus, atypical mycobacterium (e.g., *Mycobacterium kansasii*), *Nocardia, Aspergillus, Phycomycetes mucor, Candida albicans*
Chronic	Community acquired	Person to person	*Mycobacterium tuberculosis,* most common cause of chronic pneumonia. *Blastomyces dermatitides* (most common of cause of fungal pneumonia), *Histoplasma capsulatum, Coccidioides immitis, Cryptococcus neoformans*

TABLE 15-5. Common Causes of Types of Pneumonia and Important Laboratory Findings

Type of Pneumonia	Most Common Cause	Laboratory Findings
Typical	*Streptococcus pneumoniae*	Gram-positive diplococcus (lancet-shaped diplococcus), alpha hemolytic sensitive to optochin antibiotic
Interstitial (atypical)	*Mycoplasma pneumoniae*	No cell wall and cannot be Gram stained; fried-egg appearance on growth medium
Chronic	*Mycobacterium tuberculosis*	Acid-fast positive rod-shaped
Fungal	*Blastomyces dermatitidis*	Broad-based budding yeast
Aspiration (community acquired)	Oral anaerobes or *S pneumoniae*	Anaerobes can include *Prevotella, Peptostreptococcus, Bacteroides, Fusobacterium*
Aspiration (hospital acquired)	Oral anaerobes, gram-negative enterics, or *Staphylococcus aureus*	Anaerobes same as above; gram-negative enterics can include *Klebsiella pneumoniae* and *Escherichia coli*

TABLE 15-6. Comparison of Typical and Interstitial (Atypical) Pneumonias

Feature	Typical Pneumonia	Interstitial (Atypical) Pneumonia
Onset	Sudden	Gradual
Rigors	Single chill	"Chilliness"
Facies	"Toxic"	Well
Cough	Productive	Nonproductive: paroxysmal
Sputum	Purulent (bloody)	Mucoid
Temperature	39.4–40°C	<39.4°C
Pleurisy	Frequent	Rare
Consolidation	Frequent	Rare
Gram stain (sputum)	Neutrophils	Mononuclear cells
White blood cell count and differential count	>15,000/mm^3 with left shift	>15,000/mm^3
Chest radiograph	Defined density, lobar pneumonia	Nondefined infiltrate or interstitial pneumonia
Most common cause	*Streptococcus pneumoniae*	*Mycoplasma pneumoniae*

- **Q fever** due to *Coxiella burnetii* can cause pneumonia with relative bradycardia, tender hepatomegaly, endocarditis, and abnormal liver function tests. Q fever is associated with farmers who have recently birthed livestock.

- **Erythema nodosum and hilar adenopathy** can be seen in patients with pneumonia due to fungi like *Histoplasma capsulatum* (endemic in the Ohio and Mississippi river valleys) and *Coccidioides immitis* (endemic in the Southwestern United States).

- **Fungal pneumonia** is most often caused by *Blastomyces dermatitidis*. It can also produce rough verrucous skin lesions (see Chapter 3). This fungus is endemic in the Southeastern United States.

EPIDEMIOLOGY

- Two to three million cases of pneumonia are reported each year in the United States.

- Patients with pneumonia are responsible for over 10 million patient visits, 500,000 hospitalizations, and 45,000 deaths annually. Together, influenza and pneumonia are the seventh leading cause of death in the United States.

- The patient with pneumonia usually has had a previous viral upper respiratory tract infection.

- Inhalation and aspiration are the two most common means of acquiring an infectious pneumonia.

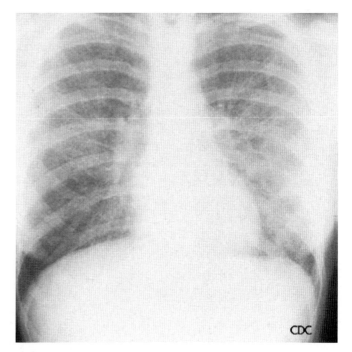

Figure 15-2. A chest radiograph of a patient with interstitial pneumonia due to *Mycoplasma pneumoniae*. Image courtesy of the Centers for Disease Control and Prevention.

- Pneumonia is more common during the winter months and in persons older than 65 years of age.

- Elderly patients are more likely to be hospitalized and die following onset of pneumonia.

- Aspiration pneumonia is an endogenous infection.

- The following conditions predispose persons to aspiration pneumonia: an altered level of consciousness, alcoholism, seizures, anesthesia, central nervous system disorders, trauma, dysphagia, esophageal disorders, and nasogastric tubes.

PATHOGENESIS

There are no resident bacteria in the lower respiratory tract of patients with pneumonia. Organisms that enter the alveoli are eliminated by alveolar macrophages, which are considered the most important means of eliminating organisms that manage to escape the defense mechanisms that occur in the upper respiratory tract and the respiratory airways (see Chapter 12).

Once a microorganism enters the alveoli, it can be opsonized by IgG in the fluid lining the alveoli and then be ingested by the macrophage via their F_c receptors.

1. If there is no specific antibody to the organism present, the macrophage can still phagocytize the invader using receptors that bind C-reactive protein or complement or by receptors to pathogen-associated molecular patterns (PAMPs). Mannan, lipopolysaccharide, lipoteichoic acid, N–formylated methionine-containing peptides, muramyl peptides, and peptidoglycan are all examples of PAMPs, which the alveolar macrophage can use to phagocytize bacterial invaders.

2. When the microorganism is phagocytized, the macrophage will destroy the organism, if possible, and present microbial antigens on the surface to awaiting B cells and T cells.

3. Once activated, the B and T cells can produce more antibody and activate macrophages. Macrophages simultaneously release factors that help carry polymorphonuclear leukocytes (PMNs) from the bloodstream and initiate an inflammatory response. PMNs, antibodies, and complement components are useful in destroying the "invaders."

Many bacteria that cause pneumonia can initially survive in the alveoli due to the following **defense mechanisms.**

1. **Capsule** (e.g., *Streptococcus pneumoniae, Haemophilus influenzae*) production prevents phagocytosis by the alveolar macrophage.

2. **Viruses and *Chlamydia*** invade host cells before the alveolar macrophages can phagocytize them.

3. ***Mycobacterium tuberculosis*** can survive in alveolar macrophages even after being phagocytized.

If the organisms survive in the alveoli, microbial growth can cause tissue injury, which stimulates the host to mount an inflammatory response. Tissue injury can occur due to exotoxins produced by a bacterium, cell lysis caused by a virus, or death of alveolar macrophages and dumping of their lysosomal contents in the alveoli due to growth of an organism in the phagocyte. Vascular permeability increases, and PMNs arrive at

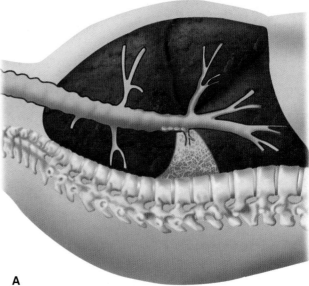

A

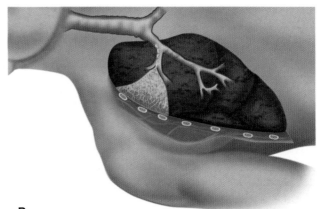

B

Figure 15-3. A schematic showing the relationship between the posture of the patient during aspiration of oral contents and the location of the infection seen in aspiration pneumonia. **A,** If a patient aspirates while lying on their back, the apical segment of the lower lobe of the lung is usually affected. **B,** If a patient aspirates while lying on their side, the lateral and posterior portions of the upper lobe of the lung are usually affected.

TABLE 15-7. Condition or Circumstance and Most Common Causative Agent of Pneumonia

Patient Profile (Condition or Circumstance)	Common Causative Agent(s)
Cystic fibrosis	*Pseudomonas aeruginosa* or *Staphylococcus aureus*
Alchohol abuse	*Klebsiella pneumoniae* or oral anaerobic bacteria (e.g., *Prevotella, Bacteroides, Peptostreptococcus, Fusobacterium*)
Nursing home resident with underlying cardiopulmonary disease; recent antibiotic therapy; or multiple medical comorbidities	Enteric gram-negative bacteria (*Enterobacter, K pneumoniae, Escherichia coli*)
Chronic obstructive pulmonary disease; alcohol abuse; elderly	*Haemophilus influenzae* and *Klebsiella pneumoniae*
Intravenous drug use	*S aureus*
Elderly; recent influenza virus infection	*S aureus*
Military recruits at basic training camp; college students living in dormitories	*Neisseria meningitidis*

the area with many of the serum components, attempting to contain and eliminate the organisms. While the microorganisms are damaging the alveoli, other alveolar macrophages are being recruited to the area of inflammation. Lymphoid tissue associated with the lungs (mediastinal lymph nodes) becomes enlarged following activation of the B and T lymphocytes. Chest radiographs may show evidence of mediastinal lymph node enlargement in the patient with pneumonia.

The accumulation of microorganisms, immune cells, and serum components can cause the alveoli to fill and spread to other alveoli that are in close proximity. This inflammatory response is described as an opacity or a consolidation seen on a chest radiograph, and is often seen in patients with pneumonia caused by *S pneumoniae*—this type of pneumonia is called typical or lobar pneumonia. The inflammatory response to the infection and the microorganisms produce factors that allow the microorganisms to leave the lung and exert systemic effects such as fever. Examples of microbial factors that can have systemic effects include endotoxin from gram-negative bacteria resulting in fever and septic shock, and cell wall components of gram-positive bacteria that can lead to fever and septic shock (see Chapter 28).

Organisms such as *Mycoplasma pneumoniae* and the influenza virus initially do not cause a large amount of fluid to accumulate in the alveoli. However, following infection with these organisms, inflammation of the interstitial spaces (walls of the alveoli) occurs, resulting in interstitial or atypical pneumonia. Chest radiographs of patients with this type of pneumonia show fine granular diffuse infiltrates.

Other organisms such as *Staphylococcus aureus*, gram-negative rod-shaped bacteria, and anaerobic bacteria produce abscesses or microabscesses. In these infections, the immune system can wall off the organisms and produce localized abscesses or microabscesses that usually show well-defined circular lesions with necrotic translucent centers on chest radiographs.

DIAGNOSIS

Patients with pneumonia may present with chest discomfort, cough (productive or nonproductive paroxysmal cough), rigors (patients with typical pneumonia) or chills (patients with interstitial pneumonia), shortness of breath, and fever. Physical examination may reveal increases in respiratory rate and heart rate and dullness to percussion over affected regions of the lungs and rales.

Chest radiographs showing new consolidations or infiltrates are definitive in helping to establish a diagnosis of pneumonia. When alveolar sacs fill with inflammatory cells and fluid, a chest radiograph will show consolidated well-defined densities that are unilateral (inhalation or aspiration pneumonia), bilateral (hematogenous spread to lungs), localized, or uniform. When a chest radiograph shows inflammation and thickening of the alveolar septa that surround the alveoli, rather than a filling of the alveolar sacs with inflammatory material, the diagnosis is more likely to be interstitial pneumonia.

Some organisms form **abscesses in the lung** (e.g., *S aureus*, Enterobacteriaceae, *Pseudomonas aeruginosa,* and anaerobic organisms); in such cases, a chest radiograph is useful in revealing abscess formation. If present, certain classic radiologic patterns may be of diagnostic value; for example,

- ***Klebsiella pneumoniae*** infection causing an upper lobar consolidation can result in a bowing fissure ("bulging fissure" sign).

- ***S aureus*** infections of the lung can cause multiple bilateral nodular infiltrates with central cavitation. In children, the chest radiograph may show ill-defined, thin walled cavities ("pneumatoceles"), bronchopleural fistulas, and empyema.

- ***P aeruginosa*** infections can result in microabscesses, which may coalesce into large abscesses.

- **Gram-negative rod infections** (e.g., *Klebsiella, Proteus, E coli*) often cause lung necrosis.

- ***M tuberculosis pneumonia*** can cause coin lesions.

- Consolidations in the dependent lung segments may indicate **aspiration pneumonia** (see Figure 15-3).

To identify the specific pathogen that is causing the pneumonia, clinical and epidemiologic data must be considered to limit the number of possible causes of the pneumonia (Table 15-8; see Tables 15-1 through 15-4 and Table15-6).

Gram stain of sputum from a patient with suspected pneumonia can be helpful in presumptive determination of the cause of the pneumonia (Figure 15-4). Some pathogens Gram stain poorly or do not Gram stain; if pneumonia is caused by one of the suspected pathogens, Dieterle silver stain (*Legionella* sp.), acid-fast stain (*Mycobacteria*), or Gomori methenamine silver stain (fungi and *Pneumocystis*) (Figure 15-5) should be ordered.

Additional laboratory tests that can aid in establishing a definitive diagnosis

- Culture of the sputum.

- Culture of blood samples for bacteria, fungi, or viruses.

TABLE 15-8. Sputum Appearance and Most Likely Cause or Type of Pneumonia

Sputum Appearance	Most Likely Cause or Type of Pneumonia
Purulent	Typical pneumonia
Mucoid	Interstitial pneumonia
Rust color	*Streptococcus pneumoniae*
Green color	*Pseudomonas aeruginosa* or *Haemophilus influenzae*
Thick currant jelly-like	*Klebsiella pneumoniae*
Large amount of blood	Cavitary tuberculosis and lung abscess
Foul smelling	Anaerobic bacterial pneumonia

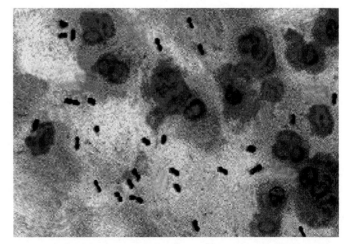

Figure 15-4. A photomicrograph of a Gram stain of sputum from a patient with pneumonia due to *Streptococcus pneumoniae*. Notice the gram-positive diplococci, which are not perfectly round, and the presence of a large number of polymorphonuclear leukocytes.

- Serology to detect antibodies produced against the pathogen or as a result of infection with the pathogen (e.g., cold agglutinins for *M pneumoniae*; detection of antibodies to the capsule of *S pneumoniae*).

- Antigen tests to detect certain antigens produced by the pathogen (e.g., polysaccharide testing for *S pneumoniae* and *H influenzae*).

- Skin tests to detect delayed-type hypersensitivity reactions to certain pathogens (e.g., *M tuberculosis*: Mantoux test, *B dermatitidis*, *H capsulatum*, *C immitis*).

- Polymerase chain reaction (PCR) performed on sputum samples to rapidly determine the cause of the pneumonia (e.g., tuberculosis).

- Urinalysis for *Legionella* antigens.

TREATMENT AND PREVENTION

Because most cases of pneumonia are caused by bacteria, treatment usually involves antibiotic therapy. Tables 15-9 and 15-10 list empiric treatment regimens for patients with pneumonia. In about one half of pneumonia patients, the etiologic agent can be determined and if the agent is known, more definitive therapy can be initiated.

There are two vaccines that can be given to adults to help prevent pneumonia. The *S pneumoniae* vaccine contains 23 capsular types of the bacterial capsule and is used in persons older

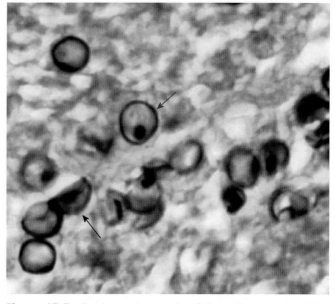

Figure 15-5. A photomicrograph of lung tissue containing methenamine silver stained cysts with cup forms (*black arrow*) and dot-like cyst wall thickenings (*blue arrow*) obtained from a patient with *Pneumocystis jiroveci* pneumonia. Image courtesy of the Centers for Disease Control and Prevention, Dr Edwin P Ewing, Jr.

TABLE 15-9. Treatment of the Pediatric Patient with Pneumonia by Age or Condition and Causative Agent

Patient Age or Condition	Causative Agent	Empiric Therapy
Neonatal pneumonia (birth to 1 month)	*Streptococcus agalactiae*, *Escherichia coli* and other coliforms, *Listeria*, *Staphylococcus aureus*, *Chlamydia trachomatis*, *Treponema pallidum*	Ampicillin + gentamicin ± cefotaxime; add vancomycin if methicillin-resistant *S aureus* is likely; if *Chlamydia* infection, treat with erythromycin
Infants (1–3 months)	*C trachomatis*, *Streptococcus pneumoniae*	Erythromycin or azithromycin **S pneumoniae:** ampicillin
Children 4 months–5 years	*Mycoplasma pneumoniae*, *Streptococcus pneumoniae*, *Haemophilus influenzae*	**Outpatient:** Amoxicillin or azithromycin **Inpatient:** Ampicillin intravenous **Inpatient ICU:** Cefotaxime
Children 5–15 years	*M pneumoniae*, *Chlamydophila pneumoniae*, *S pneumoniae* (uncommon)	**Outpatient:** Clarithromycin or azithromycin **Inpatient:** Ceftriaxone + azithromycin
Children with cystic fibrosis	*S aureus* early in disease, *Pseudomonas aeruginosa* later in *P* disease	For *S aureus*: methicillin sensitive strains: oxacillin/nafcillin; methicillin-resistant strains: vancomycin For *P aeruginosa*: tobramycin + ticarcillin or piperacillin or tobramycin + ceftazine

ICU, intensive care unit.

TABLE 15-10. Treatment of the Adult Patient with Pneumonia by Patient Profile and Causative Agent

Patient Profile	Causative Agent	Empiric Therapy
Viral pneumonia	Influenza virus, parainfluenza, adenovirus, respiratory syncytial virus, hantavirus	For influenza A and B: zanamivir or oseltamivir
Community acquired; *not* hospitalized	**No comorbidity:** *Mycoplasma pneumoniae, Chlamydophila pneumoniae,* viral, *Streptococcus pneumoniae* **Smokers:** *Streptococcus pneumoniae, Haemophilus influenzae, Moraxella catarrhalis* **Postviral bronchitis:** *S pneumonia, Staphylococcus aureus* (rare) **Alcoholic stupor:** *S pneumoniae, Klebsiella pneumoniae* and other coliforms, anaerobes (aspiration) **IV drug abuse:** *S aureus* **Airway obstruction:** Anaerobes	Azithromycin or clarithromycin or fluoroquinolones with enhanced activity against *S pneumoniae* (moxifloxacin > gatifloxacin > sparfloxacin > levofloxacin)
Community acquired; hospitalized	No comorbidity	Cephalexin + erythromycin or azithromycin or fluoroquinolones with enhanced activity against *Streptococcus pneumoniae*
Hospital acquired (nosocomial)	**Poststroke aspiration:** *S pneumoniae,* anaerobes **Water colonization:** *Legionella* sp. **Organ failure:** Coliforms **Mechanical ventilation:** Coliforms, *Pseudomonas aeruginosa, S aureus;* **Steroid use:** Yeast, *Pneumocystis jiroveci*	To cover coliforms, *S pneumoniae,* and anaerobes: Imipenem or meropenem or piperacillin *P jiroveci* pneumonia can be treated with trimethoprim/sulfamethoxazole Yeast infections can be treated with amphotericin B
Aspiration pneumonia and lung abscess	*Bacteroides, Peptostreptococcus, Fusobacterium*	Clindamycin
Chronic pneumonia with fever, night sweats, and weight loss	*Mycobacterium tuberculosis,* coccidioidomycosis, histoplasmosis	Pulmonary tuberculosis: isoniazid + rifampin + pyrazinamide Primary pneumonia due in coccidioidomycosis and histoplasmosis treatment is not usually recommended; if symptoms do not resolve within several weeks to 2 months, treat with itraconazole; for severe disease, treat with amphotericin B

than age 65. The influenza vaccine should be given yearly to all persons older than age 50 to help prevent viral pneumonia or secondary bacterial pneumonia that may occur following infection with the influenza virus. Chemoprophylaxis to prevent influenza infections is helpful in preventing secondary bacterial pneumonia (see Chapter 14).

The conjugated *S pneumoniae* heptavalent vaccine is important in preventing infection with this organism in young children. The conjugated *H influenzae* type b (Hib) vaccine prevents childhood infections with *H influenzae*. Respiratory syncytial virus infections can be prevented in premature infants, neutropenic infants, or in infants with various comorbidities with a periodic injection of respiratory syncytial virus immune globulin or humanized mouse monoclonal antibody (palivizumab). Annual immunization of children with the influenza vaccine prevents influenza infections in vaccinated children and appears to prevent spread of the virus to close contacts that may be at high risk for adverse outcomes following this viral infection.

SECTION 5

GASTROINTESTINAL TRACT AND LIVER

CHAPTER 16

THE BIG PICTURE: INFECTIONS OF THE GASTROINTESTINAL TRACT AND LIVER

OVERVIEW

Viewed in its simplest form, the gastrointestinal tract is a hollow digestive tube that extends through the center of the body from the mouth to the anus (Figure 16-1). The walls of the tube are lined with a diverse number of epithelial cells that function well at transmembrane secretion and absorption and maintain the barrier that protects the host from microbial pathogens. The barrier consists of the intact mucosal surface and a population of resident immune cells. The primary function of the gastrointestinal system is digestion and nutrient uptake.

The epithelial cells have a relatively short life, with most cells living between 48 and 72 hours. Because of mitosis (the constant turnover of cells), it is difficult for pathogens to colonize the gastrointestinal tract. However, the disadvantage of the high rate of mitosis is that the epithelial cells are more susceptible to mutagenic compounds and tumor formation.

All of the liquid and solid material ingested, along with bacteria, is carried through the tube. Bacteria colonize the areas of the tube that offer a suitable environment for growth. Soon after birth, a normal flora is established in each part of the tube. The oral cavity and the colon are at opposite ends of the tube and are heavily colonized with bacteria, and the central part of the tube, the stomach, duodenum, jejunum, and the proximal half of the ileum, are lightly colonized (Figure 16-2).

Each portion of the gastrointestinal tract has special defense mechanisms that protect it from pathogenic microorganisms. When pathogenic microorganisms or their toxins breach these defense mechanisms, disease can occur.

DEFENSE MECHANISMS OF THE GASTROINTESTINAL TRACT

The following are some of the major defense mechanisms in the gastrointestinal tract that serve to prevent infection. There are other defense mechanisms, but they will not be discussed here because they are beyond the scope of this chapter.

An **unbroken mucosal epithelium** lines all parts of the gastrointestinal system. The epithelial cells are continually sloughed off and replaced. If cell replacement is impeded (e.g., radiation therapy or cancer chemotherapy), ulceration of the mucosa can occur. The ulcer no longer is lined with epithelial cells and that surface of the ulcer can be infected. The infection can damage the blood vessels in the wall of the gastrointestinal tract, causing septicemia and fever.

The **glycocalyx** is a glycoprotein and polysaccharide layer that covers the surface of the epithelial cells. This layer presents a thick physical barrier that prevents pathogens from attaching to the epithelial cells and serves as a chemical trap that binds microorganisms of the normal flora.

Mucus plays two roles in disease prevention: (1) It acts as a physical barrier, making it more difficult for bacteria to access the epithelial cell surfaces; and (2) it coats the bacteria, making it easier to remove via peristalsis.

The normal pH of the stomach is < 4 (i.e., acidic). This **acidity** spills into the small intestine and establishes a pH gradient that prevents most bacteria from colonizing the stomach, duodenum, jejunum, and the upper half of the ileum. Therefore, most ingested pathogens never reach the intestinal tract alive.

Bile solubilizes lipids and inactivates organisms that have a lipid envelope. All enveloped viruses are inactivated, and many bacteria are unable to grow at a high bile salt concentration.

Secretory IgA helps prevent colonization by pathogens.

Peristalsis contributes to the health of the gut by aiding in fluid absorption, maintaining appropriate dilution of indigenous enteric microflora, and ridding the host of pathogenic microorganisms.

Peyer patches are unencapsulated patches of lymph follicles in the mucosa and submucosa and provide a homing site for lymphocytes. M cells lining the intestine process antigens and present antigens to the lymphocytes in the Peyer patches. The intestinal mucosa is in a constant state of "physiologic inflammation." The lamina propria is a thin layer of connective tissue that lies just below the intestinal epithelium. It contains capillaries and a central lacteal (lymph vessel) as well as numerous neutrophils, macrophages, plasma cells, and lymphocytes. After invasive infections, a vigorous inflammatory reaction ensues, resulting in many white blood cells entering the lumen of the intestine from the lamina propria.

Most of the **normal flora** in the gastrointestinal tract is composed of anaerobic bacteria, which competes with pathogens for nutrients and epithelial cell receptor sites and keeps them from causing disease (see Figure 16-2). The anaerobes in the normal flora are members of the *Bacteroides*, *Prevotella*, *Clostridium*, and *Peptostreptococcus* genera.

FACTORS THAT COMPROMISE THE GASTROINTESTINAL TRACT

The gastrointestinal tract is constantly challenged by pathogenic microorganisms that compromise the gastrointestinal tract.

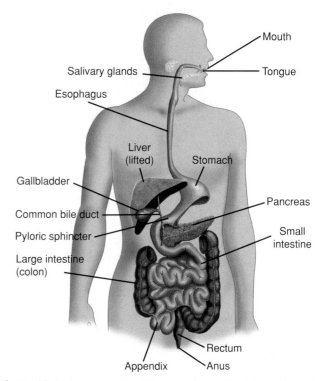

Figure 16-1. A schematic of the gastrointestinal tract, from the mouth to the anus.

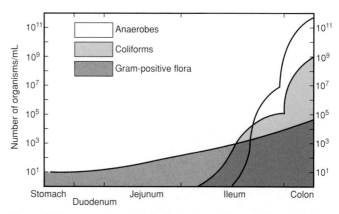

Figure 16-2. A graph showing the number of anaerobes, coliforms, and gram-positive bacteria in the gastrointestinal tract, beginning at the stomach and ending at the colon. The term "coliform" is not a taxonomic group but rather a descriptive term that defines a group of gram-negative, facultative anaerobic rod-shaped bacteria that ferment lactose to produce acid and gas. They can be found in the intestines of humans and warm-blooded animals.

Ingestion of antacids neutralizes stomach acid and allows microorganisms to proliferate in areas that have very few normal flora.

Antibiotic therapy eliminates the normal flora and allows colonization by pathogens.

Glucosteroid therapy inhibits the immune response, making it more conducive for gastrointestinal tract infections to develop.

Cancer chemotherapy and radiation therapy reduce the normal flora and the cellular and humoral immunity as well as the integrity of the intestinal epithelium.

Ingestion of preformed toxins and microorganisms produces toxins, enzymes, and immunosuppressive factors that can overcome the host defenses and cause disease.

Obstructions to the flow of liquids remove a powerful defense mechanism of the gastrointestinal tract (see above). Large diverticula and stasis of the intestines following abdominal surgery can result in severe complications for many patients.

ETIOLOGY

Many organisms cause gastrointestinal diseases, including bacteria, viruses, fungi, and parasites (Table 16-1).

MANIFESTATIONS

Despite all of the defense mechanisms that serve to prevent infection in the gastrointestinal tract, there are numerous diseases associated with the gastrointestinal and hepatobiliary systems (Figure 16-3).

AREAS AFFECTED AND MANIFESTATIONS OF DISEASES

Mouth: Ulcers on mucosal surfaces in the mouth, white or erythematous lesions on mucosa; white plague on teeth, dental caries, tooth pain and sensitivity to heat or cold, bleeding gingiva; petechia; facial pain or swelling, abscess, and cellulitis.

Salivary glands: Jaw pain when swallowing; swelling under jaw.

Esophagus: Dysphagia (difficulty in swallowing), odynophagia (painful swallowing; unique to infectious causes of esophagitis), heartburn, atypical chest pain, and regurgitation.

Stomach: Epigastric pain and tenderness that occurs 90 minutes to 3 hours after eating; vomiting, belching, indigestion, and heartburn.

Small intestine: Large volume watery diarrhea; fatty stools, increased bowel sounds, cramps, diffuse abdominal pain; *no* guarding or rebound tenderness.

Large intestine: Small volume bloody diarrhea with mucus (dysentery); cramps, diffuse abdominal pain, white blood cells frequently found in stool, and fever; *rarely* any guarding or rebound tenderness.

Liver: Upper right quadrant abdominal pain; fever, icterus, clay-colored stools, dark urine.

TABLE 16-1. Microorganisms that Cause Gastrointestinal Diseases and the Site Most Often Affected

Microbial Agent	Disease	Site Affected
Bacteria		
Corynebacterium diphtheriae	Diphtheria (see Chapter 13)	Oropharynx
Streptococcus pyogenes	Pharyngitis (see Chapter 13)	Oropharynx
Streptococcus mutans	Dental caries	Teeth
Anaerobic bacteria	Gingivitis, periodontal disease, dentoalveolar abscess, periodontal abscess, Ludwig angina	Gingiva for all but Ludwig angina Ludwig angina: sublingual and submandibular spaces
Helicobacter pylori	Gastritis, peptic ulcer disease	Stomach and duodenum
Staphylococcus aureus, enterotoxin producing	Nausea and vomiting and diarrhea	Increased serotonin release in intestine stimulates vagal afferent neurons
Bacillus cereus	Type 1 with nausea and vomiting Type 2 with diarrhea	Type 1 uncouples oxidative phosphorylation in liver mitochondria Type 2 in small intestine
Campylobacter jejuni	Diarrhea, dysentery, and fever	Intestine
Enterotoxigenic *Escherichia coli,* Enteropathogenic *E coli,* Enteroaggregative *E coli*	Diarrhea	Intestine
Enterohemorrhagic *E coli*	Diarrhea followed by bloody diarrhea, hemolytic uremic syndrome	Intestine, kidney
Enteroinvasive *E coli*	Diarrhea occasionally becoming dysentary	Intestine
Shigella sonnei, Shigella flexneri	Diarrhea followed by dysentery	Intestine
Salmonella enterica	Diarrhea followed by dysentery	Intestine
Salmonella typhi	Typhoid fever, enteric fever	Intestine, liver, spleen, blood, bone marrow, gallbladder
Salmonella paratyphi A, Salmonella schottmuelleri, Salmonella hirschfeldii	Paratyphoid fever, enteric fever	Intestine, liver, spleen, blood, bone marrow
Clostridium difficile	Diarrhea, pseudomembranous colitis, toxic megacolon	Colon
Virus		
Epstein-Barr virus	Infectious mononucleosis; pharyngitis	Oropharynx
Herpes simplex virus types 1 and 2	Gingivostomatitis	Gingiva, mucosa of mouth, lips, esophagus

TABLE 16-1. Microorganisms that Cause Gastrointestinal Diseases and the Site Most Often Affected (continued)

Microbial Agent	Disease	Site Affected
Human immunodeficiency virus	Esophagitis	Esophagus
Rotavirus	Diarrhea	Intestine
Caliciviruses (Norwalk, and Norwalk-like viruses, Norovirus)	Diarrhea	Intestine
Adenovirus	Diarrhea	Intestine
Astrovirus	Diarrhea	Intestine
Hepatitis A, B, C, D, and E viruses	Hepatitis	Liver
Fungus		
Candida albicans	Pseudomembranous candidiasis (thrush), esophagitis	Mouth, esophagus
Parasite		
Ascaris lumbricoides	Abdominal tenderness diffuse with partial or complete bowel obstruction	Intestine, appendix, bile duct, liver
Cryptosporidium parvum	Diarrhea	Intestine
Giardia lamblia	Diarrhea	Intestine
Strongyloides stercoralis	Anorexia, weight loss, nausea, chronic diarrhea or constipation, bloating	Intestine
Entamoeba histolytica	Dysentery	Colon
Enterobius vermicularis	Anal pruritus	Rectum

Peritoneum: Sharp, localized abdominal pain aggravated by motion; fever, chills, constipation, abdominal distension, decreased bowel sounds; guarding and rebound tenderness.

EPIDEMIOLOGY

Gastrointestinal diseases are the second most common cause for visits to a physician. Diarrhea is one of the most common gastrointestinal diseases among adults. Approximately 270 million cases of diarrhea in adults result in about 600,000 hospitalizations and 3000 deaths annually in the United States; an etiologic agent is identified in less than 10% of these cases. Most adults have at least one episode of diarrhea each year, and children have an average of two to three episodes per year. Many patients with diarrhea acquire the organism that causes their illness while ingesting contaminated food. Over 76 million cases of food poisoning occur each year in the United States.

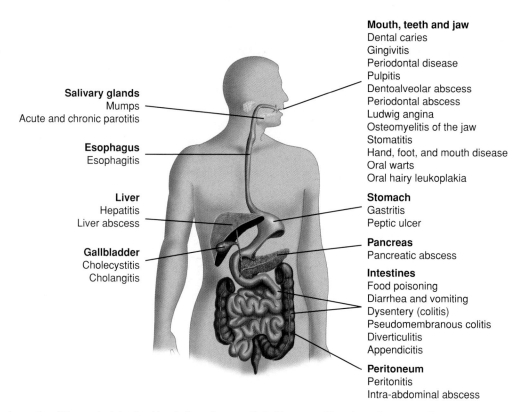

Salivary glands
Mumps
Acute and chronic parotitis

Esophagus
Esophagitis

Liver
Hepatitis
Liver abscess

Gallbladder
Cholecystitis
Cholangitis

Mouth, teeth and jaw
Dental caries
Gingivitis
Periodontal disease
Pulpitis
Dentoalveolar abscess
Periodontal abscess
Ludwig angina
Osteomyelitis of the jaw
Stomatitis
Hand, foot, and mouth disease
Oral warts
Oral hairy leukoplakia

Stomach
Gastritis
Peptic ulcer

Pancreas
Pancreatic abscess

Intestines
Food poisoning
Diarrhea and vomiting
Dysentery (colitis)
Pseudomembranous colitis
Diverticulitis
Appendicitis

Peritoneum
Peritonitis
Intra-abdominal abscess

Figure 16-3. A schematic of the gastrointestinal tract, from the mouth to the anus. Listed are the many diseases that are associated with the gastrointestinal and hepatobiliary systems.

PATHOGENESIS

The pathology associated with a particular gastrointestinal tract disease depends on the site infected or intoxicated. There are two basic mechanisms that infectious agents utilize in causing disease in these systems. One mechanism involves ingesting a preformed toxin that will cause symptoms such as food poisoning. This is called **intoxication.** The most common cause of food poisoning in the United States is due to intoxication with enterotoxin produced by *Staphylococcus aureus*. Symptoms of intoxication usually occur relatively rapidly, with an incubation period as brief as 30 minutes after ingestion of the toxin.

The other mechanism that infectious agents utilize to cause disease in the gastrointestinal tract involves **attachment to or infection of the host cells.** Some pathogens only attach to the surface of the epithelial cells and produce toxins while attached to the host cell, which causes cell damage or death. This process often results in a watery diarrhea without inflammatory cells, blood in the stools, or fever. After attaching to the cells, other pathogens enter the cells and damage or kill them. Depending on how deep the infection penetrates, symptoms can vary from a watery diarrhea (gastroenteritis), to bloody mucus-covered stool (dysentery), to invasion of the bloodstream from the intestine (enteric fever). In cases of dysentery, red blood cells and fecal leukocytes are frequently present in the feces and are a good clinical indicator of an invasive inflammatory gastrointestinal tract infection. Symptoms occur about 24–72 hours after ingestion, and if the host mounts a significant immune response, patients may have a fever. Note that the incubation period is much longer in this process than when the mechanism for causing a disease is intoxication.

DIAGNOSIS

Localizing where pathology is occurring in the gastrointestinal tract is essential to knowing how to treat the patient. Many gastrointestinal tract infections are self-limiting, whereas others require treatment to prevent severe complications. In many cases, the manifestations observed in the patient can help the physician determine the specific area of the gastrointestinal tract that is affected (e.g., diarrhea usually indicates a patient has an intestinal disease).

Once the affected area of the gastrointestinal tract is identified, procedures (e.g., endoscopy) can be performed to visualize the pathology associated with the disease and samples (e.g., stools, blood) obtained to determine the cause of the disease.

TREATMENT AND PREVENTION

The treatment and prevention of a particular infection depends on the site of the infection and the pathogen causing the disease. These topics will be discussed in more detail in Chapters 17 through 22 when the specific infections are discussed.

To prevent many gastrointestinal tract infections, patients should be encouraged to maintain good oral hygiene, properly cook and store all food, drink safe water, and take special precautions when traveling to countries outside the United States. Patients should avoid using illegal intravenous drugs, having frequent sexual contacts, and drinking excessive amounts of alcohol.

All travelers to countries where diarrheal diseases are common should observe the following recommendations. Only water that has been boiled or treated with chlorine or iodine should be used, and remember that ice is frequently made with contaminated tap water. Freezing and thawing of ice does not kill many of the organisms and is a source of infection for many travelers. Only foods that have been thoroughly cooked and are still hot and fruit that can be peeled just before eating should be consumed. All vegetables should be cooked; salads should never be eaten because vegetables are washed with tap water. Undercooked or raw fish or shellfish should not be eaten; perishable seafood should not be taken from the restaurant. Foods and beverages should not be purchased from street vendors. *A simple rule of thumb to follow when traveling overseas is to boil it, cook it, peel it, or forget it!*

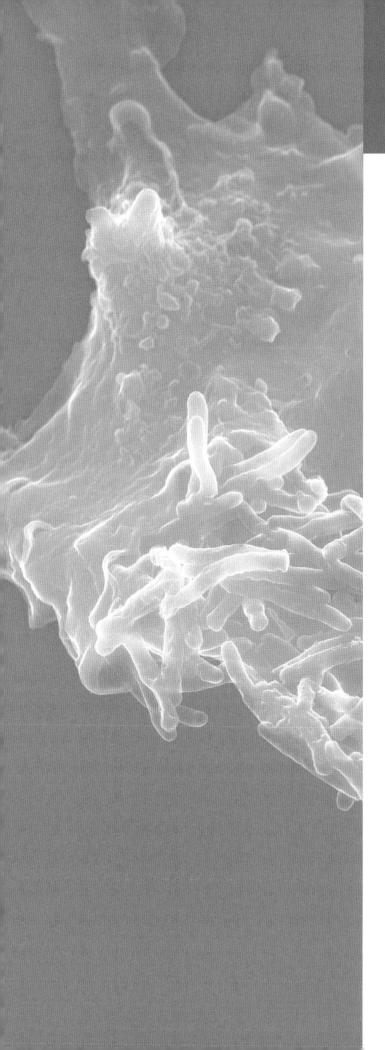

CHAPTER 17

INFECTIONS OF THE TEETH, GINGIVAE, AND JAWS

INFECTIONS OF THE TEETH AND GINGIVAE

OVERVIEW

Dental caries, gingivitis, and periodontal diseases usually are not diagnosed and treated by physicians; however, poor oral hygiene can result in infections that are of concern to physicians. Infections of the teeth and gingivae can spread to contiguous structures (e.g., sinusitis, osteomyelitis of the jaw, aspiration pneumonia). To better care for patients with these diseases, an introductory understanding of the diseases is useful. Dental caries is a lesion of the enamel and dentine of the teeth (Figure 17-1); gingivitis is an infection of the gingivae (gums); and periodontal diseases are disorders of the supporting structures of the teeth (e.g., gingivae, periodontal ligament, and supporting alveolar bone).

ETIOLOGY

Streptococcus mutans is the most common cause of dental caries. Plaque-associated periodontal disease that begins as gingivitis and develops into periodontal disease is a polymicrobial process involving the organisms listed in Table 17-1.

MANIFESTATIONS

Dental caries are small pits that form on the smooth surfaces and in the fissures of the teeth; the pits can enlarge forming necrotic centers (see Figure 17-1). Gingivitis causes the gingivae to be swollen, red, and tender, and bleed during tooth brushing (Figure 17-2). Periodontal disease results in periodontal pockets forming around the roots of the teeth and also in gingivitis (Figure 17-3).

EPIDEMIOLOGY

Dental caries, gingivitis, and periodontal disease are ubiquitous; however, with good oral hygiene and preventive dental practices, the incidence is decreasing in the Western world.

Dental caries is the leading cause of tooth loss in children younger than age 12.

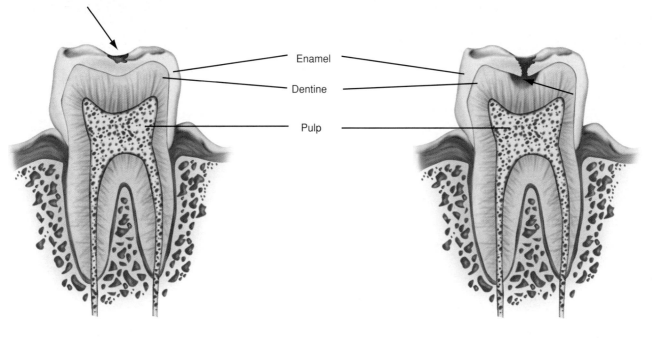

A. Enamel caries   B. Dentine caries

Figure 17-1. A schematic illustrating dental caries. **A,** Early enamel caries; **(B)** early dentine caries, neither of which usually results in pain. However, dentine caries may be sensitive to heat and cold and sweet foods and drinks.

Gingivitis and periodontal disease is the leading cause of tooth loss in adults and is present in 8–10% of the adult population.

PATHOGENESIS

Dental caries is a chronic infection of enamel or dentine due to bacteria normally found in the mouth (see Figure 17-1). A biofilm containing high numbers of *Streptococcus mutans* forms on the surface of the tooth. The bacteria in the plaque break down sugar in the saliva and produce acid that damages the enamel of the tooth and eventually forms a cavity on the surface of the tooth. If untreated, microbes can extend the lesion into the dentine and then into the pulp. If the pulp is infected, the tooth may die, and there is increased risk of development of periapical abscesses. Complications include pulpitis and dentoalveolar abscess.

Gingivitis results when increased numbers of normal flora grow in the gingival crevice and produce toxins that cause an inflammatory reaction in the gums. Plaque accumulates in the crevice resulting in an inflammatory reaction. Complications include development of periodontal disease.

Periodontal disease is an inflammation of the supporting structures of the teeth. It begins as gingivitis that spreads down to the root surface causing alveolar bone resorption and pocket formation. It can eventually lead to alveolar bone loss and damage the periodontal ligament, which causes tooth loss. Other complications include periodontal abscess and osteomyelitis of the jaws.

TABLE 17-1. Bacterial Causes of Gingivitis and Periodontal Disease

Bacteria	Gram Stain and Shape
Actinobacillus actinomycetemcomitans	Gram-negative rod
Bacteroides forsythus	Gram-negative rod
Capnocytophaga	Gram-negative rod
Eubacterium sp.	Gram-positive bacillus
Fusobacterium nucleatum	Gram-negative rod
Micromonas (Peptostreptococcus) micros	Gram-positive coccus
Porphyromonas gingivalis	Gram-negative rod
Prevotella intermedia	Gram-negative rod
Selenomonas	Gram-negative curved rod
Oral spirochetes (*Treponema denticola,* most have not been named yet)	Unable to Gram stain; spiral shape

DIAGNOSIS

Medical patients with dental caries, gingivitis, and periodontal disease are usually referred to a dentist for diagnosis, treatment, and preventive maintenance.

THERAPY AND PREVENTION

To prevent dental caries, gingivitis, and periodontal disease, patients should be encouraged to brush and floss their teeth daily, obtain professional dental examinations and cleanings twice a year, and avoid sweet and sticky foods.

INFECTIONS OF THE PERIAPICAL TISSUE AND JAW

Dentoalveolar abscesses form at the end of the tooth root. **Periodontal abscesses** form deep in the gingivae along the tooth root following advanced periodontal disease.

Ludwig angina is a cellulitis of the sublingual and submandibular spaces and can rapidly become fatal without treatment. **Osteomyelitis of the jaw** is an inflammation of the bone and the muscles around the jawbones and is more commonly seen in the mandible.

ETIOLOGY

Dentoalveolar and periodontal abscess, Ludwig angina, and osteomyelitis of the jaw are all polymicrobial infections (Table 17-2).

MANIFESTATIONS

Dentoalveolar abscesses usually cause pain in and around the affected tooth, and there may be swelling of the face over the site of the abscess. Periodontal abscess manifests similar to dentoalveolar abscess (i.e., pain and facial swelling over the site of the abscess); however, the patient with periodontal abscess also has signs of periodontal disease.

A patient with **Ludwig angina** is severely ill and has a fever, severe dysphagia, trismus, and dysphonia. The patient has brawny edema and erythema of the neck under the chin and often of the floor of the mouth that is tender to the touch (Figure 17-4). The patient will experience ***intense pain upon tongue movement***. The mouth is usually open, and the tongue is lifted upwards and backwards so that it is pushed against the roof of the mouth and the posterior pharyngeal wall. When this occurs, acute respiratory obstruction is likely to follow. Examination shows a brawny, tense swelling of the submaxillary and submental regions with enlargement of the neighboring lymphatic gland.

Osteomyelitis of the jawbone causes restricted jaw motion, pscudoparalysis, and hyperemic, warm, edematous, and tender soft tissue around the inflamed bone. Actinomycosis of the jaw may also present with a localized swelling at the angle of the mandible.

EPIDEMIOLOGY

With the advent of good oral hygiene, most infections of the periapical tissue and jaw are relatively uncommon.

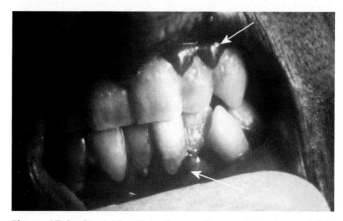

Figure 17-2. Gingivitis. Note the swollen, red gingivae of this patient. Image courtesy of the Centers for Disease Control and Prevention.

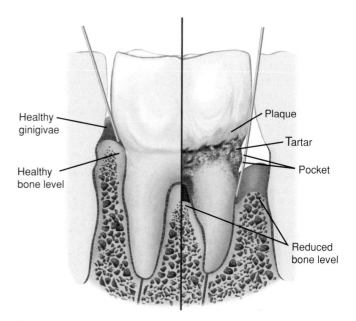

Figure 17-3. A schematic comparing healthy gingivae to the gingivae and jawbone of a person with periodontal disease.

Ludwig angina is the most commonly encountered infection of the neck space. It is uncommon but *if not treated, has a mortality rate of about 50%.*

Most cases of Ludwig angina occur following a dental infection.

PATHOGENESIS

Dentoalveolar abscess usually follows an infection of the pulp of the tooth that extends to the base of the roots. Periodontal abscesses usually are an extension of periodontal disease and form deep in the gingivae along the roots of the teeth.

Ludwig angina is a rapidly swelling cellulitis of the sublingual and submaxillary spaces, often arising from infection of the tooth roots (molars and premolars) that extend below the mylohyoid line of the mandible. Ludwig angina can also occur following infections in the floor of the mouth, the base of the tongue, and the lingual tonsils, and following salivary calculi or from intravenous injection of the internal jugular vein (especially in intravenous drug users).

DIAGNOSIS

Diagnosis of **dentoalveolar and periodontal abscesses** is usually determined based on the patient's signs and symptoms. Radiographs of the affected areas can be helpful.

Ludwig angina is usually diagnosed based on clinical signs and symptoms. CT scans and blood cultures can be helpful. The disease can quickly become life threatening; therefore, rapid diagnosis is important to the survival of patients.

Osteomyelitis can be diagnosed using radiographs; however, radiographs are not very sensitive and usually do not detect osteomyelitis early in the disease process. The patient may have an infection for up to 3 weeks before the infection is detectable on a radiograph. When detectable, the radiograph will show a "moth-eaten" appearance of the bone that is positive for osteomyelitis. CT scans are more sensitive than plane radiographs, and MRIs are more sensitive than CT scans and can detect changes even earlier. Tissue samples and culture may help to identify the causative agents. In cases of actinomycosis, needle aspiration of the abscess can be helpful. If sulfur granules are present in the aspirate, Gram stains should be performed to demonstrate gram-positive branching filamentous bacteria in the sample.

THERAPY AND PREVENTION

Patients with **dentoalveolar abscesses** should be referred to a dentist. Tooth extraction or a root canal and antibiotic therapy may be necessary. Patients with periodontal abscess should also be referred to a dentist. Tooth extraction or drainage of the abscess followed by periodontal and antibiotic treatments are usually required.

Treatment of Ludwig angina involves four principal components.

1. Adequate airway management is essential.

2. Antibiotic therapy must be designed to cover both anaerobes and *Staphylococcus aureus*. Penicillin with or without metronidazole is the first-line therapy.

TABLE 17-2. Causes of Dentoalveolar and Periodontal Abscesses, Ludwig Angina, and Osteomyelitis of the Jaw

Disease	Causative Agents
Dentoalveolar abscess	Strict anaerobes found in the oral mucosa
Periodontal abscess	Gram-negative rods, *Streptococcus* viridans group, anaerobic streptococci, spirochetes
Ludwig angina	*Streptococcus, Bacteroides, Fusobacterium, Staphylococcus aureus*
Osteomyelitis of the jaw	Gram-negative rods, anaerobic streptococci, *Actinomyces israelii*

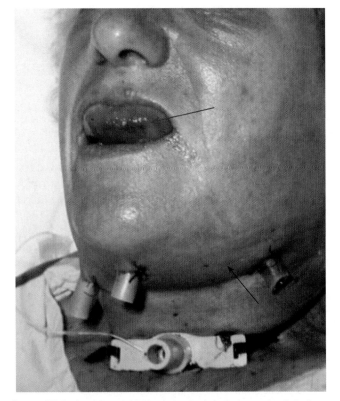

Figure 17-4. A patient with Ludwig angina that required drainage and a tracheotomy. The patient's tongue is forced up to the roof of the mouth (*blue arrow*) causing her to drool; there is erythema and swelling (*black arrow*) present below her chin and lower jaw. Image courtesy Bechara Y Ghorayeb, MD. Otolaryngology, Houston, Texas. http://www.ghorayeb.com.

3. In the past, incision and drainage of abscesses was routine. Surgical therapy now is usually reserved for cases of failure of medical treatment.

4. Attention to adequate nutrition and hydration should be given, since both are difficult to maintain in a patient with significant oropharyngeal edema.

Treatment of **osteomyelitis** consists of antibiotic therapy for an extended period (4–6 weeks). The specific antibiotic therapy depends on the cause of the infection. A bone biopsy should be obtained to determine the cause of the infection; surgical debridement maybe necessary to eliminate the infection.

Dentoalveolar and periodontal abscesses, Ludwig angina, and osteomyelitis of the jaw can usually be prevented by encouraging good oral hygiene, regularly visiting the dentist, and treating oral and dental infections promptly.

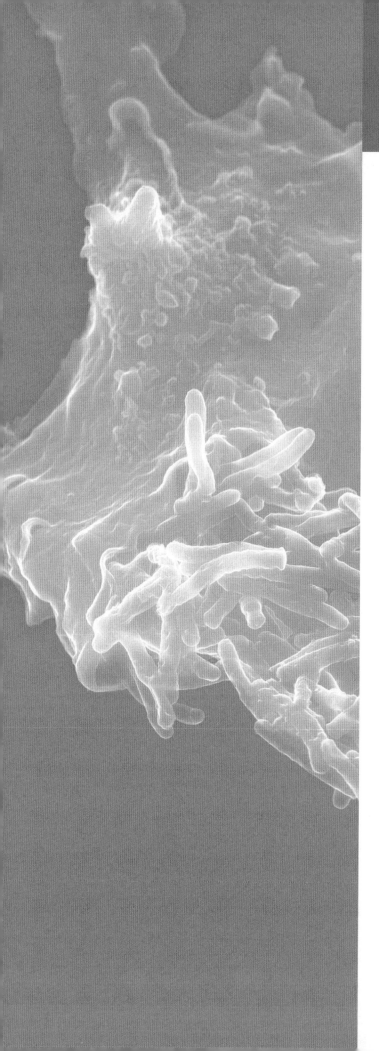

CHAPTER 18

INFECTIONS OF THE MOUTH, TONGUE, AND PAROTID GLANDS

OVERVIEW

This chapter will discuss several of the infectious diseases of the mouth, tongue, and parotid glands. These diseases include stomatitis, due to the herpes simplex viruses and to *Candida albicans,* and oral hairy leukoplakia, angular cheilitis, and parotitis.

STOMATITIS

Stomatitis is an inflammation of the mucosal surfaces in the mouth and on the tongue, and is most often caused by herpes simplex virus type 1 (HSV-1), HSV-2, and *C albicans.* If the inflammation includes the gingivae, it is called gingivostomatitis (common in HSV infections).

ETIOLOGY

The most common cause of gingivostomatitis, or oral herpes, is HSV-1, and the most common cause of candidiasis is *C albicans* (oral candidiasis). HSV-2 can also cause oral herpes, but it is less common than HSV-1.

MANIFESTATIONS

The incubation period of gingivostomatitis due to HSV-1 and HSV-2 is 1–2 days. The duration of the illness is 2–3 weeks; during this time, the patient may experience fever, fatigue, muscle aches, and irritability. Pain, burning, tingling, or itching may occur at the site of infection before sores appear; clusters of blisters then erupt (Figure 18-1). The blisters break down rapidly, appearing as tiny shallow gray ulcers on a red base. The most intense pain caused by the sores occurs at the onset, causing eating and drinking to be difficult. Sores may occur on the lips, gingivae, front of the tongue, inside of the cheeks, the throat, and the roof of the mouth (Figure 18-2) and may also extend down the chin and neck. The gingivae may become red and mildly swollen and may bleed. Cervical lymph nodes often swell and become painful. Herpes may cause pharyngitis, with shallow ulcers and a grayish coating on the tonsils of persons usually in their teens and twenties.

Types of candidiasis

1. **Acute pseudomembranous candidiasis, or thrush,** is characterized by the presence of creamy-white plaques (pseudomembranes) that consist of superficial mucosal cells, neutrophils, and yeast cells. Plaques can be found on the tongue, soft palate, cheek, gingivae, and pharynx. Lesions often begin as tiny focal areas that enlarge to white plaques, or patches (Figure 18-3). Lesions are difficult to remove when scraped with a tongue blade, resulting in an inflamed base that is painful and may bleed. In neonates and infants, there is usually a white coating in the mouth and the infant may have difficulty feeding. Candidal infection in the diaper area may accompany acute pseudomembranous candidiasis (Figure 18-4). Candidiasis may spread to the esophagus in immunocompromised hosts.

2. **Erythematous candidiasis** consists of red lesions of varying sizes that can occur on any part of the oral mucosa (Figure 18-5). If present on the tongue, lesions can be painful, fiery red, and shiny, with evidence of depapillation. This disease can be acute or chronic.

3. **Hyperplastic candidiasis, or candidal leukoplakia,** is usually an individual lesion on the oral mucosa of the cheek near the commissure, at the angles of the mouth, or on the surface of the tongue. Lesions are chronic, discrete, and raised, and may vary from a small palpable translucent or whitish area to a large dense opaque plaque that is hard and rough to the touch. Homogeneous or speckled areas, which do not rub off, can be seen. Speckled red-white lesions have an increased chance of malignant transformation.

EPIDEMIOLOGY

Oral herpes

Oral herpes is a common infection that affects about 60% of the population by 15 years of age. Mouth sores occur most commonly in children aged 1–2 years, but stomatitis can occur in persons at any age.

HSV-1 and HSV-2 infect only humans.

HSV-1 and HSV-2 are transmitted person to person following contact with infected saliva, mucous membranes, or skin, and by sharing cups or utensils. HSV-1 causes about 80% of oral herpes infections.

HSV-2 is usually transmitted to the oral cavity via oral sex and also can be transmitted orally from person to person through contact with infected saliva.

Asymptomatic shedding of HSV-1 and HSV-2 occurs periodically; it is possible for persons without herpetic lesions to infect others through shedding.

Candidiasis

C albicans is a common inhabitant of the oral flora, and any disturbance of this flora can result in overgrowth of the yeast.

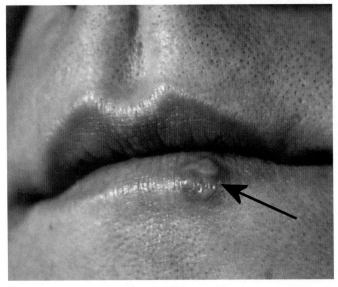

Figure 18-1. A herpetic lesion on the lower lip of a patient. Notice the blisters on the lower lip (*arrow*) of the patient. Image courtesy of the Centers for Disease Control and Prevention, Dr Hermann.

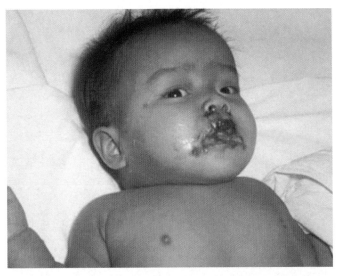

Figure 18-2. A 10-month-old child with oral herpetic lesions. Image courtesy of the Centers for Disease Control and Prevention, JD Millar.

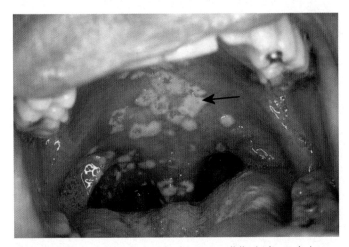

Figure 18-3. Oral pseudomembranous candidiasis (*arrow*). Image courtesy of the Centers for Disease Control and Prevention, Sol Silverman, Jr, DDS.

Candidiasis is a common endogenous disease in patients with certain predisposing conditions (Table 18-1).

Acute pseudomembranous candidiasis occurs in up to 37% of newborns. It is usually a mild and self-limiting disease and is usually seen about the fourth week of life.

The organism can also reside in the lower gastrointestinal tract; candidal diaper rash is often seen in conjunction with acute pseudomembranous candidiasis in neonates.

Acute pseudomembranous candidiasis can occur at any age in predisposed patients (see Table 18-1).

Erythematous candidiasis is most common in denture wearers.

C albicans is acquired during passage down the birth canal; by sharing drinking cups and eating utensils; during breast-feeding; and following contact with contaminated saliva.

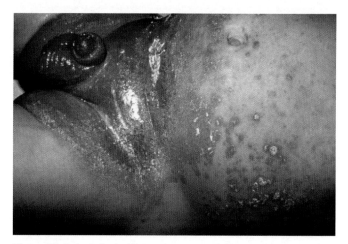

Figure 18-4. An infant with a severe case of diaper rash due to *Candida albicans*. Image courtesy of the Centers for Disease Control and Prevention.

PATHOGENESIS

Oral herpes results in painful sores on the lips, gingivae, tongue, roof of the mouth, and on the mucous membranes lining the cheeks. ***After infection,* HSV-1 and HSV-2 have the ability to progress to the following stages.**

1. During primary infection, the virus enters the skin or mucous membrane and reproduces in the mucosal cells. During this stage, oral sores and other symptoms such as fever may develop. The virus can cause asymptomatic infections, which occur twice as often as symptomatic disease.
2. The virus moves from the infected site to nerves in the region—the trigeminal root ganglion—and establishes itself latently in the host nerves. The virus reproduces and becomes inactive in the ganglion. ***HSV-1 and HSV-2 become latent in the ganglia of the host and remain in the host for a lifetime.***
3. During times of emotional or physical stress, the virus can multiply in the ganglion, and viral particles can move to the skin and cause recurrence of the vesicular lesions on the skin around the mouth and nose. ***Recurrent lesions usually are seen in the skin around the nose and mouth, and rarely inside the mouth.***

Acute pseudomembranous candidiasis results when there is a disturbance of the normal oral flora (e.g., antibiotic therapy, emotional or physical stress). *C albicans* will overgrow on the oral mucosa causing desquamation of epithelial cells and accumulation of bacteria, keratin, and necrotic tissue. This debris combines to form a pseudomembrane, which adheres closely to the mucosa.

Erythematous candidiasis can be an acute or a chronic condition. It is an inflammatory response to *Candida* overgrowth without the pseudomembrane or a candidal infection after the pseudomembrane sheds. It can occur following acute pseudomembranous candidiasis after the white plaques have shed de novo in AIDS patients, in patients receiving prolonged topical steroids or broad-spectrum antibiotic therapy, or in persons who wear dentures.

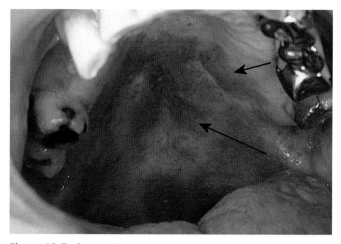

Figure 18-5. Oral erythematous candidiasis due to *Candida albicans*. Image courtesy of the Centers for Disease Control and Prevention, Sol Silverman, Jr, DDS.

TABLE 18-1. Predisposing Factors or Conditions for Candidiasis

Patients taking broad-spectrum antibiotics
Patients taking steroids (inhaled and systemic); children on inhaled steroids have increased incidence of oral candidiasis
Patients with polyendocrine disorders (e.g., diabetes mellitus)
Patients with xerostomia (dry mouth; Sjögren syndrome; after radiotherapy)
Patients with underlying immune dysfunction (e.g., HIV infection)
Persons who smoke (30–70% are more likely to have *Candida albicans* in the oral mucosa)
Persons who wear dentures
Infants and neonates

Hyperplastic candidiasis is characterized by parakeratinization of areas in the mouth with marked hyperplasia and candidal hyphae invading the parakeratinized layer at right angles and superficial to the surface. Lesions may become malignant.

DIAGNOSIS

Diagnosis of **herpes gingivostomatitis** is usually based on clinical signs and symptoms; culture and serologic tests can be performed on the virus. Scraping the base of the ulcer usually results in a positive Tzanck test (presence of multinucleated giant cells) (Figure 18-6).

Diagnosis of **candidiasis** is usually based on clinical signs and symptoms. Lesions can be swabbed and samples cultured on Sabouraud dextrose agar. The lesions can be scraped and stained with periodic acid–Schiff or Gomori methenamine silver stain to reveal the pseudohyphae of the yeast. Hyperplastic conditions should be biopsied for histology. Pseudomembranous lesions are removable; hyperplastic lesions are not.

TREATMENT AND PREVENTION

Herpes gingivostomatitis is self-limiting and usually does not require treatment; however, if severe, penciclovir or valacyclovir can be given. Treatment is not curative, and the disease can recur. Treatment of candidiasis includes use of nystatin rinses, fluconazole, or itraconazole.

ORAL HAIRY LEUKOPLAKIA

Oral hairy leukoplakia is a disease of the lateral borders of the tongue (Figure 18-7). It is most commonly seen in immunocompromised patients (e.g., human immunodeficiency virus [HIV] infection), patients with malignant tumors, and in organ transplant recipients.

ETIOLOGY

Oral hairy leukoplakia is caused by a combination of at least two important factors. One factor is that the patient is usually severely immunocompromised, and HIV infection is the most common cause of immunocompromise resulting in oral hairy leukoplakia. Another factor that is important to consider is that the patient has also been previously infected with the Epstein-Barr virus (EBV).

MANIFESTATIONS

Oral hairy leukoplakia is usually a nonpainful white plaque that occurs along the lateral borders of the tongue (see Figure 18-7). It is restricted to this region of the mouth and only rarely spreads to contiguous sites—the floor of the mouth, tonsillar pillars, ventral tongue, and pharynx.

EPIDEMIOLOGY

The incidence of oral hairy leukoplakia in intravenous drug users and homosexual men infected with HIV is about 4%.

Oral hairy leukoplakia is most common in male homosexuals infected with HIV.

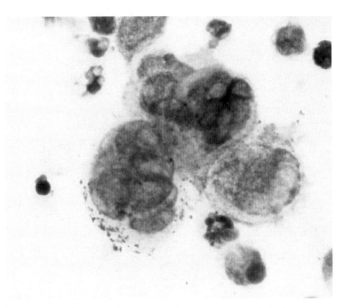

Figure 18-6. A photomicrograph of a positive Tzanck test that contains multinucleated giant cells obtained from the base of a vesicular lesion. Image courtesy of the Centers for Disease Control and Prevention, Joe Miller.

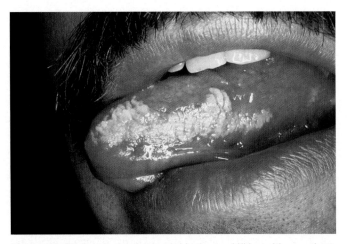

Figure 18-7. Oral hairy leukoplakia in an HIV-positive patient. Image courtesy of the Centers for Disease Control and Prevention, JS Greenspan, BDS., University of California, San Francisco, and Sol Silverman, Jr, DDS.

PATHOGENESIS

Currently, there is very little information known about the pathogenesis of oral hairy leukoplakia, but what is known is that a person with a history of infection with EBV becomes immunocompromised and the number of CD4 T lymphocytes decreases. During this time of immunosuppression, the patient who is latently infected with EBV cannot suppress EBV replication in the oral mucosa. EBV produces viral proteins important in viral replication and in tumor formation. These viral proteins contribute to the development of oral hairy leukoplakia and induction of many of the histologic features such as acanthosis (benign thickening of the mucosa) and hyperproliferation of the epithelial cells on the lateral surface of the tongue.

DIAGNOSIS

Diagnosis of oral hairy leukoplakia is based on clinical grounds (see Figure 18-7). It is quite similar in appearance to pseudomembranous candidiasis (thrush). However, the white plaques associated with oral hairy leukoplakia cannot be removed like those of pseudomembranous candidiasis. The lesions of pseudomembranous candidiasis are usually more widespread in the mouth and are painful, whereas oral hairy leukoplakia is usually seen only on the lateral surface of the tongue and is painless. The white plague can be sampled using a sterile endocervical brush, and the sample stained using the Papanicolaou technique. Cells characteristic of oral hairy leukoplakia have Cowdry type A inclusions, a ground glass appearance, and nuclear beading.

TREATMENT AND PREVENTION

Oral hairy leukoplakia is rarely treated unless the patient is infected with HIV. Patients infected with HIV are treated with highly active antiretroviral therapy (HAART), which helps to resolve the plaque. Podophyllum resin and acyclovir in combination, or podophyllum resin, acyclovir, valacyclovir, famciclovir, ganciclovir, or foscarnet alone are used when oral hairy leukoplakia is specifically treated.

ANGULAR CHEILITIS

Angular cheilitis, also known as angular stomatitis or perlèche, is an inflammation of the angles of the mouth (Figure 18-8).

ETIOLOGY

The most common cause of angular cheilitis is *C albicans*. If yellow crusting appears, *Staphylococcus aureus* is also likely to be involved.

MANIFESTATIONS

The lesions of angular cheilitis affect the angles of the mouth; soreness, erythema, and fissuring are characteristic manifestations (see Figure 18-8).

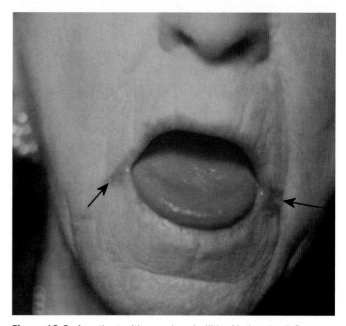

Figure 18-8. A patient with angular cheilitis. Notice the inflammation at the angles of the mouth (*arrows*) of this patient. Image courtesy of the Centers for Disease Control and Prevention.

EPIDEMIOLOGY

Angular cheilitis is usually seen in elderly persons because they are more likely to have sagging facial muscles and ill-fitting dentures, which produce a fold in the angle of the mouth. It may also be seen in persons with HIV infection.

Children who suck their fingers or thumbs and traumatize their lips are more likely to develop angular cheilitis.

Other causes of angular cheilitis include vitamin B deficiency and iron deficiency anemia.

PATHOGENESIS

Angular cheilitis involves erythema and maceration of the skin adjacent to the angle of the mouth.

DIAGNOSIS

Diagnosis of angular cheilitis is usually determined based on signs and symptoms. The lesion can be swabbed and cultured to determine the organisms involved.

TREATMENT AND PREVENTION

Treatment of angular cheilitis includes topical application of hydrocortisone 1% and clioquinol 3%. Prevention can include proper nutrition and referral to a dentist for proper fitting dentures.

PAROTITIS

The mumps virus and *S aureus* can cause inflammation in any of the salivary glands. However, because the parotid gland is affected most frequently, these two infections are called benign viral parotitis (mumps) and acute bacterial parotitis.

Benign viral parotitis (mumps)
Mumps is a common childhood inflammatory disease of the salivary glands with occasional serious complications. Although infection of the parotid glands is the most common manifestation, many other organs can be involved (e.g., epididymoorchitis, oophoritis, aseptic meningitis). The incidence of mumps has decreased dramatically since the introduction of the mumps vaccine.

ETIOLOGY

Mumps is caused by an RNA virus in the paramyxovirus family, called the mumps virus.

MANIFESTATIONS

Mumps is usually asymptomatic. If a clinically apparent case of mumps occurs, a prodrome of myalgia, anorexia, malaise, and a low-grade fever usually precedes the parotitis. The parotitis can include swollen and tender salivary glands, with the parotid gland most commonly affected (Figure 18-9). The patient may also complain of earaches, which last about 1 week and are usually bilateral. The orifices of the submandibular (Wharton duct) and parotid (Stensen duct) ducts become red and swollen with pinpoint petechial hemorrhages. Obstruction of these inflamed

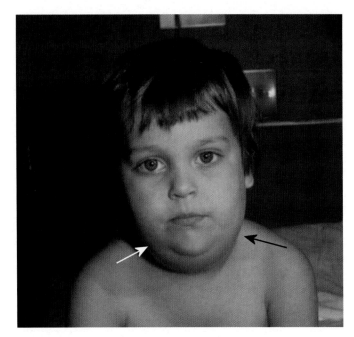

Figure 18-9. A child with parotitis (*arrows*) due to the mumps virus. Image courtesy of the Centers for Disease Control and Prevention.

ducts by edema or cellular debris causes pain when chewing or drinking. The mumps virus can also infect and cause inflammation of the pancreas, thyroid, prostate, and lacrimal glands.

Other systems infected by the mumps virus include the central nervous system (CNS) and the male and female reproductive systems. Mumps virus infection of the CNS results in **aseptic meningitis.** Symptoms include fever, headache, nausea and vomiting, and lethargy, and usually subside within 3–10 days after onset. The virus can cause permanent damage to the vestibulocochlear nerve, which results in unilateral deafness in most cases. Mumps virus infection of the epididymis and the testis causes a bilateral inflammation of the testis called **epididymoorchitis.** Epididymoorchitis occurs abruptly and includes bilateral testicular swelling, tenderness, nausea and vomiting, elevated temperature, and chills. Sterility due to mumps orchitis is rare. The condition is usually seen in adolescent patients.

Mumps virus infection of the ovaries causes an inflammation of the one or both ovaries. Symptoms of **oophoritis** include abdominal tenderness and pain that can mimic appendicitis if the right ovary is involved. There is no evidence that the mumps virus causes impaired fertility in females. However, if a pregnant woman acquires the mumps virus during the first trimester of pregnancy, there is an increased chance of fetal death and abortion. If the mother acquires the mumps virus during the second or third trimester, there is little risk of congenital disease. Neonatal mumps infection is extremely rare.

EPIDEMIOLOGY

- Distribution of the mumps virus is worldwide, and humans are the only known reservoir.

- Before introduction of the mumps vaccine (measles-mumps-rubella [MMR]) in 1967, about 50% of children contracted the disease. Currently, about 1500 cases of mumps are reported each year. The male to female ratio is 1:1.

- Before universal vaccination of children with the MMR vaccine, mumps was one of the leading causes of childhood deafness (1:15,000 cases of mumps). Deafness was unilateral in 75% of cases.

- **Mumps** is primarily a childhood disease, with about 95% of all cases occurring in children younger than 15 years of age.

- The mumps virus infects the CNS in about 50% of patients and can result in **aseptic meningitis.** Symptoms are seen in 10% of cases, and males are more likely to be symptomatic than females (male to female ratio is 3:1). Severe encephalitis may occur and is seen in 2.6 per 1000 cases; in 1.4% of those cases, it is fatal.

- **Epididymoorchitis** occurs in about 20% of postpubertal males who contract mumps.

- **Oophoritis,** or ovarian mumps, occurs in 5% of postpubertal females.

- Viral transmission of mumps occurs through inhalation of respiratory droplets or by direct person-to-person contact. Patients are infectious 2–3 days before symptoms appear until 9 days after symptoms disappear. ***The mumps virus is***

highly contagious. One third of cases are subclinical, yet they are also infectious to other susceptible individuals.

PATHOGENESIS

The mumps virus usually enters the body through the upper respiratory tract and infects regional lymph nodes. A viremia occurs and disseminates the virus to the meninges, salivary glands, testes, pancreas, ovaries, kidneys (most patients have impaired renal function), thyroid, eyes, and mammary glands. The mumps virus has a tropism for glandular tissue and is neurotropic causing meningitis, encephalitis, myelitis, polyneuritis, polyradiculitis, and cranial neuritis.

DIAGNOSIS

The clinical signs and symptoms of mumps usually suffice for diagnosis of mumps parotitis. The parotid gland feels jelly-like; the overlying skin usually *is not warm* to the touch as occurs in bacterial parotitis. Orchitis, pancreatitis, and aseptic meningitis are often associated with high total white cell counts (above 20,000/mm^3 with a high number of polymorphonuclear leukocytes). Rapid diagnosis can be made directly on pharyngeal cells or on urine sediment using an immunofluorescence assay for viral antigen.

THERAPY AND PREVENTION

Symptomatic treatment of mumps is recommended to alleviate distress associated with the patient's symptoms. A live attenuated mumps vaccine is available for infants 12–15 months of age and is given in the MMR vaccine. A second dose of the MMR vaccine should be given to children at 4–6 years of age. ***The vaccine should NOT be given during pregnancy because the viruses in the MMR vaccine are live attenuated viruses that can cross the placenta, causing fetal damage.***

Acute bacterial parotitis

Acute bacterial parotitis is an infection of the salivary glands. Previously, it was a frequent cause of mortality in terminally ill dehydrated patients and had a high mortality rate; however, with the advent of antibiotic and intravenous fluid therapy, the disease is now relatively uncommon.

ETIOLOGY

The most common cause of acute bacterial parotitis is *S aureus*.

MANIFESTATIONS

Patients with acute bacterial parotitis experience progressively painful swelling of the salivary glands. Chewing increases the pain. The swollen glands are tender to the touch, and the skin overlying the swollen glands is erythematous and warm (Figure 18-10). Massage of the affected glands results in purulent saliva.

EPIDEMIOLOGY

Acute bacterial parotitis is more common in elderly patients who are more likely to be taking medications with an

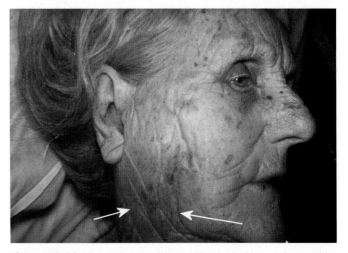

Figure 18-10. An elderly patient with staphylococcal parotitis. Notice the erythema and swelling under the patient's jaw (*arrows*). Image courtesy of the Centers for Disease Control and Prevention, Dr Thomas F Sellers, Emory University, Atlanta, GA.

atropine effect, which retards salivary flow and predisposes the patient to ascending infection.

Patients who are dehydrated, chronically ill, or postoperative, or patients who have dry mouth are more likely to develop acute bacterial parotitis.

PATHOGENESIS

If the flow of saliva is affected, bacteria can enter the ducts and ascend to the salivary gland, causing inflammation and pain.

DIAGNOSIS

Clinical presentation is helpful in determining the diagnosis of the patient with acute bacterial parotitis. In mumps, the glands are tender to the touch but the overlying skin is not erythematous, nor is it warm to the touch as it is in acute bacterial parotitis. Massaging the patient's inflamed salivary glands expresses purulent saliva. The purulent saliva can be Gram stained and cultured to identify the causative agent.

THERAPY AND PREVENTION

Treatment of acute bacterial parotitis involves intravenous antibiotics (e.g., empiric therapy, vancomycin) and rehydration of the patient. The choice of antibiotics can be changed based on the results of culture and antibiotic sensitivity. If antibiotic treatment fails to resolve the infection, incision and drainage may be necessary. This infection can be prevented by ensuring proper hydration of chronically ill patients, elderly patients, and postoperative patients.

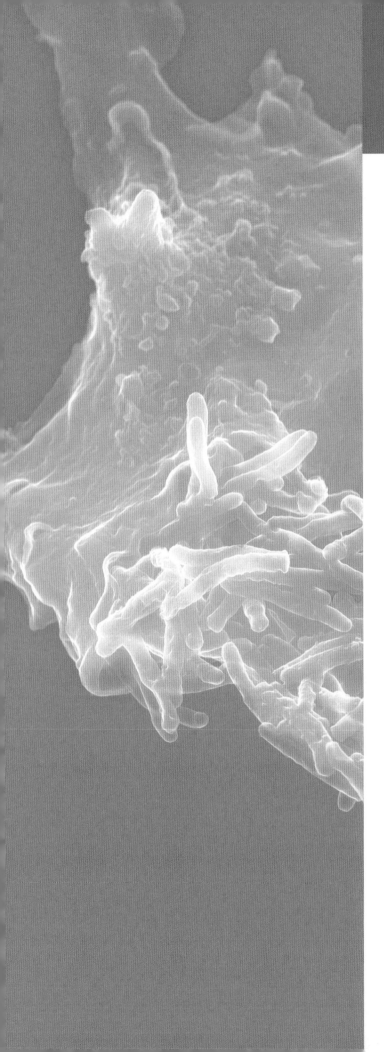

CHAPTER 19

INFECTIONS OF THE ESOPHAGUS, STOMACH, AND UPPER DUODENUM

OVERVIEW

This chapter will discuss infectious diseases of the esophagus (esophagitis), the stomach (gastritis and gastric ulcers), and the upper duodenum (duodenal ulcers). A general term used when referring to ulcers of the stomach and duodenum is peptic ulcer disease. Esophagitis usually occurs in immunocompromised persons.

ESOPHAGITIS

Infectious esophagitis is an infection and inflammation of the esophagus that results in dysphagia and odynophagia.

ETIOLOGY

Many different microorganisms can cause infectious esophagitis; however, *the most common infectious cause of esophagitis is Candida albicans*. Other important causes include cytomegalovirus (CMV), herpes simplex virus (HSV), varicella-zoster virus (VZV), and human immunodeficiency virus (HIV).

MANIFESTATIONS

A patient with esophagitis has acute onset of dysphagia (difficulty swallowing), odynophagia (painful swallowing), heartburn, retrosternal discomfort or pain, nausea and vomiting, fever, abdominal pain, epigastric pain, anorexia, weight loss, and cough (Figure 19-1). See Table 19-1 for unique manifestations of infectious esophagitis listed by causative agent.

EPIDEMIOLOGY

Esophagitis is most common in immunocompromised patients. Symptomatic infection is increased in patients with acquired immunodeficiency syndrome (AIDS), leukemia, and lymphoma, but uncommon in the general population.

C albicans esophagitis is an AIDS-defining condition in a patient infected with human immunodeficiency virus (HIV).

Approximately 8–28% of AIDS patients with dysphagia and odynophagia have been found to have cultures positive for CMV.

Major predisposing factors of esophagitis include antibiotic use, radiation therapy or chemotherapy, hematologic malignancies, and AIDS.

PATHOGENESIS

Infectious esophagitis usually occurs in immunosuppressed persons. A wide range of abnormalities in host defense may predispose a person to this opportunistic infection such as neutropenia, impaired chemotaxis, phagocytosis, alteration in humoral immunity, and impaired T-cell lymphocyte function. Corticosteroids, cytotoxic agents, radiation, and immune modulators may also contribute to impaired host immune function. Disruption of mucosal protective barriers and antibiotics that suppress the normal bacterial flora can also contribute to invasion of the esophagus by organisms in the normal flora.

Patients with HIV and persistently low CD4 counts are more likely to develop fungal esophagitis. Illnesses that interfere with esophageal peristalsis such as achalasia, progressive systemic sclerosis, and esophageal neoplasias can increase the likelihood of developing fungal esophagitis. Patients with systemic diseases such as diabetes mellitus, adrenal dysfunction, and alcoholism, and the elderly are also more likely to develop infectious esophagitis.

DIAGNOSIS

Odynophagia (painful swallowing) is a symptom that is unique to infectious esophagitis. If a patient with dysphagia (difficulty swallowing) also mentions odynophagia, esophagogastroduodenoscopy (EGD) is the preferred procedure to confirm the diagnosis because it allows direct visualization and sampling of the mucosal tissue (Figure 19-2).

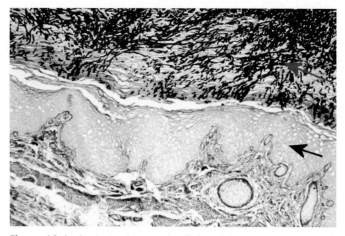

Figure 19-1. A photomicrograph of *Candida* esophagitis stained with methenamine silver stain and digitally colorized. Notice the large number of black pseudohyphae in the pseudomembranous material (*red arrow*) on the surface of the esophagus (*black arrow*). Image courtesy of the Centers for Disease Control and Prevention.

TABLE 19-1. Unique Manifestations of Esophagitis by Causative Agent

Causative Agent	Manifestation(s)
Candida albicans	Patients usually also have acute pseudomembranous candidiasis (see Figure 19-2; see Chapter 18)
Herpes simplex virus (HSV)	Abrupt onset of symptoms Earliest esophageal lesions are 1- to 3-mm round vesicles located in the middle to distal esophagus Multinuclear giant cells are present (identified by Tzanck test in biopsy material)
Cytomegalovirus (CMV)	Gradual onset of symptoms No cases of CMV esophagitis have been reported in hosts with normal immune function Large solitary shallow ulcers or multiple discrete lesions at the distal end of the esophagus are often present
Human immunodeficiency virus (HIV)	Early lesions are small and aphthoid (thrush-like) and occur during a period of transient fever, chills, malaise, and the rash seen in early HIV infection Later, giant deep ulcers as large as several centimeters in diameter can be seen Fistula formation, perforation, hemorrhage, or superinfection may complicate large ulcers
Varicella-zoster virus	Patients usually have dermatologic lesions consistent with chickenpox or shingles

TREATMENT AND PREVENTION

Infectious esophagitis due to *C albicans* can be treated with clotrimazole. Patients with infectious esophagitis due to HSV or CMV can be treated with ganciclovir. Corticosteroids can be given to reduce the inflammatory response. Patients should avoid situations that cause immunosuppression or destroy the composition of the normal flora (e.g., broad-spectrum antibiotic therapy).

INFECTIONS OF THE STOMACH AND UPPER DUODENUM

Chronic active gastritis, gastric ulcer disease, and duodenal ulcer disease are inflammatory diseases that are usually caused by *Helicobacter pylori*. Chronic active gastritis is an inflammation or irritation of the stomach lining; gastric ulcer disease develops in the stomach; and duodenal ulcer disease is chronic and recurrent and results in deep and sharply demarcated ulcers within the first 3 cm of the duodenum. The more general term used is peptic ulcer disease (PUD), which includes both gastric and duodenal ulcer disease (Figure 19-3).

ETIOLOGY

The most common cause of infectious chronic active gastritis and PUD is *H pylori*, a short, spiral-shaped, microaerophilic gram-negative bacillus. Most cases of gastric carcinoma are the consequence of lifelong *H pylori* infection and the effect that this chronic infection has on mucosal carcinogenesis.

MANIFESTATIONS

Chronic active gastritis is usually asymptomatic; however, when symptoms do exist, they include pain or discomfort, with the pain usually located in the upper central portion of the abdomen (the "pit" of the stomach) (Table 19-2). Symptoms can occur suddenly, which is particularly true in persons older than 65 years of age.

The most common symptom of PUD is gnawing or burning pain in the epigastrium, which typically occurs when the stomach is empty (90 minutes to 3 hours after a meal), between meals, and in the early morning hours (see Table 19-2). The duration of pain may be minutes to hours. Symptoms of PUD may last for weeks to months, with remissions that may last months to years followed by recurrence of the symptoms.

EPIDEMIOLOGY

Approximately 50% of the world's population is infected with *H pylori*; prevalence of the infection in the United States is about 35–40%.

In the United States, *H pylori* is most prevalent among adults older than 60 years of age and in African Americans, Hispanics, and lower socioeconomic groups.

Chronic active gastritis

About 20% of individuals infected with *H pylori* develop chronic active gastritis.

The male to female ratio of chronic active gastritis is 1:1.

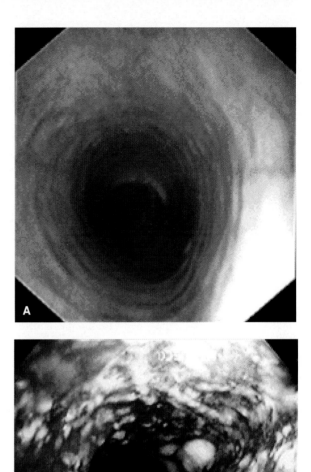

Figure 19-2. Endoscopic images of (**A**) a normal esophagus (*top panel*) and (**B**) an esophagus with a severe *Candida albicans* esophagitis (*bottom panel*). Note the white pseudomembranous growth on the surface of the esophagus in the image on the bottom. Image courtesy of Robert D Fusco, MD, Three Rivers Endoscopy Center, Moon Township, PA. http://www.gihealth.com.

PUD

Over 25 million Americans will suffer from PUD during their lifetime. Each year, there are 500,000 to 850,000 new cases of PUD and more than one million ulcer-related hospitalizations.

Most cases of PUD are caused by H pylori, NOT by spicy foods, acid, or stress.

The primary factor predisposing people to PUD is colonization with *H pylori*; genetic factors also may be important predisposing factors for PUD. About 50% of children with duodenal ulcer disease have a first- or second-degree relative with duodenal ulcer disease.

Persons with blood group O have a higher incidence of duodenal ulcer disease.

Duodenal ulcerative disease usually occurs in persons 25–75 years of age.

Gastric ulcerative disease usually occurs in persons 55–65 years of age.

The male to female ratio for gastric and duodenal ulcer disease is 2:1.

There is an association between long-term infection with *H pylori* and the development of gastric adenocarcinomas or lymphomas.

Transmission of *H pylori* is person to person, and humans are the only known reservoir.

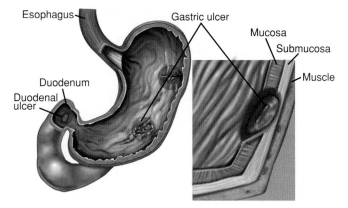

Figure 19-3. A schematic showing peptic ulcer disease. Note the location of the gastric ulcer and the duodenal ulcer.

TABLE 19-2. Manifestations of Gastritis and Peptic Ulcer Disease (PUD)

Disease	Manifestations
Chronic active gastritis	Pain usually located in the upper central portion of the abdomen or the "pit" of the stomach, may feel like it is "going right straight through" as it travels from the belly to the back Pain is a burning, aching, gnawing, or sore Urge to belch, but belching either does not relieve the pain or relieves it only briefly Nausea and vomiting (vomitus may be clear, green, or yellow and blood-streaked or completely bloody)
Critically ill patient with chronic active gastritis	All the symptoms listed above for chronic active gastritis and in addition patients may become pale and sweaty, and experience tachycardia Vomit blood, have bloody stools or dark sticky, foul-smelling stools
PUD (includes gastric and duodenal ulcers)	Gnawing or burning pain in the epigastrium Bleeding that may result in anemia, weakness, and fatigue Hematemesis, hematochezia, or melena

Unique characteristics of gastric and duodenal ulcerative disease

Gastric ulcer	Pain is made worse by eating
Duodenal ulcer	Pain is usually relieved by eating or by antacids

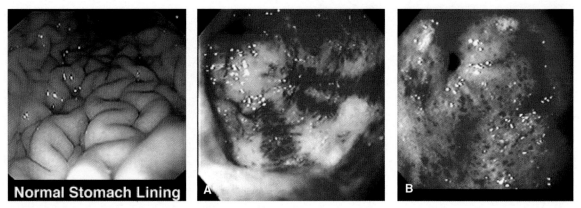

Figure 19-4. Endoscopic images of the stomach lining of three different patients. The first image (*left panel*) shows the stomach lining of a patient with no inflammation in the stomach (normal). Notice the healthy pink tissue and the many rugae. Images **A** and **B** are taken from two patients with gastritis. Notice the change in color due to the inflammation of the stomach lining. Image courtesy of Robert D Fusco, MD, Three Rivers Endoscopy Center, Moon Township, PA. http://www.gihealth.com.

PATHOGENESIS

Infection with *H pylori* is associated with virtually all ulcers not induced by nonsteroidal antiinflammatory drugs (NSAIDs). *H pylori* cells colonize the deep layers of the mucosal gel that coats the gastric mucosa and disrupts its protective properties. The bacterium is motile and uses its "corkscrew"-like motility to migrate within the gastric and duodenal mucosa.

Researchers do not understand completely the pathogenesis of *H pylori* bacteria and the formation of ulcers. However, the ability of the bacteria to sense pH, produce flagella, urease, cytotoxic protein called vac A (vacuolating toxin), and the *cagA* gene product are important in the pathogenesis of ulcer formation. The bacteria produce large amounts of urease allowing them to generate ammonium ions, which buffer the gastric acid. The vac A protein causes vacuoles to form in certain cells and has been demonstrated to cause pore formation in human cells. The *cagA* gene product is injected in host cells by the bacteria, which causes several changes in host cell signaling.

Colonization of *H pylori* in the stomach and duodenum is associated with an accumulation of inflammatory cells in the lamina propria. The inflammatory cells release cytokines that reduce somatostatin levels and cause an increase in gastrin levels. Damage to tissues results in gastritis and eventually causes an ulcer. The ulcers are usually less than 1 cm in diameter and penetrate through the mucosa and submucosa and into the muscularis propria (Figure 19-3). The ulcer floor has no intact epithelium; it normally contains a zone of eosinophilic necrosis resting on a base of granulation tissue surrounded by variable amounts of fibrosis. Researchers believe that *H pylori* infects virtually all patients who are diagnosed with chronic active gastritis.

DIAGNOSIS

Diagnosis of gastritis and PUD involves recognizing the common signs and symptoms and determining that *H pylori* infection is present; this can be determined with a serologic test, a C_{13}-labeled urea breath test, and by endoscopy with tissue biopsy. Endoscopy allows direct visualization of gastritis (Figure 19-4), ulcers (Figures 19-5 and 19-6), and carcinomas.

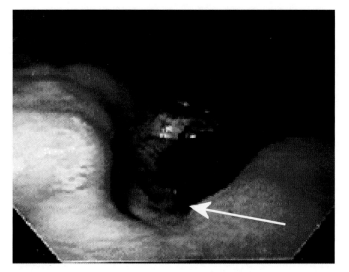

Figure 19-5. Endoscopic image of a deep gastric ulcer (*arrow*). Image courtesy of Robert D Fusco, MD, Three Rivers Endoscopy Center, Moon Township, PA. http://www.gihealth.com.

Biopsy specimens can be tested for *H pylori* urease activity and examined for inflammation and abnormal tissue.

TREATMENT AND PREVENTION

Treatment of chronic gastritis and ulcerative disease involves three drugs: a proton pump inhibitor (e.g., lansoprazole or omeprazole) and two antibiotics (e.g., amoxicillin and clarithromycin). Some patients may also be treated with bismuth (Pepto-Bismol), or bismuth may be used instead of a proton pump inhibitor. Unfortunately, about 10–30% of the clinical isolates of *H pylori* are resistant to at least one of the antimicrobial agents used to treat these diseases, and treatment failures are common.

No prevention methods or vaccines have been discovered thus far for *H pylori* infection. Treatment of chronic gastritis appears to reduce the risk of the patient developing gastric carcinoma, but it does not eliminate the risk entirely.

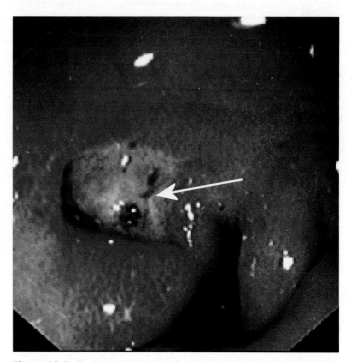

Figure 19-6. Endoscopic image of a duodenal ulcer (*arrow*). Image courtesy of Robert D Fusco, MD, Three Rivers Endoscopy Center, Moon Township, PA. http://www.gihealth.com.

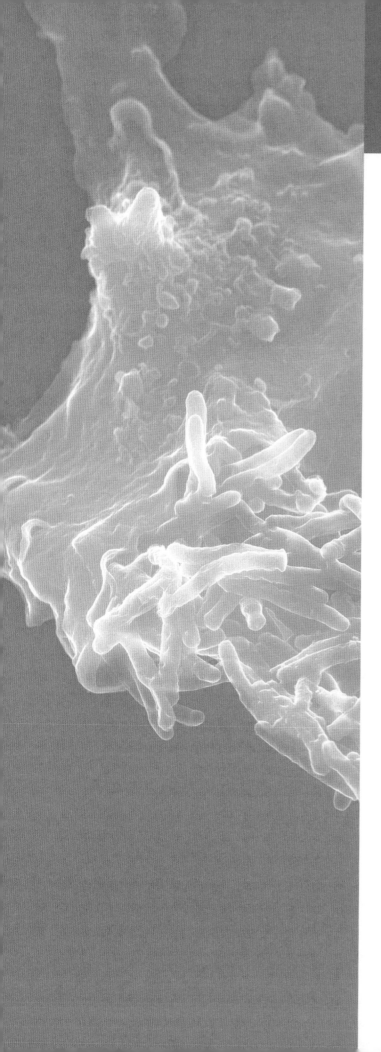

CHAPTER 20

LIVER: VIRAL HEPATITIS

OVERVIEW

The most common liver infection in the United States is viral hepatitis. Viral hepatitis is divided into two major groups: fecal-borne hepatitis and blood-borne hepatitis.

FECAL-BORNE HEPATITIS

Viral hepatitis is transmitted by contaminated fecal material. It is a serious inflammatory disease of the liver that is associated with poor sanitation and is common in underdeveloped countries. Two different viruses are commonly associated with fecal-borne hepatitis: hepatitis A virus (HAV) and hepatitis E virus (HEV).

ETIOLOGY

HAV is common in the United States, whereas HEV is usually acquired by travelers to countries outside the United States. Both viruses are single-stranded RNA nonenveloped viruses. Several other viruses can cause viral hepatitis (see below, blood-borne hepatitis).

MANIFESTATIONS

HAV infections have an incubation period of 14–45 days, with an average of 28 days. During this time, *some patients who smoke may develop distaste for cigarettes.* Most children with HAV infections are asymptomatic, whereas only a small number of adults are asymptomatic. Most symptomatic patients with HAV infection have jaundice.

The initial symptoms of HAV include fever (about 39°C), malaise, fatigue, headache, anorexia, nausea and vomiting, pain in the right upper quadrant, and hepatosplenomegaly. Classic symptoms of hepatitis that may develop later include cholestasis (dark urine and clay-colored stools) followed within 1–5 days by clinical jaundice (yellowing of skin and whites of eyes). The liver is enlarged and tender. Liver damage causes increased blood levels of aspartate aminotransferase (AST), alanine aminotransferase (ALT), and bilirubin. Groups or settings where people are at higher risk of acquiring an HAV infection are listed in Table 20-1.

EPIDEMIOLOGY

About 44% of cases of cases of viral hepatitis are caused by HAV, 49% by hepatitis B (HBV), and 7% by hepatitis C (HCV).

TABLE 20-1. Groups at High Risk of Acquiring Hepatitis A Viral (HAV) Infection

Group	Comments	Settings	Comments
Travelers to countries with high rates of HAV	HAV remains one of the most common vaccine-preventable diseases of travelers	**Food-service establishments**	8% of food handlers have HAV
Men who have sexual activity with men (MSM)	HAV-infected MSMs report more frequent oral-anal contact, longer duration of sexual activity, and more sex partners than MSMs without serologic evidence of infection	**Child care centers**	Many children shed virus and are asymptomatic while shedding
Illicit drug users (injection and noninjection drugs)	Usually involves users of methamphetamine	**Health-care institutions**	

About 4500 cases of HAV are reported each year.

Natural hosts for HAV and HEV are humans and lower primates.

The highest incidence of HAV infection is among children 5–9 years of age and young adults 25–35 years of age. The prevalence of prior HAV infection among the general population in the United States is estimated to be 22–39%.

HEV is not endemic in the United States; however, residents of the United States who acquire HEV usually have a history of foreign travel. HEV epidemics have been reported in India, Pakistan, Nepal, Burma, North Africa, and Mexico.

The incidence of HAV and HEV infections is higher in persons living in crowded conditions and in areas of low socioeconomic development. More than 90% of the population in developing countries has been infected with HAV, whereas less than 50% of the population in developed countries has been infected with HAV.

A chronic carrier state does not occur in patients infected with HAV or HEV. These two types of hepatitis are maintained in a population by serial transmission from subclinically infected persons to susceptible persons.

Persons infected with HAV shed virus up to 10 days before symptoms begin. About 90% of children and 25–50% of adults shed virus and are asymptomatic.

Vaccination for HAV has significantly reduced the number of cases of HAV in the United States (Figure 20-1).

Mortality rates are very low in cases of HAV infection (0.1–0.2%). The mortality rate of HEV infection is higher than HAV infection in the general population (1–2%) and *is even* **higher in pregnant women (20%) who have been infected with HEV in the third trimester.**

Person-to-person transmission via the fecal-oral route is the primary means of HAV and HEV transmission. Transmission occurs most frequently among close contacts in households and extended family settings, and can be transmitted following ingestion of fecally contaminated water or food.

HAV infection is rarely transmitted following transfusion of blood or blood products that were collected from donors during the viremic phase of HAV infection.

Sporadic outbreaks of HAV infection occur following ingestion of shellfish harvested from fecally contaminated waters.

PATHOGENESIS

After ingestion, HAV and HEV can withstand the harsh conditions in the stomach and intestines. These viruses replicate in the oropharynx and epithelial lining of the intestines, where they initiate a transient viremia and infect the liver. HAV and HEV bind to and replicate primarily within liver parenchymal cells. The viruses are released into bile and eventually into stool. HAV and HEV may be shed in feces for 10 days before clinical symptoms appear.

Although most infections are subclinical, lymphoid infiltration, Kupffer cell proliferation, and necrosis of the parenchyma cells can occur. Antibody-antigen complexes and complement fixation contribute to inflammation and tissue damage. All HAV infections are acute and are self-limited by the production of immunoglobulin M (IgM) and IgG reactive with the virus. These anti-HAV antibodies result in long-lasting immunity to future HAV exposure. Mortality rates are very low following HAV infection (0.1–0.2%), although high mortality rates (20%) are observed in pregnant woman infected with HEV during the third trimester of pregnancy.

DIAGNOSIS

Diagnosis of viral hepatitis includes identifying clinical signs and symptoms including malaise, liver enlargement, jaundice, and icterus. Blood studies reveal elevated liver enzyme levels (ALT and AST). Serologic testing aids in confirmation of the clinical diagnosis (Table 20-2).

THERAPY AND PREVENTION

Supportive care and rest are currently the only treatment for patients with viral hepatitis. Immunoglobulin (Ig) given within 2 weeks of infection lessens the severity of symptoms or prevents symptoms. Ig is of no value once symptoms have appeared.

In the United States, immunization with the HAV vaccine is recommended for all children at 1 year of age. Vaccination of children 1 year of age and older and adolescents and adults at the age-appropriate dose is preferred for those who plan to travel repeatedly or reside for long periods in intermediate or high-risk areas. All HAV vaccines contain inactivated (killed) virus and should be given in two doses at least 6 months apart.

Ig is recommended for travelers younger than 1 year of age and for persons 1 year of age and older who need only short-term protection. The HAV vaccine or Ig is recommended for all susceptible persons traveling or working in countries with intermediate or high rates of HAV infection.

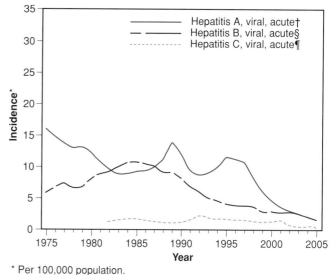

* Per 100,000 population.
† Hepatitis A vaccine was first licensed in 1995.
§ Hepatitis B vaccine was first licensed in June 1982.
¶ An anti-Hepatitis C virus (HCV) antibody test first became available in May 1990.

Figure 20-1. A graph showing the incidence of viral hepatitis from 1975 to 2005 in the United States. Notice the declines in the incidence of hepatitis A and hepatitis B viral infections, which are due in part to vaccination. Image courtesy of the Centers for Disease Control and Prevention.

TABLE 20-2. Serologic Tests for Hepatitis A Virus (HAV)

Stage of Hepatitis Infection	Immunoglobulin M (IgM)	Immunoglobulin G (IgG)
Acute HAV infection	+	−
Previous HAV infection	−	+

BLOOD-BORNE VIRAL HEPATITIS

A severe and sometimes chronic form of viral hepatitis, known as blood-borne viral hepatitis, is transmitted via blood transfusions, blood products, needle sticks, shared drug paraphernalia, breast-feeding, and sexual contact.

ETIOLOGY

There are three different viruses that infect the liver and result in blood-borne viral hepatitis: **hepatitis B virus** (HBV), **hepatitis C virus** (HCV), and **hepatitis D virus** (HDV). HBV is an enveloped partially double-strand DNA virus in the hepadnavirus family. HCV is an enveloped single-strand RNA virus in the flavivirus family. HDV is a single-strand RNA viroid called the delta agent. The HDV agent is a defective virus that cannot infect a hepatocyte without the hepatocyte also being infected with HBV. To infect a hepatocyte, HDV must be coated with HBsAg. HBV and HDV can coinfect a person simultaneously (coinfection) or HDV can infect a patient after infection with HBV (superinfection). Thus, delta agent is found only in concurrent HBV infections.

MANIFESTATIONS

The incubation period for HBV infection is longer than that for HAV infection and is anywhere from 7 to 160 days in duration. Asymptomatic infections occur about 65% of the time. Most children do not have any symptoms of HBV infection; however, when symptoms occur in children, they are usually less severe than symptoms in adults. Early symptoms of acute infection include fatigue, anorexia, nausea, pain and fullness in the upper right quadrant, and fever. Manifestations that develop later may include arthritis, rash, and cholestasis (jaundice and icterus), and tend to be more severe than in patients infected with HAV.

Fulminant HBV hepatitis occurs in 1% of acutely infected individuals, and it is more likely to become fulminant if the patient is coinfected with HBV and HDV. Manifestations are more severe and can be fatal. Patients have severe liver damage with abdominal ascites and bleeding; the liver shrinks rather than swells.

Chronic infections are *NOT* seen in patients infected with HAV and HEV, but are observed in patients with HCV and HBV infections. Chronic hepatitis usually follows mild or asymptomatic initial infection. Most chronically infected patients are asymptomatic for many years; however, in time, liver damage can result in cirrhosis and liver failure. Chronic viral hepatitis is usually detected by elevated liver enzyme levels (AST and ALT) obtained on a routine blood analysis.

Patients with chronic HBV infection are more likely to develop fulminant hepatitis or a more severe hepatitis when superinfected with HDV. Primary hepatocellular carcinoma (HCC) can occur in patients with chronic HBV or HCV infection. HCC can develop in a patient who has been infected with HBV or HCV anywhere from 9 to 35 years later.

EPIDEMIOLOGY

HBV, HCV, and HDV

   Humans and other primates are the only hosts, with chronic carriers serving as reservoirs.

   Distribution for HBV, HCV, and HDV is worldwide.

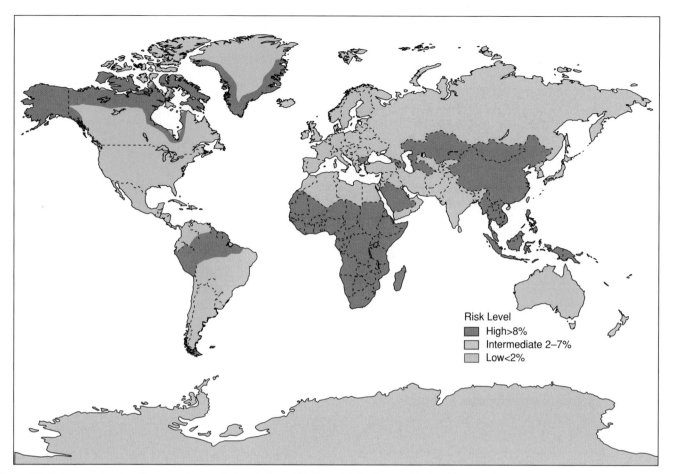

Figure 20-2. A map showing the prevalence of chronic hepatitis B viral infection worldwide. Note the high prevalence in Asia, Africa, some countries in South America, and Alaska.

HBV

HBV infection is the tenth leading cause of death worldwide and results in 500,000 to 1.2 million deaths per year due to chronic hepatitis, cirrhosis, and HCC. About 1.25 million Americans are chronically infected with HBV.

Approximately 15–40% of patients chronically infected with HBV will develop cirrhosis, liver failure, or HCC. HCC accounts for 320,000 deaths per year.

About 5–15% of persons in tropical countries are chronically infected with HBV, whereas only 0.1–0.5% of persons in the United States are chronically infected (Figure 20-2).

In the United States, about 20% of patients with HCC are chronically infected with HBV.

HBV is present in blood, saliva, semen, vaginal secretions, and menstrual blood, and to a lesser extent in perspiration, breast milk, tears, and the urine of infected individuals. Table 20-3 lists persons at high risk for acquiring HBV infection.

HBV is transmitted through contact with infected body fluids. In areas of high endemicity, the most common route of transmission is perinatal or the infection is acquired during the preschool years.

The route of transmission has important clinical implications because there is a very high probability of developing

TABLE 20-3. Persons at High Risk for Hepatitis B (HBV) Infection

Intravenous drug users
Patients undergoing blood transfusions or hemodialysis
Personnel in contact with blood and blood products
Persons with multiple sexual contacts (heterosexual and homosexual)
Immunosuppressed persons
Infants born to mothers with chronic HBV
Residents and staff members of institutions for the mentally handicapped
Persons from endemic regions (e.g., China, parts of Africa, Alaska, Pacific islands)

chronic HBV if the infection is acquired perinatally or in the preschool years. Chronic HBV infection occurs in 90% of infants infected at birth, 30% of children infected at ages 1–5 years, and 6% of persons infected after 5 years of age.

The virus can be spread percutaneously (e.g., needle sharing, acupuncture, ear piercing, tattooing, transfusion of whole blood or blood products) and through very close personal contact involving the exchange of blood or secretions (e.g., sexual intercourse, child birth). *The most common means of transmission of HBV in the United States is via sexual contact.*

The pattern of transmission of HBV varies with chronic HBV prevalence. In areas where chronic infections (chronic hepatitis) are highly endemic (East and Southeast Asia and Sub-Saharan Africa), transmission is usually perinatal (from a carrier mother to her newborn) or by close contact between children (horizontal transmission). Perinatal transmission of HBV usually occurs during or soon after delivery following contact of the infant with maternal blood and other body fluids.

In areas of low endemicity (Western Europe and North America), perinatal transmission of HBV is less common and transmission occurs mainly through percutaneous routes and by sexual contact between adults.

HCV

There are 26,000 new cases of HCV infection each year in the United States, and 25–30% of cases are symptomatic.

Chronic hepatitis is more common in HCV infections (85%) than in HBV infections (5–10%).

About 70% of persons infected with HCV develop chronic liver disease; about 20% of patients with chronic HCV develop cirrhosis of the liver, and 20% of cirrhotic patients experience liver failure. Only 10% of patients with chronic HBV develop cirrhosis of the liver and liver failure.

In the United States, about 30% of patients with HCC had a previous chronic HCV infection.

Infection with HCV is the leading infectious indication for liver transplantation.

About 4.1 million Americans, or 1.6%, have been infected with HCV; of this number, 3.2 million are chronically infected.

HCV infections are mainly transmitted via blood transfusion (90% of cases) and hemodialysis and renal transplantation (20% of cases). HCV can also be transmitted by sexual contact; however, the efficiency of sexual transmission is quite low.

The risk for perinatal HCV transmission is about 4%.

HDV

HDV infection can be acquired either as a coinfection with HBV or as a superinfection of patients with chronic HBV infection.

Patients with HBV-HDV coinfection may have more severe acute disease and a higher risk of fulminant hepatitis

(2–20%) compared with patients infected with only HBV (1%). Chronic HBV infection appears to occur less frequently in persons with HBV-HDV coinfection.

Chronic HBV carriers who acquire HDV superinfection usually develop chronic HDV infection. In chronic HBV carriers with HDV superinfection, 70–80% have developed evidence of chronic liver diseases with cirrhosis compared with 15–30% of patients with chronic HBV infection alone.

HDV infections are usually due to percutaneous exposures and are usually seen in intravenous drug users.

PATHOGENESIS

HBV enters the bloodstream and infects the cells of the liver by replicating within the cells. Symptoms may not be observed for 45 days or more, depending on the dose of HBV, the route of infection, and the individual. HBV genomes integrate into host chromosomes during replication and are the basis of chronic infections. Large amounts of **HBV surface antigen** (HBsAg) and virions are released in the blood.

Immune complexes formed by HBsAg and antibody are responsible for hypersensitivity reactions that occur in some patients (e.g., arthritis, rash, liver damage, vasculitis, or arthralgia). Liver parenchymal cell degeneration results from cellular swelling and necrosis; resolution of the infection allows the liver parenchyma to regenerate. Fulminant HBV infection, activation of chronic infection, or coinfection with the delta agent can lead to permanent liver damage or cirrhosis. Both cell-mediated immunity and inflammation are responsible for the resolution of HBV infection and its symptoms. Acute cases of HBV disease are usually of short duration with significant symptomology.

After chronic HBV infection, the immune system attempts to clear the HBV by destroying infected hepatocytes, which leads to increasing circulatory blood levels of ALT. Most patients will clear HBeAg (hepatitis B envelope antigen), produce antibodies to HBeAg (anti-HBe), and achieve a state of nonreplicative infection that is characterized by low or undetectable serum levels of HBV DNA and normal ALT levels. Figure 20-3 shows a graphic representation of the pathogenesis of an acute HBV infection.

Chronic HBV infection is defined as the presence of HBsAg in the bloodstream following infection by HBV for at least 6 months (Figure 20-4). The early phase of chronic HBV infection is characterized by the presence of HBeAg and high serum levels of HBV DNA (referred to as HBeAg-positive chronic HBV).

Over time, 25% of persons who acquire HBV as children will develop cirrhosis or HCC as adults. Cirrhosis may develop as a consequence of repeated immune system attacks in which the normal hepatocytes are destroyed and replaced with fibrous tissue. **_Once established, cirrhosis cannot be cured;_** however, its progress may be stopped if the cause is removed. Without treatment, the typical progression is from compensated cirrhosis to decompensated cirrhosis. Decompensated cirrhosis is characterized by cessation of enzymatic processes in the liver and subsequent severe clinical complications such as fluid retention in the abdomen (ascites), jaundice, internal bleeding, and hepatic encephalopathy. Patients with decompensated cirrhosis are

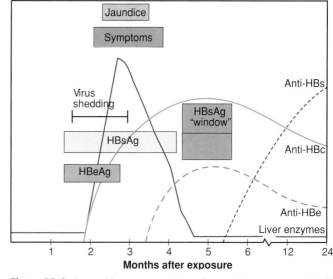

Figure 20-3. A graphic representation of a typical acute hepatitis B viral infection. Note the appearance of the viral antigens HBsAg, HBeAg, and the timing of the host's humoral response to the viral infection. Also notice the "window" period when anti-HBs and HBsAg are not detectable in the serum. HBsAg, HBV surface antigen; HBeAg, HBV envelope antigen; anti-HBs, antibody to HBsAg; anti-HBc, antibody to HBV core antigen; anti-HBe antibody to HBeAg.

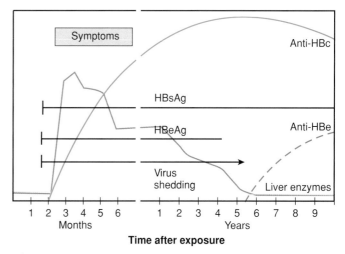

Figure 20-4. Graphic representation of a chronic hepatitis B viral infection. Notice the prolonged time of viral shedding and the lack of HBsAg antibody production. HBsAg, HBV surface antigen; HBeAg, HBV envelope antigen; anti-HBe antibody to HBeAg.

candidates for liver transplantation; without transplantation, death results from end-stage liver disease.

Hepatocytes that have been damaged due to excessive alcohol use, chronic HBV and HCV infections, hematochromatosis, and exposure to aflatoxin can become malignant and result in HCC. About 80% of people with HCC have preexisting cirrhosis of the liver.

DIAGNOSIS

Initial diagnosis of HBV, HCV, and HDV infection is usually determined clinically if signs and symptoms are present. Laboratory evaluation of the blood for elevations in ALT, AST, alkaline phosphatase, and bilirubin aids in making an initial diagnosis. A confirmatory diagnosis can be determined following reactivity in various serologic tests for HBV (Table 20-4; see Figure 20-3), HCV (see Table 20-4), and HDV.

Blood tests for HBV infections are somewhat more complicated than most serologic tests. Tests for HBV infection detect both viral antigens and antibodies to viral antigens. To confirm whether a patient has HBV infection, three blood tests are usually ordered: HBV surface antigen (HBsAg), antibody to HBV core antigen (anti-HBcAg), and antibody to HBsAg (anti-HBsAg) (see Figure 20-3 and Table 20-4).

During the **acute phase** of HBV infection, the virus is actively dividing and infectious and incomplete viral particles are being produced. These infectious and incomplete viral particles enter the bloodstream with enough HBsAg present in the

TABLE 20-4. Hepatitis Panel for Hepatitis B (HBV) and Hepatitis C (HCV) Infections

Stage of Hepatitis Infection	HBsAg	Anti-HBsAg	Anti-HBc IgM	Anti-HBc IgG	HBeAg	Anti- HBeAg	Anti-HCV
Early acute HBV	+	−	+	−	+	−	−
"Window period" HBV	−	−	+	−	+/−	+/−	−
Convalescent HBV	−	+	−	+	−	+	−
Late convalescent HBV	−	−	−	+	−	+	−
Chronic active hepatitis	Positive for >6 months	−	−	+	+	−	−
Chronic persistent hepatitis	Positive for >6 months	−	−	+	−	+	−
Vaccinated for HBV	−	+	−	−	−	−	−
Compatible for HCV	−	−	−	−	−	−	+

HBsAg, hepatitis B virus surface antigen; anti-HBsAg, antibody to HBsAg; anti-HBc IgM, immunoglobulin M antibody to HBV core antigen; anti-HBc IgG, immunoglobulin G antibody to HBV core antigen; HBeAg, HBV envelope antigen; anti-HBeAg, antibody to HBeAg; anti-HCV, antibody to hepatitis C virus.

blood to be detected in samples. Patients who are positive for HBsAg have early acute HBV infection (see Figure 20-4 and Table 20-4).

Within 3–4 weeks following HBV infection, patients who recover from the infection will produce antibodies to HBsAg and HBcAg. The anti-HBsAg produced by the patient removes the HBsAg from the bloodstream. HBV infected patients become negative for both HBsAg and anti-HBsAg, making diagnosis of HBV infection impossible if assay is obtained for only these two molecules. Fortunately, IgM antibody to HBcAg (IgM anti-HBcAg) continues to be detectable in the bloodstream. The period when HBsAg and anti-HBsAg are no longer detectable but IgM anti-HBcAg is detectable is called the "window period" (see Figure 20-3 and Table 20-4).

Within 5–6 weeks following infection, as virus replication is stopped by the immune response, enough HBsAg is eliminated from the blood and anti-HBsAg is detectable. By this time, patients will also be producing IgG to HBcAg (IgG anti-HBcAg). A patient infected with HBV who is negative for HBsAg but positive for anti-HBsAg and IgG anti-HBcAg is entering convalescence (see Table 20-4). Eventually, anti-HBsAg is not detectable but most persons with a previous HBV infection will be positive for IgG anti-HBcAg (see Figure 20-3 and Table 20-4).

If a patient becomes chronically infected with HBV, HBsAg is not eliminated from the bloodstream and can be detected for long periods of time. By definition, any patient who has detectable HBsAg for 6 months or longer has a chronic HBV infection (see Figure 20-4 and Table 20-4).

An HBeAg test is used to determine if a patient infected with HBV is infectious (see Figure 20-4); patients with anti-HBeAg are not considered infectious. Patients who have chronic HBV hepatitis with HBeAg are infectious and usually have a much worse prognosis (chronic active hepatitis), whereas patients with chronic HBV infection and anti-HBeAg (chronic persistent hepatitis) are less likely to have serious infections and are not considered as infectious.

Serologic tests are available to detect antibody production to HCV and HDV and confirm a diagnosis of viral hepatitis.

THERAPY AND PREVENTION

Treatment of acute infections with HBV, HCV, and HDV involves supportive care. Treatment of chronic HBV infections can include human interferon alpha (IFNα), lamivudine (3TC), or adefovir dipivoxil (given for 4–12 months). Adefovir dipivoxil and lamivudine are nucleoside-nucleotide analogues that suppress HBV replication through inhibition of HBV-DNA polymerase. Patients with chronic hepatitis who are HBeAg positive usually are more responsive to therapy than patients with chronic hepatitis who are HBeAg negative. Treatment with conventional IFNα not only results in loss of viremia and normalization of liver enzymes, but it also improves long-term outcomes and survival and alters the natural history of the disease.

Two different treatment strategies exist for treating chronic HCV patients: (1) immediate treatment with Peginterferon alfa-2a and ribavirin for up to 48 weeks; or (2) watchful waiting with liver biopsy performed every 3 years and drug therapy initiated if hepatitis progresses to a moderate stage of liver damage or cirrhosis.

To prevent infection of both HBV and HDV, immunization with the HBV vaccine is recommended for all children. ***This vaccine was called the first "cancer vaccine" because of its ability to prevent chronic HBV infection and the resultant HCC that occurs in some chronically infected HBV patients.*** The vaccine contains purified recombinant HBsAg. Persons who have been successfully vaccinated will produce anti-HBs and may be confused as having had a prior HBV infection; however, persons who have been vaccinated do *NOT* produce anti-HBc. Persons who have had a prior HBV infection will produce anti-HBc; thus vaccinated persons can be differentiated from persons with a prior infection by assaying for antibody to both HBsAg and HBcAg. HBV immunoglobulin prepared from plasma with a high titer of anti-HBsAg but no detectable HBsAg is used in combination with vaccination for infants born to HBV-positive mothers and for susceptible persons who were exposed to HBV.

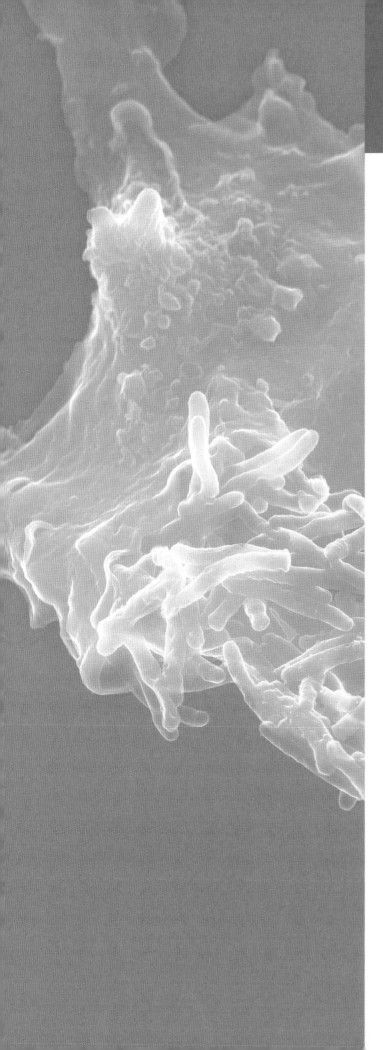

INFECTIONS OF THE SMALL INTESTINE

OVERVIEW

Numerous bacteria, viruses, and parasites cause diseases in the intestines that result in diarrhea or dysentery, nausea and vomiting, and abdominal cramping (Table 21-1). If the infection is in the small intestine, symptoms include watery diarrhea and vomiting. Infections in the large intestine usually result in dysentery (small fecal volume with mucus and blood).

Not all of the diseases occur after an infection, but they can occur after ingestion of preformed toxin. Usually symptoms of intoxication such as nausea, vomiting, and diarrhea occur soon after ingestion of the toxin (1–8 h). Symptoms of an intestinal infection tend to occur much later (24–72 h) than symptoms following intoxication (Table 21-2).

Diarrhea is an important symptom of intestinal disease and is the most common cause of death in developing countries (2.5 million deaths per year). Over 211 million cases of diarrhea occur in the United States every year. Pathogens causing diarrhea can be transmitted to humans three basic ways: in food, in water, and person to person. Many of these infections are self-limiting and do not require treatment; however, some can spread to other sites in the body and require treatment to prevent complications (e.g., bacteremia).

This chapter will include discussion of diseases that primarily affect the small intestine and will be divided into the following topics: food poisoning, viral gastroenteritis, bacterial gastroenteritis, and parasitic gastroenteritis. Invasive gastroenteritis, which primarily involves the large intestine, will be discussed in Chapter 22.

FOOD POISONING

Food poisoning is an intoxication associated with the ingestion of preformed microbial toxins. *It is not an infection.* Since the toxins are ingested preformed and no microbial growth within the body is required, the incubation times are very short (within 2–12 h) and there is no fever. Botulism has an incubation time (>12 h) that is longer than the incubation times seen with the other causes of food poisoning (usually <12 h).

ETIOLOGY

Food toxemia is primarily due to bacteria, which include *Staphylococcus aureus* (gram-positive aerobic coccus), *Bacillus cereus* (gram-positive aerobic rod), *Clostridium perfringens* type A (gram-positive anaerobic rod), and *Clostridium botulinum* (gram-positive anaerobic rod).

MANIFESTATIONS

In cases of gastroenteritis caused by food poisoning, it is important to differentiate toxemia from infectious diarrhea. The key features that are unique to toxemia are rapid onset of symptoms following ingestion of contaminated food or drink, lack of fever, and absence of fecal leukocytes. Symptoms of toxemia usually occur within 12 hours after toxin ingestion, compared to an incubation period of 24–72 hours for infections.

Some unique aspects of causes of food poisoning

S aureus produces toxins that cause vomiting (often projectile) but little or no diarrhea. Symptoms occur within 1–4 hours after ingestion of contaminated food.

B cereus can cause two different types of food poisoning. Type I occurs when the organism grows in starchy foods (especially fried rice), and an emetic illness is seen within 2–3 hours after ingestion. Type II *B cereus* food poisoning occurs when the organism grows in meat, vegetables, and sauces, producing a heat-labile enterotoxin. When ingested, the enterotoxin can cause profuse diarrhea within 10–12 hours after ingestion of the toxin.

C perfringens causes abdominal cramping and watery diarrhea that usually occurs within 8–12 hours after ingestion of its toxin; the diarrhea generally lasts less than 24 hours.

C botulinum toxin produces symptoms 1–2 days after ingestion of improperly home-canned vegetables or sausage. Botulism is the only intoxication that has an incubation period of over 12 hours because of the amount of time required for the toxin to spread from the intestine to the nerve synapses. Initial symptoms include blurred vision with fixed and dilated pupils, dry mouth, constipation, and abdominal pain. A bilateral descending weakness of the peripheral muscles develops resulting in flaccid paralysis. Death is usually attributed to respiratory failure. Patients maintain a clear sensorium throughout the illness.

EPIDEMIOLOGY

Staphylococcal food poisoning is the most common cause of food poisoning in the United States. It occurs most often in foods that require hand preparation such as potato salad, ham salad, and sandwich spreads.

B cereus outbreaks are relatively uncommon and are associated with many foods. Fried rice is a leading cause of emetic food poisoning (*B cereus* type I) in the United States. Other starchy foods such as potato, pasta, and cheese products have also been associated with this form of food toxemia. Meats, milk, vegetables, and fish have been associated with the diarrheal *B cereus* type II food toxemia.

TABLE 21-1. Organisms that Cause Intestinal Disease

Type of Organism	Organism
Bacteria	*Staphylococcus aureus*
	Bacillus cereus
	Clostridium perfringens
	Clostridium botulinum
	Vibrio cholerae
	Escherichia coli
	Salmonella
	Shigella
	Campylobacter
	Clostridium difficile
	Listeria monocytogenes
Viruses	Rotaviruses
	Norwalk virus
	Noroviruses (Norwalk-like viruses)
	Adenoviruses
	Astroviruses
Parasites	*Cryptosporidium parvum*
	Giardia lamblia
	Entamoeba histolytica

TABLE 21-2. Organisms that Cause Intoxication or Infection

Intoxications	*Staphylococcus aureus*
	Bacillus cereus
	Clostridium perfringens
	Clostridium botulinum
Infections	*Escherichia coli*
	Salmonella
	Shigella
	Campylobacter
	Clostridium difficile
	Vibrio cholerae
	Listeria monocytogenes
	Rotaviruses
	Norwalk virus
	Adenoviruses
	Astroviruses
	Caliciviruses
	Noroviruses
	Cryptosporidium parvum
	Giardia lamblia
	Entamoeba histolytica

C perfringens is found in soil and dust and in the gastro-intestinal tract of animals and humans. This organism produces heat-resistant spores that can survive cooking and grow to large numbers if the cooked food is held between 4°C and 60°C for an extensive amount of time. Meat and poultry dishes and sauces and gravies are foods most frequently associated with this form of food toxemia.

C botulinum is relatively rare, with only 15–40 cases of botulism diagnosed yearly in the United States. Botulism causes death in approximately 30% of patients. Botulism usually occurs in home-canned foods. Recent use of botulinum toxin for cosmetic purposes has resulted in several cases of botulism when improperly diluted unlicensed concentrated toxin preparations have been used.

PATHOGENESIS

S aureus produces eight distinct antigenic types of enterotoxin. They are water-soluble, low-molecular weight proteins that are heat stable (resist boiling for 30 minutes). Staphylococcal enterotoxins cause 5-hydroxytryptamine (serotonin) to be released in the intestine, which then binds to 5-hydroxytryptamine receptors on vagal afferent neurons and causes emesis.

B cereus produces several different enterotoxins during spore germination, which cause either vomiting or diarrhea. The type of toxin produced is dependent on the type of food in which the spore germinates. In high-carbohydrate foods such as rice or pasta, an emetic heat-stable enterotoxin is produced causing nausea and vomiting or *B cereus* type I food poisoning. The heat-stable enterotoxin depsipeptide cereulide causes vomiting through an unknown mechanism.

The diarrheal form of *B cereus* type II, which results from the heat-labile enterotoxins hemolysin BL (HBL) and non-hemolytic enterotoxin, is produced as the bacteria grow in the food or in the intestine. In a high-protein food, the diarrheal heat-labile enterotoxins result in diarrhea. These enterotoxins stimulate the adenyl cyclase-cyclic adenosine monophosphate system in intestinal epithelial cells and cause fluid accumulation in the intestine.

C perfringens enterotoxin binds to the brush-border membrane in the small intestine and disrupts ion transport in the ileum and jejunum, altering membrane permeability. Excess amounts of ions and water enter the lumen, resulting in a watery diarrhea. The toxin is formed when the vegetative cells become spores; conditions in the small intestine cause spore formation. Meat products contaminated with large numbers of organisms are needed to cause disease. Refrigeration prevents growth of organisms in meat, and reheating meat destroys the heat-labile enterotoxin.

C botulinum produces seven antigenically distinct types of neurotoxin; human disease is associated with toxin types A, B, E, and F. If the spores of *C botulinum* are not destroyed during the canning process, when cooled sufficiently, the spores will germinate and the resulting vegetative cells will produce toxin. This large toxin is an A-B type toxin. The B portion protects the toxin from being inactivated by stomach acid and forms a pore in the membrane of the nerve cell to allow entry of the A portion into the cell. The A portion is a metalloproteinase that blocks neurotransmission of cholinergic synapses by preventing the release of acetylcholine at the neuromuscular junction and causing a flaccid paralysis that remains until the nerve endings regenerate.

DIAGNOSIS

Except for botulism, diagnosis of the source of food intoxication usually is not sought. Most food intoxications rarely cause significant long-term problems and are self-limiting. The only reason to determine the food source and cause is in the case of food poisonings resulting from food eaten at public institutions such as restaurants or elder-care facilities. In such cases, the contaminated food is often cultured or immunoassays are performed to detect the enterotoxins in the food. Certain foods are more likely to be contaminated with a particular pathogen. Table 21-3 lists foods and the pathogens they are likely to contain.

The only fatal food poisoning is botulism. Emphasis should be placed on ruling out botulism in the diagnosis. Presumptive diagnosis of botulism is determined by the presence of a rapidly descending paralysis. A history of ingestion of home-canned food or honey is helpful. Anaerobic culture of the organism from the food source and demonstration of toxin production using a mouse bioassay can be performed, but the sample must be sent to a public health laboratory for analysis.

TREATMENT AND PREVENTION

There is usually no treatment given for toxemia due to *S aureus*, *B cereus*, or *C perfringens*. If the patient becomes dehydrated, intravenous replenishment of fluids and electrolytes are administered.

Patients with signs or symptoms compatible with botulism or patients who are known to have eaten food shown by laboratory testing to contain the toxin should be admitted to an intensive care unit to permit monitoring of respiratory and cardiac function. Patients should be induced to vomit; gastric lavage should be performed if exposure has occurred within several hours and patients should be given trivalent (A, B, E) botulinum antitoxin to neutralize unabsorbed toxin in the bloodstream.

Good personal hygiene while handling foods will help prevent *S aureus* from contaminating foods, and refrigeration of raw and cooked foods will prevent the growth of these bacteria. To prevent food toxemia caused by *C perfringens*, hot foods should be served immediately or held above 46°C. After cooking, large quantities of food should be divided into smaller portions and refrigerated immediately. The food should be reheated to 60°C prior to serving. Adhering to these methods will also prevent food poisonings due to *B cereus*. Botulism can be prevented by proper canning of foods, by avoiding tasting of canned food before cooking, and by boiling canned foods for 10 minutes before eating to destroy any neurotoxins that may have been produced.

VIRAL GASTROENTERITIS

Viral gastroenteritis is one of several common causes of diarrhea in the United States, and can be caused by rotavirus, adenovirus, astrovirus, and caliciviruses.

TABLE 21-3. Organisms that Commonly Cause Food Poisoning

Food Source	Organism
Dairy	*Campylobacter, Salmonella*
Eggs	*Salmonella*
Meats	*Clostridium perfringens, Bacillus cereus, Campylobacter, Salmonella*
Ground beef; leafy green vegetables	*E coli* O157:H7
Poultry	*Campylobacter*
Pork	*Clostridium perfringens*
Seafood	Astrovirus, *Vibrio*
Oysters	Calicivirus, *Vibrio*
Vegetables	*Clostridium perfringens*
Foods that require more handling (e.g., salads such as egg, tuna, chicken, potato, and macaroni; sandwich fillings; bakery products such as cream-filled pastries, cream pies, and chocolate eclairs)	*Staphylococcus aureus*
Rice; starchy foods	*Bacillus cereus*
Home-canned foods; honey (in children <1 year of age)	*Clostridium botulinum*

ETIOLOGY

Rotavirus is a naked double-stranded RNA virus. The Caliciviridae family contains several naked single-stranded RNA-containing viruses that cause gastroenteritis The viruses in the Caliciviridae family that cause gastroenteritis are Norwalk virus and noroviruses (formerly called Norwalk-like viruses). The Astroviruses are naked positive-sense, single-stranded RNA viruses that are similar in appearance to a five- or six-pointed star. Adenoviruses serotypes 40 and 41 are the only DNA viruses that cause gastroenteritis.

MANIFESTATIONS

Following infection with any of the viruses mentioned above (i.e., rotavirus, adenovirus, astrovirus, and caliciviruses), symptoms of viral gastroenteritis include low-grade fever, abdominal pain, watery diarrhea, and nausea and vomiting (Table 21-4).

EPIDEMIOLOGY

Each year, more than 3.5 million infants develop acute viral gastroenteritis resulting in more than 500,000 office visits, 55,000 hospitalizations, and 30 deaths.

Of a total of 13.8 million cases of food-related illness from all causes, rotavirus, adenovirus, astrovirus, and caliciviruses cause 9.2 million cases of illness each year.

Rotavirus

Rotavirus is the most common cause of severe diarrhea among children younger than 2 years of age, resulting in the hospitalization of approximately 55,000 children per year in the United States and mortality in over 600,000 children per year worldwide. Rotavirus infections are more common in the winter. In adults, the disease tends to be mild.

Rotaviruses replicate in the intestine of most domestic and many wild animals.

The most common mode of transmission of rotavirus is via the fecal-oral route. The virus is stable in the environment, and transmission can occur through ingestion of contaminated water or food and contact with contaminated surfaces.

Norwalk virus and noroviruses

Norwalk virus infection affects older children and adults.

Norwalk virus replicates in the intestines of most domestic and many wild animals.

Noroviruses are the most common cause of outbreaks of gastroenteritis in industrialized countries. Gastroenteritis caused by norovirus infection is a highly seasonal syndrome, and is often referred to as "winter vomiting disease."

Noroviruses are found in the stool or vomit of infected persons. It is highly contagious and can spread rapidly.

The Norwalk virus and noroviruses are transmitted via the fecal-oral route by food handlers directly from person to person, through contaminated food or water, or by contact with contaminated surfaces or fomites.

TABLE 21-4. Organisms that Cause Viral Gastroenteritis

Organism	Comments
Rotaviruses	Usually cause disease in children <2 years of age **Most common cause of infant diarrhea** The incubation period being is 2–4 days Diarrhea can last 4–8 days, resulting in dehydration Most common in the winter
Norovirus	Symptoms last 12–60 hours Incubation period is 12–48 hours **Most common cause overall of viral gastroenteritis** Infect children and adults Most common in the winter (winter vomiting syndrome)
Norwalk virus	Symptoms similar to norovirus infections Causes symptoms in children and adults Most common in summer
Astroviruses	Usually cause symptoms in children <5 years of age (vomiting is uncommon) Most common in the winter
Adenoviruses	Cause symptoms similar to rotavirus infections except that the infants tend to be older Complications can include intussusception.

Astroviruses

Astroviruses have been isolated from birds, cats, dogs, pigs, sheep, cows, and humans.

Like rotaviruses, astrovirus infections occur throughout the year, with peaks during the winter months.

Most astrovirus infections are detected in children younger than 5 years of age, with the majority of children younger than 1 year of age.

Adenoviruses

Transmission of adenoviruses can be by direct contact, fecal-oral route, or occasionally they are waterborne.

PATHOGENESIS

Rotavirus, adenovirus, astrovirus, and caliciviruses invade and destroy mature epithelial cells in the middle and upper villus, causing decreased absorption of sodium and water from the bowel lumen.

DIAGNOSIS

Diagnostic tests usually are not performed to identify the causes of viral gastroenteritis. However, a rapid antigen test of stool, either by enzyme immunosorbent assay or the latex agglutination test, can be used to aid in the diagnosis of rotavirus infection.

THERAPY AND PREVENTION

Viral gastroenteritis is a self-limiting disease, but it is often necessary to administer fluids and electrolytes to patients to prevent dehydration. Oral rehydration therapy is recommended for preventing and treating early dehydration. Shock, severe dehydration, and decreased consciousness require intravenous therapy. Administering antiemetics and antidiarrheal agents to small children is not recommended.

Natural immunity is usually incomplete, and multiple episodes of viral gastroenteritis can occur in infants. In time, the episodes become less severe. Two highly effective rotavirus vaccines are currently available and should be given to infants at 2, 4, and 6 months of age. Persons who are infected with norovirus should not prepare food while they are symptomatic and for 3 days after they recover from the illness.

BACTERIAL GASTROENTERITIS

Bacterial gastroenteritis results in large volume watery diarrhea and abdominal cramps. Although vomiting is common in viral gastroenteritis, it is much less common in bacterial gastroenteritis. The bacteria that cause bacterial gastroenteritis colonize the surface of the small intestine but do not invade the mucosa. Bacterial gastroenteritis is a noninflammatory diarrhea; fecal specimens do *NOT* contain any fecal leukocytes.

ESCHERICHIA COLI INFECTION

Bacterial gastroenteritis due to *E coli* is a common malady of people traveling outside the United States and is caused by three different types of *E coli*: enterotoxigenic *E coli* (ETEC), enteroaggregative *E coli* (EAEC), and enteropathogenic *E coli* (EPEC).

ETIOLOGY

ETEC and EAEC both cause what is commonly known as traveler's diarrhea. ETEC can also cause diarrhea in infants; EPEC thus far has been incriminated only in mild diarrheal disease in infants primarily younger than 6 months of age.

MANIFESTATIONS

Severe disease caused by ETEC and EAEC is characterized by abrupt onset of watery diarrhea and abdominal cramping. The duration of diarrhea caused by ETEC is about 24 hours after initiation of fluid replacement therapy. The duration of diarrhea caused by EAEC is several days before resolution.

PATHOGENESIS

ETEC strains colonize the small intestine and produce two enterotoxins called LT (heat labile toxin) and ST (heat stable toxin). Both toxins ultimately stimulate the secretion of chloride by the host cells, which results in a watery diarrhea. LT is an A-B toxin similar to the cholera toxin—it is composed of one A subunit and five B subunits. The B subunits bind to GM_1 ganglioside on the host cell. Following endocytosis of the bound toxin, the A subunit is released into the cytoplasm and adenosine diphosphate ribosylates the guanosine triphosphate (GTP)-binding protein. The GTP-binding protein then activates adenylate cyclase, resulting in increased intracellular levels of cyclic adenosine monophosphate (AMP). Cyclic AMP activates cyclic AMP-dependent protein kinase (A kinase), causing supranormal phosphorylation of chloride channels. The stimulation of chloride ion secretion from secretory crypt cells and inhibition of sodium chloride absorption by villus tip cells causes an increase in luminal ion content, drawing water passively through the paracellular pathway and resulting in an osmotic diarrhea.

ST is quite different from LT. ST is a peptide of 18 or 19 amino acids and binds to a membrane-spanning enzyme called guanylate cyclase. Guanylate cyclase is located in the apical membrane of intestinal epithelial cells, and binding of ST to the extracellular domains of the protein stimulates its intracellular enzymatic activity. This causes increases in intracellular cyclic guanosine monophosphate, which ultimately stimulates chloride ion secretion or inhibition of NaCl adsorption, or both. Once again, an osmotic diarrhea occurs.

EPEC produces no demonstrable toxin. EPEC strains cause what is termed an attaching-and-effacing histopathology in the small intestine. These *E coli* strains are adherent to the epithelial cells and then disrupt the microvilli (effacement). They then intimately adhere to the host cells and inject, by a type III secretory system (Figure 21-1), bacterial factors into the host cells and cause alterations in the glycocalyx of the epithelial cells in the small bowel. EPEC express rope-like bundles of filaments, termed bundle-forming pili, which create a network of fibers that bind the individual organisms together and are used to bind the bacterial cells to the surface of the intestinal epithelial cells.

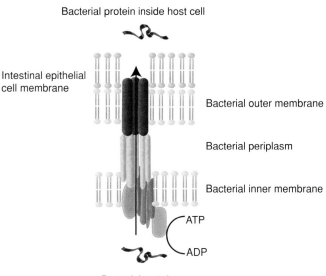

Figure 21-1. A schematic of the type III bacterial secretory system. Contact between the bacteria and host cell induces the bacterial cell to produce the proteins needed to construct the type III bacterial secretion system. EPEC produces the proteins that form a channel between the cytoplasm of the bacterium and the cytoplasm of the host cell so that bacterial proteins can be placed in the host cell. Some of these bacterial proteins cause alterations in the glycocalyx of the epithelial cells in the small bowel. ATP, adenosine triphosphate; ADP, adenosine diphosphate.

EAEC infection involves three stages that include adherence to the intestinal mucosa. Stage 1 is enhanced mucus production that encases the bacteria in a biofilm on the surface of the intestinal mucosa; stage 2 is elaboration of a cytotoxin, which kills the intestinal cells; and stage 3 is when damage causes the watery diarrhea.

EPIDEMIOLOGY

E coli is the most common cause of traveler's diarrhea, resulting in 50 million cases in persons traveling to developing countries. It is believed that there are about 50,000 cases of traveler's diarrhea each day worldwide.

ETEC is the most common bacterial cause of a type of bacterial gastroenteritis called traveler's diarrhea. EAEC causes about 25% of cases of traveler's diarrhea.

Persons traveling to high-risk areas worldwide are more likely to acquire traveler's diarrhea (Figure 21-2). An average of 30–50% of travelers to high-risk areas will develop traveler's diarrhea during a 1- to 2-week stay.

Traveler's diarrhea is a clinical syndrome resulting from microbial contamination of ingested food and water. It can occur during or shortly after travel, and usually affects persons traveling from an area with a well-developed hygiene and sanitation infrastructure to a less developed one.

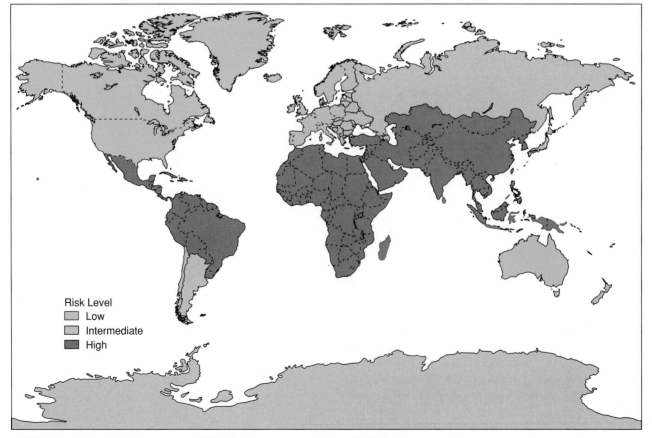

Figure 21-2. A map showing risk areas worldwide that are common for traveler's diarrhea.

TABLE 21-5. Stool Characteristics Useful in the Diagnosis of Intestinal Diseases

Stool Characteristics	Small Bowel	Large Bowel
Appearance	Watery	Mucous and/or bloody
Volume	Large	Small
Frequency	Increased	Increased
Blood	May be positive but not visibly bloody	Can be visibly bloody
pH	<5.5	>5.5
White blood cells	<5 cells per high power field	>10 cells per high power field
Serum leukocytes	Normal	Can have a leukocytosis if an invasive infection
Organisms	**Viral** Rotavirus Adenovirus Calicivirus Astrovirus Norwalk virus Noroviruses	**Invasive bacteria** *Escherichia coli* *Shigella* species *Salmonella* species *Campylobacter* species *Yersinia* species
	Toxic bacteria *Escherichia coli* *Clostridium perfringens* *Vibrio cholerae* *Bacillus cereus*	**Toxic bacteria** *Clostridium difficile*
	Parasites *Giardia lamblia* *Cryptosporidium parvum*	**Parasites** *Entamoeba histolytica*

DIAGNOSIS

Bacterial gastroenteritis is usually a self-limiting disease, and diagnosis is determined on clinical grounds. Definitive diagnosis of ETEC infections can be made by isolating the bacteria from stool samples on MacConkey agar and assaying for the toxins by enzyme-linked immunoassay (ELISA) or with a DNA probe to detect the toxin genes. Knowing the characteristics of the fecal sample can be useful in distinguishing between infections of the small intestine (Table 21-5) and infections of the large intestine (see Chapter 22).

TREATMENT AND PREVENTION

Treatment of gastroenteritis caused by *E coli* usually involves oral replacement of the fluid and electrolytes lost in feces. Per-oral therapy is almost always adequate; however, if severe, intravenous treatment may be necessary. If antibiotics are needed, ciprofloxacin or levofloxacin are usually prescribed. Rifaximin has been approved for the treatment of traveler's diarrhea caused by noninvasive strains of *E coli*. Bismuth subsalicylate may provide symptomatic relief, with less severe abdominal cramps and less frequent stools.

For travelers to high-risk areas, several approaches should be encouraged to minimize the risk of getting traveler's diarrhea. These include instructions regarding food and beverage selection, use of bismuth subsalicylate for prophylaxis, and use of prophylactic antibiotics (e.g., rifaximin). Other means of preventing these infections include eating foods that are freshly cooked and served piping hot and avoiding water, ice, milk, beverages diluted with water (e.g., reconstituted fruit juices), and foods washed in water, such as salads. Other foods that are considered risky include raw or undercooked meat and seafood and raw fruits and vegetables. Prophylactic antibiotics are not recommended for most travelers, but may be considered for short-term travelers who are high-risk hosts (immunosuppressed or immunocompromised patients) or persons taking critical trips (e.g., trips due to family deaths, essential business trips, rescue efforts after a catastrophe) during which even a short bout of diarrhea could adversely affect the purpose of the trip.

TABLE 21-6. Manifestations of Cholera

- Profuse watery diarrhea
- Vomiting may occur after diarrhea

Severe cases of cholera

- The patient may be cyanotic and have sunken eyes and cheeks, a scaphoid abdomen, poor skin turgor, and thready or absent peripheral pulses
- The voice may be high pitched or inaudible
- Vital signs include tachycardia, tachypnea, and low or unobtainable blood pressure
- Heart sounds are distant and can oftentimes be inaudible
- Bowel sounds are indicative of hypoactive intestines

CHOLERA

The *Vibrio cholerae* organism is ingested with water or food and causes an acute illness due to an enterotoxin elaborated by *V cholerae*, which have colonized the small bowel. In its most severe form, there is rapid loss of liquid and electrolytes from the gastrointestinal tract, resulting in hypovolemic shock, metabolic acidosis, and death.

ETIOLOGY

V cholerae is a slightly curved gram-negative rod. This organism produces lipopolysaccharide (LPS) and is subdivided into 140 serogroups (O1 to O140) based on differences in LPS. Only the O1 and O139 serogroups produce cholera toxin and cause the most severe form of cholera. The O1 serogroup is further subdivided into serotypes (Inaba, Ogawa, and Hikojima) and biotypes (classical and el tor).

MANIFESTATIONS

The onset of cholera is abrupt and results in large amounts of watery diarrhea (Table 21-6). Several liters of liquid may be lost within a few hours, rapidly leading to profound shock.

EPIDEMIOLOGY

- Cholera is endemic in Louisiana and in India, West Bengal, and Bangladesh.

- Only about 1–10 cases of cholera occur each year in the United States, and patients usually have a history of travel to countries with endemic cholera.

- The organism is usually ingested in contaminated water or food (e.g., shellfish and crabs).

PATHOLOGY

V cholerae is acid sensitive, and most ingested organisms are killed by stomach acidity. About 10^8–10^{10} bacterial cells must be ingested to cause disease. The organisms that survive passage through the stomach attach to the microvilli of the glycocalyx of epithelial cells of the jejunum and ileum, where they multiply and liberate cholera enterotoxin, mucinase, and endotoxin. They do not invade the mucosa. All signs, symptoms, and metabolic derangements in cases of cholera result from rapid loss of liquid from the small intestine.

The enterotoxin (cholera toxin) consists of a binding moiety (B) and an activating moiety (A). Five equal subunits comprise the B moiety. On exposure to small bowel epithelial cells, each B subunit rapidly binds to GM_1 monosialoganglioside in the gut cell wall. Following binding, the A moiety migrates through the epithelial cell membrane. The A moiety contains adenosine diphosphate (ADP) ribosyltranferase activity and catalyzes the transfer of ADP-ribose from nicotinamide adenine dinucleotide (NAD) to a GTP-binding protein that regulates adenylate cyclase activity. The ADP-ribosylation of GTP-binding protein inhibits the GTP turnoff reaction and causes a sustained increase in adenylate cyclase activity. The resultant increased intracellular cyclic AMP acts at two sites to cause net secretion of isotonic liquid within the small bowel lumen. First, the increased cyclic AMP inhibits sodium chloride absorption across the glycocalyx via the cotransport mechanism; and second, the increase in cyclic AMP stimulates active chloride secretion into the gut lumen. Water in the tissues follows the ions, causing the profuse watery diarrhea. There is no significant damage to the cells lining the intestine.

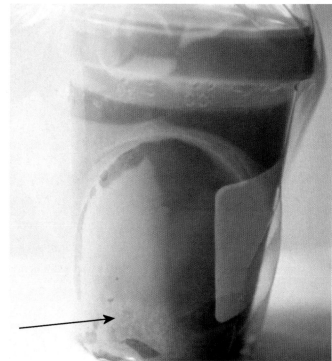

Figure 21-3. "Rice-water" fecal sample obtained from a cholera patient showing flecks of mucus that have settled to the bottom of the sample (*black arrow*). The odor of the stool is inoffensive, with a faint fishy odor. Stools are isotonic with plasma and contain high levels of sodium, potassium, and bicarbonate, and numerous *Vibrio cholerae* bacterial cells. Image courtesy of the Centers for Disease Control and Prevention.

DIAGNOSIS

In endemic or epidemic areas, the diagnosis of cholera is determined based on the clinical presentation, especially the presence of "rice water" stools (Figure 21-3). Definitive diagnosis is determined by plating a fecal sample on TCBS (thiosulfate-citrate-bile salt-sucrose) agar, which is selective for *Vibrio* and differentiates *V cholerae* (yellow on TCBS) from the other vibrios (green on TCBS) (Figure 21-4). An adrenal cell assay can also be used to detect the toxin.

TREATMENT AND PREVENTION

Successful therapy of cholera requires prompt replacement of fluids and electrolytes. Oral rehydration therapy is usually the first therapy attempted; however, if the dehydration cannot be corrected by oral administration of fluids, intravenous administration of fluids can be given. Tetracycline reduces the severity and length of disease.

INFANT BOTULISM

Botulism in infants younger than 1 year of age can follow either ingestion of the preformed toxin, as discussed above (see food poisoning), or after ingesting *C botulinum* spores.

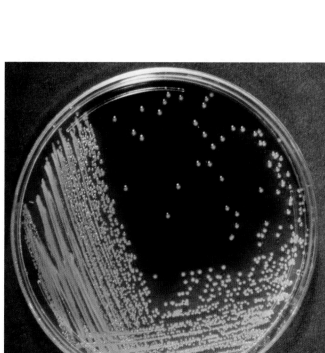

Figure 21-4. *Vibrio cholerae* growing on thiosulfate-citrate-bile salt-sucrose agar. Notice the yellow color of the colonies. Other colonies of *Vibrio* species will appear green on this medium. Image courtesy of the Centers for Disease Control and Prevention.

ETIOLOGY

C botulinum can colonize the gastrointestinal tract of an infant younger than 1 year of age, producing the botulism toxin in the intestines.

MANIFESTATIONS

Constipation is the first sign of disease, followed by the same neurologic signs discussed in the section on food poisoning.

EPIDEMIOLOGY

About 70–100 cases of infant botulism occur each year in the United States.

It is **most common in infants younger than 1 year of age.**

A common source of *C botulinum* spores is honey, which is used to sweeten the infant's milk or water.

PATHOLOGY

The *C botulinum* spores are ingested. Because of the lower acidity of the infant's stomach, spores can survive passage into the intestines. The spores geminate in the infant's small intestine, colonize it, and produce botulinum toxin in the intestine. The toxin then travels to the myoneural junctions and inhibits release of acetylcholine, causing a flaccid paralysis (Figure 21-5).

DIAGNOSIS

Presumptive diagnosis of botulism is determined by the presence of a rapidly descending paralysis. A history of ingestion of honey is helpful. Culture of the organism from the food and demonstration of toxin production can be performed (see food poisoning).

TREATMENT AND PREVENTION

Antibiotics generally are not effective and may exacerbate the illness by elimination of normal flora. Therapy is the same as for adult botulism (see food poisoning), except that antitoxin is generally not used because the disease is milder in children.

PARASITIC GASTROENTERITIS

Giardia lamblia and *Cryptosporidium parvum* are protozoan parasites that cause watery diarrhea worldwide.

Giardiasis

Acute infections of giardiasis can be asymptomatic or they can result in bloating, flatulence, and watery diarrhea. Chronic infections can lead to malabsorption and steatorrhea (fatty diarrhea).

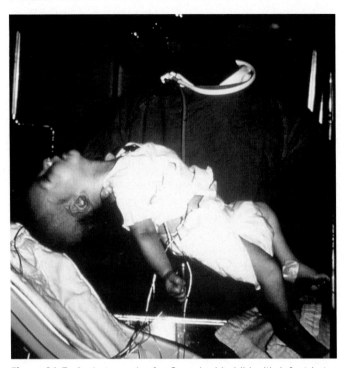

Figure 21-5. A photograph of a 6-week old child with infant botulism. Notice the loss of muscle tone in the head and neck region. Image courtesy of the Centers for Disease Control and Prevention.

ETIOLOGY

G lamblia (also called *G intestinalis*) is a protozoan flagellate that produces both a cyst to survive harsh environmental conditions and a trophozoite, which is only viable in the intestine. The cyst germinates in the intestine to produce the trophozoites. The teardrop-shaped trophozoites have a smooth dorsal surface with a concave ventral surface and a prominent anterior adhesive disk (Figure 21-6). The cysts are ellipsoidal (Figure 21-7).

MANIFESTATIONS

Giardiasis can result in asymptomatic or symptomatic disease that ranges from mild watery diarrhea to severe malabsorption syndrome. The incubation period ranges from 1 to 4 weeks. Disease onset is sudden and consists of foul-smelling watery diarrhea, abdominal cramps, flatulence, and steatorrhea. Spontaneous recovery can occur within 10 to 14 days; however, a chronic disease with multiple relapses can develop.

EPIDEMIOLOGY

Giardiasis is the most common intestinal protozoan parasite of humans in the United States. About 5000–7000 cases of giardiasis occur each year in the United States.

The parasite lives in the intestines of humans and in domestic and nondomesticated mammals.

Ingestion of water containing *G lamblia* cysts can cause infection (Figure 21-8). The cyst is the infectious form of the parasite.

Most persons are infected via the fecal-oral route of transmission.

PATHOLOGY

Ingestion of water containing *G lamblia* cysts causes infection. The cyst then develops into a trophozoite in the duodenum. The trophozoites adhere to the epithelium of the microvillus using their adhesive disks. Adherence of the parasite to the wall of the intestine does not cause a significant amount of damage; however, the parasite does cause a disaccharidase deficiency in the small intestine. The epithelial cells lining the microvilli do not absorb ingested disaccharides, causing an osmotic diarrhea with bloating, flatulence, and watery diarrhea.

Severe *G lamblia* infections can result in malabsorption and steatorrhea. Pathologic changes are mild in most cases, but shortening and thickening of the villi associated with acute focal inflammatory changes in the mucosal epithelium may be seen initially and are followed by chronic inflammatory infiltrates in the lamina propria.

DIAGNOSIS

Presumptive diagnosis is made on the basis of a history of drinking water that has not been chlorinated and the expression of classic clinical symptoms. Confirmative diagnosis requires detecting *G lamblia* trophozoites or cysts in feces. Because the parasite is not consistently shed in feces, a fecal sample collected on each of three consecutive days should be

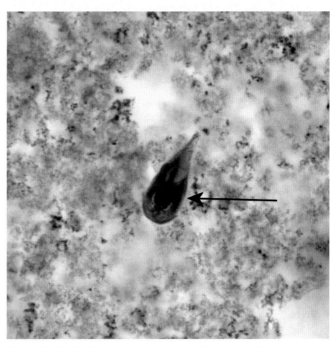

Figure 21-6. A photomicrograph of a *Giardia lamblia* trophozoite (*black arrow*). Notice the teardrop shape of this protozoan parasite (trichrome stain). Image courtesy of the Centers for Disease Control and Prevention, DPDx, Melanie Moser.

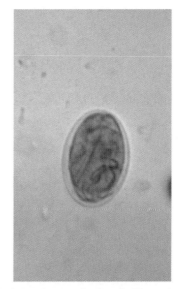

Figure 21-7. A photomicrograph of an iodine stain of *Giardia lamblia* cyst in a stool sample. Notice the elliptical shape of the cyst. Image courtesy of the Centers for Disease Control and Prevention.

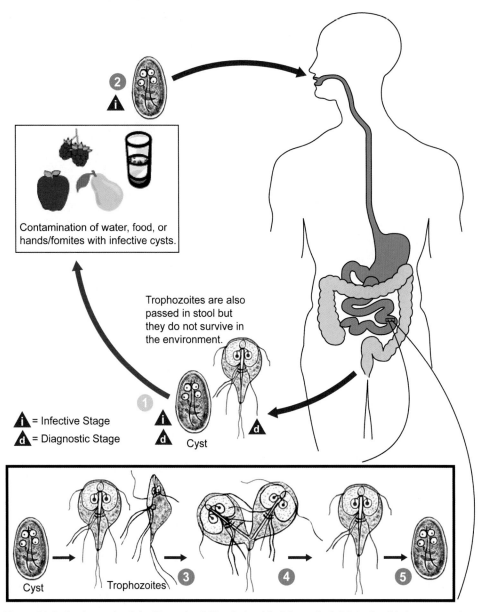

Figure 21-8. A schematic of the life cycle of *Giardia lamblia* (also called *G intestinalis*). Image courtesy of the Centers for Disease Control and Prevention, Alexander J da Silva, PhD, and Melanie Moser.

examined for cysts and trophozoites. If neither cysts nor trophozoites are found, the duodenum can be sampled by duodenal aspiration, string test (Entero-Test), or biopsy of the upper small intestine.

TREATMENT AND PREVENTION

Asymptomatic carriers and persons with symptoms of giardiasis infection should be treated with metronidazole, nitazoxanide, or quinacrine hydrochloride for 10 days. All drinking water should be boiled when on extended outdoor trips. Chlorination will not kill the cysts. Proper maintenance of filtration systems at water plants is essential.

Cryptosporidiosis

Cryptosporidium parvum is a protozoan parasite that primarily affects immunocompromised persons. *C parvum* can cause a severe and chronic diarrhea in HIV-infected patients and is an AIDS-defining condition.

ETIOLOGY

C parvum is a coccidium parasite that stains red using the acid-fast staining technique (Figure 21-9).

MANIFESTATIONS

In persons with normal immune function, an asymptomatic carrier state can occur as well as a self-limiting watery diarrhea. Spontaneous remission usually occurs in about 10 days. However, in the immunocompromised person, the diarrheal disease can be severe and chronic ($\geq$ 50 stools a day for months to years) and result in large amounts of fluid loss.

EPIDEMIOLOGY

C parvum occurs worldwide and inhabits the intestines of a variety of animals, fish, mammals, and reptiles, and is a common contaminant in water (Figure 21-10).

Ingestion of oocysts of *C parvum* in immunocompromised persons is more likely to result in a persistent chronic diarrhea. Only 150 oocysts can cause diarrhea in humans.

It is a frequent cause of diarrhea in daycare centers and among male homosexuals.

Autoinfections and person-to-person spread (fecal-oral and anal-oral) is common.

PATHOGENESIS

The pathogenesis of *C parvum* is not completely understood; however, it is known that the parasite affects intestinal ion transport and causes inflammatory damage of the microvilli, which results in malabsorption of the small intestine. Loss of cell-mediated immunity increases the risk of infection and is a common cause of chronic diarrhea in AIDS patients.

DIAGNOSIS

The cysts of *C parvum* are acid-fast positive; a stool smear stained with Kinyoun acid-fast stain can be used to visualize the parasites (see Figure 21-9).

TREATMENT AND PREVENTION

C parvum infection is usually self-limiting in persons with normal immune functioning and does not require medication; however, immunocompromised individuals with chronic

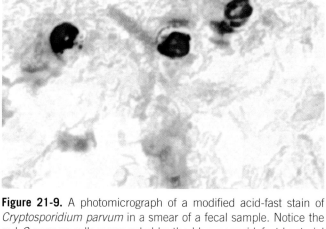

Figure 21-9. A photomicrograph of a modified acid-fast stain of *Cryptosporidium parvum* in a smear of a fecal sample. Notice the red *C parvum* cells surrounded by the blue nonacid–fast bacterial cells. Image courtesy of the Centers for Disease Control and Prevention, DPDx, Melanie Moser.

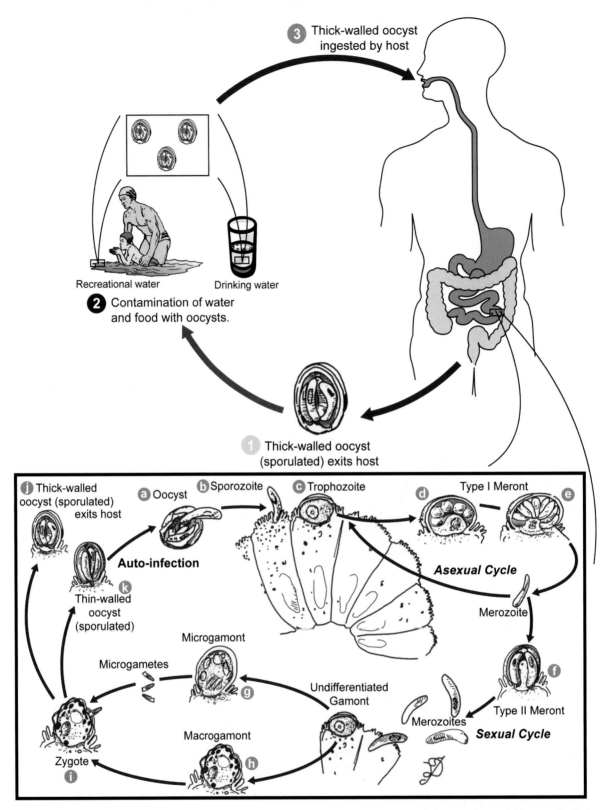

Figure 21-10. A schematic of the life cycle of *Cryptosporidium parvum*. Note that the infectious form of this parasite is the oocyst. Contaminated water is the most common means of acquiring this organism. Image courtesy of the Centers for Disease Control and Prevention, Alexander J da Silva, PhD, and Melanie Moser.

C parvum infection can be treated with nitazoxanide. Nonspecific antidiarrheal agents may provide temporary relief for patients where the infection will resolve without antiparasitic treatment. Contaminated water sources should be avoided.

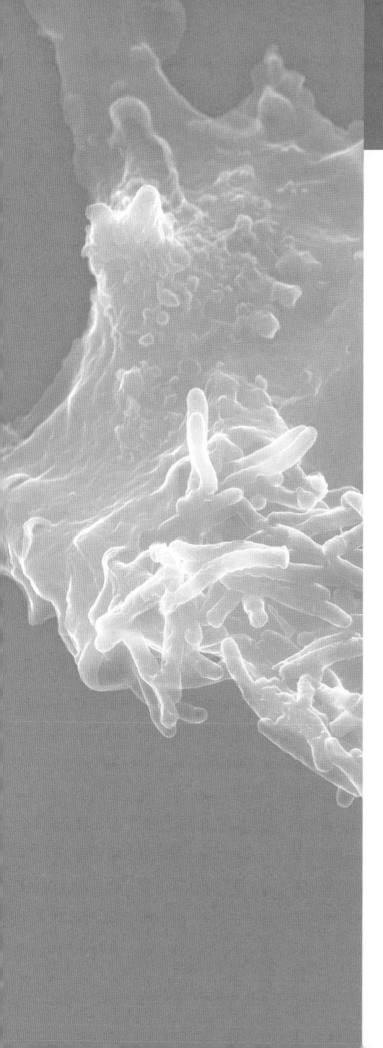

CHAPTER 22

INFECTIONS OF THE LARGE INTESTINE

OVERVIEW

The major infections discussed in this chapter include pseudomembranous colitis, bacterial dysentery (which includes campylobacteriosis, shigellosis, salmonellosis, *Escherichia coli* dysentery), and amebiasis (known as parasitic dysentery). These infections occur primarily in the large intestine and can invade the surrounding tissues. Invasion of the intestine can result in blood in feces and cause an inflammatory response (leukocytosis).

PSEUDOMEMBRANOUS COLITIS

Pseudomembranous colitis usually occurs after long-term antibiotic treatment and is due to overgrowth of *Clostridium difficile* in the colon and production of toxin by this bacterium.

ETIOLOGY

C difficile is an anaerobic gram-positive, spore-forming rod that produces toxin A and toxin B. Both toxins are cytophilic, but only toxin A is active against intestinal epithelial cells.

MANIFESTATIONS

Symptoms of pseudomembranous colitis vary from an asymptomatic carrier state to fulminant colitis. Watery diarrhea is the most common symptom. Other symptoms include crampy bilateral lower quadrant pain that decreases after bowel movements, low-grade fever, and mild peripheral blood leukocytosis. Usually the diarrhea begins 5–10 days after the initiation of antibiotic therapy; however, symptoms may be delayed as long as 10 weeks after completion of antibiotic therapy. Patients who develop pseudomembranous colitis have similar symptoms except that pseudomembranes can be observed on the mucosal surface of the colon when viewed during colonoscopy.

A fulminant colitis develops in 2–3% of patients. Patients with pseudomembranous colitis have a severe morbidity and high mortality rate. Diarrhea is usually present; however, the patient can be constipated. There is diffuse, severe abdominal

225

pain associated with hypoactive bowel sounds, abdominal distension, and guarding. A marked peripheral blood leukocytosis is common. Perforation of the colon can result. Development of lactic acidosis usually signals impending bowel perforation and irreversible bowel damage that requires surgical intervention. Complications can include toxic megacolon and bowel perforation. Toxic megacolon results in a persistently high fever, marked leukocytosis, lack of response to antibiotics, and marked bowel thickening seen on CT scan.

EPIDEMIOLOGY

About 3 million cases of *C difficile* diarrhea or pseudomembranous colitis occur in the United States annually.

C difficile is a bacterium that is resistant to most broad-spectrum antibiotics and is present in the intestine of about 5% of humans. Long-term systemic antibiotic therapy reduces the number of viable bacteria in the intestine but allows *C difficile* to become the predominate organism in the gastrointestinal tract.

Diarrhea due to *C difficile* and antibiotic use develops in up to 30% of hospitalized patients. The most common antibiotics implicated include second- and third-generation cephalosporins, ampicillin and amoxicillin, and clindamycin.

Pseudomembranous colitis is primarily a disease of hospitalized patients.

The intestines of patients with pseudomembranous colitis are colonized by *C difficile* via the fecal-oral route.

PATHOGENESIS

Systemic antibiotic treatment reduces the normal flora and interferes with the bacterial breakdown of carbohydrates. The increased amounts of undigested carbohydrates increase the osmotic load in the colon by preventing water resorption and causing watery diarrhea.

If *C difficile* is present in the colon, it will overgrow and produce toxins A and B, which bind to and kill cells in the bowel wall. The organism produces small amounts of these toxins, which only achieve cytotoxic levels when it is the predominant organism. Disease severity is related to the number of receptors for the bacterial toxin on the epithelial cells lining the colon. These toxins cause the epithelial cells to become more round in shape (or round up) and die by stimulating host cell mitogen-activated protein kinases (MAP-kinases) and inactivating proteins that regulate actin filament assembly (small guanosine triphosphate [GTP]-binding Rho proteins). The toxins cause depolymerization of actin filaments, which cause the cells to round up and detach and shallow ulcers to form. Acute inflammation with pus and mucus formation results in pseudomembrane formation. Inflammation can extend through the full thickness of the bowel.

DIAGNOSIS

Diagnosis of pseudomembranous colitis generally is determined on the basis of a history of antibiotic therapy within the past month. Culture usually is not performed due to its expense and difficulty. An enzyme-linked immunoassay (ELISA) for toxins A and B can be performed on the fecal specimen. In about 50% of cases, fecal samples contain leukocytes and are heme positive. Endoscopy revealing the pseudomembranes can confirm the diagnosis if the patient is unable to produce a fecal sample or if an immediate diagnosis is required.

TREATMENT AND PREVENTION

Withdrawal of the antibiotic and replacement of the intestinal flora generally suffices in the treatment of pseudomembranous colitis. If dehydrated, the patient should be given intravenous fluids and electrolytes. ***Antimotility drugs should not be given because they increase the likelihood of full-blown colitis and toxic megacolon.***

If antibiotic treatment is necessary, metronidazole will eradicate *C difficile;* however, asymptomatic persons should not be treated with this drug. Except in cases of severe disease, oral vancomycin should be avoided to prevent selecting for vancomycin-resistant enterococci. Patients with toxic megacolon should be treated surgically; bowel resection and ileostomy are recommended.

Standard infection control measures must be meticulously followed to prevent the spread of the bacterial spores from patient to patient. Thorough hand washing should be emphasized, and prolonged use of broad-spectrum antibiotic treatment should be avoided. The use of clindamycin, a common antibiotic that can cause overgrowth of *C difficile,* should be limited.

BACTERIAL DYSENTERY

Bacterial dysentery can occur in the large and small intestine. Organisms that cause bacterial dysentery and are discussed in this chapter include *Campylobacter, Shigella, Salmonella,* and *E coli.* These organisms are invasive and cause the host to mount an inflammatory response. The stool volume frequently is small and contains mucus and leukocytes; if invasion is deep enough, the stool can be heme positive. The patient usually has a fever and complains of abdominal pain and pain while attempting to defecate (tenesmus).

In most cases, antimicrobial treatment of bacterial dysentery is beneficial. Treatment with antimotility drugs to stop the bacterial dysentery is contraindicated. ***The three most common causative organisms of bacterial dysentery are Campylobacter, Shigella, and Salmonella.*** Campylobacter, Shigella, *Salmonella,* and the invasive *E coli* (enterohemorrhagic *E coli* [EHEC] and enteroinvasive *E coli* [EIEC]) are discussed below.

CAMPYLOBACTERIOSIS

Campylobacter species are gram-negative slender, curved motile rods. These organisms are comma- or S-shaped (or seagull-shaped).

ETIOLOGY

There are eight different species of *Campylobacter* that cause gastrointestinal infections; *C jejuni* is the most common species associated with human infection. *Campylobacter* are gram-negative S-shaped or gull wing–shaped rods that commonly occur in pairs and are microaerophilic and motile (Figure 22-1). *Campylobacter* are relatively fragile, and are sensitive to environmental stresses (e.g., 21% oxygen, drying, heating, disinfectants, and acidic conditions). The organisms require reduced oxygen and increased carbon dioxide and hydrogen concentrations for optimal growth. The optimal temperature for growth is 42°C.

MANIFESTATIONS

Most cases of campylobacteriosis are mild and subside within 7 days; some cases may last for 2 weeks or longer. Symptoms include periumbilical cramping, intense abdominal pain that mimics appendicitis, malaise, myalgias, headache, and vomiting. Watery diarrhea is the most common manifestation.

Inflammatory bowel disease may occur in some patients with campylobacteriosis. Manifestations include malaise, fever, abdominal cramps, tenesmus, and bloody stools; fecal leukocytes are observed with light microscopy. The inflammation and pathology that is due to *C jejuni* is indistinguishable from the inflammation and pathology due to *Shigella*, *Salmonella*, and *E coli*. Clinical findings are not diagnostic. Complications are rare, but infections have been associated with reactive arthritis (persons with HLA-B27), hemolytic uremic syndrome (HUS), Guillain-Barré syndrome, and septicemia.

EPIDEMIOLOGY

C jejuni is a leading cause of bacterial diarrheal illness in the United States, with about 2 million cases per year. It is the second most common cause of invasive dysentery; *Salmonella* infections are the most common cause.

C jejuni is *not* carried by healthy individuals in the United States or Europe but can be isolated from healthy cattle, chickens, birds, and even flies. Between 20% and 100% of chicken meat sold in retail food markets is contaminated with this organism.

It is present in some nonchlorinated water sources such as streams and ponds.

Ingestion of undercooked or raw meat (e.g., poultry), unpasteurized milk, and nonchlorinated water contaminated with *Campylobacter* are the most common means of transmission.

About 1 million bacterial cells must be ingested to cause disease.

PATHOGENESIS

C jejuni adheres to intestinal epithelial cells and M cells. Depending on the bacterial strain, it can produce a heat-labile toxin or cause host cells to ingest bacterial cells. If a heat-labile enterotoxin is produced, a watery diarrhea occurs. If organisms induce the host cells to ingest the bacteria, an inflammatory colitis will usually occur. After adhering to the host cells, the bacteria use a type III secretory system to inject bacterial proteins into the host cells (Figure 22-2). These bacterial proteins cause the host cells to ruffle and ingest the bacterial cells.

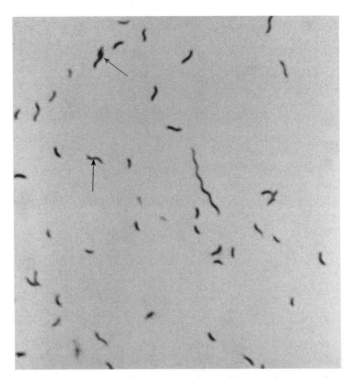

Figure 22-1. A photomicrograph of *Campylobacter* demonstrating the S-shaped (*black arrow*) and gull wing-shaped (*blue arrow*), gram-negative rod (Gram stain). Image courtesy of the Centers for Disease Control and Prevention.

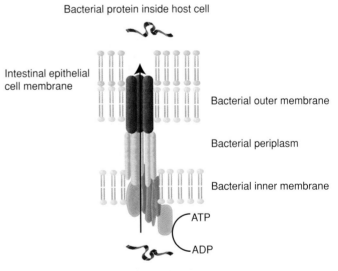

Figure 22-2. A schematic of the type III bacterial secretory system. Contact between the bacteria and the host cell induces the bacterial cell to produce the proteins needed to construct the type III bacterial secretion system. *Shigella* and *Salmonella* produce these proteins that form a channel between the cytoplasm of the bacterium and the cytoplasm of the host cell, so that bacterial proteins can be placed in the host cell. Some of the bacterial proteins cause the host cell to ruffle and then engulf the bacterial cell.

Some strains of *C jejuni* produce a toxin called shiga toxin or verotoxin that enters the cytoplasm of the host cells and interrupts protein synthesis by removing an adenine residue from the 28S rRNA in the 60S ribosomal unit. Shiga toxin kills the host cells and results in the formation of superficial ulcers in the bowel mucosa and induces an acute inflammatory response.

Immunocompromised patients, patients with chronic illnesses, and persons at the extremes of ages are more likely to develop a bacteremia that may be transient and resolve without treatment or may infect other sites (e.g., meninges, lungs, heart, blood vessels). The clinical manifestations following *C jejuni* infection are similar to those caused by *Shigella* and EIEC.

DIAGNOSIS

Presumptive diagnosis of campylobacteriosis is based on the finding of gull wing–shaped bacteria in watery, bloody, leukocyte-filled feces. These bacteria have a characteristic darting motility. Definitive diagnosis requires isolation of the organism from stool or from other sites of infection. Isolation requires the use of campy-BAP or Skirrow media. These media contain antibiotics that reduce the growth of other enteric microorganisms.

TREATMENT AND PREVENTION

Most *C jejuni* infections are mild and self-limited. They usually do not require antibiotic therapy, and correction of electrolyte abnormalities and oral rehydration is sufficient. Treatment is reserved for compromised hosts or persons with fever, increasingly bloody diarrhea, or symptoms that last longer than 1 week. *C jejuni* is usually sensitive to erythromycin, gentamicin, tetracycline, ciprofloxacin, and clindamycin. Properly cooking chicken, pasteurizing milk, and chlorinating drinking water will kill the bacteria and prevent infections with these bacteria.

SHIGELLOSIS

Shigella is a common contaminant of water sources. A small number (200) of these bacteria can cause diseases in humans. Fortunately, *Shigella* rarely invades the bloodstream.

ETIOLOGY

There about 50 *Shigella* species that can be classified into one of four serologic groups. Only two serologic groups are common in the United States: Group B, which contains *S flexneri*, is a species commonly isolated in the United States; and Group D, which contains *S sonnei*, is the most commonly isolated cause of shigellosis in the United States. *Shigella* is a nonmotile, nonlactose fermenting gram-negative rod that is closely related to *E coli* and shares antigens and toxin-producing capability with them.

MANIFESTATIONS

After an incubation period of 36–72 hours, the initial nonspecific symptoms of shigellosis are prominent and include fever

(38–39°C) and cramping abdominal pain. Watery diarrhea usually appears after 48 hours, with dysentery (e.g., bloody small volume stools containing mucus; tenesmus) supervening about 2 days later. Abdominal tenderness is usually general, and the abdominal wall is not rigid. Sigmoidoscopy reveals intense hyperemia (Figure 22-3), multiple small bleeding sites, loss of transverse mucosal folds, and thick, purulent mucus secretions. Tenesmus is present, and feces are bloody, mucoid, and small volume. Fluid and electrolyte loss may be relatively significant, particularly in pediatric and geriatric populations. Septicemia caused by *E coli* may be initiated by shigellosis.

EPIDEMIOLOGY

Shigella is found only in humans and monkeys. About 300,000 cases of shigellosis occur each year in the United States.

Shigella is quite resistant to eradication by stomach acid. As few as 200 organisms can infect the large intestine, and about 1 million organisms must infect the large intestine to cause campylobacteriosis and salmonellosis.

Shigellosis is mainly a disease of children between the ages of 1 and 4 years.

It is more common in closed population groups that have substandard sanitation (e.g., prisoner-of-war camps, homes for mentally retarded, American Indian reservations).

Shigellosis is primarily transmitted by the fecal-oral route. Contaminated drinking water and person-to-person transmission are common means of spreading this bacterial infection.

PATHOLOGY

Shigella adheres to intestinal epithelial cells and M cells. After adhering to the host cells, the bacteria use a type III secretory system to inject bacterial proteins into the host cells (see Figure 22-2). These bacterial proteins cause the host cells to ruffle and ingest the bacterial cells. Once in the cells, the bacteria use a surface hemolysin to lyse the phagosome membrane and escape into the cytoplasm. The bacteria then use the host cell's actin to move around inside the cell (actin rocket tails). When bacteria reach the periphery of the cell, the cell pushes outward to form membrane projections, which are then ingested by adjacent cells.

Some strains of the *Shigella* genus produce the shiga toxin or verotoxin, which is similar to the verotoxin of *E coli* O157:H7. The shiga toxin or verotoxin enters the cytoplasm of the host cells and stops protein synthesis by removing an adenine residue from the 28S rRNA in the 60S ribosomal unit. This toxic activity results in death of the host cells.

The cell-to-cell travel and toxin activity produces superficial ulcers in the bowel mucosa and induces an extensive acute inflammatory response. The inflammatory response usually prevents entry of the bacteria into the bloodstream. Unlike certain species of *Salmonella* (e.g., *S typhi*, *S paratyphi* A), *Shigella* only rarely enters the bloodstream.

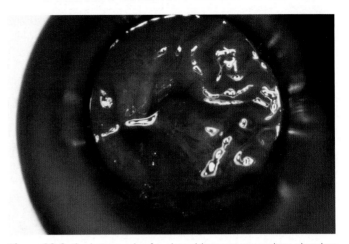

Figure 22-3. A photograph of a sigmoidoscopy procedure showing the interior mucosal surface of the rectum of a patient with bacillary dysentery, or shigellosis. Examination of the sigmoid colon with a sigmoidoscope revealed an inflamed and engorged mucosa. Image courtesy of the Centers for Disease Control and Prevention.

DIAGNOSIS

Presumptive diagnosis of shigellosis is based on acute onset of fever and diarrhea with bloody and mucoid feces. Definitive diagnosis requires the isolation of *Shigella* from feces. Microabscesses in a rectal biopsy are suggestive of shigellosis. Diffuse involvement of the mucosa with multiple shallow ulcers 3–7 mm in diameter is suggestive of shigellosis. A rectal swab of an ulcer will reveal clumps of neutrophils, macrophages, and erythrocytes. Stool usually contains white blood cells and is positive for lactoferrin. *Shigella* is commonly isolated on *Salmonella-Shigella* agar (S-S agar).

TREATMENT AND PREVENTION

Shigellosis is usually a self-limited disease; however, to shorten the course of the illness and prevent person-to-person spread, treatment with trimethoprim-sulfamethoxazole or ciprofloxacin usually is recommended. Fluid and electrolyte replacement is necessary in severe cases. ***Antidiarrheal compounds that inhibit peristalsis are CONTRAINDICATED.***

To avoid acquiring shigellosis, the following precautions should be taken: drinking contaminated water or foods washed with contaminated water should be avoided; utensils and drinking glasses should not be shared with persons who are ill; hands should always be washed after changing diapers; and easy to reach hand-washing facilities should be provided in day-care centers.

SALMONELLOSIS

Several different strains of *Salmonella* cause human disease. For example, some strains such as *S enterica* invade the tissues of the intestine but remain there and do not disseminate via the bloodstream to other organs of the body. *S enterica* causes enteritis, which is the most common form of disease due to *Salmonella*. However, other strains of *Salmonella*, including *S typhi, S paratyphi* A, *S schottmuelleri,* and *S hirschfeldii,* can invade the tissues of the intestine and are disseminated via the bloodstream to other parts of the body. *S typhi, S paratyphi* A, *S schottmuelleri, S hirschfeldii* cause enteric fevers and are less common than enteritis.

ETIOLOGY

Salmonella are gram-negative motile, rod-shaped facultative anaerobes that produce hydrogen sulfide (H_2S) gas and do not ferment lactose. Table 22-1 lists the species of *Salmonella* that can cause human infections.

MANIFESTATIONS

S enterica is the most common form of salmonellosis. It causes enteritis, a disease that results in diarrhea, fever, and abdominal cramps. Symptoms appear about 24–48 hours after ingestion of contaminated food or water. Initially the patient experiences nausea and vomiting, abdominal cramps, and nonbloody diarrhea. There may be signs of systemic involvement because patients will have fever, headache, and

TABLE 22-1. Diseases Caused by *Salmonella*

Bacteria	Disease Caused
Salmonella enterica	Enteritis
S enterica serovar *choleraesuis*	Bacteremia
S paratyphi A	Paratyphoid fever (enteric fever), bacteremia
S schottmuelleri (formerly *S paratyphi* B)	Paratyphoid fever (enteric fever), bacteremia
S hirschfeldii (formerly *S paratyphi* C)	Paratyphoid fever (enteric fever), bacteremia
S typhi	Typhoid fever (enteric fever), bacteremia

myalgias. Symptoms last from 2 days to 1 week and usually resolve spontaneously.

All salmonellae can cause bacteremia. However, *S paratyphi* A, *S schottmuelleri, S hirschfeldii, S enterica* serovar *choleraesuis,* and *S typhi are* strains that are more likely to cause bacteremia. The clinical presentation is similar to other cases of gram-negative sepsis (see Chapter 28). The risk of bacteremia is higher in pediatric, geriatric, and immunocompromised patients.

Enteric fevers are caused by *S typhi* (typhoid fever), *S paratyphi A, S schottmuelleri, and S hirschfeldii* (paratyphoid fever). About 10 to 14 days after ingestion, patients experience a gradually increasing fever with headache, myalgias, malaise, and anorexia. The symptoms persist for about 1 week and are followed by diarrhea. These manifestations correspond to an initial bacteremic phase, followed by colonization of the gallbladder and then reinfection of the intestines. Symptoms of *S typhi* tend to be more severe than symptoms seen in patients with paratyphoid fever. *S typhi* can cause skin lesions called rose spots (Figure 22-4). The strains of *Salmonella* responsible for enteric fevers can chronically colonize the gallbladder and serve as an infectious reservoir. Patients can be colonized and can be infectious for up to 1 year following resolution of symptoms.

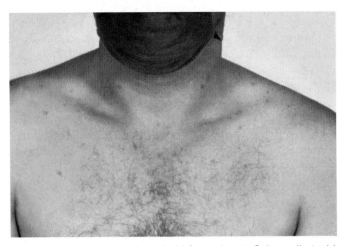

Figure 22-4. A patient with typhoid fever due to *Salmonella typhi.* Note the rose-colored spots on the patient's chest. Image courtesy of the Centers for Disease Control and Prevention. Armed Forces Institute of Pathology, Charles N Farmer.

EPIDEMIOLOGY

About 2–4 million cases of salmonellosis occur in the United States each year, and the incidence appears to be increasing.

About 1 million bacterial cells must be ingested to cause disease. Because large numbers of organisms are required to cause infection, most infections occur following ingestion of heavily contaminated foods.

Salmonellosis is more common in the summer months when warmer temperatures allow for rapid growth of the organisms in contaminated foods.

Almost all strains of *Salmonella* (except *S paratyphi* A, *S schottmuelleri, S hirschfeldii,* and *S typhi*) colonize virtually all animals. Salmonella are commonly found inhabiting the intestines of chickens, reptiles, birds, and humans.

S paratyphi A, *S schottmuelleri, S hirschfeldii* and *S typhi* are found only in humans.

Some humans infected with these organisms become chronic carriers after *S paratyphi* A, *S schottmuelleri, S hirschfeldii,* or *S typhi* colonize the gallbladder. These carriers transmit the infection via fecal-oral routes.

Transmission from animals (e.g., turtles, iguanas) to humans and from animal food products to humans (e.g., raw meats, poultry, eggs, milk and dairy products, fish, shrimp, cream-filled desserts and toppings, peanut butter, cocoa, and chocolate) is common.

PATHOGENESIS

Salmonella are sensitive to killing by gastric acid. Therefore, *Salmonella* requires large numbers of organisms to cause an infection of the intestines. If the acid in the stomach is reduced or neutralized, fewer organisms are required. If the organisms survive the stomach's acidity, the bacteria attach to the epithelial cells in the small intestine and colon. Once attached to the host cells, *Salmonella* bacteria use a type III secretory system to inject bacterial proteins into the host cells (see Figure 22-2). These bacterial proteins cause the host cells to ruffle and ingest the bacterial cells in large vacuoles. In the vacuoles, the bacteria replicate and eventually cause the cells to lyse. Following host cell lysis, the bacteria escape into the extracellular environment and gain entry into the mesenteric lymph nodes and some enter the bloodstream. Most infections result in fever, abdominal pain, and diarrhea. One of the few serovars of *S enterica* that can enter the bloodstream and cause nontyphoidal bacteremia is *S enterica* serovar *choleraesuis*.

The strains of *Salmonella* that cause enteric fevers can rapidly enter the bloodstream. These strains cause only minimal damage in the intestine (little, if any, diarrhea). *S paratyphi* A, *S schottmuelleri*, *S hirschfeldii*, and *S typhi* are most invasive. These bacteria pass through the cells lining the intestines and are engulfed by macrophages. They survive in the macrophages and are carried by the macrophages to the liver, spleen, and bone marrow where they replicate. Manifestations of the disease correspond to an initial bacteremic phase (gradually increasing fever with headache, myalgias, malaise, and anorexia), followed by colonization of the gallbladder and reinfection of the intestines (diarrhea).

DIAGNOSIS

Salmonella cause less inflammation than do *Shigella*. In *Salmonella* infections, there are fewer fecal leukocytes, and isolation of the organisms from a fecal sample using S-S agar is necessary for a definitive diagnosis.

THERAPY AND PREVENTION

Enteritis is self-limiting in most people. Treatment prolongs carriage of the bacteria and does not shorten the course of the illness. However, certain patients should be treated because of their increased likelihood of developing bacteremia, endocarditis, and osteomyelitis. These groups include neonates, persons older than 50 years of age, immunocompromised patients, patients with sickle-cell disease, and patients with prosthetic valves or vascular grafts. Fluid and electrolyte replacement is necessary in severe cases. ***Antidiarrheal compounds that inhibit peristalsis are CONTRAINDICATED.***

Patients with enteric fevers warrant immediate antibiotic therapy (e.g., ciprofloxacin or ceftriaxone) and in severe cases, fluid and electrolyte replacement is necessary. ***Antidiarrheal compounds that inhibit peristalsis are also contraindicated in enteric fevers.***

Persons traveling to countries with high rates of typhoid fever should be vaccinated. Two typhoid vaccines are available for use in the United States: an oral live attenuated vaccine and a Vi capsular polysaccharide vaccine that is injected.

DYSENTERY DUE TO *E COLI*

The *E coli* strains normally resident in the human intestine have minimal or no invasive ability. However, enterohemorrhagic

E coli (EHEC) and enteroinvasive *E coli* (EIEC) have acquired certain genetic traits from *Shigella* that allow them to possess the same invasive capabilities that *Shigella* possesses.

EHEC strains, also called shiga toxin-producing *E coli* (STEC), have acquired shiga toxin, which causes cell death, edema, and hemorrhage in the lamina propria. The blood from the lamina propria can enter the lumen of the intestine and cause hemorrhagic colitis. The shiga toxin in kidneys can cause hemolytic uremic syndrome (HUS). The most common cause of hemorrhagic colitis and HUS is EHEC serotype O157:H7; however, non-O157:H7 serotypes of *E coli* can produce shiga toxin and cause hemorrhagic colitis and HUS.

ETIOLOGY

EHEC *E coli* serotypes are O157:H7 and non-O157:H7. EIEC strains *of E coli* can also cause dysentery. EHEC and EIEC are facultative gram-negative, motile rod-shaped bacteria. ***E coli O157:H7 does not ferment sorbitol, and thus can be differentiated from non-O157:H7 serotypes of E coli, which do ferment sorbitol.***

MANIFESTATIONS

EHEC causes hemorrhagic colitis. Manifestations include severe crampy abdominal pain and watery diarrhea followed by grossly bloody diarrhea; there usually is ***no fever.*** The symptomology of HUS includes the triad of acute renal failure, thrombocytopenia, and microangiopathic hemolytic anemia. Hemorrhagic colitis usually precedes HUS. EIEC infection produces a watery diarrhea, which can result in dysenteric stools (small volume, mucous-containing bloody feces).

EPIDEMIOLOGY

- About 500–700 cases of EHEC infection are reported each year in the United States.

- EHEC can live in the intestines of healthy cattle. Meat can be contaminated during slaughter, and organisms can be mixed into beef when it is ground.

- ***The most common means of infection is consumption of insufficiently cooked ground beef.*** Only a minimal number of organisms are necessary to cause infection.

- The second most common source of EHEC infection occurs following consumption of fresh leafy green vegetables (e.g., spinach, sprouts, lettuce). Other sources of infection involve consumption of salami and unpasteurized milk and juice and ingestion of sewage-contaminated water or swimming in contaminated water.

- In some persons, especially children younger than 5 years of age and the elderly, infection with EHEC can also cause HUS. About 2–7% of EHEC infections lead to HUS.

- In the United States, HUS is the principal cause of acute kidney failure in children; most cases of HUS are caused by *E coli* O157:H7.

- Infected persons can transmit the infection from person to person if hygiene or handwashing habits are inadequate, which is particularly likely among toddlers who are not toilet trained.

Family members and playmates of these children are at high risk of becoming infected. Young children typically shed the organism in feces for 1–2 weeks after the illness has resolved.

PATHOGENESIS

Most pathology in EHEC infections occurs in the lamina propria of the ascending and transverse colons. Colonic biopsy specimens show focal necrosis and infiltration of neutrophils. Damage to the kidneys is due to the shiga toxin and results in swollen glomerular epithelial cells, fibrin deposition, and infiltrates of inflammatory cells. The pathology of EIEC infections is similar to that of most *Shigella* infections.

DIAGNOSIS

Isolation and identification of the etiologic agent is necessary for definitive diagnosis of *E coli* dysentery. To grow EHEC O157:H7, the carbohydrate sorbitol must be included in the medium.

THERAPY AND PREVENTION

Antimotility drugs and antibiotics should NOT be given to patients to treat EHEC infections. Administration of antibiotics kills the bacteria and releases additional toxin, increasing the likelihood that the patient will develop HUS. To prevent EHEC infections, individuals should be advised to properly cook all food and to drink only pasteurized fruit juices.

EIEC infections are usually self-limiting; however, in severe cases, patients can be given trimethoprim-sulfoxazole or a fluoroquinolone or ciprofloxacin. ***Antimotility drugs should NOT be given.*** EIEC infections can be prevented by drinking from safe potable water sources.

PARASITIC DYSENTERY: AMEBIASIS

Entamoeba histolytica is the ***only*** parasite that causes dysentery, and it is relatively uncommon in the United States. However, it does cause infections worldwide and can invade tissues contiguous to the colon.

ETIOLOGY

E histolytica is a protozoan parasite. It is an amoeba that exists in two forms: the trophozoite form and the cyst form. The motile amoeboid trophozoite is the only form present in tissue. The cyst form is the infectious form of the parasite (Figure 22-5).

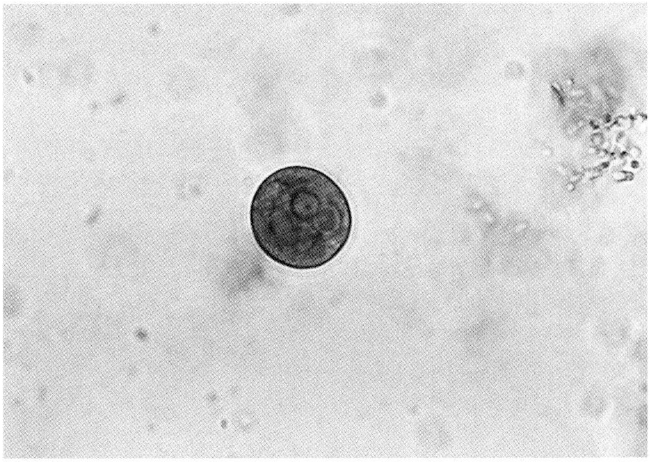

MANIFESTATIONS

After an incubation period of 1–5 days, amebiasis begins with a prodromal episode of diarrhea, abdominal cramps, nausea and vomiting, and tenesmus. Feces may be watery; in dysentery, feces are generally watery and contain mucus and blood.

Trophozoites of *E histolytica* can penetrate the colon and infect the liver, causing amebic liver abscess. Symptoms of amebic liver abscess include abrupt onset of high fever and right upper quadrant abdominal pain. The pain is constant and may radiate to the right scapula and shoulder. It may become

Figure 22-5. A photomicrograph of a cyst of *Entamoeba histolytica* (iodine stain). Image courtesy of the Centers for Disease Control and Prevention, Dr LLA Moore, Jr.

pleuritic and increase when the patient lies on the right side. An abscess of the left lobe of the liver may cause predominantly epigastric pain that radiates to the left shoulder. Anorexia and nausea and vomiting may occur.

Involvement of nonhepatic extraintestinal organs is much less frequent in amebiasis. Trophozoites may disseminate to other organs, especially when there is a liver abscess, by direct extension into the lung, pleural cavity, or pericardium or through the bloodstream to the lung or brain. Cutaneous lesions may result from direct invasion of macerated epithelium in the perianal area when trophozoite-containing liquid feces contaminate the skin (Figure 22-6).

EPIDEMIOLOGY

- The distribution of the parasite *E histolytica* is worldwide, with higher incidence in developing countries.

- In industrialized countries, high-risk groups include male homosexuals, travelers outside the United States, recent immigrants, and institutionalized populations (e.g., prison inmates).

- **The liver is the most common site of extraintestinal amebic disease**.

- Amebiasis is transmitted by fecal contamination of drinking water and foods, but can also be transmitted by direct contact with fecally contaminated hands or objects as well as by sexual contact.

PATHOGENESIS

E histolytica exists in two different forms: an infectious cyst and a tissue-dwelling trophozoite. The cyst of *E histolytica* is ingested and passes through the stomach and small intestine. The cyst then excysts and produces the trophozoite in the intestine, which adheres to the surface-exposed lectins of intestinal epithelial cells. After adherence, trophozoites invade the colonic epithelium. The trophozoites of *E histolytica* lyse the target cells using the parasite's ionophore-like protein to induce leakage of ions (Na^+, K^+, Ca^+) from the cytoplasm of the target cell, which causes watery diarrhea. Ameboid movement and amebic enzymes such as proteases, hemolysins, cysteine kinase, hyaluronidase, and mucopolysaccharidases facilitate penetration into the wall of the intestine. After penetrating the wall of the intestine, *E histolytica* will produce flask-shaped ulcers in the intestines (Figure 22-7). **These ulcerations are characteristic of this disease and usually occur in the cecum, appendix, and ascending colon**.

E histolytica can also produce hepatic abscess, brain abscess, and rectal ulcerations. The trophozoites eventually penetrate the venules and lymphatics in the wall of the intestine, and gain access to the liver via the portal vein. The organisms in the hepatic microcirculation produce necrosis of the endothelium and penetrate into the periportal sinusoids, where they can digest pathways into the hepatic lobules. There is no initial inflammatory reaction; however as necrosis progresses, polymorphonuclear leukocytes gradually surround the lesion without formation of a definite wall. The lesions may remain focal or progress to form large solitary abscesses. Lung and brain abscesses are less

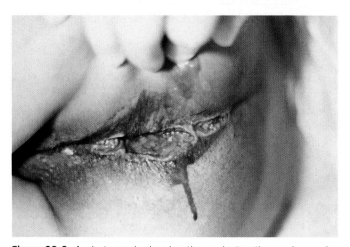

Figure 22-6. A photograph showing tissue destruction and granulation of the anoperineal region due to *Entamoeba histolytica* infection. In more serious cases of amebiasis, amoebae can cause an infection of tissue outside of the intestinal tract, as shown in this photograph. Image courtesy of the Centers for Disease Control and Prevention.

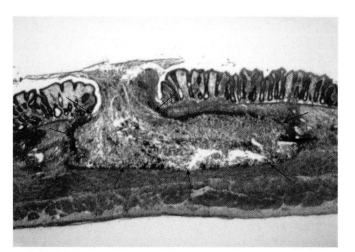

Figure 22-7. A photomicrograph of a cross-section of the wall of the large intestine showing a flask-shaped ulcer caused by *Entamoeba histolytica*. Image courtesy of the Centers for Disease Control and Prevention, Dr Mae Melvin.

common and are similar to those seen in the liver. Skin ulcerations are usually perirectal and have only minimal inflammation.

DIAGNOSIS

The diagnosis of amebiasis is confirmed by identifying *E histolytica* in feces or in tissues obtained from lesions. If the cytoplasm of the trophozoite contains red blood cells, the diagnosis of amebiasis is definitive (***the presence of intracytoplasmic red blood cells is pathognomonic for E histolytica***) (Figure 22-8). Leukocytosis without eosinophilia is common. ELISA assays are used to detect cysts in feces.

Serology for antibodies to the parasite is useful in extraintestinal infections. Chest radiograph, CT scan, and MRI are useful in visualizing extraintestinal amebic abscesses. A brown milkshake-like (anchovy paste-like) material is often aspirated from liver abscesses (Figure 22-9).

THERAPY AND PREVENTION

Asymptomatic intestinal *E histolytica* infections can be treated with paromomycin or iodoquinol. Mild to moderate disease that includes diarrhea or dysentery can be treated with metronidazole followed by either paromomycin or iodoquinol. If the pleura surrounding the lungs are involved, drainage via a chest tube or thoracotomy may be necessary. Only large liver abscesses (>12 cm in diameter), should be treated surgically. Contaminated water sources and behaviors that result in fecal-oral spread of the organism should be avoided.

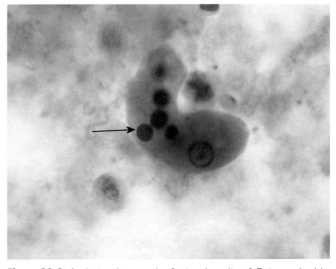

Figure 22-8. A photomicrograph of a trophozoite of *Entamoeba histolytica*. The trophozoite contains intracytoplasmic erythrocytes (*arrow*) obtained from the host (trichrome stain). Image courtesy of the Centers for Disease Control and Prevention, Dr N J Wheeler, Jr.

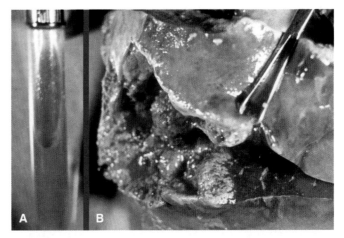

Figure 22-9. A, A tube of chocolate-colored pus drained from a liver abscess caused by *Entamoeba histolytica*. **B,** A photograph of a liver with extensive destruction due to *Entamoeba histolytica* infection. Images courtesy of the Centers for Disease Control and Prevention, Dr Mae Melvin and Dr E West, Mobile, AL.

SECTION 6

HEMATOPOIETIC AND LYMPHORETICULAR SYSTEMS

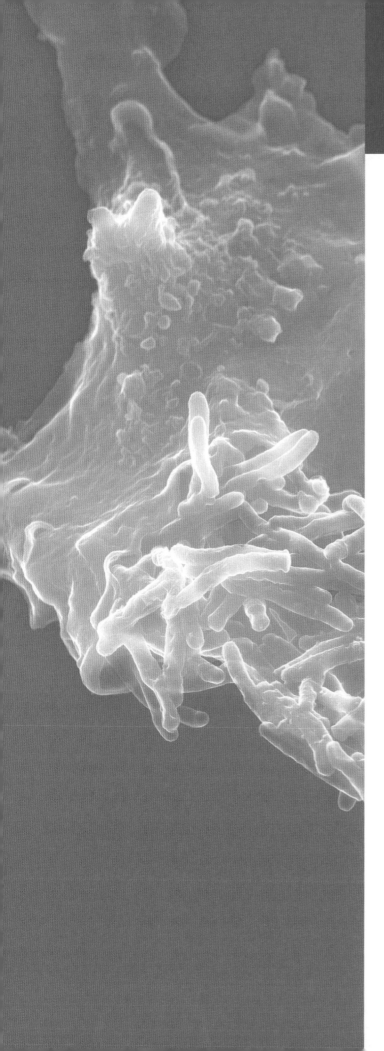

CHAPTER 23

THE BIG PICTURE: INFECTIONS OF THE HEMATOPOIETIC AND LYMPHORETICULAR SYSTEMS

OVERVIEW

The hematopoietic system consists of organs and tissues involved in the production of the cellular components of blood—lymphocytes, phagocytes, and erythrocytes. Infections of these cellular components of blood will be discussed in Chapters 24, 25, 26, and 27. The organs and tissues in the hematopoietic system include bone marrow, liver, lymph nodes, spleen, and thymus. The lymphoreticular system consists of the tissues of the lymphoid system and the mononuclear phagocyte system (reticuloendothelial system). The lymphoid system includes the thymus, bone marrow, lymph nodes, spleen, and the lymphoid tissues associated with the gastrointestinal tract (e.g., tonsils, Peyer patches) (Figure 23-1). The mononuclear phagocyte system includes monocytes, macrophages, endothelium lining the sinusoids of the spleen, lymph nodes, bone marrow, and the fibroblastic reticular cells of hematopoietic tissues. The lymphoreticular and mononuclear phagocytic systems respond to infections and produce cells (e.g., bone marrow) or house cells (e.g., spleen, lymph nodes) that are part of the innate and acquired immune system.

The lymphoreticular system and the hematopoietic system share common components and, as a result, symptoms associated with many of the diseases of these systems are similar, including splenomegaly, hepatomegaly, fever (recurring or constant), malaise, anorexia, and regional or generalized lymphadenopathy (Table 23-1; see Chapters 24–27). Human immunodeficiency virus (HIV), Epstein-Barr virus, and cytomegalovirus infections can all cause flu-like symptoms (e.g., malaise, fever, and anorexia); unfortunately, symptoms usually are not specific and diagnosis of many of these infections can be difficult.

Some symptoms, however, can be relatively unique and help considerably in determining the causative agent. For example, inflammation of the lymph nodes can be a helpful clinical feature because certain infectious agents (e.g., infectious mononucleosis) tend to cause cervical lymphadenopathy. Other infections (e.g., HIV) cause generalized lymphadenopathy (see Table 23-1; *note that several of the diseases mentioned in Table 23-1 are discussed in detail in other chapters in the book*). The pathology observed in the lymph nodes can also be helpful in narrowing down the cause of a particular lymphadenopathy (Table 23-2).

Infectious agents such as the *Plasmodium* sp. infect erythrocytes and cause lysis of the cells, resulting in recurrent fevers and in some cases in severe anemia. The periodicity of recurring fevers in malaria, babesiosis, and relapsing fever can be helpful in determining a diagnosis. For example, a patient with relapsing fever tends to have a fever that lasts about 7 days, followed by the temperature returning to normal for about 7 days. The fever then returns for about 7 days and so on, for about three or four recurrences. On the other hand, a patient infected with the malaria parasite will have a fever for about 24 hours. Depending on the species of *Plasmodium* involved, the temperature will return to normal for 3 or 4 days, then the fever will recur and last 24 hours, with several recurrences.

Some organisms such as *Rickettsia rickettsii*, the agent that causes Rocky Mountain spotted fever, infect and damage the endothelial cells, resulting in hemorrhage into the skin. *Bartonella henselae* also can infect endothelial cells but will cause bacillary angiomatosis, a systemic disease resulting in multiple subcutaneous nodules. It is characterized histologically by vascular proliferation in immunocompromised hosts (e.g., acquired immunodeficiency syndrome [AIDS] patients).

The infectious diseases that involve the hematopoietic and lymphoreticular systems are discussed in Chapters 24, 25, 26, and 27 according to the predominant host cell infected (Table 23-3). Some organisms infect several of the cells in these systems, making this division of diseases somewhat arbitrary.

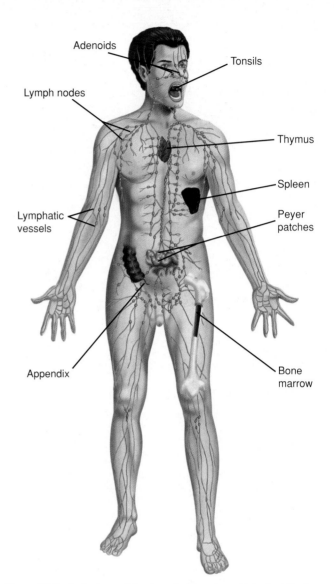

Figure 23-1. A diagram of the lymphoid system. Note that the bone marrow is important in the production of erythrocytes and leukocytes. The thymus is important in lymphocyte selection and maturation. The spleen, tonsils, adenoids, lymph nodes, Peyer patches, and appendix are important in aiding presentation of antigens to the leukocytes.

TABLE 23-1. Distribution of Lymphadenopathy of Various Diseases

	Disease	Microorganism(s)	Regional	Generalized	Systemic Manifestations
Bacterial	Pyogenic	*Streptococcus pyogenes* or *Staphylococcus aureus*	Yes; depends on site of inoculation	No	Prominent
	Cat-scratch disease	*Bartonella henselae*	Yes; depends on site of cat scratch or bite	No	Occasional; mild
	Plague	*Yersinia pestis*	Yes; usually inguinal	No	Prominent
	Tularemia	*Francisella tularensis*	Yes; depends on site of inoculation		
	Chancroid	*Haemophilus ducreyi*	Yes; usually inguinal	No	No
	Lymphogranuloma venereum	*Chlamydia trachomatis*	Yes; usually inguinal	No	Common; moderate
	Rocky Mountain spotted fever	*Rickettsia rickettsii*	No	Yes	Prominent
	Miliary tuberculosis	*Mycobacterium tuberculosis*	No	Yes	Prominent
	Syphilis	*Treponema pallidum*	Yes; during primary stage; usually inguinal	Yes; during secondary stage and in congenital disease	Variable
Viral	Infectious mononucleosis	EBV, CMV	Yes; cervical	No	Common; mild to moderate
	Genital herpes	HSV-2, usually	Yes; inguinal	No	Common; mild to moderate
	Epidemic keratoconjunctivitis	Adenovirus 8, 19, 37	Yes; ipsilateral preauricular	No	Occasional; mild
	Persistent generalized lymphadenopathy	HIV	No	Yes	Variable
	Rubella	Rubella virus	Yes	Yes	Common; mild
Fungal	Histoplasmosis	*Histoplasma capsulatum*	Yes	Yes	Uncommon
	Coccidioidomycosis	*Coccidioides immitis*	Yes	No	Uncommon
Protozoan	Toxoplasmosis	*Toxoplasma gondii*	Yes	No	Uncommon

EBV, Epstein-Barr virus; CMV, cytomegalovirus; HSV, herpes simplex virus; HIV, human immunodeficiency virus.

TABLE 23-2. Some Causes of Lymphadenitis and Pathology Observed in Lymph Nodes

Pathology	Disease
Acute suppurative	Pyogenic infections, plague
Caseating necrosis	Tuberculosis and atypical mycobacterial infections
Necrotizing granulomatous	Cat-scratch disease, tularemia, lymphogranuloma venereum
Nonnecrotizing granulomatous	Histoplasmosis, coccidioidomycosis

TABLE 23-3. Diseases of the Hematopoietic and Lymphoreticular Systems Listed by Chapter where Discussed

Chapter	Cell Type Infected	Diseases	Etiology
24	Lymphocytes	AIDS Infectious mononucleosis CMV infections	HIV EBV CMV
25	Phagocytic cells	Cat-scratch disease Tularemia Ehrlichiosis Q fever Brucellosis (Malta fever)	*Bartonella henselae* *Francisella tularensis* *Ehrlichia* and *Anaplasma* *Coxiella burnetii* *Brucella*
26	Erythrocytes	Malaria Babesiosis	*Plasmodium* *Babesia microti*
27	Endothelial cells	Bacillary angiomatosis Relapsing fever Human pulmonary syndrome	*Bartonella henselae* and *Bartonella quintana* *Borrelia* Sin Nombre virus (hantavirus)

AIDS, acquired immunodeficiency disease syndrome; HIV, human immunodeficiency virus; EBV, Epstein-Barr virus; CMV, cytomegalovirus.

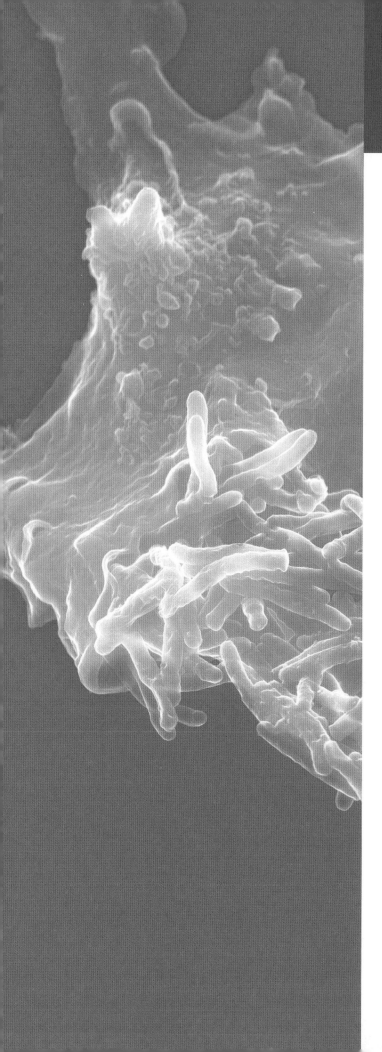

CHAPTER 24

LYMPHOCYTES

OVERVIEW

The organisms discussed in this chapter can infect several different cell types, including neurons, epithelial cells, salivary glands, lymphocytes, macrophages, and monocytes. The ability of these viruses to infect lymphocytes is discussed in relationship to the dramatic effects the viruses have on the immune response.

There are two basic types of human lymphocytes: B lymphocytes and T lymphocytes. When activated, B lymphocytes become plasma cells that produce antibodies. B lymphocytes require two different signals to become plasma cells: They must bind antigen with their surface bound antibody, and they must be exposed to cytokines (interleukin 4 [IL-4] and IL-5) produced by T lymphocytes (T-helper cells). Antibody production to foreign antigens is called the humoral immune response.

There are two types of T lymphocytes: T-helper cells (CD4$^+$ cells) and T-cytotoxic cells (CD8$^+$ cells). When activated, the T-cytotoxic cells can eliminate the host cells infected with virus, *Mycobacteria*, certain intracellular bacteria, fungi, parasites, and tumor cells. The cellular immune response occurs when cells kill other cells. The T-cytotoxic cells require two signals to become activated: They must bind antigen with their T-cell receptor, and they must be exposed to cytokine (interferon γ [IFN-γ]) from T-helper cells.

There are two basic types of T-helper cells: Th1 and Th2. These cells are essential in helping the body mount a humoral and a cellular immune response. Th1 T-helper cells produce IFN-γ to activate the T-cytotoxic cells. Th2 T-helper cells produce IL-4 and IL-5 to activate B lymphocytes. Without T-helper cells, the patient's adaptive immune systems (i.e., humoral and cellular immune responses) become much less effective at eliminating microbial invaders.

The diseases discussed in this chapter are acquired immunodeficiency syndrome (AIDS), infectious mononucleosis, and cytomegalovirus (CMV) infections. Human immunodeficiency virus (HIV) causes AIDS, and the AIDS virus infects T-helper lymphocytes. CMV causes several different diseases, depending on the host infected because CMV can infect many different cell types (e.g., epithelial cells, T cells, macrophages). The infection is spread through the body and establishes a latent infection in T lymphocytes and macrophages. EBV causes infectious mononucleosis and infects B lymphocytes.

ACQUIRED IMMUNODEFICIENCY SYNDROME

AIDS is an epidemic that has caused significant morbidity and mortality in most countries worldwide. Destruction of CD4$^+$ T lymphocytes (T-helper lymphocytes) predisposes infected individuals to a wide range of opportunistic infections, tumors, dementia, and death.

ETIOLOGY

HIV type 1 (HIV-1) and HIV-2 are human retroviruses in the lentivirus subfamily. The most common cause of AIDS is HIV-1.

MANIFESTATIONS

Untreated HIV infection involves three stages of disease, as shown in Figure 24-1, and is ultimately fatal. In many patients,

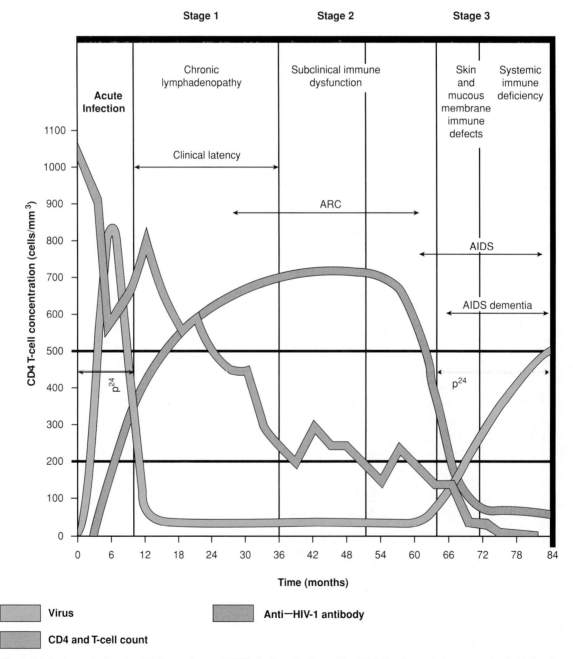

Figure 24-1. A graph showing the three stages of HIV infection. Notice as the CD4 T-cell count decreases, patients begin to manifest the signs and symptoms of AIDS. ARC, AIDS-related complex; AIDS, acquired immunodeficiency syndrome.

symptoms of HIV infection do not occur until stage 3 of the infection.

Stage 1, or primary HIV infection, has an incubation period of 1–3 weeks before symptoms begin (Table 24-1). This stage ends with the production of high titers of anti-HIV antibodies at 2–3 months postinfection.

Stage 2 HIV infection is usually **asymptomatic** and in most cases persists for 6 years or longer. Patients produce large amounts of anti-HIV antibody. HIV is detectable in blood, semen, and cervical secretions. If symptoms occur, the patient presents with persistent generalized lymphadenopathy or AIDS-related complex (ARC) (Table 24-2).

Stage 3 is usually a period when **symptoms of various opportunistic infections or spontaneous neoplasms** begin. The severity and frequency of these infections and neoplasms is directly related to the decline of CD4$^+$ T cells.

EPIDEMIOLOGY

- HIV-1 infection is found worldwide, and HIV-2 infection is found mainly in West Africa. Table 24-3 lists the prevalence of HIV and AIDS in adults by region of the world.

- Two principal genetic groups of HIV-1, designated M (main) and O (outlier), have currently been identified. Genetic group M is highly prevalent and is further classified into 10 established envelope subtypes, A through J.

- HIV-1 subtype B is found predominately in Europe and in North and South America; HIV-1 subtype C is commonly seen in sub-Saharan Africa (see Table 24-3).

- *HIV-positive persons are infectious during both asymptomatic and symptomatic stages of infection.*

- In 2003, AIDS was the sixth leading cause of death in persons 25–44 years of age in the United States.

- In 2005, the total number of adults and adolescents diagnosed with AIDS was 42,466; 31,024 cases were males and 11,442 cases were females.

- In the United States, most persons infected with HIV are males aged 30–44 years who live in the most populous cities and states (Figure 24-2; Table 24-4).

- *The most common mode of transmission of HIV worldwide is heterosexual contact* (Table 24-5). HIV is **NOT** transmitted by casual contact or by touching, hugging, kissing, coughing, sneezing, insect bites, water, food, utensils, toilets, and swimming pools or public baths.

- *In 2005, the most common mode of transmission of HIV in males in the United States was male-to-male sexual contact; in females, the most common mode of transmission was heterosexual contact.*

PATHOGENESIS

The ability of HIV to infect and destroy CD4-expressing T cells (T-helper cells or T-helper lymphocytes) and macrophages induces immunosuppression in patients with AIDS. When large numbers of T-helper cells are destroyed, the body eventually

TABLE 24-1. Symptoms of Stage 1 (Primary) HIV Infection

Patients may have NO symptoms OR they may have any or all of the following:

- "Mononucleosis-like symptoms" (malaise, pharyngitis, low-grade fever, cervical lymphadenopathy)
- Myalgia
- Arthralgia
- Lymphadenopathy
- Hepatosplenomegaly
- Headache
- Meningitis
- Encephalitis rash (small pink papules or macules over much of the body)

TABLE 24-2. Symptoms of AIDS-related Complex (ARC)

- Fever
- Fatigue
- Diarrhea
- Weight loss
- Night sweats
- Immunologic abnormalities
- Dementia
- Spontaneous neoplasms

TABLE 24-3. Prevalence of Living Adults with HIV/AIDS in 2006

Region	Prevalence (% of population infected)
Sub-Saharan Africa	5.9 %
Caribbean	1.2 %
Eastern Europe and Central Asia	0.9 %
North America	0.8 %
South and Southeast Asia	0.6 %
Latin America	0.5 %
Oceania	0.4 %
Western and Central Europe	0.3 %
East Asia	0.1 %

HIV, human immunodeficiency virus; AIDS, acquired immunodeficiency syndrome.

is unable to mount an immune response to infectious agents and to eliminate tumor cells. The severity of the HIV infection is closely aligned with the reduction in CD4 T cells (T-helper cells) and the increase in HIV virus particles in the blood (Figure 24-3).

During anal and vaginal intercourse, HIV can bind to the surface of antigen-presenting cells called Langerhans and dendritic cells, and can infect CD4 T cells in the lamina propria just beneath the epithelia of the vaginal wall or colon (see Figure 24-3). The virus can reach these cells following trauma that disrupts the protective epithelium and by binding to the surface of Langerhans cells, which have portions of the cell surface exposed to the lumen of the vagina and colon. The likelihood of HIV infection being transmitted during anal or vaginal intercourse is higher if the person exposed to an HIV-contaminated secretion already has a sexually transmitted infection such as syphilis, gonorrhea, or genital herpes, which can produce mucosal ulceration and inflammation.

HIV binds to dendritic cells via a lectin called DC-SIGN (dendritic cell-specific intercellular adhesion molecule 3-grabbing nonintegrin) or CD209, a C-type lectin receptor. The Langerhans cells, dendritic cells, and infected CD4 T cells then transport HIV to the regional lymph nodes and present HIV to CD4 T cells in the lymph nodes. HIV then infects the CD4 T cells in the node.

HIV binds with glycoprotein 120 (gp120) to CD4 T cells and uses gp41 to fuse to the host cell's cytoplasmic membrane. To infect a CD4 T cell, gp120 must bind to two host cell surface receptors (Figure 24-4). All HIV viruses must bind to the CD4 host cell receptor to infect the host cells. However, depending on the strain of HIV virus, one of two other host CD4 T-cell chemokine receptors, known as CCR5 and CXCR4, must be present on the cell to be infected by the virus.

T cell-tropic HIV (T-tropic HIV) requires CD4 and CXCR4 host cell receptors to infect the host cell. T-tropic viruses are usually transmitted via blood and blood products, and are syncytia-inducing viruses that infect CD4 T cells. Macrophage tropic HIV (M-tropic HIV) requires CD4 and CCR5 host cell receptors to infect the host cell. M tropic viruses are usually transmitted via sexual contact. They infect macrophages and some CD4 T cells, but are not syncytia-inducing viruses.

If HIV is transmitted via percutaneous injection, it can infect dendritic and monocyte-macrophage lineage cells. The macrophage lineage cells produce CD4, CCR5, and CXCR4, which can be infected by M-tropic and T-tropic HIV viruses. The HIV-infected macrophages and dendritic cells can then transport HIV to the regional lymph nodes through the lymph or the bloodstream. Once in the lymph nodes, HIV infects CD4 T cells.

When HIV reaches the lymph node, it continuously replicates in CD4 T cells. The virus and infected CD4 T cells are released from the nodes into the blood and then transmitted to other areas of the body (e.g., lymph nodes, brain, spleen) (Figure 24-5). HIV can destroy CD4 T cells in several different ways, including accumulation of the nonintegrated DNA copies of the viral genome, increased permeability of the plasma membrane, syncytia formation, and induction of apoptosis. The host can produce large numbers of CD4 T cells to replace the cells that are destroyed by HIV. Without treatment, however, the ability of the host to

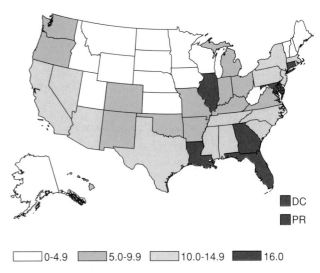

■DC
■PR

□ 0-4.9   ■ 5.0-9.9   □ 10.0-14.9   ■ 16.0

Figure 24-2. A map of the United States showing the incidence of AIDS by state in 2005. Image courtesy of the Centers for Disease Control and Prevention. AIDS, acquired immunodeficiency syndrome.

TABLE 24-4. Estimated Number of HIV-infected Persons by Age in 2005

Age	Number of Cases in 2005
<13	168
13–14	43
15–19	1213
20–24	3876
25–29	4581
30–34	5123
35–39	6123
40–44	6054
45–49	4396
50–54	2790
55–59	1535
60–64	768
≥65 and older	660

TABLE 24-5. Modes of Transmission of Human Immunodeficiency Virus (HIV)

Type of Transmission	Mode of Transmission	Comments
Sexual	Anal Vaginal Homosexual Heterosexual	Homosexual routes of transmission occur in male homosexuals and are the ***most common route of transmission in the United States*** Heterosexual routes of transmission are the ***most common routes worldwide and in females in the United States***
Inoculation in blood	Transfusion of blood or blood products Needle sharing among intravenous drug users and mucous-membrane exposure to health care workers (e.g., dentists, oral surgeons) Needlestick, open wound, Tattoo needles	Needle sharing in intravenous drug users is the second most common route of transmission in the United States
Perinatal	Transplacental (intrauterine transmission) Peripartum transmission (during labor and delivery) Breast milk ingestion in neonates	Peripartum transmission and ingestion of breast milk together are the ***most common means of transmission to children <5 years of age***

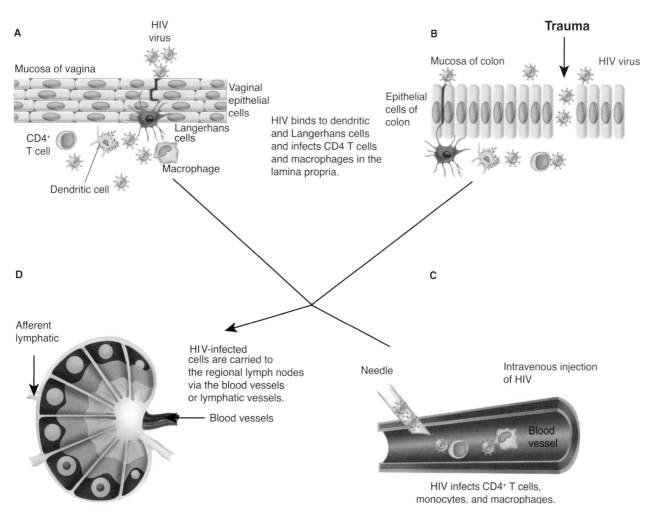

Figure 24-3. A schematic of the human immunodeficiency virus (HIV) and the cell types infected following exposure to the host and at the vaginal mucosa (**A**), colonic mucosa (**B**), and after intravenous injection of an illicit drug (**C**). After infecting host cells, the virus is carried to the regional lymph nodes via the bloodstream or the lymphatic vessels (**D**).

replace these cells slows and the number of CD4 T cells decreases within 6–10 years.

CD8 T cells are critical in controlling the progression of HIV disease. However, to become activated and kill HIV-infected cells or release factors that suppress viral replication, CD8 T cells must be activated by CD4 T cells. As the number of CD4 T cells decreases, so does the number of activated CD8 T cells. Virus replication is no longer inhibited, and infected cells are not eliminated. The amount of virus in the blood increases, reaching 5000–10,000 viral particles per mL of blood.

As the number of CD4 T cells decreases, the ability of the patient to fight certain infections and eliminate malignant cells also is reduced (see Figure 24-1). CD4 T cells are essential in the activation of CD8 T cells. CD8 T cells are important in delayed-type hypersensitivity (DTH) responses, which eliminate viral, fungal, and mycobacterial infections as well as malignant cells. CD4 T cells also regulate antibody production by B cells. The ability to produce antibodies in response to an infection is reduced, making bacterial infections more common. As the number of CD4 T cells decreases, HIV-infected monocytes and microglial cells in the brain die and release neurotoxic substances or chemotactic factors that promote inflammation in the brain.

Reservoirs of HIV infection are established early in macrophages and resting T cells during mucosal infection. A pool of latently infected memory CD4 T cells develops during the very earliest stages of acute HIV infection. These infected cells are able to persist in the patient's body for extremely long periods of time, possibly decades.

DIAGNOSIS

There are no unique signs and symptoms of HIV infection, which makes diagnosis difficult unless laboratory tests are performed (Table 24-6). A history of high-risk behaviors and complaints of malaise, generalized lymphadenopathy, fever, or rash may be grounds for serologic testing for HIV infection. HIV antibodies are usually detectable with an ELISA within 3–4 weeks after infection. However, false positives occur, and a second ELISA must be performed; if positive, a Western blot test for HIV is necessary to confirm the diagnosis of HIV infection.

Detection of HIV in the blood using reverse transcriptase polymerase chain reaction (RT-PCR) is also considered a confirmatory test for HIV infection. RT-PCR can be used to detect HIV RNA in plasma during the first 2–4 weeks of infection when patients may be seronegative and yet are infective. To determine if a neonate born to an HIV-infected mother is infected with HIV, an ELISA to detect HIV protein p24 is performed. Antibodies from an HIV-infected mother cross the placenta, making diagnosis of neonatal infections using serology impossible. RT-PCR of neonatal plasma can also be used to detect HIV infection in neonates.

HIV-infected patients do not receive a diagnosis of AIDS until they have met the clinical definition of AIDS, which was developed in 1993 and is useful in treatment decisions and in determining the prognosis of the patient. Tables 24-7 through 24-10 contain information necessary to determine if an HIV-infected patient has AIDS.

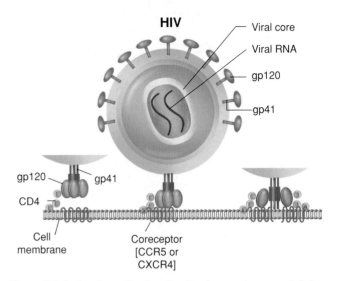

Figure 24-4. A schematic showing the human immunodeficiency virus (HIV) gp120 binding to CD4 and a chemokine receptor (CCR5 or CXCR4). Binding of gp120 to its two receptors brings the virus close enough to allow gp41 to bind to the host cell membrane and cause fusion of HIV with the host cell membrane.

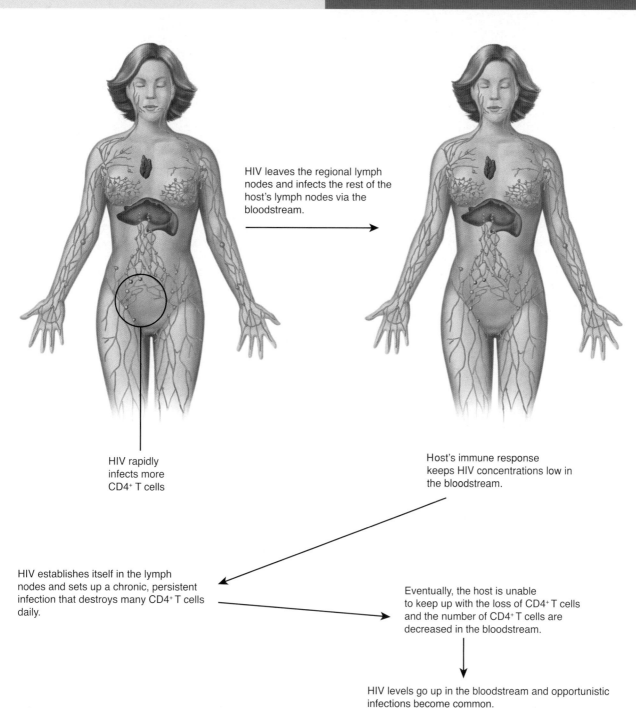

HIV leaves the regional lymph nodes and infects the rest of the host's lymph nodes via the bloodstream.

HIV rapidly infects more CD4+ T cells

Host's immune response keeps HIV concentrations low in the bloodstream.

HIV establishes itself in the lymph nodes and sets up a chronic, persistent infection that destroys many CD4+ T cells daily.

Eventually, the host is unable to keep up with the loss of CD4+ T cells and the number of CD4+ T cells are decreased in the bloodstream.

HIV levels go up in the bloodstream and opportunistic infections become common.

Figure 24-5. A schematic showing the spread of the human immunodeficiency virus (HIV) from the regional lymph nodes to other lymph nodes and the progression of the viral infection.

THERAPY AND PREVENTION

Eradication of HIV infection cannot be achieved with currently available antiretroviral regimens; therefore, lifelong treatment to suppress the virus is necessary. Highly active antiretroviral therapy (HAART) available since 1995 has resulted in durable antiviral responses however, and many benefits of long-term therapy are being reported. Successful HAART results in suppression of viral replication and halts damage to the immune system. It also partially restores the immune system, leading to partial restoration of immune function. Clinical benefits accompanying these immunologic benefits include fewer opportunistic infections and a longer lifespan for patients. The five different classes of antiretroviral drugs that are currently available are listed in Table 24-11.

HAART therapy is a complex treatment regimen and requires a strong lifelong commitment from the patient. HAART should be offered to any patient with established HIV infection and a confirmed plasma HIV-1 RNA level of more than 5000–10,000 copies per mL of blood. There are currently three combination regimens employed as initial HAART, which are listed in Table 24-12. Plasma viremia is a strong prognostic indicator in HIV infection. The higher the HIV RNA levels in the bloodstream, the worse the patient's prognosis. Real time PCR is used to determine HIV-1 RNA levels in the blood and is useful in determining a patient's prognosis and the effectiveness of antiviral treatment.

Prevention methods that have reduced the incidence of HIV infections include safe-sex practices (condom use), safe use of needles (no needle sharing), and early screening for HIV infection. Circumcised men are less likely to acquire HIV infections than uncircumcised men. Circumcision reduces female-to-male transmission by about 50%; however, circumcision does not appear to prevent HIV transmission in homosexual males. Treatment of HIV-1 infected pregnant women, as indicated above, can prevent most infections of the fetus or infant (Table 24-13). ***There is no vaccine currently available to prevent HIV-1 infection or the progression from HIV infection to AIDS.***

INFECTIOUS MONONUCLEOSIS

Infectious mononucleosis is a common infection that results in fever, sore throat, and cervical lymphadenopathy accompanied by a lymphocytosis.

ETIOLOGY

The causative agent of infectious mononucleosis is Epstein-Barr virus (known as EBV or human herpes virus 4 [HHV-4]).

TABLE 24-6. Diagnostic Tests Used to Detect HIV Infection

Test	Purpose
ELISA	Initial screening; two different ELISA results must be positive before a confirmatory test is performed
Latex agglutination	Initial screening
Western blot analysis	Confirmatory test
p24 antigen	Early marker of infection (detection of a recent infection)
RT-PCR	Detection of virus RNA in blood (detection of a recent infection) and to confirm treatment efficacy
CD4:CD8 T-cell ratio	Staging the disease and to confirm treatment efficacy
Isolation and culture of virus	Only available in research laboratories

HIV, human immunodeficiency virus; ELISA, enzyme-linked immunosorbent assay; RT-PCR, reverse transcriptase polymerase chain reaction.

TABLE 24-7. The 1993 Revised Classification System for the Diagnosis of HIV Infection and AIDS*

| CD4 T-Cell Count | CLINICAL CATEGORIES | | |
	(A) Asymptomatic, Acute (primary) HIV or PGL**	(B) Symptomatic, Neither Category A nor C Conditions†	(C) AIDS-indicator Conditions ††
>500/μL	A1	B1	**C1**
200–499/μL	A2	B2	**C2**
<200/μL	**A3**	**B3**	**C3**

HIV, human immunodeficiency virus; AIDS, acquired immunodeficiency syndrome.

*All patients who can be classified in the bolded cells of the table have AIDS. Persons with AIDS-indicator conditions (category C; see Table 24-10) as well as those with CD4+ T-lymphocyte counts <200/μL (categories A3 or B3) were reportable as AIDS cases in the United States and territories effective January 1, 1993.

**PGL, persistent generalized lymphadenopathy. See Table 24-8 for clinical category A conditions.

†See Table 24-9 for clinical category B conditions.

††See Table 24-10 for AIDS indicator conditions.

MANIFESTATIONS

Infectious mononucleosis has a prodrome that includes headache, malaise, and fatigue for 4–5 days. Following the prodrome, there is usually a triad of symptoms—fever, pharyngitis, and lymphadenopathy (Table 24-14). Most young children with infectious mononucleosis are asymptomatic; symptoms are more pronounced in previously uninfected young adults.

Major complications occur in 1–5% of cases of infectious mononucleosis. Most common complications are lymphocytic meningitis, encephalitis, encephalomyelitis, polyneuritis, mononeuritis, and Guillain-Barré syndrome. Guillain-Barré syndrome is a condition that can lead to respiratory paralysis and death. Splenic rupture can occur, but is rare. Severe tonsillitis may lead to airway obstruction if a tracheotomy is not performed.

EPIDEMIOLOGY

- Infection with EBV occurs worldwide among humans and usually occurs as a subclinical infection in early childhood.

- Infectious mononucleosis is most commonly seen in young adults 15–25 years of age.

- The incubation period is 1–2 months. Many patients cannot recall being exposed to EBV.

- About 70% of persons in the United States are infected with EBV by 30 years of age.

- Because EBV is only minimally contagious, a person must be exposed to an infected person several times before becoming infected with the virus.

- After recovery, the virus remains in the saliva for months. More than 90% of EBV-infected persons intermittently have lifelong shedding of virus even when asymptomatic.

- EBV is acquired by contact with infected cervical and oral secretions. Transmission can be via blood transfusions.

PATHOGENESIS

Epithelial cells of the oropharynx are the portals of EBV infection. The virus is transmitted primarily by repeated contact with oropharyngeal secretions, and is primarily transmitted by adults 30–50 days after infection or by children 10–14 days after infection. EBV can be isolated from saliva, blood, and lymphatics. EBV invades B lymphocytes by means of their CD21 receptors; within 18–24 hours, EBV antigens are detectable within the lymphocyte nucleus.

The signs and symptoms of infectious mononucleosis are the result of viral replication and the host immune response to viral antigens. Infected B lymphocytes spread the infection throughout the reticuloendothelial system (e.g., liver, spleen, and peripheral lymph nodes). EBV infection of B lymphocytes results in a humoral and cellular response to the virus. It initiates B lymphocyte proliferation (plasma cells) and immortalization (memory B lymphocyte) without the role of T-helper cells. EBV is a B-cell mitogen that can cause many B lymphocytes to become antibody-producing plasma cells.

Many of the antibody-producing plasma cells produce antibodies that do not react with EBV antigens. Some of the plasma cells produce antibodies that react with red blood cells from

TABLE 24-8. Clinical Category A Conditions for Diagnosis of HIV Infections*

Consists of one or more of the conditions listed below in an adolescent or adult with documented HIV infection (i.e., two positive ELISA results for HIV and a positive Western blot)

- Acute primary HIV infection
- Asymptomatic HIV infection
- Persistent generalized lymphadenopathy
- Accompanying illness or history of acute HIV infection

*Conditions listed in clinical categories B (see Table 24-9) and C (see Table 24-10) must NOT have occurred.
HIV, human immunodeficiency virus; ELISA, enzyme-linked immunoabsorbent assay; ELISA, enzyme-linked immunosorbent assay.

TABLE 24-9. Clinical Category B Conditions for Diagnosis of HIV Infections*

Symptomatic conditions in an HIV-infected adolescent or adult and that are *not* included among conditions listed in clinical category C and that meet at least 1 of the following criteria:

- The conditions are attributed to HIV infection or are indicative of a defect in cell-mediated immunity, or
- The conditions are considered by physicians to have a clinical course or to require management that is complicated by HIV infections.
- Category B conditions take precedence over those in category A. For example, someone previously treated for oral or persistent vaginal candidiasis (and who has not developed a category C disease) but who is symptomatic should be classified in clinical category B.

Examples of conditions in clinical category B include but are not limited to:

- Bacillary angiomatosis
- Candidiasis, oropharyngeal (thrush)
- Candidiasis, vulvovaginal; persistent, frequent or poorly responsive to therapy
- Cervical dysplasia (moderate or severe)
- Cervical carcinoma in situ
- Constitutional symptoms, such as fever (38.5°C) or diarrhea lasting >1 month
- Hairy leukoplakia, oral
- Herpes zoster (shingles), involving at least 2 distinct episodes or >1 dermatome
- Idiopathic thrombocytopenia purpura
- Listeriosis
- Pelvic inflammatory disease, particularly if complicated by tubo-ovarian abscess
- Peripheral neuropathy

*Conditions listed in category C (see Table 24-10) must *not* have occurred.
HIV, human immunodeficiency virus.

TABLE 24-10. Clinical Category C Conditions for Diagnosis of HIV Infections*

Includes the clinical conditions listed in the AIDS surveillance case definition. For classification purposes, once a category C condition has occurred, the person will remain in category C and is considered to be a patient with AIDS.

Category C conditions include:

- Candidiasis of the trachea, bronchi, or lungs
- Candidiasis of the esophagus
- Cervical carcinoma, invasive
- Coccidioidomycosis, disseminated or extrapulmonary
- Cryptococcoses, extra pulmonary
- Cryptosporidiosis, chronic intestinal (>1 month duration)
- Cytomegalovirus (CMV) disease (other than liver, spleen, nodes), CMV retinitis (with loss of vision)
- Encephalopathy, HIV related
- Herpes simplex virus: Chronic ulcer(s) (>1 month duration) or bronchitis, pneumonitis, or esophagitis
- Histoplasmosis, disseminated or extra pulmonary
- Isosporiasis, chronic intestinal (>1 month duration)
- Kaposi sarcoma
- Lymphoma, primary brain
- Lymphoma (immunoblastic or equivalent term)
- *Mycobacterium avium* complex or *Mycobacterium kansasii,* disseminated or extrapulmonary
- Mycobacterium tuberculosis, any site (pulmonary or extrapulmonary)
- *Mycobacterium,* other species or unidentified species disseminated or extrapulmonary
- *Pneumocystis jiroveci* pneumonia (PCP pneumonia)
- Progressive multifocal leukoencephalopathy
- Pneumonia, recurrent
- *Salmonella* septicemia, recurrent
- Toxoplasmosis of brain
- Wasting syndrome due to HIV

*A patient with any one of these conditions is defined as an AIDS patient regardless of CD4 T-cell count.
HIV, human immunodeficiency virus; AIDS, acquired immune deficiency syndrome.

other mammals such as cattle and sheep. This humoral immune response, called the heterophile response, is the basis for the serologic tests used to screen for infectious mononucleosis (e.g., heterophil antibody test [Monospot test]). Other plasma cells produce antibodies that react with EBV antigens and can be used to confirm a diagnosis of infectious mononucleosis. As with many viral infections, the T-lymphocyte response is essential in the control of EBV infection; natural killer (NK) cells and predominantly CD8 cytotoxic T cells control proliferating B lymphocytes infected with EBV.

During the acute phase of infectious mononucleosis, as many as 20% of the circulating B lymphocytes will produce EBV antigens, whereas only 1% will produce antigens during convalescence. The virus usually is not found free in the blood but is present as immune complexes, which may cause the arthralgias and urticarial rashes that occur during the acute phase of the disease.

B lymphocytes that produce complete virions are killed by viral-directed cytolysis, whereas infected B lymphocytes that do not produce complete virions are the target of cytotoxic T cells that control their proliferation. Lymphocytosis associated with infectious mononucleosis is caused by an increase in the number of circulating activated T and B lymphocytes (also

TABLE 24-11. Antiretroviral Drugs Used in HAART*

Class of Drug	Mechanism of Action	Name of Drug
Nucleoside or nucleotide reverse transcriptase inhibitors (NRTIs)	NRTIs inhibit HIV reverse transcriptase and can be placed within the viral DNA When the NRTIs are placed in the viral DNA by the reverse transcriptase, transcription of the viral genes is inhibited. This prevents virus replication and subsequent spread of the viral infection.	Abacavir, emtricitabine (FTC), zidovudine (AZT), didanosine (DDI), zalcitabine (DDC), lamivudine (3TC), tenofovir (disoproxil fumarate), reverset (d4FC), and stavudine (D4T)
Nonnucleoside reverse transcriptase inhibitors (NNRTIs)	These drugs also inhibit reverse transcriptase, which prevents virus multiplication and spread	Efavirenz (EFV), nevirapine, and delavirdine
Protease inhibitors (PIs)	HIV produces its own protease, which is important in the production of infective viral particles. The protease cleaves the viral proteins to the correct sizes so that a mature viral particle can form (viral assembly). PIs inhibit the retroviral protease from cleaving the viral proteins. These drugs help to slow the spread of the virus to other uninfected cells.	Amprenavir, atazanavir, fosamprenavir, ritonavir, indinavir, nelfinavir (NFV), saquinavir, and tipranavir
Fusion entry inhibitors	A peptide that interferes with the viral gp41 protein and prevents fusion of HIV with the host cell.	Enfuvirtide
CCR5 entry inhibitors	These inhibitors bind to the CCR5 receptor on the host CD4 cells and block binding of the HIV virion to the surface of the CD4 cells.	Maraviroc

*HAART, highly active antiretroviral therapy. *Note: This list is likely to be incomplete because new antiretroviral drugs are rapidly being approved.*

known as Downey cells because of their atypical presence in peripheral blood). EBV can be recovered from oropharyngeal washings 12–18 months after the disappearance of circulating Downey cells and the patient has recovered from the illness. **Infection with the EBV virus is lifelong.**

DIAGNOSIS

Diagnosis of infectious mononucleosis involves identifying atypical lymphocytes in peripheral blood smears (Figure 24-6). During acute EBV disease, the number of lymphocytes increases to 50–60% of the total leukocytes in the peripheral blood (a count of 20,000–50,000/μL), of which 10% are atypical lymphocytes (95% are T lymphocytes, 5% are B lymphocytes), or Downey cells. The presence of atypical lymphocytes is probably the earliest indication of EBV infection, but is not specific for it. Atypical lymphocytes can be seen in patients with lymphoproliferative disorders (e.g., common variable immune deficiency, Chédiak-Higashi syndrome, Wiskott-Aldrich syndrome, X-linked lymphoproliferative disorders), hepatitis, CMV, rubella, and roseola. Modest leukocytosis is seen, and an elevated erythrocyte sedimentation rate (ESR) is also frequently reported.

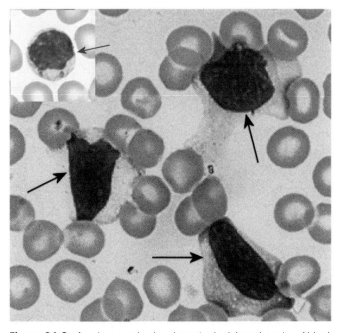

Figure 24-6. A micrograph showing atypical lymphocytes (*black arrows*) from a patient with infectious mononucleosis. For comparison, notice the normal lymphocyte in the upper left corner of the image (*blue arrow*).

TABLE 24-12. HAART Regimens for a Naïve HIV-infected Patient

HAART Regimen	Drugs
NNRTI-based regimens that are PI sparing	1 NNRTI and 2 NRTIs (e.g., efavirenz + zidovudine + lamivudine)
PI-based regimens that are NNRTI sparing	1 or 2 PIs + 2 NRTIs (e.g., lopinavir/ritonavir (coformulation) + lamivudine + zidovudine)
Triple NRTI regimens that are both PI- and NNRTI-sparing	Abacavir + lamivudine + zidovudine

HAART, highly active antiretroviral therapy; NNRTI, nonnucleoside reverse transcriptase inhibitor; NRTI, nucleoside or nucleotide reverse transcriptase inhibitors; PI, protease inhibitor.

As mentioned above, EBV is a B-lymphocyte mitogen that causes many different types of B lymphocytes to produce antibodies (immunoglobulin). Some plasma cells induced to multiply and produce immunoglobulin will produce immunoglobulin M (IgM), which does not react with EBV-specific antigens but recognizes antigenic determinants on sheep, horse, and cattle erythrocytes. The IgM antibodies are called heterophile antibodies because they react with something other than EBV viral proteins. The EBV heterophile antibody titers are highest during the first 4 weeks of disease, and the heterophile antibody tests are frequently used to detect the antibodies that react with sheep, horse, or cattle erythrocytes rather than EBV proteins. False-negative reactions occur in 10% of adults and 50% of children. About 60–90% of adults are positive for heterophile antibodies when tested during the first 2 weeks of the illness. Most children younger than age 2 are negative for the heterophile antibodies. If heterophile antibodies cannot be detected, the diagnosis of infectious mononucleosis can be obtained by testing serum for EBV-specific antibodies (Table 24-15).

THERAPY AND PREVENTION

Most cases of infectious mononucleosis are mild or moderate. Therefore, supportive therapy including bed rest and analgesics is the primary form of treatment for acute infectious mononucleosis. Symptoms of infectious mononucleosis are very similar to bacterial pharyngitis (caused by *Streptococcus pyogenes*). If a physician treats a patient with strep throat based solely on clinical signs and symptoms, the physician may give antibiotic treatment to a patient who has infectious mononucleosis. Patients with infectious mononucleosis who are prescribed ampicillin or amoxicillin can develop a rash. The best means of preventing most complications of infectious mononucleosis is exposure to the virus early in life, since the syndrome in children is milder than the disease in adults.

CYTOMEGALOVIRUS INFECTIONS

At least 80% of adults worldwide carry antibody to the CMV virus. CMV causes asymptomatic infections, serious congenital infections, heterophile antibody-negative mononucleosis in adults, and fever hepatitis syndrome in neonates and transplant recipients.

TABLE 24-13. Treatment to Prevent Transmission of HIV from an HIV-infected Mother to the Fetus or Infant

Period of Zidovudine (ZDV) Administration	Regimen
Antepartum	Oral administration of ZDV to the mother initiated 14–34 weeks' gestation and continued throughout the pregnancy
Intrapartum	Intravenous administration of ZDV to the mother during labor and until delivery and single dose of nevirapine during labor
Postpartum	A single dose of nevirapine to the newborn after birth and oral administration of ZDV to the newborn for the first 6 weeks of life, beginning 8–12 hours after birth

HIV, human immunodeficiency virus.

ETIOLOGY

CMV, or HHV-5, is a herpes virus; as with all herpes viruses, infection is lifelong.

MANIFESTATIONS

A fetus can be infected with CMV via the mother's bloodstream during a primary infection of the mother or by virus ascending from the cervix following reactivation of a prior infection. Symptoms of a congenital infection are usually less severe or can be prevented in the fetus of a seropositive mother (reactivation). Approximately 10–15% (4000 per year) of infants infected in utero via a primary maternal infection exhibit CMV inclusion disease and may exhibit teratogenesis (Table 24-16). *Healthy infants who acquire CMV at birth usually exhibit NO symptoms of disease.*

Neonates also can acquire CMV via blood transfusions. Of all seronegative neonates exposed to a seropositive donor, 13.5% acquire CMV. Significant clinical disease can occur in premature neonates who acquire CMV by blood transfusion. The most common manifestations include pneumonia and hepatitis.

Young adults who are infected with CMV are generally asymptomatic, but they may develop a disease resembling infectious mononucleosis called **heterophile-negative mononucleosis syndrome.** Symptoms of this disease include sore throat without exudative tonsillitis, fever, and atypical lymphocytosis. The results of liver function tests are abnormal.

Patients who have undergone transplantations and had post-transfusion infections usually experience asymptomatic infections. Manifestations of disease include mononucleosis-like syndrome, pneumonia, or hepatitis in adults.

Both reactivation and primary CMV infections can cause disease in immunocompromised patients. Interstitial pneumonia is a common outcome in the immunocompromised and can be fatal if not treated. Other manifestations include hepatitis, encephalitis, esophagitis (in 10% of AIDS patients), colitis (in 10% of AIDS patients), pancreatitis, cholecystitis, chorioretinitis (in 10–15% of AIDS patients), and necrotizing adrenalitis.

EPIDEMIOLOGY

- Infection rates are highest in children younger than age 6 and increased for young adults.

- The rate of CMV infection in adolescents in industrialized countries is about 10–15%, increasing to about 50% by 35 years of age.

- CMV has been isolated from urine, blood (harbored within leukocytes), stool, amniotic fluid, most bodily secretions (e.g., saliva, breast milk, semen), as well as tissues harvested for transplantation.

- *CMV is the most common viral cause of congenital defects* in the United States, with 0.2–2% of all newborns infected with CMV.

- Up to 20% of pregnant women harbor CMV in the cervix at term and are likely to experience reactivation of CMV during the pregnancy. About 50% of the neonates exposed to an infected cervix acquire CMV and become excreters of the

TABLE 24-14. Signs and Symptoms of Infectious Mononucleosis

- Fever: Adults 38.3–38.9°C; children may not have fever
- Cervical lymphadenopathy
- Pharyngitis with diffuse pharyngeal inflammation and tonsillar swelling; can be exudative or nonexudative
- Bilateral edema of the upper eyelids (palpebral edema)
- Early in illness, appearance of faint evanescent nonpruritic maculopapular rash
- Petechiae on hard and soft palates may occur later in disease (30% of symptomatic patients)
- Swelling of anterior and posterior cervical lymph nodes plus axillary, epitrochlear, mediastinal, and mesenteric nodes
- Splenomegaly (occurs in 50% of cases with acute mononucleosis and is a late finding)
- Hepatomegaly (occurs in about 10% of patients)
- Increased ALT, AST, and lactic acid dehydrogenase levels in blood
- Jaundice (occurs in about 5% of cases)
- Early in illness, cutaneous anergy and decreased cellular immune responses to mitogens and antigens

ALT, alanine transaminase; AST, aspartate transaminase.

TABLE 24-15. Serology Specific for EBV

Stage of EBV Disease	EBV Antibody Responses			
	Heterophile Antibody	Anti-VCA		Anti-EBNA
		IgM	IgG	
Acute EBV mononucleosis	+ or −	+	+	−
Past EBV infection	−	−	+	+

EBV, Epstein-Barr virus; EBNA, EBV nuclear antigen; VCA, viral capsid antigen; anti-VCA IgM, immunoglobulin M antibody to viral capsid antigen; anti-VCA IgG, immunoglobulin G antibody to viral capsid antigen.

TABLE 24-16. Manifestations of Congenital Cytomegalovirus Inclusion Disease

- Microcephaly
- Thrombocytopenia with petechiae or purpura
- Intracerebral calcification
- Hepatosplenomegaly
- Chorioretinitis
- Rash
- Seizure disorders
- Jaundice
- Mental retardation and hearing loss (1–3% of cases)
- Interstitial pneumonia

virus at 3–4 weeks of age. Neonates may also acquire a CMV infection from maternal milk or colostrum.

■ *The most common means of transmission of CMV includes heterosexual and homosexual contact, transfusions, and transplantations.*

PATHOGENESIS

CMV infections are usually subclinical. The virus infects epithelial cells, macrophages, and T lymphocytes. CMV is highly cell-associated and spreads to coalescing cells. The close cell interaction protects the virus from antibody inactivation. Cell-mediated immunity is required for resolution of symptoms and contributes to symptoms. CMV eventually becomes latent within T lymphocytes, endothelial cells, and monocyte-derived macrophages. Suppression of cell-mediated immunity allows recurrence of symptoms and can result in severe disease. The virus has the ability to induce immunosuppression during primary infections and reactivation of latent infections.

DIAGNOSIS

Diagnosis of a CMV infection can be confirmed by detection of CMV-induced large inclusion bodies present in urine sediment. The owl's eye appearance of CMV-infected cells can easily be seen in tissue or organ preparations from any part of the body (Figure 24-7). Cells are enlarged and contain intranuclear and intracytoplasmic inclusions and peripheralized chromatin. An atypical lymphocytosis is also present in a complete blood count (see Figure 24-6). The ability to culture CMV from the patient is the most reliable diagnosis.

CMV can be found in most body fluids and cultured on eukaryotic diploid fibroblast cells. Viral growth in tissue culture can be visualized 16–36 hours after inoculation by applying monoclonal antibodies and immunofluorescent staining. Patients infected with *CMV who have symptoms of mononucleosis (e.g., fever, cervical lymphadenopathy, pharyngitis) do not have a heterophile antibody response. Patients who are positive for heterophile antibodies have mononucleosis due to EBV and not to CMV.* Complement fixation can be used to detect CMV-IgM antibodies in infants infected with CMV in utero.

THERAPY AND PREVENTION

The most effective treatment for CMV infections is ganciclovir and foscarnet. Hyperimmune human anti-CMV immunoglobulin has been used to reduce CMV disease associated with renal transplantations. Safe-sex practices as well as blood and tissue screening will help limit the spread of CMV.

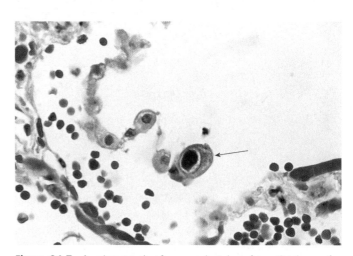

Figure 24-7. A micrograph of a sample taken from the lung of a patient with active cytomegalovirus pneumonia shows a cytomegalic pneumocyte (*blue arrow*) containing characteristic intranuclear inclusion (owl's eye inclusion). Image courtesy of the Centers for Disease Control and Prevention, Dr Edwin P Ewing, Jr.

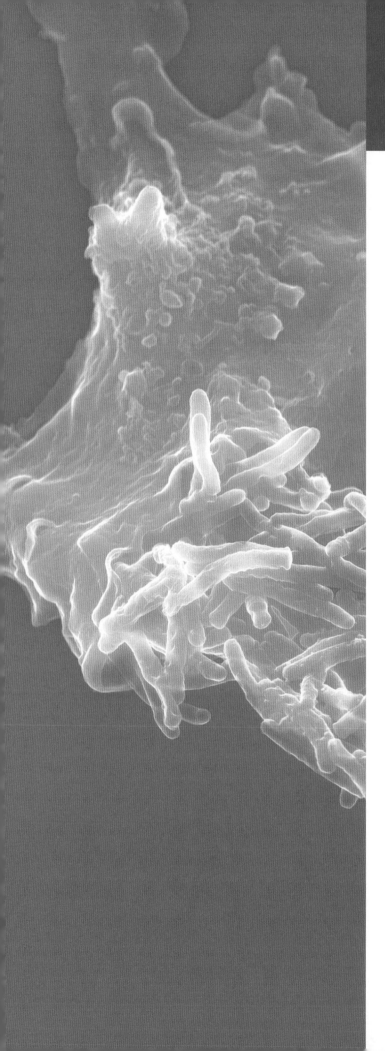

CHAPTER 25

PHAGOCYTIC CELLS

OVERVIEW

The bacterial diseases that will be discussed in this chapter are listed in Table 25-1, which summarizes the diseases, the causative agents, and the host cells parasitized by the bacteria. The organisms that cause the diseases are either facultative intracellular pathogens or obligate intracellular pathogens that survive in phagocytes of the host.

CAT-SCRATCH DISEASE

Cat-scratch disease is a slowly progressive, self-limiting, chronic lymphadenopathy that usually occurs in children. Cat-scratch disease, as its name implies, is transmitted to humans by the scratch or bite of a cat that has *Bartonella henselae* in its saliva and on its nails.

ETIOLOGY

B henselae (formerly *Rochalimaea henselae*) is a rod-shaped, gram-negative organism that causes cat-scratch disease.

MANIFESTATIONS

B henselae can cause several different diseases depending on the status of a person's immune system (Figure 25-1). However, individuals with a normally functioning immune system who acquire this organism usually manifest classic cat-scratch disease with fever and a regional lymphadenopathy (Figure 25-2). Occasionally, the organism can cause symptoms associated with its ability to infect the brain and retina. Immunocompromised hosts can develop the diseases illustrated in Figure 25-1 as well as bacillary angiomatosis and peliosis hepatica.

Classic cat-scratch disease has an incubation period of 1–2 weeks. In 50–90% of cases, a brownish papule or pustule forms at the site of the scratch or bite and is considered an indicator of cat-scratch disease. Regional lymphadenopathy follows within 3–10 days and is often accompanied by fever, malaise, and anorexia. Generally, the lymph nodes are 1–5 cm in diameter and proximal to the site of *B henselae* inoculation (see Figure 25-2). The most commonly involved nodes are in the axillary, epitrochlear, cervical, and supraclavicular areas. Over a period of weeks to months, lymph nodes may become fluctuant or suppurative or may spontaneously regress. Full resolution generally occurs within 1 month, with or without treatment. A biopsy of

TABLE 25-1. Summary of Bacterial Diseases, Their Causative Agents, and the Host Cells*

Disease	Bacteria	Facultative or Obligate Intracellular Pathogen	Host Cell
Cat-scratch disease	*Bartonella henselae*	Facultative	Macrophages
Tularemia	*Francisella tularensis*	Facultative	Monocytes
Human anaplasmosis	*Anaplasma phagocytophilum*	Obligate	Neutrophils
Human monocytic ehrlichiosis	*Ehrlichia chaffeensis*	Obligate	Monocytes
Canine granulocytic ehrlichiosis	*Ehrlichia ewingii*	Obligate	Neutrophils
Q fever	*Coxiella burnetii*	Obligate	Macrophages
Brucellosis (undulant fever, or Malta fever)	*Brucella*	Facultative	Macrophages and neutrophils

*The table includes the bacterial diseases discussed in this chapter.

lymph nodes will reveal hyperplasia, granuloma formation, and suppuration.

An increasing number of atypical manifestations of *B henselae* infections are now being recognized as atypical cat-scratch disease. These include complications in the retina (Leber neuroretinitis), conjunctiva, and preauricular lymph nodes (Parinaud oculoglandular syndrome) and central nervous system (cat-scratch disease encephalopathy and neuropathy), heart (endocarditis), and skin (erythema nodosum).

Leber neuroretinitis, or idiopathic stellate neuroretinitis, results in a loss of visual acuity and a macular star (Figure 25-3). Patients with Parinaud oculoglandular syndrome have conjunctival inflammation with preauricular adenopathy and a characteristic granulomatous lesion in the conjunctiva.

The most serious but rare complication of classic catch-scratch disease is cat-scratch encephalopathy. Manifestations include headache, tonic-clonic seizures, combative behavior, and coma. These symptoms typically occur suddenly, usually 1–8 weeks after the onset of lymphadenopathy. Recovery is usually complete.

B henselae does not remain in the regional lymph nodes of immunocompromised patients and can spread to other parts of the body through the bloodstream, resulting in bacillary angiomatosis (see Chapter 27) and peliosis hepatica. Liver biopsies reveal cystic blood-filled spaces in patient with peliosis hepatica.

EPIDEMIOLOGY

▨ There are about 25,000 cases of cat-scratch disease diagnosed each year.

▨ Most cases of cat-scratch disease occur during the late summer and early winter months.

▨ About 80–90% of cases of cat-scratch disease occur in patients younger than 21 years of age.

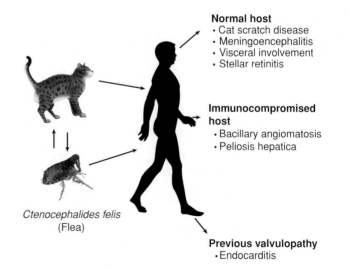

Normal host
• Cat scratch disease
• Meningoencephalitis
• Visceral involvement
• Stellar retinitis

Immunocompromised host
• Bacillary angiomatosis
• Peliosis hepatica

Ctenocephalides felis
(Flea)

Previous valvulopathy
• Endocarditis

Figure 25-1. A schematic of the transmission cycle of cat-scratch fever and the diseases caused by *Bartonella henselae*.

- *B henselae* infects kittens and can remain in the bloodstream for up to 1 year. Bacteremic cats are more likely to infect their owners following bites or scratches.

- Cats living in the warmer humid climates of the United States (e.g., the southeast) are more likely to be infected with *B henselae*.

- Fleas (*Ctenocephalides felis*) carry *B henselae* and can transmit the bacterium from cat to cat.

- Exposure to kittens is a greater risk factor for contracting human *B henselae* infection than exposure to adult cats.

- *B henselae* can be transmitted to humans following contact with cats (scratches, bites).

PATHOGENESIS

Cats are infected with *B henselae* following the bite of a flea that carries the bacteria and then transmits the bacteria to humans through a bite or a scratch. *B henselae* enters the cat's bloodstream, where it can live in the erythrocytes for several months to a year. The cat appears to be asymptomatic while *B henselae* is in the bloodstream. How the organism is transmitted from the cat's bloodstream to the saliva is not understood; however, it is likely that the nails are contaminated with saliva that contains *B henselae* after they groom themselves with the tongue.

Once in the tissue of an immunocompetent human, *B henselae* are phagocytized by macrophages but are not killed by the macrophage. The bacteria are transported to the lymph nodes that are in the region of the bite or scratch. The macrophages produce several proinflammatory cytokines (e.g., interleukin 1, [IL-1] and tumor necrosis factor alpha [TNF-α]), which recruit neutrophils and macrophages to the lymph node causing the node to swell. The inflammatory reaction within the node is granulomatous and consists of a central zone of necrosis, an inner rim of palisading macrophages, and an outer rim of lymphocytes and nonpalisading macrophages. IL-1 induces the fever associated with cat-scratch disease and activates T-helper lymphocytes in the node following presentation of *B henselae* antigens to the T-cell receptors. The activated T-helper lymphocytes produce TNF-γ which induces the macrophages in the lymph node to produce nitric oxide. Nitric oxide intermediates are produced following a reaction with oxygen in the tissues; the nitric oxide intermediates then kill the *B henselae* in the lymph node and eliminate the infection. The inflammation in the node eventually resolves and the swelling regresses.

B henselae occasionally can escape the lymph node of immunocompetent hosts and invade the central nervous system, heart, or skin via the bloodstream, causing the atypical manifestations mentioned above. There is very little known about the pathogenesis of these complications; however, the complications all resolve completely with few or no sequelae following treatment.

DIAGNOSIS

To confirm a clinical diagnosis of classic cat-scratch disease, three of the following four criteria must be met.

- History of contact with a cat resulting in a scratch or a papular or pustular lesion near the scratch in the dermis or mucous membrane or a macular star in the retina.

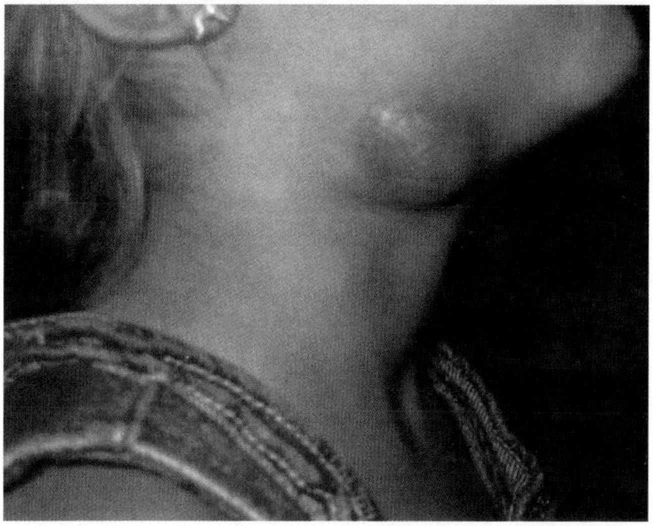

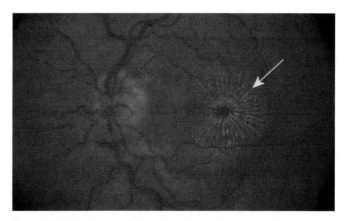

Figure 25-2. A photograph of a patient with regional lymphadenopathy due to cat-scratch disease. The patient was scratched by a cat on the cheek above the area of lymph node swelling.

Figure 25-3. An image of the retina that reveals an edematous optic disc and a macular star that can be seen in atypical cases of cat-scratch disease (Leber neuroretinitis). Image courtesy of G Arunagiri MD, FRCS, Ind Medica (http://www.indmedica.com/).

- Positive cat-scratch disease skin-test or positive indirect fluorescent antibody assay to detect *B henselae*.

- Negative results of laboratory investigations for unexplained lymphadenopathy (e.g., purified protein derivative [PPD] skin test and cultures of aspirated pus or lymph nodes).

- Characteristic lymph node lesions (necrotizing granulomatous).

THERAPY AND PREVENTION

The efficacy of antibiotic therapy currently has not been proven for classic cat-scratch disease in immunocompetent hosts. Symptomatic care for most patients is indicated. Swollen lymph nodes will resolve within 1–6 months. The infection usually will resolve in 90% of patients without treatment; however, there may be some clinical benefit to treatment with antibiotics such as azithromycin if lymph node swelling is extensive. Table 25-2 lists treatment recommendations for classic and atypical cat-scratch disease.

Disposal of the cat to prevent the disease is not recommended since the cat will only carry *B henselae* for a limited period of time. Declawing appears to make no difference. Flea control measures should be undertaken if there is a cat in the home environment.

TULAREMIA

Tularemia is a general term for several forms of disease caused by *Francisella tularensis*. The most common form of the disease is an indolent, febrile condition manifested by a skin ulcer and enlarged, tender regional lymph nodes. *F tularensis* is a hardy non–spore-forming organism that is capable of surviving for weeks at low temperatures in water, moist soil, hay, straw, or decaying animal carcasses. It is on the United States Centers for Disease Control's list of category A biological weapons.

ETIOLOGY

All forms of tularemia are caused by *F tularensis*, a gram-negative coccobacillus.

MANIFESTATIONS

F tularensis can cause several different forms of disease, depending on how the organism is acquired and include ulceroglandular, oculoglandular, pneumonia, typhoidal, and oropharyngeal. Each type of disease and its manifestations will be discussed below.

Ulceroglandular tularemia is the most common form of the disease and has an incubation period following inoculation in the skin of about 48 hours. Initially, a papule (erythematous, pruritic bump) forms at the inoculation site. The overlying skin becomes taut, thin, and shiny, but not fluctuant (movable and compressible). About 96 hours later, the enlarging papule ulcerates leaving an ulcer in the skin (Figure 25-4). Many patients will also have a fever with abrupt onset that can last up to 1 month in the absence of treatment. Patients may experience headache and occasionally photophobia and may also develop a regional lymphadenopathy in the area that drains the wound site.

TABLE 25-2. Recommended Treatments for Diseases Caused by *Bartonella henselae*

Disease	Treatment
Classic cat-scratch disease	None If lymph node swelling is extensive, azithromycin
Leber neuroretinitis, Parinaud oculoglandular syndrome	Doxycycline and rifampin
Cat-scratch disease encephalopathy	Doxycycline and rifampin
Endocarditis	Doxycycline and gentamicin

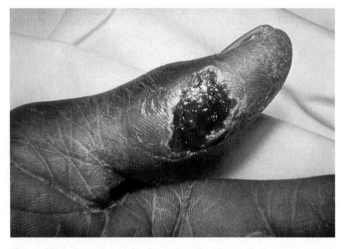

Figure 25-4. A photograph of an ulcer that formed on a patient with ulceroglandular tularemia. Image courtesy of the Centers for Disease Control and Prevention, Dr Thomas F Sellers, Emory University, Atlanta, GA.

Pneumonic tularemia is the most serious form of tularemia and is often a complication of the typhoidal and ulceroglandular forms of tularemia. Signs and symptoms include a nonproductive cough, substernal burning, and rhonchi. Nausea, vomiting, diarrhea, and abdominal pain are common in pneumonic tularemia and in pneumonia due to *Legionella pneumophila* (Legionnaire disease) but are rare in the more common bacterial causes of pneumonia (e.g., *Streptococcus pneumoniae*). Chest radiographs may be normal or may show peribronchial patchy infiltrates, effusions, and hilar adenopathy. Apprehension and toxicity are marked and shock is common.

Typhoidal tularemia can result in an endotoxemia produced by the bacilli lysing in the blood. Symptoms include a continuous fever (without chills or sweats), myalgia, severe headache, and hepatosplenomegaly.

Oropharyngeal tularemia is an acute exudative or membranous pharyngotonsillitis with cervical lymphadenopathy.

Oculoglandular tularemia is the rarest form of tularemia. Symptoms include pain, photophobia, intense ocular congestion, itching, lacrimation, edema of the ocular conjunctiva, and mucopurulent discharge.

EPIDEMIOLOGY

- Tularemia is a sporadic disease that occurs in areas of high endemicity.
- There are about 500,000 cases per year worldwide. About 300 cases are reported annually in the United States.
- The highest number of cases in the United States occurs in the Midwest during the summer months when ticks are common and east of the Mississippi during the winter months when cottontail rabbits are hunted (Figure 25-5).
- Tularemia can occur following
  - Handling of infected cottontail rabbit tissue.
  - Handling of body fluids or pelts of infected cottontail rabbits.
  - Bites of the ticks and deer flies.
  - Handling specimens or cultures in the clinical laboratory.
  - Ingestion of water contaminated with the bacteria.
  - Ingestion of improperly cooked meat from animals infected with the bacteria.
  - Inhalation of aerosols contaminated with *F tularensis.*
- *F tularensis* can be aerosolized several ways, including running over animals that have died from tularemia with a lawnmower or release of *F tularensis* as a biological weapon.

PATHOGENESIS

F tularensis is able to enter through unbroken skin and has an incubation period of infection of 1–21 days. If the organism enters the skin, a papule forms at the site of entry, which develops into an ulcer and is accompanied by fever and lymphadenopathy. If organisms enter the bloodstream, they are entrapped in the reticuloendothelial organs, where they

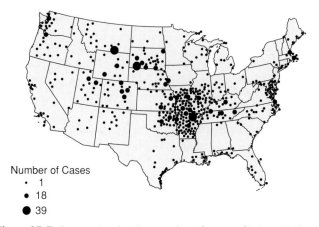

Number of Cases
- · 1
- ● 18
- ⬤ 39

Figure 25-5. A map showing the number of cases of tularemia from 1990 to 2000 in the United States. Notice that the disease is most prevalent in the central midwestern parts of the United States. Image courtesy of the Centers for Disease Control and Prevention.

proliferate and induce abscesses and granulomata. Bacilli survive inside monocytes, which contributes to relapses.

If the organisms are inhaled, multiple necrotizing granulomata form and destroy alveolar septa, resulting in bronchopneumonia, bronchitis, or tracheitis. Bacteremia can occur when alveolar macrophages containing *F tularensis* enter the hilar lymphatics.

About 1 million bacilli are required to cause disease following ingestion. Patients usually develop pharyngitis and cervical lymphadenopathy. Wiping the eye with contaminated hands can result in infection of the conjunctival sac and nearby lymph nodes (oculoglandular tularemia).

DIAGNOSIS

Tularemia is an acute febrile illness that rarely produces a leukocytosis. The erythrocyte sedimentation rate and the C-reactive protein are elevated. Contact with rabbits, ticks, or deer flies are informative, but not required. Smears of aspirates from enlarged lymph nodes usually contain the organisms. Patients who present with skin ulcers and enlarged regional lymph nodes accompanied by fever must be diagnosed as having tularemia until proven otherwise. An agglutination test is positive 10–14 days after infection. The agglutination test has some cross reactivity with *Brucella* antigens. Polymerase chain reaction (PCR) can also be used to identify *F tularensis* infections.

The severe forms of tularemia (pneumonic and typhoidal) are more difficult to diagnose. Gram stain of the sputum is usually not helpful in visualizing *F* tularensis. An immunofluorescent reagent is available for use directly on smears of sputum. Culture of *F tularensis* from sputum, from bronchial or gastric washings, or from blood is possible in guinea pigs or on glucose-cystine-blood agar containing cycloheximide and penicillin G to suppress normal flora, but is usually not done because of the highly contagious nature of *F tularensis,* which has resulted in several documented laboratory infections while handling patient samples. A skin test (Foshay test) is available that will produce a positive reaction in most patients within the first 7 days of the disease.

THERAPY AND PREVENTION

The drug of choice for treatment of tularemia is streptomycin; however, gentamicin is also effective. Without therapy, fatality rates range from 5% (ulceroglandular) to 30% (pneumonic). Infection provides lifelong partial immunity. An attenuated strain of *F tularensis* is available as a vaccine for persons at risk of acquiring tularemia (e.g., veterinarians, hunters). Gloves should be worn when dressing rabbits. Insect repellents should be applied to prevent tick and deer fly bites. Ticks should be removed promptly.

EHRLICHIOSIS AND ANAPLASMOSIS

After the bacterium *Ehrlichia* or *Anaplasma phagocytophilum* is injected into the bloodstream by a tick, it enters either a monocyte or granulocyte, depending on the species of the bacterium.

It replicates in the phagosome of the cell and destroys it. Two species of *Ehrlichia* (*E chaffeensis* and *E ewingii*) and one species of *Anaplasma* (*A phagocytophilum*) that cause disease in humans have been identified in the United States.

Three basic types of ehrlichiosis have been observed in the United States: *E chaffeensis,* the agent of human monocytic ehrlichiosis; *E ewingii,* the agent of canine granulocytic ehrlichiosis; and *A phagocytophilum,* the agent of human anaplasmosis (formerly called human granulocytic ehrlichiosis). The symptoms of these diseases are similar to those of Rocky Mountain spotted fever, with the exception that a rash is less common in ehrlichiosis or anaplasmosis.

ETIOLOGY

All three of these bacteria are obligate intracellular parasites. *E chaffeensis* infects primarily mononuclear cells (monocytes and macrophages); *A phagocytophilum* infects primarily neutrophils; and *E ewingii* primarily infects neutrophils and occasionally eosinophils.

MANIFESTATIONS

Many infections are so mild that infected individuals who are asymptomatic do not consult a physician; if patients are symptomatic, the symptoms begin 5–10 days after a tick bite.

Symptoms of **human monocytic ehrlichiosis** include fever, headache, malaise, and muscle aches. In children particularly, a maculopapular or petechial rash can be seen later in the disease process; about 40–50% of adults will develop the rash. Other manifestations may include nausea, vomiting, diarrhea, cough, joint pain, and mental confusion. Important laboratory findings include **leukopenia, thrombocytopenia,** and **elevated liver enzymes.** If untreated, the disease can be severe, and as many as 50% of all patients require hospitalization. Severe manifestations of the disease may include prolonged fever, renal failure, disseminated intravascular coagulopathy, meningoencephalitis, adult respiratory distress syndrome, seizures, or coma. Approximately 2–3% of untreated patients die due to the infection.

Symptoms of **canine granulocytic ehrlichiosis** are similar to those of human monocytic ehrlichiosis. Disease usually is not seen in immunocompetent individuals. Most symptomatic infections are seen in people who have other medical conditions that cause immunosuppression (e.g., HIV infection, splenectomy, transplantation patients, patients receiving immunosuppressive drugs).

Symptoms of **human anaplasmosis** are similar to those of human monocytic ehrlichiosis and canine granulocytic ehrlichiosis; the rash is less common than in human monocytic ehrlichiosis and occurs in only 10% of patients. Severe illness, as seen with human monocytic ehrlichiosis and canine granulocytic ehrlichiosis, can also occur, especially if the disease is untreated. As many as 50% of all patients with human anaplasmosis require hospitalization. Without treatment, the fatality rate can be as high as 1%.

Patients with compromised immunity caused by immunosuppressive therapies (e.g., corticosteroids or cancer chemotherapy), HIV infection, or splenectomy are more likely to develop severe disease following infection with any of these three pathogens.

EPIDEMIOLOGY

- There are about 200 cases of anaplasmosis and 200 cases of human monocytic ehrlichiosis each year in the United States (Figures 25-6 and 25-7). The incidence of *E ewingii* infection is uncertain because there is serologic cross-reactivity between it and *E chaffeensis*.

- About 80–90% of cases of ehrlichiosis occur from April to September.

- Rates of reported cases of ehrlichiosis increase with age; most patients are older adults (usually >40 years). This pattern contrasts with age-specific incidence of Rocky Mountain spotted fever, which occurs most frequently in children.

- Canine granulocytic ehrlichiosis primarily causes infections in canines.

- Ehrlichiosis and anaplasmosis are all transmitted from mammalian reservoirs to humans by hard ticks.

- The mammalian reservoirs for *E chaffeensis* and *E ewingii* include white-tailed deer, elk, rodents, coyote, fox, wolves, raccoon, opossum, and dogs.

- Mammalian reservoirs for *A phagocytophilum* include small mammals such as mice, chipmunks, and voles.

- The distribution of the tick determines where human infections occur. The lone star tick, which transmits both *E chaffeensis* and *E ewingii,* is found in the southeastern, middle atlantic, midwestern, and south central United States. *A phagocytophilum* is transmitted by the black-legged tick, *Ixodes scapularis*, found in the eastern United States, and by the western black-legged tick, *Ixodes pacificus*, found in the western United States (Figure 25-8).

PATHOGENESIS

The hematopoietic system is the main organ system infected in patients with ehrlichiosis and human anaplasmosis. The bacteria are obligate intracellular parasites that multiply in the phagosome of the host cell. ***The organisms produce mulberry-shaped vacuole-bound intracytoplasmic inclusions in the leukocyte called morulae, which aids in diagnosing these diseases*** (Figure 25-9). The immune response to the organisms is beneficial in eliminating the bacteria, but is harmful in that most of the damage to the host results from the immune response to the infection.

DIAGNOSIS

Ehrlichiosis and human anaplasmosis are difficult diseases to diagnose because they are similar to many other diseases. The clinical clues (e.g., laboratory test results and signs and symptoms) and the epidemiologic clues (e.g., history of tick bite) can aid in the initial diagnosis. Microscopy of Wright or Giemsa stained peripheral blood samples is of limited value in detecting the morulae in human monocytic ehrlichiosis but can be of value in diagnosing patients with human anaplasmosis (see Figure 25-9). Morulae-containing cells can be detected in only 10% of patients with human monocytic ehrlichiosis; however, 20–80% of patients with human anaplasmosis show visible morulae in stained peripheral blood smears.

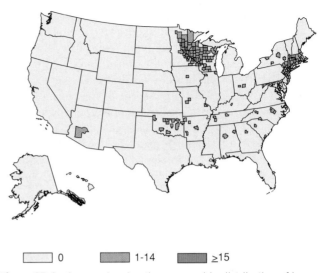

0   1-14   ≥15

Figure 25-6. A map showing the geographic distribution of human granulocytic ehrlichiosis (now known as human anaplasmosis) in 2005 in the United States. Notice the large number of reported cases in Minnesota and Wisconsin. Image courtesy of the Centers for Disease Control and Prevention.

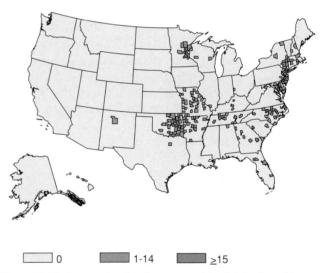

0   1-14   ≥15

Figure 25-7. A map showing the geographic distribution of human monocytic ehrlichiosis in 2005 in the United States. Image courtesy of the Centers for Disease Control and Prevention.

The most common means of confirming a clinical diagnosis of ehrlichiosis and human anaplasmosis is by PCR and serology. Serologic evaluations are conducted using indirect immunofluorescence assay. Antibodies in the serum bind to the organisms on a slide and are detected by a fluorescein-labeled conjugate. Amplification of the bacterial DNA by PCR is the next most frequently used method for detecting infection. This test is available through the Centers for Disease Control and Prevention and some state health laboratories, as well as a number of research and commercial laboratories.

Direct isolation of the organism remains the gold standard for confirmatory diagnosis, but it is the most difficult and time-consuming approach. Both *E chaffeensis* and *A phagocytophilum* have been recovered from the blood of acutely ill patients by using canine DH82 and human HL-60 cells, respectively. *E chaffeensis* has been observed within 7–36 days in culture. *A phagocytophilum* may be seen within 7–12 days after inoculation of cells with patient blood.

THERAPY AND PREVENTION

The drug of choice in treating all patients with ehrlichiosis and human anaplasmosis is doxycycline. Due to the serious consequences of untreated infections, treatment should not be postponed until the diagnosis is confirmed.

Infections can be prevented by limiting exposure to ticks. In persons exposed to tick-infested habitats, prompt, careful inspection and removal of crawling or attached ticks is an important method of preventing disease. Bacteria are transmitted from the tick to humans after several hours of attachment.

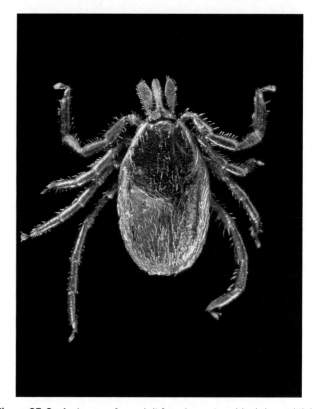

Figure 25-8. An image of an adult female western black-legged tick, *Ixodes pacificus*, which transmits *Borrelia burgdorferi*, the agent of Lyme disease, and *Anaplasma phagocytophilum*, the agent of human granulocytic anaplasmosis. Image courtesy of the Centers for Disease Control and Prevention, Dr Amanda Loftis, Dr William Nicholson, Dr Will Reeves, Dr Chris Paddock.

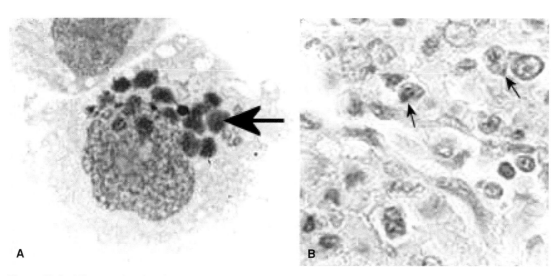

A

B

Figure 25-9. Micrographs showing neutrophils that contain *Anaplasma phagocytophilum*. **A**, A micrograph of a neutrophil containing the morulae (*black arrow*), which is sometimes seen in stained peripheral blood smears. **B**, Micrograph showing intracellular bacteria detected by an immunohistochemical technique. Image courtesy of JS Dumler et al. Human granulocytic anaplasmosis and *Anaplasma phagocytophilum*. Emerg Infect Dis [serial on the Internet]. 2005 Dec [*date cited*]. Available from http://www.cdc.gov/ncidod/EID/vol11no12/05-0898.htm.

Q FEVER

Q fever is a zoonotic bacterial infection that is worldwide in distribution.

ETIOLOGY

Coxiella burnetii is an obligate intracellular, gram-negative bacterium that dwells in the phagolysosome of phagocytes and causes Q fever.

MANIFESTATIONS

About 50% of patients with infections caused by *C burnetii* are asymptomatic. After an incubation period of 2–3 weeks, patients who develop symptoms have a rapid onset of high fever (up to 40°C), malaise, myalgia, confusion, sore throat, chills, sweats, nonproductive cough, nausea, vomiting, diarrhea, abdominal pain, and chest pain. If untreated, the fever will last 1–2 weeks. About 30–50% of symptomatic patients will develop pneumonia, if untreated. Liver function tests are usually abnormal; some patients may develop hepatitis. Most patients with acute Q fever recover in about 2 months without complications. The mortality rate for acute Q fever is 1–2%.

Patients who have had acute Q fever may develop a chronic form of this bacterial infection from 1 to 20 years after the initial infection. Endocarditis is a serious complication of chronic Q fever. The aortic valve is the most commonly affected valve, with the mitral valve being the second most commonly affected. Patients who develop chronic Q fever usually have preexisting valvular heart disease or a history of vascular graft. Transplant recipients and patients with cancer or chronic kidney disease are also at risk of developing chronic Q fever. The mortality rate is quite high (65%) for patients who have chronic Q fever.

EPIDEMIOLOGY

▢ Q fever is an uncommon cause of infection in the United States, with only 50–150 cases of the disease reported each year (Figure 25-10).

▢ The main reservoirs for human infection are domesticated ruminants, primarily cattle, sheep, and goats, although other domesticated animals and pets can also transmit the bacterium to humans.

▢ Most infected animals are asymptomatic; however, abortions in sheep and goats have been associated with the infection. The organisms are excreted in milk, urine, and feces of infected animals.

▢ Large numbers of *C burnetii* are seen in amniotic fluid and in the placenta of animals. The dried excreta and amniotic fluid containing the organisms becomes aerosolized and is inhaled by persons working in these environments. Most cases of Q fever occur during animals' birthing times.

▢ A few cases of Q fever have occurred following aspiration of unpasteurized milk contaminated with *C burnetii*.

▢ *C burnetii* is capable of living for long periods in the environment and is infectious even after extended periods of drying. Certain occupations are at higher risk of being infected with the organism, including veterinarians; workers in meat processing plants; persons who have contact with sheep, cattle, and goats; and researchers at facilities housing sheep.

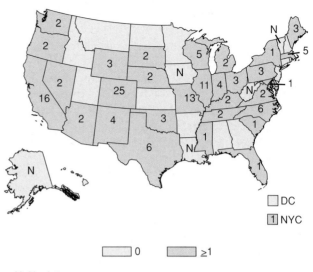

Figure 25-10. A map showing the number of cases of Q fever reported in the United States in 2005. Image courtesy of the Centers for Disease Control and Prevention.

PATHOGENESIS

C burnetii is transmitted to humans via aerosols. The organism can exist in an endospore-like form and live for long periods of time in the environment. Once in the lungs, the bacteria are carried in the bloodstream to the liver and bone marrow and are then phagocytosed by macrophages. In spite of phagosome-lysosome fusion, the bacteria survive. Growth in the macrophages can result in T-lymphocyte–mediated granulomas. Elimination of the infection requires release of interferon gamma and a T-lymphocyte response.

DIAGNOSIS

There are no unique signs or symptoms of Q fever that would aid in making a definitive diagnosis. Many patients with Q fever do have a transient thrombocytopenia, but that is not unique to the disease. The only method of determining a definitive diagnosis is by serology. Most laboratories use an indirect immuno-fluorescence assay; other assays involve DNA testing and immunohistochemical staining.

   C burnetii exists in two antigenic forms (phase I and phase II), which aids in determining the difference between acute and chronic infection. Antibodies form early to phase II antigens and much later to phase I antigens. Therefore, patients with acute Q fever infections usually have high levels of antibody to phase II antigens and low levels of antibody to phase I antigens (IgG antibodies to phase II and IgM antibodies to phases I and II). Patients with chronic infections usually have high levels of antibody to phase I antigens and low or decreasing levels of antibody to phase II antigens. Increased levels of IgG and IgA to phase I antigens are predictive of Q fever endocarditis.

THERAPY AND PREVENTION

Doxycycline is the drug of choice for treating Q fever, although quinolones are also effective. Treatment outcomes are most effective if therapy begins within the first 3 days of symptomatic disease. Relapses are not uncommon, and if relapse occurs, the patient must begin a second round of treatment.

   Chronic Q fever is much more difficult to treat than acute Q fever. Endocarditis caused by *C burnetii* usually requires the use of two different antimicrobial agents for extended periods of time. Two treatment regimens currently have been examined: The first is doxycycline given in combination with quinolones for at least 4 years. The second regimen, which results in fewer relapses, is doxycycline given in combination with hydroxy-chloroquine for 1½ to 3 years.

   Prevention includes instruction on proper disposal of placenta, birth products, fetal membranes, and aborted fetuses at facilities housing sheep and goats. Only pasteurized milk and dairy products should be used. Imported animals should be quarantined.

BRUCELLOSIS

Brucellosis, which is also called undulant or Malta fever, is a prolonged recurring febrile disease involving the reticuloendothelial system and is transmitted to humans from a genitourinary infection of sheep, cattle, and pigs.

TABLE 25-3. Some Diseases with Recurring Fever: Causative Agents, Periodicity, and Duration of Fever

Disease	Causative Agent	Periodicity of Fever	Duration of Fever
Malaria	*Plasmodium*	Every 3 to 4 days (except *P falciparum,* where fever can be continuous)	Fever lasts 24 hours with the fever ending in a drenching sweat
Brucellosis (undulant fever, or Malta fever)	*Brucella*	Daily	Fever recurs in the evening and is gone by morning following a drenching sweat
Relapsing fever	*Borrelia*	Every 7–10 days	Fever lasts 7–10 days

ETIOLOGY

Brucella abortus, B melitensis, B suis, and *B canis* are gram-negative coccobacilli.

MANIFESTATIONS

There are three types of brucellosis: inapparent, acute (lasting <1 month), and chronic (lasting >1 month). The incubation period is about 7–21 days after contact, inhalation, or ingestion of the organisms. Symptoms include malaise, chills, daily fevers (39–40°C), weakness, headache, backache, and anorexia and weight loss. Especially in cases of infection due to *B melitensis,* the fever and drenching sweats recur in late afternoon or evening. Other symptoms include splenomegaly with lymphadenopathy and hepatomegaly. Brucellosis can continue for weeks to years and can be confused with other recurring febrile illnesses (e.g., malaria and relapsing fever). Table 25-3 lists the differences in the length of the fever and fever periodicity.

EPIDEMIOLOGY

- There are 150–200 cases of brucellosis per year, with 50–60% occurring in handlers of livestock or meat products.

- Patients range in age from 20 to 50 years; the disease is five times more common in men than in women.

- The disease has been reported in every state in the United States; however, more cases occur in states that are heavily involved in the livestock industry (Figure 25-11).

- Infection results from occupational exposure to infected animals (e.g., feral swine) or consumption of unpasteurized products (e.g., milk or cheese). Organisms gain entry by contact through mucous membranes or broken skin or by inhalation or ingestion.

PATHOGENESIS

The *Brucella* organisms penetrate the skin or mucous membranes, are engulfed by polymorphonuclear leukocytes, and then enter the lymphatics and the bloodstream. *Brucella* multiplies within the polymorphonuclear leukocytes and lyses them (facultative intracellular parasite). It can also multiply within the macrophages of the reticuloendothelial system inducing small granulomas and abscesses. Periodic release of *Brucella* into the bloodstream induces recurrent chills and fever. Antigen-specific activated macrophages are able to kill *Brucella* with T lympho-

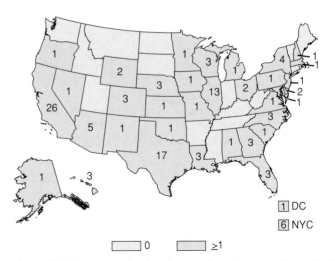

Figure 25-11. A map showing the number of cases of brucellosis reported in the United States in 2005. Image courtesy of the Centers for Disease Control and Prevention.

cytes. *B melitensis* infections are usually the most severe. *B abortus* is associated with less frequent infection and a greater proportion of subclinical cases. The virulence of *B suis* strains for humans varies but is generally intermediate in severity.

DIAGNOSIS

Brucellosis should be suspected in patients with typical manifestations and a history of exposure. Definitive diagnosis requires isolation of *Brucella* from the blood or from reticuloendothelial tissue biopsies (bone marrow). The gram-negative coccobacilli require 2–3 days of incubation at 37°C and 5–10% carbon dioxide to produce visible colonies on blood agar. A positive tube agglutinin assay using *B abortus* antigen has a titer of 160–640.

THERAPY AND PREVENTION

Treatment of brucellosis includes tetracycline plus gentamicin or streptomycin for 4–6 weeks; fever may persist 2–7 days after therapy is initiated. About 10% of cases relapse within 3 months of therapy. Infections can be prevented by minimizing occupational exposure, pasteurizing dairy products, immunizing livestock, and destroying infected livestock.

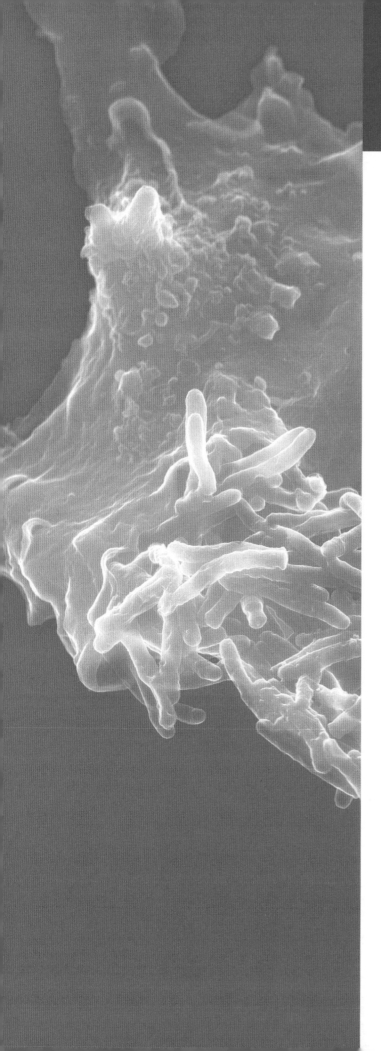

CHAPTER 26

ERYTHROCYTES

OVERVIEW

The two diseases that will be discussed in this chapter are malaria and babesiosis. Both diseases are caused by protozoan parasites that infect erythrocytes and are transmitted by arthropod vectors; malaria is transmitted by a mosquito, and babesiosis is transmitted by a tick.

MALARIA

Malaria is a febrile disease that causes anemia. It was once endemic in the United States and is currently one of the most common infections worldwide, infecting 300–500 million people annually.

ETIOLOGY

Malaria is caused by obligate intracellular protozoan parasites of the genus *Plasmodium.* The four species of human malarial parasites are *P vivax, P falciparum, P malariae,* and *P ovale.*

MANIFESTATIONS

The incubation period for malaria is 2 weeks or longer. There is a brief prodromal period with symptoms of fever, headache, and myalgia. Symptoms begin with a cold stage (a shaking chill), followed by a fever stage (40–41°C) that lasts about 24 hours, and finally a wet stage. The wet stage occurs several hours after the fever, when the body temperature drops quickly to normal and profuse sweating begins. The patient is exhausted but well until the next cycle of fever begins. Other symptoms include splenomegaly and anemia.

Three basic types of malaria
1. **Benign tertian** (*P vivax* and *P ovale*) with a fever every third day.
2. **Benign quartan** (*P malariae*) with a fever every fourth day.
3. **Malignant tertian** (*P falciparum*), in which the cold stage is less pronounced and the fever stage is more prolonged and intensified. The fever is continuous or only briefly remittent. There is no wet stage. This type of malaria is more dangerous because of the complications caused by capillary blockage (i.e., convulsion, coma, acute pulmonary insufficiency, and cardiac failure). Large numbers of erythrocytes

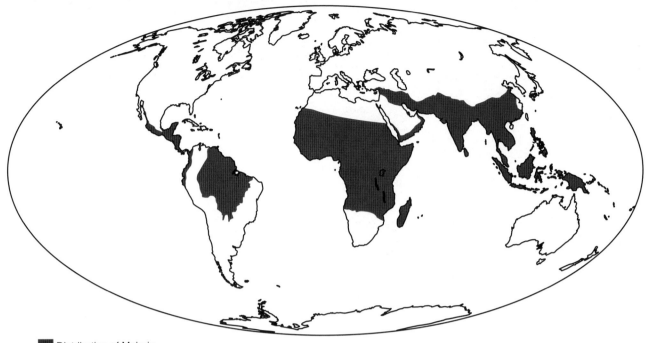

Distribution of Malaria

Figure 26-1. A world map showing the countries where malaria is endemic. Image courtesy of the Centers for Disease Control and Prevention.

are parasitized and destroyed, which may result in dark-colored urine (blackwater fever, manifested by intravascular hemolysis, hemoglobinuria, and kidney failure).

Two species of *Plasmodium, P vivax* and *P ovale,* can remain in the liver if the patient is not treated properly. The organisms leave the liver and re-infect erythrocytes, causing the symptoms described above. Relapsing malaria occurs when there are relapses many years after the initial episode of malarial disease.

EPIDEMIOLOGY

- About 700,000–2.7 million people die of malaria each year; 75% of deaths are African children.

- The highest transmission rates are found in countries in sub-Saharan Africa (Figure 26-1).

- About 41% of the world's population lives in areas where malaria is transmitted (e.g., parts of Africa, Asia, the Middle East, Central and South America, Hispaniola, and Oceania).

- *P vivax* is the most common cause of malaria and is found in subtropical and temperate areas of the world. *P vivax* and *P ovale* cause relapsing malaria.

- *P falciparum* is found in tropical regions and causes the most severe and fatal disease.

- *P malariae* is limited entirely to subtropical areas. The species is less common than *P falciparum* or *P vivax.*

- *P ovale* is the least common malarial species and is endemic in Africa.

- Although malaria is no longer endemic in the United States, about 1200 cases are reported each year because of travel to countries where malaria is endemic.

- *P falciparum* is the most common species of malarial parasite diagnosed in the United States, followed by *P vivax, P malariae,* and then *P ovale.*
- Malaria is transmitted primarily by the bite of an infected *Anopheles* mosquito (Figure 26-2).

PATHOGENESIS

The general features of the following parasitic life cycle apply to all *Plasmodium* species. ***Sporozoites are the infective form,*** transmitted during the blood meal of a female *Anopheles* mosquito feeding on a human (Figure 26-3). The sporozoites invade and reside within hepatocytes, where they increase. Several days after the initial infection, some of the sporozoite progeny (called merozoites) leave the liver and enter the bloodstream to infect erythrocytes and form the trophozoite, or ring-cell stage, of the parasite.

The **erythrocyte stage** begins when merozoites infect the red blood cells. The parasites attach to specific red blood cell receptors and are endocytosed to initiate infection. The Duffy blood group protein is the red blood cell receptor that *P vivax* uses to bind to the surface of erythrocytes. A person who is negative for the Duffy antigen (FyFy rather than Fy^a or Fy^b) is resistant to infection by *P vivax.* Asexual reproduction (schizogony) proceeds through a series of stages resulting in the rupture of the erythrocyte and the release of up to 25 merozoites per erythrocyte.

Fever is the hallmark symptom of malaria and is induced when the erythrocytes rupture and merozoites are released. Vasodilation and hypotension occur in response to the high fever. Anemia results following erythrocyte destruction and indirectly from increased phagocytosis of red blood cells, capillary hemorrhage, thrombosis, and decreased marrow function. The most severe anemia is associated with *P falciparum* infection. A brown to black pigmentation of organs occurs when the malarial pigment hemozoin is ingested by phagocytes in lymphoid tissue, the liver and spleen, and bone marrow. Hemozoin is a partially digested form of human hemoglobin produced in the digestive food vacuole of the parasite while it dwells in the erythrocyte.

Hepatomegaly and splenomegaly occur following dilation of the sinuses and are due to the increased numbers of macrophages in these organs, especially the spleen. Parasitized red blood cells in immune complexes occlude capillaries and cause local hemorrhaging and anoxia in many tissues, with the brain being the most severely affected. In severe disease, intravascular hemolysis in the kidney can cause hemoglobinemia and hemoglobinuria and dark-colored urine called blackwater fever. After the immune response has terminated the erythrocytic cycle, *P vivax* and *P ovale* hypnozoites can remain dormant in the liver and cause relapse months to years later.

After one or more asexual cycles in the erythrocytes, some intraerythrocytic merozoites develop into male and female **gametocytes,** which are the sexual forms of the parasite. Gametocytes are ingested by the mosquito and can fuse within the mosquito's gut to form a zygote, which initiates the sexual reproductive cycle (sporogony). After several developmental stages in the mosquito, the parasite migrates to the salivary glands of the mosquito as a sporozoite.

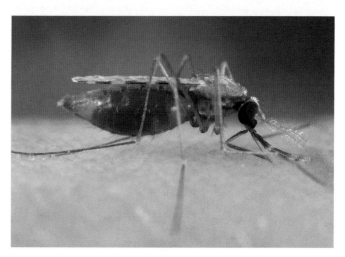

Figure 26-2. A photograph of an *Anopheles* mosquito while it is obtaining a blood meal from a human. Image courtesy of the Centers for Disease Control and Prevention, James Gathany.

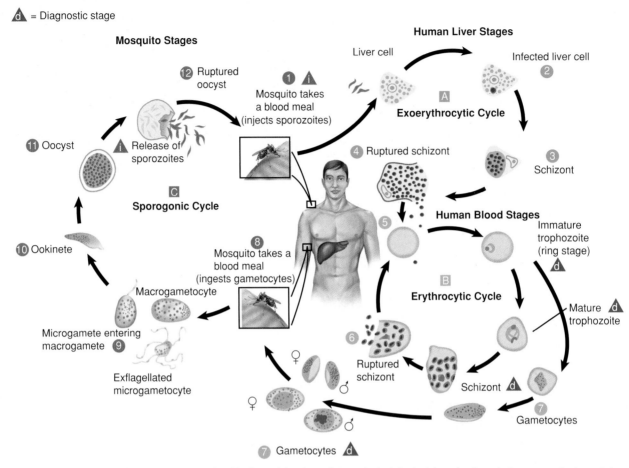

Figure 26-3. The life cycle of *Plasmodium* species. During a blood meal, a malaria-infected female *Anopheles* mosquito inoculates sporozoites into the human host ❶. Sporozoites infect liver cells ❷ and mature into schizonts ❸, which rupture and release merozoites ❹. In *P vivax* and *P ovale* infections, a dormant stage (hypnozoites) can persist in the liver and cause relapses by invading the bloodstream weeks, or even years later. After replication in the liver (exoerythrocytic schizogony), Ⓐ the parasites undergo asexual multiplication in the erythrocytes (erythrocytic schizogony Ⓑ). The merozoites released from the liver infect red blood cells ❺. The ring-cell stage occurs when trophozoites mature into schizonts in the red blood cells, which rupture and release merozoites ❻. Some parasites differentiate into sexual erythrocytic stages (gametocytes) ❼. The gametocytes, male (microgametocytes) and female (macrogametocytes), are ingested by an *Anopheles* mosquito during a blood meal ❽. The parasites' multiplication in the mosquito is known as the sporogonic cycle Ⓒ. While in the mosquito's stomach, the microgametes penetrate the macrogametes generating zygotes ❾. The zygotes in turn become motile and elongated (ookinetes) ❿, which invade the midgut wall of the mosquito where they develop into oocysts ⓫. The oocysts grow, rupture, and release sporozoites ⓬, which make their way to the mosquito's salivary glands. Inoculation of the sporozoites into a new human host allows the malaria life cycle to continue ❶. Image courtesy of the Centers for Disease Control and Prevention.

DIAGNOSIS

Diagnosis of malaria is obtained following visualization of parasitized erythrocytes in thick or thin peripheral blood smears stained with Wright or Giemsa stain (Figure 26-4). Serology includes agar diffusion, passive hemagglutination, immunofluorescence, and ELISA. Malaria-specific antibody is not detectable until after symptoms begin, and is useful for patients who have negative blood smears and for detecting carriers of *P vivax* and *P ovale* in blood used for transfusions. This recurring febrile disease can be confused with other recurring febrile illnesses (e.g., brucellosis and relapsing fever; see Chapter 25). Table 26-1 lists the differences in the periodicity and duration of the fever.

THERAPY AND PREVENTION

Once a diagnosis of malaria has been confirmed, appropriate anti-malarial treatment must be initiated immediately (Table 26-2). Malarial infections can be prevented using mosquito control measures and mosquito netting treated with insecticide. Chemoprophylaxis includes taking chloroquine when in chloroquine-sensitive areas. In areas with chloroquine-resistant *P falciparum*, quinine sulfate, mefloquine, or atovaquone-proguanil is suggested. Because these chemoprophylactic agents do not eliminate *P vivax* and *P ovale* (forms of the parasite that remain in the liver), primaquine phosphate treatment is recommended when living in endemic areas.

BABESIOSIS

Babesiosis is a protozoan infection of the erythrocytes that is transmitted by ticks, and is most commonly seen in northeastern parts of the United States.

ETIOLOGY

There are over 100 species of *Babesia;* however, only *B microti* and variants of the protozoan parasite are endemic in the United States. *B microti* is endemic in the northeastern and midwestern parts of the United States. *Babesia* WA-1 is a variant of *B microti* and has been reported in California and Washington. Another *B microti* variant, MO-1, has been isolated from patients living in Missouri.

MANIFESTATIONS

Babesia inhabits the erythrocytes and causes a hemolytic anemia that results in a variety of symptoms associated with this infection. In regions where malaria is endemic, babesiosis has been misidentified as malaria. Symptoms include fatigue, myalgia, arthralgia, nausea and vomiting, and dark urine. Physical signs include fever, shaking chills, hepatosplenomegaly, and jaundice. Most persons who have been infected by this parasite are asymptomatic and improve without treatment. Persons who develop symptoms tend to be elderly, immunocompromised, or have been splenectomized.

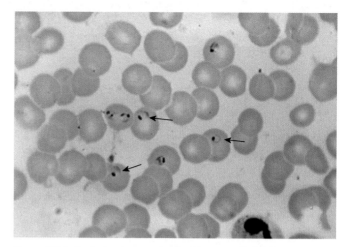

Figure 26-4. A photomicrograph of a Giemsa-stained thin blood film that reveals the ring-cell stage of the *Plasmodium falciparum* trophozoites (*black arrows*). Image courtesy of the Centers for Disease Control and Prevention, Steven Glenn, Laboratory & Consultation Division.

TABLE 26-1. Some Diseases with Recurring Fevers: Causative Agents and Periodicity and Duration of Fever

Disease	Causative Agent	Periodicity of Fever	Duration of Fever
Malaria	*Plasmodium*	Every 3–4 days (except *P falciparum* where fever can be continuous)	Fever lasts 24 hours, with the fever ending in a drenching sweat
Brucellosis	*Brucella*	Daily	Fever recurs in the evening and is gone by morning, ending in a drenching sweat
Relapsing fever	*Borrelia*	Every 7–10 days	Fever lasts 7–10 days

TABLE 26-2. Treatment of *Plasmodium* Infections (Listed by Species and Chloroquine Resistance)

Species	Chloroquine Resistance	Therapy
P falciparum	No	Chloroquine
P falciparum	Yes	Quinine sulfate **plus** doxycycline, tetracycline, or clindamycin **OR** atovaquone-proguanil **OR** mefloquine
P vivax	No	Chloroquine **plus** primaquine phosphate*
P vivax	Yes	Quinine sulfate **plus** doxycycline or tetracycline **plus** primaquine phosphate* **OR** Mefloquine **plus** primaquine phosphate*
P malariae	No	Chloroquine
P ovale	No	Chloroquine **plus** primaquine phosphate*

*The other drugs used to treat malaria only eliminate the parasites in the erythrocytes. *P vivax* and *P ovale* produce hypnozoites that dwell in the liver. Relapses of malaria will be more likely to occur if primaquine phosphate, a drug that eliminates the liver forms (hypnozoites) of the parasite, *is not used* in treating patients with these diseases due to infections by the *Plasmodium* species.

EPIDEMIOLOGY

- Babesiosis is endemic in the northeastern and midwestern United States and in California and Washington.

- About 25% of patients infected with *B microti* are also infected with the Lyme disease bacteria *Borrelia burgdorferi*, and usually have more severe symptoms for longer periods of time than if infected with either one of these agents alone.

- *Babesia* is a protozoan parasite that is transmitted to humans by the *Ixodes* tick (Figure 26-5) and can be acquired from transfusion of blood infected with the parasite.

PATHOGENESIS

Unlike malaria, which infects hepatocytes initially and then infects erythrocytes, *B microti* trophozoites only infect erythrocytes. Damage to red blood cells causes a hemolytic anemia and thrombocytopenia. Increases in atypical lymphocytes are seen in complete blood counts of peripheral blood samples. The changes in the membrane of the erythrocytes cause the cells to be less likely to change shape as they move through the capillaries, making the cells much more adherent. This can lead to the development of acute respiratory distress syndrome in severely affected patients.

DIAGNOSIS

A complete blood count of a peripheral blood sample can aid in the diagnosis of babesiosis, revealing a hemolytic anemia, thrombocytopenia, atypical lymphocytes, and leukopenia. Thick and thin Giemsa-stained peripheral blood smears should be performed, similar for patients with malaria. Blood smears of

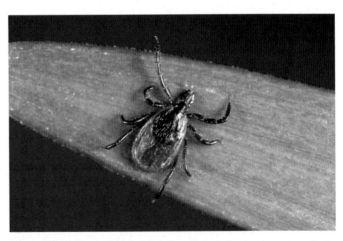

Figure 26-5. A photograph of the deer tick, *Ixodes scapularis*, which transmits babesiosis. Image courtesy of the Centers for Disease Control and Prevention, Michael L Levin, PhD.

patients with babesiosis will frequently show ring-cell forms that contain no pigment, similar to patients with malaria. ***Some erythrocytes may contain the pathognomonic tetrad of trophozoites, frequently called the Maltese cross*** (Figure 26-6). Liver function tests usually reveal mildly elevated hepatic transaminases, lactic dehydrogenase, and serum bilirubin. The patient's urine may be dark, and urinalysis may reveal hemoglobinuria and proteinuria. In severe cases, the patient may have hypoxia.

In patients who have negative peripheral blood-stained specimens, there are a variety of serologic assays that may help, including an immunofluorescent antibody assay, ELISA, and immunoblot assays. Polymerase chain reaction (PCR) can be used to confirm the diagnosis.

TREATMENT AND PREVENTION

Treatment of babesiosis usually includes clindamycin and quinine. However, the treatment regimen of atovaquone and azithromycin results in fewer side effects. Prevention of babesiosis involves identification of persons most at risk of developing severe disease and encouraging them to avoid exposure to ticks as well as educating them about methods of tick prevention. Disease transmission requires about 24 hours; therefore, prompt removal of any attached ticks is helpful in preventing infections.

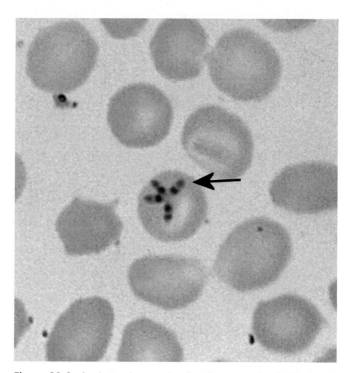

Figure 26-6. A photomicrograph of a Giemsa-stained thin blood smear containing the tetrad of trophozoites showing the Maltese cross (*black arrow*), characteristic of babesiosis. Image courtesy of the Centers for Disease Control and Prevention, Steven Glenn, Laboratory & Consultation Division.

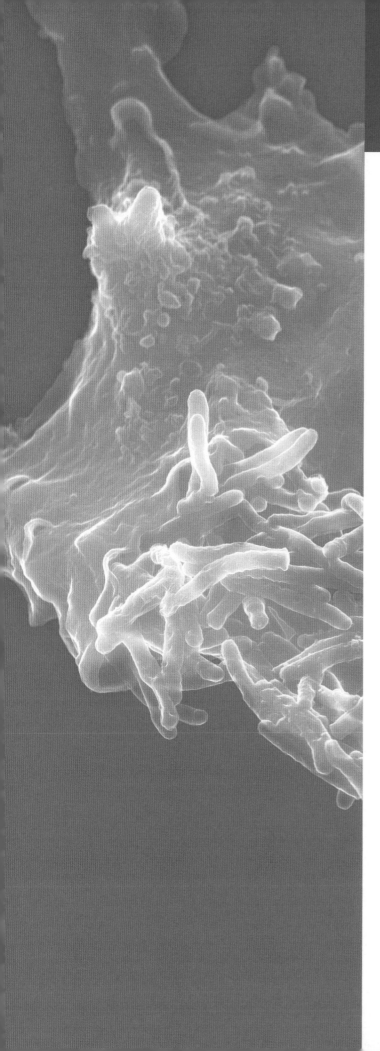

CHAPTER 27

ENDOTHELIAL CELLS

OVERVIEW

This chapter discusses the infectious diseases that occur following infection or destruction of the endothelial cells that line the blood vessels. Damage to endothelial cells can cause hemorrhage (e.g., Rocky Mountain spotted fever) or increases in capillary permeability (e.g., hantavirus pulmonary syndrome), and in some diseases can result in death. Other organisms infect the endothelial cells to escape the host's immune reaction (e.g., relapsing fever), and others produce factors that induce angiogenesis (e.g., bacillary angiomatosis).

The three diseases that will be discussed in this chapter are bacillary angiomatosis (caused by *Bartonella henselae* and *Bartonella quintana*), relapsing fever (caused by *Borrelia*), and hantavirus pulmonary syndrome (caused by *Hantavirus*). A fourth disease, Rocky Mountain spotted fever (caused by *Rickettsia rickettsii*), infects the endothelium and causes macules and petechia of the skin. It was discussed in Chapter 2 and will not be discussed in this chapter.

BACILLARY ANGIOMATOSIS

Bacillary angiomatosis is a systemic disease diagnosed in immunocompromised patients. It results in numerous subcutaneous nodules and is characterized by vascular proliferation. These nodules have also been observed postmortem in the larynx, gastrointestinal tract, peritoneum, and diaphragm. Bacillary angiomatosis is classified as a category B condition in patients infected with human immunodeficiency virus (HIV).

ETIOLOGY

B henselae and *B quintana* cause bacillary angiomatosis.

MANIFESTATIONS

Nearly all cases of bacillary angiomatosis are seen in immunocompromised patients, with the most cases reported in patients with AIDS. Immunocompetent persons can also develop the disease, but it is rare.

Patients with bacillary angiomatosis usually report having scattered cutaneous papules and nodules or a subcutaneous nodule resembling a common bacterial abscess. Some of the nodules can be rather large (up to 10 cm in diameter). Patients may have only one lesion or hundreds of lesions. The four different skin

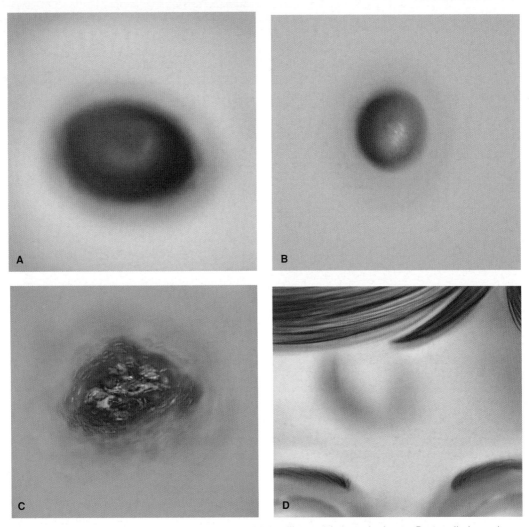

Figure 27-1. Drawings of skin lesions in patients with bacillary angiomatosis due to *Bartonella henselae* or *Bartonella quintana*. **A,** A violaceous nodule resembling Kaposi sarcoma; **B,** a nodule resembling pyogenic granuloma; **C,** a lichenoid violaceous plaque; and **D,** a subcutaneous nodule.

lesions seen in this disease are (1) globular angiomatous papules or nodules resembling pyogenic granuloma, (2) violaceous nodules resembling Kaposi sarcoma, (3) a lichenoid violaceous plaque, or (4) a subcutaneous nodule with or without ulceration (Figure 27-1).

Because the disease can cause pathology in other parts of the body besides the skin, a patient may have weight loss and lymphadenopathy. *B henselae* can also infect the liver causing hepatica peliosis, which results in nausea, vomiting, diarrhea, and fever with hepatosplenomegaly.

EPIDEMIOLOGY

▪ About 50% of patients with bacillary angiomatosis are infected with *B henselae,* and the remaining cases are infections caused by *B quintana*.

▪ The disease is primarily seen in immunocompromised patients, predominately in patients with acquired immunodeficiency syndrome (AIDS) with CD4 cell counts below 200.

▪ Bacillary angiomatosis can be transmitted to humans following a cat scratch or bite.

■ *B quintana* can also be transmitted to humans by the body louse *Pediculus humanus* (Figure 27-2).

PATHOGENESIS

Trauma to the dermis that is associated with a cat bite or scratch can expose an individual to *B henselae* or *B quintana*. *B quintana* can also be transmitted to humans by body lice. Once in the dermis, *Bartonella* will be phagocytized by macrophages and taken to the regional lymph nodes. *Bartonella* are contained within the regional lymph nodes of immunocompetent patients. If symptomatic, patients will manifest signs and symptoms of classic cat-scratch disease (Chapter 25). However, immuno-compromised individuals are unable to contain the bacteria, and *Bartonella* will enter the bloodstream and infect endothelial cells throughout the body. The infected endothelial cells produce monocyte-macrophage chemoattractant protein 1 (MCP-1), which attracts macrophages to the site of infection. The macrophages are activated at the site of endothelial cell infection to secrete vascular endothelial growth factor (VEGF) and other endothelial cell mitogens to induce vascular proliferation. The *Bartonella* infected endothelial cells will upregulate proangiogenic factors, inhibit apoptosis through inhibition of caspases, and upregulate adhesion molecules, which promote vascular proliferation as well.

DIAGNOSIS

A physical examination of the patient for the characteristic lesions and biopsy of the lesions helps to confirm the diagnosis of bacillary angiomatosis. Hematoxylin and eosin (H&E) stained slides show sections with many blood vessels of varying dimensions lined by swollen endothelial cells containing bacilli. The bacteria can be stained more clearly with Warthin-Starry silver stain. Infiltrates of acute and chronic inflammatory cells as well as fibrin deposits may also be seen.

THERAPY AND PREVENTION

Treatment of patients who have bacillar angiomatosis with oral erythromycin for 3 months usually results in the skin lesions gradually fading. Disposal of the cat is not recommended since it will carry the bacillus for only a limited period of time; declawing appears to make no difference in cat to human transmission rates. Flea-control measures should be undertaken on a regular basis.

RELAPSING FEVER

Relapsing fever is a recurring febrile disease transmitted to humans by ticks (endemic form). It is caused by several different *Borrelia* species.

ETIOLOGY

Endemic relapsing fever is caused by at least 15 different *Borrelia* species. Soft ticks of the genus *Ornithodorus* spread the tick-borne variety (Figure 27-3). The *Borrelia* species that cause endemic relapsing fever are named according to the species of the tick that transmits the bacterium to humans; for example, *B parkeri* is transmitted by *Ornithodoros parkeri* and *B hermsii* is transmitted by *Ornithodoros hermsii*.

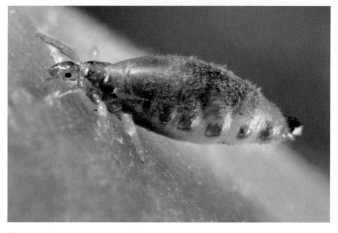

Figure 27-2. A photograph of the female body louse *Pediculus humanus* var. *corporis* as it obtains a blood meal from a human host. This louse can transmit *Bartonella quintana*. Image courtesy of the Centers for Disease Control and Prevention, Frank Collins, PhD.

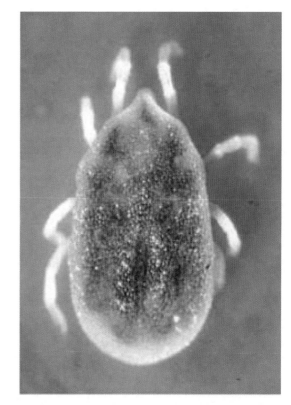

Figure 27-3. A soft-shelled nymph of *Ornithodoros hermsi*. Image courtesy of TG Schwan et al. Tick-borne Relapsing Fever Caused by *Borrelia hermsii*, Montana. Emerg Infect Dis [serial online] 2003 Sept [*date cited*]. Available from URL http://www.cdc.gov/ncidod/EID/vol9no9/03-0280.htm.

MANIFESTATIONS

In endemic relapsing fever, an abrupt onset of symptoms is usually seen with high fever, rigors, severe headache, muscle pains, weakness, anorexia, weight loss, and cough. Systemic complications can include nausea and vomiting, upper abdominal pain due to liver and spleen involvement, and a dry cough. Other manifestations include splenomegaly, hepatomegaly, jaundice, rash, respiratory symptoms, and central nervous system involvement.

A primary febrile episode ends within 3–6 days and can culminate in fatal shock. Patients who survive will appear well for about 7–10 days; after a period without fever, the fever will relapse and last 3–6 days. Subsequent relapses tend to be less severe. In most cases of endemic relapsing fever, there are 3–10 relapses.

EPIDEMIOLOGY

- Endemic relapsing fever occurs worldwide; however, only a few cases of endemic relapsing fever are reported in the United States each year.

- Most cases of endemic relapsing fever occur in the late spring and summer in the western mountainous states, south into Texas, and northwest into Washington.

- Clusters of cases of endemic relapsing fever are reported, for example, in groups of campers sharing a rustic facility infested with rodents on which the ticks feed.

- Endemic relapsing fever is transmitted by soft ticks (Ornithodoros sp.) from a rodent reservoir to humans (see Figure 27-3).

PATHOGENESIS

In endemic relapsing fever, *soft ticks feed for short periods during the night and then fall off the host. A patient can be infected with Borrelia within minutes after the tick attaches to the host.* This is an important distinction from other tick-borne diseases, such as Lyme disease, in which ticks feed for longer periods of time and it can take several hours before the bacterium that causes Lyme disease, *Borrelia burgdorferi*, infects the host.

Large numbers of *Borrelia* are present in the bloodstream (spirochetemia) following transmission from the tick. During the spirochetemia, *Borrelia* invades the endothelium. After multiplying in the endothelial cells, the bacteria are released into the bloodstream and patients develop symptoms that include fever. Symptoms resolve when the host's immune system produces antibodies to the proteins on the outer surface of the *Borrelia* and eliminates the bacteria from the bloodstream. However, *Borrelia* that remains in the endothelial cells are not killed and can change the proteins on their outer surface. *Borrelia* producing new outer membrane proteins can avoid destruction by antibodies directed against the original infecting bacteria. Thus, the patient clinically improves until the *Borrelia*, with different surface proteins, multiplies sufficiently to cause another relapse. This period of bacterial multiplication can take from 7 to 10 days. Specific immunoglobulin-complement–mediated lysis and the release of endotoxin accounts for some symptoms. Relapses continue until the *Borrelia* no longer produce novel antigenic variations of their surface proteins. If untreated, most organs of the body are infected; mortality is usually associated with myocarditis.

TABLE 27-1. Some Diseases with Recurring Fevers: Causative Agents and Periodicity and Duration of Fever

Disease	Causative Agent	Periodicity of Fever	Duration of Fever
Malaria	*Plasmodium*	Every 3–4 days (except *P falciparum* where fever can be continuous)	Fever lasts 24 hours, with the fever ending in a drenching sweat
Brucellosis	*Brucella*	Daily	Fever recurs in the evening and temperature is normal by morning, with the fever ending in a drenching sweat
Relapsing fever	*Borrelia*	Every 7–10 days	Fever lasts 7–10 days

DIAGNOSIS

The signs and symptoms of relapsing fever can be very similar to those of typhoid fever. However, in relapsing fever, the patient's pulse rate is rapid in proportion to the fever. A relative bradycardia occurs in typhoid fever and helps to differentiate relapsing fever from typhoid fever. Relapsing fever can be mistaken for brucellosis or malaria; however, the periodicity of the fevers differs (Table 27-1). A peripheral blood smear stained with Giemsa or Wright stain will demonstrate the spirochetemia in 70% of patients during the febrile period and result in a definitive diagnosis (Figure 27-4).

THERAPY AND PREVENTION

The mortality rate of endemic relapsing fever is 1% with treatment and 30–70% without treatment. Tetracycline is effective in the treatment of relapsing fever. As is seen in the treatment of syphilis, patients treated for relapsing fever may also experience a Jarisch-Herxheimer reaction. This reaction produces apprehension, diaphoresis, fever, tachycardia, and tachypnea, with an initial pressor response followed rapidly by hypotension. Erythromycin or chloramphenicol can be used in the treatment of pregnant women and children. It should be noted that **chloramphenicol can cause serious and sometimes fatal blood dyscrasias** (e.g., aplastic anemia, hypoplastic anemia, thrombocytopenia, granulocytopenia) and **should only be given to seriously ill children.**

To prevent endemic relapsing fever, it is important to wear proper clothing that keeps ticks from gaining access to the skin and apply N,N-diethyl-*m*-toluamide (DEET) in tick-laden areas. Cabins in endemic regions should be treated with insecticide, and rodents should be controlled for endemic disease.

HANTAVIRUS PULMONARY SYNDROME

Hantavirus pulmonary syndrome is a relatively new disease reported in the United States. The first cases of hantavirus pulmonary syndrome occurred in 1993 and were in the four-corner region of the United States in Arizona, Utah, Colorado, and New Mexico. This viral infection can cause significant pulmonary edema, and although relatively rare has a high mortality rate (35%).

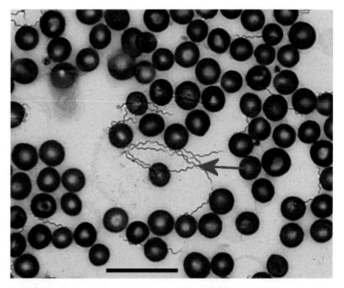

Figure 27-4. A photomicrograph of *Borrelia hermsii* (*blue arrow*) in a thin smear of mouse blood stained with Wright-Giemsa stain. Image courtesy of TG Schwan et al. Tick-borne Relapsing Fever Caused by *Borrelia hermsii*, Montana. Emerg Infect Dis [serial online] 2003 Sept [*date cited*]. Available from: URL: http://www.cdc.gov/ncidod/EID/vol9no9/03-0280.htm.

TABLE 27-2. Signs and Symptoms of Hantavirus Pulmonary Syndrome

Stage of Disease	Signs and Symptoms	Comments
Prodrome (lasts 3–5 days)	Fever, myalgias, headache, chills, dizziness, and nausea and vomiting	Respiratory tract symptoms are minimal or absent; thus, the physician may conclude that the patient has viral gastroenteritis
Late or cardiopulmonary phase (lasts 24–48 hours)	Shortness of breath, cough, fever, tachypnea, tachycardia, and rales Chest radiographs usually show a pattern of noncardiac pulmonary edema: ● Cardiac silhouette is *NOT* enlarged ● Perihilar haziness ("shaggy-heart" sign) is characteristic ● Interstitial edema due to pulmonary capillary leak, which manifests as peribronchial cuffing or Kerley B lines	Cough and tachypnea generally do not develop until about day 7 Most patients with pulmonary edema require mechanical ventilation
Convalescence	Resolution of cardiopulmonary stage is heralded by onset of significant diuresis	Following diuresis, the patient improves quite rapidly

ETIOLOGY

The virus responsible for hantavirus pulmonary syndrome is a new-world hantavirus called Sin Nombre virus.

MANIFESTATIONS

Sin Nombre virus causes manifestations of cardiopulmonary disease called hantavirus pulmonary syndrome (Table 27-2).

EPIDEMIOLOGY

- Cases of hantavirus pulmonary syndrome have been reported in 31 states.
- A total of 465 cases of the disease were reported in the United States from 1993 to March 2007 (Figure 27-5).
- Sin Nombre virus is present in animal urine or feces from mice. The virus is transmitted to humans following aerosolization of murine urine or feces.

PATHOGENESIS

Portals of entry for the Sin Nombre virus include the respiratory and digestive tracts. Viral multiplication occurs in the endothelial cells. Viremia and fever occur 2–14 days after infection.

Viral antigens can be seen within the endothelium of capillaries throughout various tissues of the patient with hantavirus pulmonary syndrome. High concentrations of hantaviral antigens are seen in the pulmonary microvasculature and in follicular dendritic cells within the lymphoid follicles of the spleen and lymph nodes. Typical hantaviral inclusions are frequently seen in pulmonary endothelial cells. Antibodies produced to the hantaviral antigens damage the endothelial cells and increase capillary permeability. The increased capillary permeability in the lungs results in leakage of protein-rich plasma from the capillaries into the lungs and the pleura. This leakage causes the cardiopulmonary signs and symptoms listed in Table 27-2.

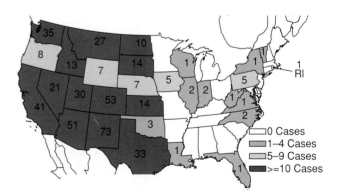

Figure 27-5. A map of the United States showing hantavirus pulmonary syndrome cases by state from 1993 to March 2006. The blue arrow points to the four corner region of the United States where the first outbreak of hantavirus pulmonary syndrome occurred. Image courtesy of the Centers for Disease Control and Prevention.

TABLE 27-3. Clinical Definition of Hantavirus Pulmonary Syndrome

Hantavirus pulmonary syndrome is an illness characterized by one or more of the following clinical features:

- A febrile illness (>38.3°C) with bilateral diffuse interstitial edema that may radiographically resemble ARDS, with respiratory compromise requiring supplemental oxygen, developing within 72 hours of hospitalization, and occurring in a previously healthy person.

- An unexplained respiratory illness resulting in death, with an autopsy examination indicating noncardiogenic pulmonary edema without an identifiable cause.

- Laboratory criteria for diagnosis include detection of hantavirus-specific IgM or rising titers of hantavirus-specific IgG, or detection of hantavirus-specific RNA sequence by PCR in clinical specimens, or detection of hantavirus antigen by immunohistochemistry.

ARDS, adult respiratory distress syndrome; IgM, immunoglobulin M; IgG, immunoglobulin G; RNA, ribonucleic acid; PCR, polymerase chain reaction.

DIAGNOSIS

A clinical case definition has been developed for diagnosis of patients with hantavirus pulmonary syndrome and is described in Table 27-3. The white blood cell count of patients with hantavirus pulmonary syndrome is usually elevated, with a marked left shift (bandemia). White blood cell precursors (band cells) may be as high as 50%, and atypical lymphocytes are frequently present (Figure 27-6). Atypical lymphocytes usually are observed at the onset of pulmonary edema. The platelet count in about 80% of individuals with hantavirus pulmonary syndrome is below 150,000. A dramatic decrease in the platelet count indicates a transition from the prodrome to the pulmonary edema phase (cardiopulmonary phase) of the illness. Early in the disease, chest radiographs show interstitial pulmonary edema, which progresses to alveolar edema with severe bilateral involvement (see Figure 27-7). Pleural effusions are common and can be large enough to be seen on chest radiographs.

THERAPY AND PREVENTION

Treatment of hantavirus pulmonary syndrome involves supportive care. Ribavirin may be useful if given early in the course of the disease. Improved sanitation standards and control of the rodent populations is important in preventing this disease.

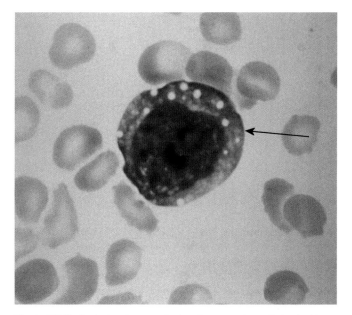

Figure 27-6. A photomicrograph showing an enlarged atypical lymphocyte (*black arrow*) found in a peripheral blood smear from a patient with hantavirus pulmonary syndrome. Hematologic findings are important in the diagnosis of hantavirus pulmonary syndrome. The large atypical lymphocyte combined with a bandemia and a decreasing platelet count are characteristic of this disease. Image courtesy of the Centers for Disease Control and Prevention.

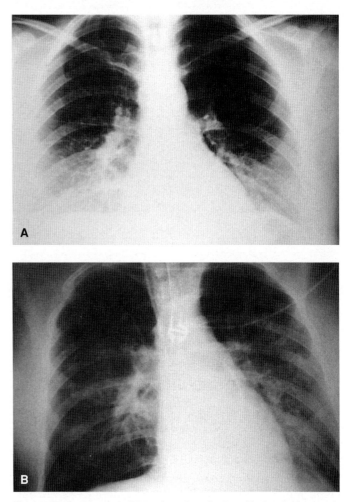

Figure 27-7. Chest radiographs of patients with hantavirus pulmonary syndrome. **A,** A chest radiograph of a patient in the early stages of bilateral pulmonary effusion. **B,** A chest radiograph of the midstage bilateral pulmonary effusion due to hantavirus pulmonary syndrome. Image courtesy of the Centers for Disease Control and Prevention, D Loren Ketai, MD.

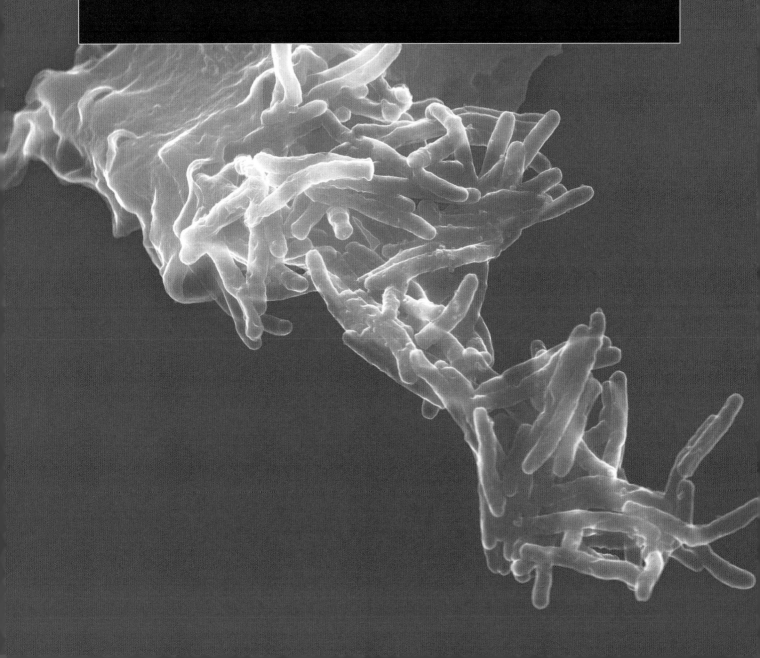

SECTION 7

CIRCULATORY SYSTEM

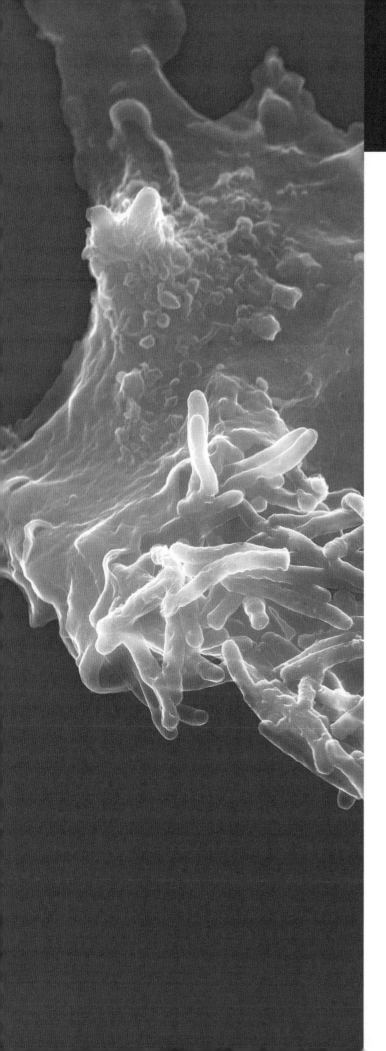

CHAPTER 28

THE BIG PICTURE: INFECTIONS OF THE CIRCULATORY SYSTEM: SEPSIS AND SEPTIC SHOCK

OVERVIEW

Sepsis is a systemic response that is caused by the presence of pathogenic microorganisms or their toxins, or both, in the bloodstream. During sepsis, the body mounts an immune response to the infection or the microbial toxins, or both. In the early stages of sepsis, the immune response can be characterized as a systemic inflammatory response syndrome (SIRS) (Figure 28-1). In the later stages of sepsis, the immune system can mount a response that results in an unbalanced state, with inflammation overwhelming the factors that control the inflammatory response. This unbalanced inflammatory state causes leakage of blood from the vascular space into the interstitial spaces in the tissues, resulting in hypotension and hypoperfusion of the organs (severe sepsis or septic shock) (Table 28-1). Hypoperfusion of the organs can result in organ failure (multiple organ dysfunction syndrome [MODS]).

The timing of clinical intervention is essential to the survival of septic patients. Early identification of sepsis with appropriate treatment significantly increases the chances that the patient will survive. However, even with appropriate and aggressive treatment, 50–60% of patients with septic shock will die if the process is identified too late (Figure 28-2).

SEPSIS AND SEPTIC SHOCK

ETIOLOGY

Most cases of sepsis occur as the result of an infection of the urinary tract, lungs, or the peritoneum. Other sources of sepsis include skin, soft tissue, and central nervous system (CNS) infections. Approximately 50% of cases of sepsis are due to gram-negative bacteria, and slightly less than 50% are caused by gram-positive bacteria. Less common causes of sepsis include fungi, viruses such as the human immunodeficiency virus (HIV), and protozoa.

Sepsis in the neonate

Sepsis in the neonate (<1 month old) is usually caused by *Streptococcus agalactiae* (group B *Streptococcus*) and less commonly by *Escherichia coli*. During labor or delivery, the neonate can become infected with *E coli* or *S agalactiae*. Infection with these organisms may initially manifest as pneumonia or meningitis. Other causes of neonatal sepsis include *Klebsiella* and *Enterobacter*.

Pediatric sepsis

The most common causes of sepsis in the pediatric age group include *Streptococcus pneumoniae*, *Neisseria meningitidis*, and *Staphylococcus aureus*. Antecedent infections that may cause sepsis in this group of patients include meningitis, skin infections, bacterial rhinosinusitis, and otitis media. Common causes of meningitis include *S pneumoniae* and *N meningitidis*. *S aureus* is a common cause of skin infections, and *S pneumonia* is frequently the cause of bacterial rhinosinusitis and otitis media. Other causes of sepsis in the pediatric population include *E coli*, *S agalactiae* (Group B *Streptococcus*), *Klebsiella*, and *Enterobacter*.

Sepsis in adults

An antecedent infection usually serves as the source of sepsis in adults. The most common sites of infection in adults are the urinary tract, the respiratory tract, and the abdomen. Urinary tract infections are common in sexually active women and can ascend from the bladder to the kidneys and into the bloodstream. Males with benign prostatic hyperplasia are more likely to be diagnosed with urinary tract infections, which can also ascend to the kidneys and then into the bloodstream.

Many adults are diagnosed with pneumonia each year. Bacteria are the most common cause of pneumonia in adults, and frequently bacteria leave the lungs and enter the bloodstream.

Many older adults develop diverticulosis. The diverticula can occasionally release bacteria into the peritoneum, causing peritonitis or intra-abdominal abscesses. The rich vascular supply of the peritoneum allows bacteria to enter the bloodstream. More details on the causes of sepsis in adults are listed in Table 28-2.

Special concerns

Elderly patients are more susceptible to sepsis, have less physiologic reserve to tolerate the insult from infection, and are more likely to have underlying diseases, all of which adversely impact survival. Elderly patients also are more likely to have atypical presentations, such as hypothermia rather than a fever, or nonspecific presentations when septic. The common causes of sepsis in the elderly are the same as those seen in younger adults (see Table 28-2).

EPIDEMIOLOGY

■ Sepsis causes 9.3% of all deaths in the United States each year. There are about 400,000 cases of sepsis diagnosed per year, and approximately 50% of these patients progress to septic shock (see Figure 28-2).

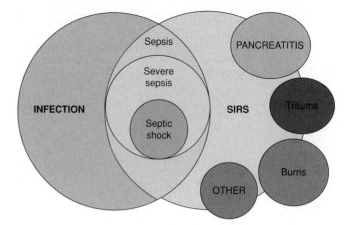

Figure 28-1. A Venn diagram showing the relationships between the causes of systemic inflammatory response syndrome (SIRS) and infection and between SIRS, sepsis, severe sepsis, and septic shock.

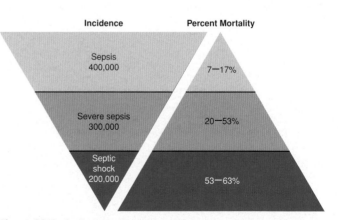

Figure 28-2. A diagram illustrating the incidence of sepsis, severe sepsis, and septic shock and the percent mortality as the severity of the patient's condition increases.

TABLE 28-1. Clinical Definitions of the Progression from SIRS to MODS

Disease Stage	Clinical Definition	Signs and Symptoms	Comments
SIRS	Two or more of the signs and symptoms	Chills	
		Alteration in body temperature	Body temperature >38°C or <36°C
		Alteration in mental status	
		Tachycardia	Tachycardia (>90 beats/min)
		Tachypnea	Tachypnea (>20 respirations per min or $PaCO_2$ <32 mm Hg)
		Altered WBC count	WBC count (leukocyte count >12,000/mm^3, <4,000/mm^3)
		"Left shift"	Increase in the number of immature neutrophils or band cells (>10% immature [band] cells)
		Thrombocytopenia	
		Decreased perfusion	Decreased perfusion: mottled skin, poor capillary refill
		Increased blood glucose concentration	
		Petechiae and purpura	
Sepsis	At least 2 signs and symptoms of SIRS plus a documented site of infection	See SIRS signs and symptoms Hypoperfusion abnormalities, hypotension	Must include laboratory isolation of a microorganism from the bloodstream or from another site of infection that can lead to an infection of the bloodstream.
Severe sepsis	Sepsis with organ dysfunction	Hypotension and hypoperfusion abnormalities	Examples of hypoperfusion abnormalities include lactic acidosis [>4 mmol/L (36 mg/dL) lactate], oliguria, and acute alteration in mental status. A hypotensive patient has a mean arterial pressure <70 mm Hg. Resuscitation with IV fluids increases blood pressure to normal levels.
Septic shock	Sepsis-induced hypotension, despite fluid resuscitation, plus hypoperfusion abnormalities	Hypotension and hypoperfusion abnormalities	In contrast to severe sepsis, a patient with septic shock remains hypotensive despite fluid resuscitation. Hypoperfusion abnormalities are as mentioned in severe sepsis.
MODS	Presence of altered organ functions that cannot be normalized without intervention		

SIRS, systemic inflammatory response syndrome; WBC, white blood cell; IV, intravenous; MODS, multiple organ dysfunction syndrome.

TABLE 28-2. Bacterial Causes of Adult Sepsis and the Common Sites of Infection

Bacterial Agents Gram-negative Bacteria	Common Infection(s)	Comments
Escherichia coli	UTI; prostatitis	Most common cause of UTIs and prostatitis in adults
Klebsiella pneumoniae	UTI; pneumonia	Common cause of pneumonia in chronic alcoholics
Enterobacter	UTI	
Pseudomonas aeruginosa	Infected burn wounds and pneumonia in patients with cystic fibrosis	Sepsis due to *P aeruginosa* has the highest mortality rate
Proteus	UTI	UTI due to these organisms have an elevated urine pH
Bacteroides fragilis	Peritonitis	Most common cause of anaerobic sepsis

Bacterial Agents Gram-positive bacteria	Common Infection(s)	Comments
Streptococcus pneumoniae	Pneumonia; meningitis	Most common cause of pneumonia and meningitis in adults
Streptococcus pyogenes	Skin and soft tissue	Produces superantigens (pyrogenic exotoxins) that cause streptococcal TSS; bacteria are usually present in the bloodstream
Staphylococcus aureus	Skin and soft tissue	Produces a superantigen toxin called TSS toxin, which causes TSS in menstruating women or in patients with an infected wound
Enterococcus	UTI	

UTI, urinary tract infection; TSS, toxic shock syndrome.

- Sepsis is the seventh leading cause of death in children aged 1–4 years and is the ninth leading cause of death in children aged 5–14 years.

- Approximately 2 of 1000 live-born infants are infected by *S agalactiae* (group B streptococcal sepsis), with a case fatality of 5–10%.

- **Bacteria are the most common cause of sepsis.** Gram-negative bacteria cause 50% of cases of septic shock, resulting in 115,000 deaths per year. Gram-negative bacteria cause more deaths due to sepsis than do gram-positive bacteria.

- **Septic shock** caused by gram-positive bacteria (<50% of cases) is now more common because of the increased incidence in cases of pneumonia and the use of intravascular devices.

- **Septic shock** is the most common cause of mortality in the intensive care unit. In 2004, it was the tenth leading cause of death in the United States. About 50–60% of patients with septic shock die each year.

- Mortality increases as the number of symptoms of SIRS increases and as the severity of the disease process increases.

TABLE 28-3. Suspected Sources of Sepsis

Source	Pneumonia	Peritonitis	Skin and Soft Tissue Infections	Urinary Tract Infections	Bacterial Meningitis
Major community-acquired pathogens	*Streptococcus pneumoniae* *Haemophilus influenzae* *Legionella* sp. *Chlamydia pneumoniae*	*Escherichia coli* *Bacteroides fragilis*	*Streptococcus pyogenes* *Staphylococcus aureus* *Clostridium* sp. Polymicrobial infections Aerobic gram negative bacilli *Pseudomonas aeruginosa* Anaerobes *Staphylococcus* sp.	*Escherichia coli* *Klebsiella sp.* *Enterobacter* sp. *Proteus* sp.	*Streptococcus pneumonie* *Neisseria meningitidis* *Listeria monocytogenes* *Escherichia coli* *Haemophilus influenzae*
Major nosocomial pathogens	Aerobic gram negative bacilli	Aerobic gram negative bacilli Anaerobes *Candida* sp.	*Staphylococcus aureus* Aerobic gram negative bacilli	Aerobic gram negative bacilli *Enterococcus* sp.	*Pseudomonas aeruginosa* *Escherichia coli* *Klebsiella* sp. *Staphylococcus* sp.

SOURCES OF INFECTION

The most frequent infectious sources of septic shock include pneumonia, peritonitis, and urinary tract infections. Other sources of infection include the skin and soft tissues, intestinal tract, central nervous system (CNS), oropharynx, instrumentation sites, contaminated inhalation therapy equipment, and intravenous fluids (Table 28-3). The source of the infection is an important determinant of clinical outcome. Certain cases of sepsis are more likely to develop into severe sepsis; for instance, severe sepsis is most likely to occur in patients with nosocomial pneumonia. Severe sepsis is more likely to occur in patients with intra-abdominal infection and polymicrobial bacteremia or postoperative wound infections and bacteremia. However, patients with bacteremia associated with intravascular catheters or indwelling urinary catheters have a lower risk of developing severe sepsis.

Patients at increased risk of developing sepsis

▪ Patients with **underlying diseases,** including neutropenia, solid tumors, leukemia, dysproteinemias, cirrhosis of the liver, diabetes mellitus, acquired immune deficiency syndrome (AIDS), and other serious chronic conditions.

▪ **Antecedent surgery or instrumentation,** including catheters and prosthetic devices.

▪ **Prior drug therapy:** Immunosuppressive drugs, especially broad-spectrum antibiotics.

▪ **Men older than age 50** are more likely to develop benign prostatic hyperplasia, which makes them more susceptible to development of cystitis and pyelonephritis. These infections can lead to sepsis, and the most common cause is *E coli.*

▪ **Sexually active women aged 20–45 years of age** are much more likely to develop urinary tract infections, which can lead to sepsis. The most common cause is *E coli.*

▪ During labor and delivery, **neonates** can be infected with *E coli* and *S agalactiae,* resulting in neonatal sepsis.

- **Other conditions associated with an increased risk of developing sepsis** are childbirth, septic abortion, trauma, widespread burns (*Pseudomonas aeruginosa* and *S aureus*), and intestinal ulceration (*Bacteroides* and gram-negative rods).

MANIFESTATIONS

Symptoms of sepsis are usually nonspecific and include fever, chills, and constitutional symptoms of fatigue, malaise, anxiety, or confusion. Symptoms may be absent in serious infections, especially in elderly patients. There is a continuum of clinical manifestations that usually begin with SIRS and can end with MODS. See Table 28-1 for details concerning the signs and symptoms associated with sepsis. *Remember,* **patients treated early in this disease continuum have fewer complications and have a much better chance of survival.**

Organ dysfunction associated with severe sepsis and septic shock

Perfusion of the organs is reduced in patients with severe sepsis to septic shock. Some of the organ dysfunctions that result from this reduced perfusion are listed below. Severe sepsis and septic shock can simultaneously affect several organs, resulting in a mixture of signs and symptoms.

- **Lung:** Decrease in arterial PO$_2$; acute respiratory distress syndrome (ARDS) due to leakage of the contents of the capillaries into alveoli; tachypnea.
- **Kidney:** Acute renal failure and proteinuria.
- **Liver:** Elevated levels of serum bilirubin and alkaline phosphatase; cholestatic jaundice.
- **Gastrointestinal tract:** Nausea and vomiting, diarrhea, ileus.
- **Heart:** Cardiac output is initially normal or elevated. Later, impaired cardiac contractility can occur.
- **Brain:** Confusion.
- **Skin:** Some organisms are more likely to cause changes in the skin. Some organisms produce toxins that can cause dilatation of the blood vessels in the skin, resulting in a rash or erythroderma. Other organisms damage the endothelial cells, which line the blood vessels and cause leakage of the blood from the vascular space into the skin, resulting in petechiae or purpuras. Yet other organisms enter the skin from the bloodstream and cause erythema and necrosis (ecthyma gangrenosum).
  1. **Petechiae or purpura:** Usually due to infections with *N meningitidis* or *Rickettsia rickettsii* (Figure 28-3).
  2. **Generalized erythroderma:** Toxic shock syndrome (TSS) presents with a sunburn-like rash, which then causes skin peeling. It is due to either *S aureus* or *Streptococcus pyogenes* (Figure 28-4).
  3. **Ecthyma gangrenosum:** The most common cause of this skin damage is due to *P aeruginosa* infection (Figure 28-5).

Complications associated with septic shock

The reported incidence of the complications in SIRS (listed below) and sepsis is most frequently CNS dysfunction followed by liver failure, acute renal failure, disseminated intravascular coagulation (DIC), and then ARDS. Patients with septic shock

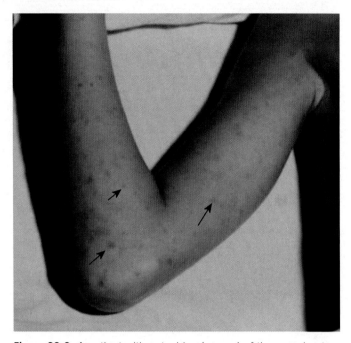

Figure 28-3. A patient with petechiae (*arrows*) of the arm due to a *Rickettsia rickettsii* infection. Image courtesy of the Centers for Disease Control and Prevention.

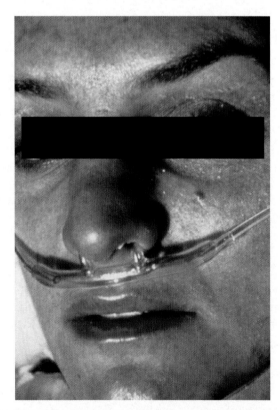

Figure 28-4. A patient with the characteristic sunburn-like rash of the face due to toxic shock syndrome. Image courtesy of the Centers for Disease Control and Prevention.

are most likely to develop acute renal failure followed by DIC and then ARDS. Complications include ARDS, DIC, acute renal failure, intestinal bleeding, liver failure, CNS dysfunction, and heart failure.

PATHOGENESIS

The systemic response to sepsis is a complex sequence of events that can be defined as a spectrum of clinical conditions caused by the immune response of a patient to an infection characterized by systemic inflammation, hypotension, and hypoperfusion of the organs.

Immunologic response to sepsis

Following a microbial infection or a microbial intoxication, the immune response triggers a complex series of events that cause an overwhelming inflammatory response. Dilation of the peripheral vasculature occurs and becomes "leaky," resulting in peripheral pooling of the blood, hypotension, and hypoperfusion of organs.

1. Various **microbial triggers** cause the white blood cells to produce large amounts of proinflammatory cytokines.

   - Gram-negative bacteria produce endotoxin, also known as lipopolysaccharide (LPS). LPS is the most common gram-negative bacterial trigger of cytokine release. This microbial trigger binds to cell receptors on the host's macrophages and activates regulatory proteins such as nuclear factor kappa B (NFκB). LPS activates the regulatory proteins by interacting with several receptors. The CD receptors pool the LPS-LPS–binding protein complex on the surface of the cell, and the Toll-like receptors (TLR) translate the signal into the cells (Figure 28-6).

   - The most common gram-positive bacterial triggers include superantigens such as TSS toxin (TSST) and staphylococcal enterotoxin produced by *S aureus* and streptococcal pyrogenic exotoxin A (SpeA) produced by *S pyogenes*. Instead of binding in the groove of the major histocompatibility complex (MHC) (Figure 28-7), superantigens bind on the outer surface of the antigen-presenting cells' MHC class II molecule as well as on the outer surface of certain T-cell receptors present on T cells (Figure 28-8). Superantigen binding causes T-cell activation and massive proinflammatory cytokine production and release, which can cause fever, endothelial cell damage, dilation of the peripheral vasculature, peripheral pooling of blood in the interstitial space, organ hypoperfusion, organ dysfunction, shock, and death. Unlike most antigens that activate only a few T cells (1 in 10,000 T cells) to cause an immune response, superantigens activate many T cells (one in five T cells), causing a much more vigorous and sometimes life-threatening immune response.

2. With either type of microbial trigger, the immune response begins with an overwhelming inflammatory response due to increased production of proinflammatory cytokines, which include tumor necrosis factor (TNF), interleukin-1 (IL-1), IL-12, interferon gamma (IFN-λ), and IL-6 (see Figure 28-6).

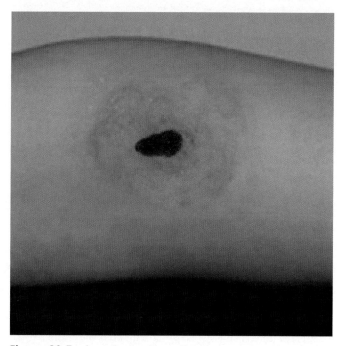

Figure 28-5. A patient with ecthyma gangrenosum due to *Pseudomonas aeruginosa* sepsis. Note the necrotic center and the erythema surrounding the necrosis.

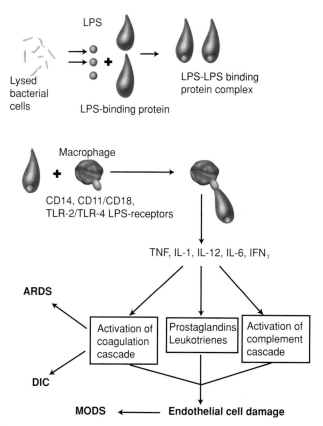

Figure 28-6. The basic mechanism by which lipopolysaccharide (LPS) stimulates the inflammatory response and activates the coagulation and complement cascades. ARDS, adult respiratory distress syndrome; DIC, disseminated intravascular coagulation; MODS, multiple organ dysfunction syndrome; TNF, tumor necrosis factor; IL, interleukin.

3. Proinflammatory cytokines can act directly or indirectly through secondary mediators to affect organ function. The secondary mediators include nitric oxide, thromboxanes, leukotrienes, platelet-activating factor, prostaglandins, and complement.

4. The primary and secondary mediators cause the activation of the complement cascade, production of prostaglandins and leukotrienes, and activation of the coagulation cascade.

DIAGNOSIS

The diagnosis of sepsis requires a high index of suspicion, a thorough history and physical examination, appropriate laboratory studies, and a close follow-up of the patient's hemodynamic status.

A through **history** helps to determine if the infection causing the sepsis was community acquired or nosocomially acquired and if the patient is immunocompromised. Important details include exposure to animals, travel, tick bites, occupational hazards, alcohol use, seizures and loss of consciousness, medications, and underlying diseases that may predispose the patient to specific infectious agents. Some clues to a septic event include fever, hypotension, oliguria (diminished excretion of urine), or anuria (no urine excreted); tachypnea and hypothermia without obvious cause; and bleeding.

In all neutropenic patients and in patients with a suspected pelvic infection, the physical examination should include rectal, pelvic, and genital examinations. Such examinations may reveal rectal, perirectal, or perineal abscesses, pelvic inflammatory disease or abscesses, or prostatitis.

Numerous laboratory tests are usually ordered for patients suspected of having sepsis (Table 28-4). *Cultures of suspected sites of infection are important so that the causative organism(s) can be identified and antibiotic sensitivities can be determined to guide appropriate antimicrobial therapy.* Laboratory tests can be useful to alert the physician of the potential for the increasing severity of the patient's condition. Some of these tests can be helpful in indicating whether SIRS is due to processes other than microbial infection.

THERAPY AND PREVENTION

Early diagnosis and **intervention** are highly effective in stopping the sequence of events leading to septic shock. There are *three priorities when treating the septic patient.*

1. **Immediate stabilization of the patient.** The immediate concern when treating patients with severe sepsis is reversal of life-threatening abnormalities (ABCs: airway, breathing, circulation). Patients with severe sepsis should be admitted to an intensive care unit and vital signs (i.e., blood pressure, heart rate, respiratory rate, and temperature) should be monitored.

2. **The blood must be rapidly cleared of microorganisms.** Prompt and early institution of empiric treatment with **antimicrobial agents** is essential and decreases the development of shock and reduces the mortality rate. The choice of drugs administered depends on the source of the infection (Table 28-5).

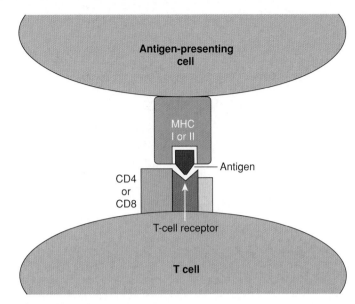

Figure 28-7. The interaction of an antigen with the major histocompatability complex (MHC) and T-cell receptor.

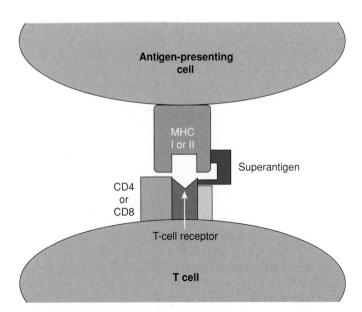

Figure 28-8. The interaction of a superantigen with the major histocompatability complex (MHC) and T-cell receptor.

TABLE 28-4. Laboratory Studies Useful in Assessing a Septic Patient

Laboratory Study	Comments
Blood chemistry, blood lactic acid level, and electrolytes	Respiratory alkalosis signals impending shock that is reversible with fluid resuscitation. Metabolic acidosis can develop just prior to hypotension or can occur simultaneously. Hyperbilirubinemia and proteinuria are often present. Hyperventilation commonly induces respiratory alkalosis.
Cultures of blood, sputum, urine, CSF, and from other obviously infected sites should be performed	At least two sets of blood cultures should be obtained over a 24-h period. During intermittent fever spikes, bacteremia is most prominent 0.5 h before the spike, and blood drawn at this time is more likely to contain detectable bacteria.
CBC with differential	In early stages of disease process, leukocytosis with left shift and thrombocytopenia are frequently observed. Leukopenia may occur in certain patients (elderly). Neutrophils may contain toxic granulations, Döhle bodies, or cytoplasmic vacuoles. Later in the disease process, thrombocytopenia worsens.
Procalcitonin (PCT)	Good nonspecific marker for differentiating systemic bacterial inflammatory responses from nonbacterial systemic inflammatory responses.
C-reactive protein	A nonspecific marker for inflammation.
BUN and creatinine	Later in the disease process, azotemia is more prominent.
Coagulation profile	Later in the disease process, there is a prolongation of PT and PTT times, decreased fibrinogen, and the presence of D-dimers and fibrin split products, suggesting DIC.
Blood glucose	Diabetics can develop hyperglycemia.
Liver function tests	Serum bilirubin and alkaline phosphatase levels can become elevated, and cholestatic jaundice may develop later in the disease process as liver function is affected.
Arterial blood gas	ARDS can result in lower O_2 levels in the bloodstream.
Imaging studies	Chest radiograph to determine if antecedent pneumonia, CT of abdomen may reveal presence of abdominal abscesses if the source of the infection is still unknown, MRI may reveal hard to find sites of infection in the head or abdomen.

CSF, cerebrospinal fluid; CBC, complete blood cell count; BUN, blood urea nitrogen; DIC, disseminated intravascular coagulation; ARDS, adult respiratory distress syndrome; O_2, oxygen.

3. **The original focus of infection must be treated.** Foreign bodies should be removed; purulent exudate should be drained; infected organs should be removed; and gangrenous tissue should be débrided or amputated.

Prevention of sepsis

Avoid trauma to mucosal surfaces that are normally colonized by gram-negative bacteria.

- Use **trimethoprim-sulfamethoxazole** prophylactically in children with leukemia.

- Use topical silver nitrate, silver sulfadiazine, or sulfamylon prophylactically in burn patients.

- Sterilization of the bowel aerobic flora with polymyxin or gentamicin with vancomycin and nystatin is effective in reducing gram-negative sepsis in neutropenic patients.

- Indwelling catheters should be properly cared for and frequently examined for the possibility of infection.

Detection and treatment of **pregnant patients** with vaginal colonization by *S agalactiae* reduces neonatal morbidity and mortality rates from group B streptococcal sepsis. Vaginal and perianal swab samples should be obtained from the pregnant patient at 35–37 weeks' gestation; cultures of these samples should be obtained to determine if the patient is colonized with *S agalactiae*. Pregnant patients who are colonized with *S agalactiae* should be treated with intrapartum penicillin to reduce the chances of neonatal sepsis.

TABLE 28-5. Antimicrobial Agents Used to Treat Septic Patients

Clinical Situation	Antimicrobial Agent(s)
Community-acquired pneumonia	Third- (ceftriaxone) or fourth- (cefepime) generation cephalosporin given with an aminoglycoside (gentamicin)
Nosocomial pneumonia	Cefepime or imipenem-cilastatin and an aminoglycoside
Abdominal infection	Imipenem-cilastatin or piperacillin-tazobactam and aminoglycoside
Nosocomial abdominal infection	Imipenem-cilastatin and aminoglycoside or piperacillin-tazobactam and amphotericin B
Skin and soft tissue infection	Vancomycin and imipenem-cilastatin or piperacillin-tazobactam
Nosocomial skin and soft tissue infections	Vancomycin and cefepime
Urinary tract infection	Ciprofloxacin and aminoglycoside
Nosocomial urinary tract infection	Vancomycin and cefepime
CNS infection	Vancomycin and third-generation cephalosporin or meropenem
Nosocomial CNS infection	Meropenem and vancomycin

CNS, central nervous system.

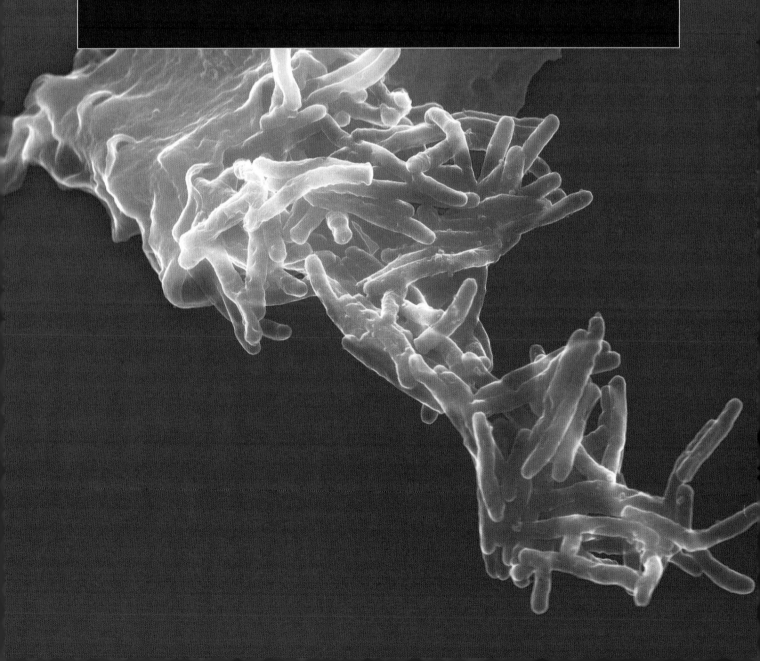

SECTION 8

CARDIOVASCULAR SYSTEM

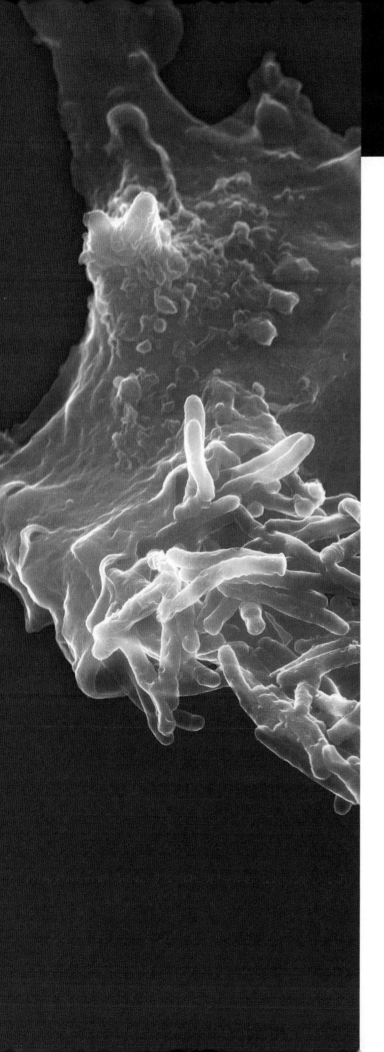

CHAPTER 29

THE BIG PICTURE: INFECTIONS OF THE CARDIOVASCULAR SYSTEM

OVERVIEW

This section of the book will discuss pericarditis, myocarditis, endocarditis, and rheumatic heart disease, all diseases of the cardiovascular system. Pericarditis, myocarditis, and endocarditis are due to infections of the pericardial space, the heart myocytes, and the endothelial lining of the heart valves, respectively (Figures 29-1 and 29-2). Rheumatic heart disease is the result of an autoimmune reaction to cross-reactive antigens produced by *Streptococcus pyogenes* following pharyngitis due to infection by *S pyogenes* (see Figure 29-1).

Cross-reactive antigens are antigens produced by a microorganism that causes the host to produce antibodies. These antibodies react with the microbial antigen and will also react with the host's tissues, causing an autoimmune reaction. The autoimmune reaction is called rheumatic fever, which can cause inflammation in the joints, heart, heart valves, nerves, skin, and subcutaneous tissues. The most severe complication of rheumatic fever is rheumatic heart disease, which causes inflammation of the heart and can irreversibly damage the heart valves.

Pericarditis is an infection of the pericardium, a barrier that protects the heart from infections that occur in nearby tissues (see Figure 29-2A). The pericardium consists of an outer fibrous layer and an inner serous layer (see Figure 29-2B). The fibrous pericardium is a tough sac that is attached to the diaphragm, sternum, and costal cartilage. The serous layer is thin and is the layer that is closest to the surface of the heart.

The pericardial space between the fibrous and serous layers of the pericardium contains about 20 mL of fluid (Figure 29-2B), which is similar to plasma in protein and electrolyte composition. In most cases, 120 mL of additional fluid can accumulate in the pericardium without an increase in pressure on the heart. However, if more fluid accumulates in the pericardial space, marked increases in pericardial pressure can occur (see Figure 29-2C). This increase in pericardial pressure can prevent the ventricles of the heart from filling properly with blood, which decreases cardiac output causing hypotension. Cardiac tamponade occurs when cardiac output is decreased due to increases in pericardial pressure. Infections of the pericardium can cause accumulation of fluid in the pericardial space, resulting in cardiac tamponade.

Three different types of pericarditis will be discussed in Chapter 30: viral, purulent, and chronic pericarditis (Table 29-1). Viral pericarditis is the most common cause of pericardial infection in the United States.

Myocarditis is defined as inflammation of the myocardium and is characterized by myocyte necrosis (see Figure 29-1). Myocarditis can occur following infection (e.g., virus), toxic exposure (e.g., zidovudine; hypersensitivity to penicillin), and autoimmune reactions (e.g., systemic lupus erythematosus). Infections of the heart that result in myocarditis will be discussed in Chapter 30. Just as viruses are the most common cause of pericarditis, they are also the most common cause of myocardial infection (see Table 29-1).

Endocarditis is an inflammation of the inner surface, or endothelium of the heart. The surfaces most commonly affected in endocarditis are the surfaces of the heart valves. Endocarditis can be classified as infective or noninfective. Noninfective endocarditis is very rare and can follow autoimmune reactions (e.g., Libman-Sacks endocarditis) or can occur in patients with mucinous adenocarcinoma. Infective endocarditis can be further

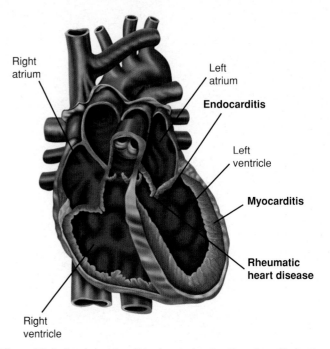

Figure 29-1. A schematic of the heart showing the sites of infection in endocarditis and myocarditis and the sites of inflammation in rheumatic heart disease.

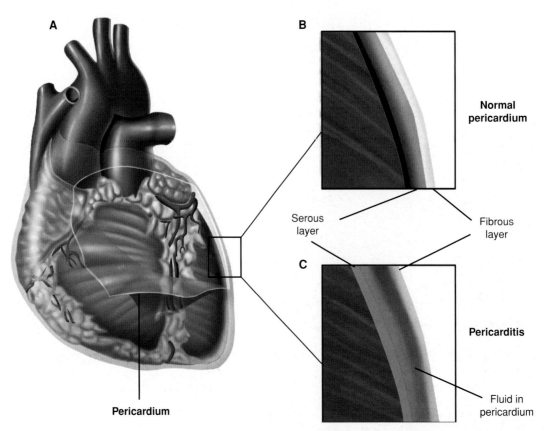

Figure 29-2. A schematic of the heart surrounded by the pericardial sac (**A**); **B**, serous and fibrous layers of the pericardium; **C**, the pericardium, the site where fluid accumulates in a patient with pericarditis.

TABLE 29-1. Common Infectious Causes of Heart Disease

Disease	Infectious Cause(s)	Infection or Inflammatory Reaction to Infection
Viral pericarditis	Enteroviruses: coxsackieviruses A and B; echovirus	Infection
Purulent pericarditis	*Staphylococcus aureus; Streptococcus pneumoniae*	Infection
Chronic pericarditis	*Mycobacterium tuberculosis*	Infection
Myocarditis	Coxsackievirus B	Infection
Subacute infective endocarditis	*Streptococcus* sp.	Infection
Acute infective endocarditis	*S aureus*	Infection
Acute rheumatic heart disease	*S pyogenes*	Inflammatory reaction to infection

subdivided into subacute and acute endocarditis (discussed in Chapter 30). Bacteria are the most common causes of both subacute and acute endocarditis (see Table 29-1).

Acute rheumatic fever is an autoimmune reaction with the heart, joints, central nervous system, skin, and subcutaneous tissues following untreated pharyngitis caused by *Streptococcus pyogenes*. The most serious complication of acute rheumatic fever is rheumatic heart disease, which causes carditis and valvulitis. Both acute rheumatic fever and rheumatic heart disease will be discussed in Chapter 30. Although rheumatic heart disease is rare, it is still the leading cause of mitral valve insufficiency and stenosis in the United States This autoimmune reaction is always a concern in children with untreated pharyngitis caused by *S pyogenes* (see Table 29-1).

PERICARDITIS, MYOCARDITIS, ENDOCARDITIS, AND RHEUMATIC HEART DISEASE

OVERVIEW

This chapter will discuss four different infectious diseases that affect the heart. Three of the diseases, namely pericarditis, myocarditis, and endocarditis, are directly caused by microorganisms that infect the pericardial space, the heart myocytes, and the endothelium that lines the heart valves, respectively. Viruses are the most common cause of pericarditis and myocarditis; endocarditis is usually caused by bacteria. The fourth disease, rheumatic heart disease, is *NOT* due to an infection of the heart, but rather to an autoimmune reaction of the host to the heart and its valves following an antecedent bacterial infection of the pharynx caused by *Streptococcus pyogenes*.

PERICARDITIS

Pericarditis is an inflammation of the fibroserous sac enclosing the heart and has multiple infectious and noninfectious causes (Figure 30-1). There are three different types of infectious pericarditis: viral pericarditis, purulent pericarditis (also called acute bacterial pericarditis), and chronic pericarditis (also called tuberculous pericarditis).

ETIOLOGY

As mentioned above, viruses are the most common cause of pericarditis. ***The viruses that most commonly cause viral pericarditis are the Enteroviruses*** (i.e., coxsackieviruses A and B and echovirus). Less common causes of viral pericarditis include herpes viruses, adenoviruses, influenza virus, human immunodeficiency virus (HIV), and mumps virus.

Purulent pericarditis is quite rare, and the most common causes are *Staphylococcus aureus* and *Streptococcus pneumoniae*

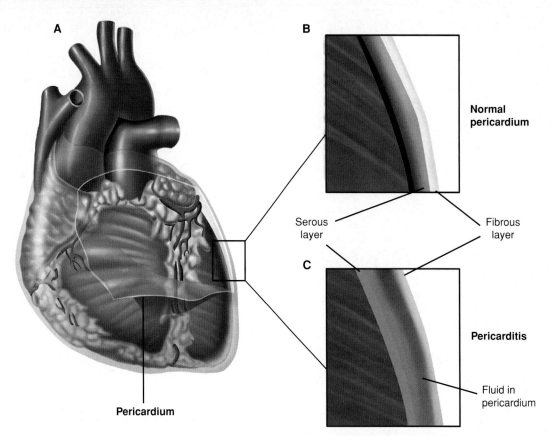

Figure 30-1. A schematic of the heart surrounded by the pericardial sac (**A**); the serous and fibrous layers of the pericardium (**B**); and the site where fluid accumulates in the pericardium during pericarditis (**C**).

and other streptococci. Chronic pericarditis also is rare and is caused most commonly by *Mycobacterium tuberculosis.* Fungi can also cause chronic pericarditis but are much less common causes than *M tuberculosis* (e.g., *Candida albicans*).

MANIFESTATIONS

Manifestations of pericarditis vary depending upon the cause of the infection. Physical findings in all three types of pericarditis depend on how much exudate accumulates in the pericardial space (Tables 30-1 and 30-2).

Viral pericarditis usually presents with sharp substernal chest pain that worsens upon inspiration. Pain is also worsened in the supine position. Therefore, patients with viral pericarditis tend to prefer to sit up and lean forward to lessen the pain.

The signs and symptoms of **purulent pericarditis** develop suddenly and include fever and dyspnea. Only about one third of patients have the chest pain described as a symptom of viral pericarditis. Unfortunately, in many cases there are no specific symptoms, and the infection is often misdiagnosed.

Tuberculous pericarditis has the most insidious clinical onset. The patient may have vague dull chest pain, weight loss, night sweats, cough, and dyspnea.

EPIDEMIOLOGY

Pericarditis is a relatively common disease. Autopsy findings reveal that 2–6% of patients have pericardial inflammation but in most cases the cause of death is not due to pericarditis.

TABLE 30-1. Signs that May Be Present in Viral, Purulent, or Chronic Pericarditis

Sign(s)	Comments
Friction rub	Usually auscultated early when there is little fluid in the space; as more fluid accumulates, the sound disappears
Pulsus paradoxicus	Drop in peak systolic blood pressure of >20 mm Hg on inspiration; finding associated with cardiac tamponade
Kussmaul sign	Paradoxic increase in venous distention and pressure during inspiration; finding associated with cardiac tamponade
Jugular venous distention and abnormal jugular venous pulsations	Finding associated with cardiac tamponade
Ewart sign	Area of dullness to percussion at the tip of the left scapula
Decreased or muffled heart sounds	More common when large amounts of fluid are in the pericardium
Abnormal electrocardiographs (ECG)	ECGs from a patient with pericarditis can be quite similar to patients with an acute myocardial infarction or with normal-variant repolarization abnormality. In pericarditis, the ST segment is elevated in all leads. The ST-segment elevation shows upward concavity (so-called "smiling face"). The PR interval is depressed. (For a list of the differences in the ECG in these three conditions, refer to Table 30-2.)

TABLE 30-2. ECG Segment or Shape Changes in Acute Pericarditis, Acute MI, and Normal-Variant Repolarization Abnormality

ECG Segment or Shape Change	Acute Pericarditis	Acute MI	Normal-variant Repolarization Abnormality
ST-segment	ST-segment elevation in all leads, with no ST-segment depression	ST-segment elevation in anatomically contiguous leads, with reciprocal ST-segment depression	ST-segment elevation in middle and left precordial leads, but may be widespread with no reciprocal ST-segment depression
ST-segment shape	Upward concave ST-segment elevation ("smiling face")	Upward convex ST-segment elevation	Upward convex ST-segment elevation
T-wave	No T-wave inversion in leads with ST-segment elevation	T-wave inversion in leads with ST-segment elevation as MI evolves	May have T-wave inversion in leads with ST-segment elevation
PR-segment	PR-segment depression	No PR-segment depression	No PR-segment depression
Q waves	Q waves during evolution	May have Q waves during evolution	No Q waves

ECG, electrocardiograph; MI, myocardial infarction.

- Only 1 of every 1000 hospital admissions is diagnosed clinically as pericarditis.

- Many cases of idiopathic pericarditis are believed to be viral in origin and occur in the spring and autumn coincident with outbreaks of enteroviral disease.

- The mortality rate is higher in acute purulent pericarditis than in viral pericarditis and exceeds 50% in untreated acute purulent pericarditis. With appropriate therapy, the mortality rate is about 30%.

- **Viral pericarditis** is usually acquired following ingestion of fecally contaminated food or water.

- **Purulent pericarditis** can occur following spread of a localized infection to the pericardium (e.g., lung infections), surgery, or as a result of a bacteremia.

- **Chronic pericarditis** can be acquired following inhalation of *M tuberculosis* and spread of the organism from the lungs to the bloodstream and then to the pericardium. About 5% of patients with pulmonary tuberculosis also have pericardial involvement.

PATHOGENESIS

In most cases of pericarditis, the microorganisms reach the pericardium through the bloodstream. Rarely, the organism will enter the pericardium by direct extension from the lungs or by direct inoculation during surgery or invasive medical procedures or from trauma.

Viruses that cause **viral pericarditis** produce a relatively mild inflammatory reaction that is associated with focal damage to the adjacent myocardium. Pericardial and myocardial damage is the result of direct cellular damage by the infecting virus, destruction of virally infected cells by sensitized T lymphocytes, or antibody-dependent cell-mediated cytotoxicity. The organism colonizes the pericardium and stimulates an inflammatory reaction, which results in the accumulation of serous exudate. The amount of serous exudate in the pericardial space can vary from a small amount of exudate containing many mononuclear cells and elevated amounts of fibrinogen to a large amount of neutrophil-rich, bloody effusion fluid. If large amounts of fluid accumulate, cardiac tamponade (the exertion of pressure or compression of the heart) can occur, resulting in circulatory failure.

Mild fibrosis and occasional adhesions between visceral and parietal surfaces of the pericardium may occur following resolution of the viral pericarditis. However, such a fibrotic reaction rarely gives rise to a constrictive pericarditis. *The disease is self-limiting and rarely fatal*.

In **purulent pericarditis,** bacterial pathogens such as *S pneumoniae* usually infect the pericardium following extension from an adjacent pneumonia. The common causes of bacteremias are *S aureus, Neisseria meningitidis,* and *Haemophilus influenzae* and reach the pericardium through the bloodstream. Postoperative infections of the pericardium are usually caused by *S aureus* or gram-negative aerobic rods. The bacteria that cause purulent pericarditis usually invoke a strong, rapidly progressing purulent immune reaction. The purulent exudate in the pericardial space contains many polymorphonuclear leukocytes in a large volume of effusion fluid. Pericardial and myocardial tissue injury results from toxin and enzyme production by the bacteria and is also due to the rapidly progressing cardiac tamponade. Healing is associated with extensive fibrosis, which may progress to a chronic, constrictive pericarditis.

Chronic pericarditis results from hematogenous spread during primary infections due to *M tuberculosis*. The bacteria can spread to the pericardium by lymphatic drainage from the respiratory tract or via direct spread from the lungs or pleura. The early granulomatous stages of this infection are associated with large pericardial effusions (>300 mL) that are typically serosanguinous and contain a predominance of mononuclear cells. As the disease evolves, the inflammatory process becomes chronic; fusion of the serous and fibrous pericardial layers frequently occurs, causing constrictive pericarditis and circulatory failure.

DIAGNOSIS

Determining the cause of viral pericarditis is difficult and is not usually sought. Pericardiocentesis can be used in some cases to culture for the infecting agent (e.g., purulent pericarditis with cardiac tamponade). The unique presentation of substernal pain that is worse during inspiration or when the patient is supine and is relieved by the patient leaning forward is helpful in making the diagnosis. Chest radiographs may reveal the flask-shaped, enlarged cardiac silhouette due to large amounts of fluid present in the pericardial space. Echocardiography can detect pericardial thickening and pericardial fluid accumulation.

Electrocardiographs (ECGs) of patients with acute purulent pericarditis can appear similar to those of patients with acute myocardial infarction or normal-variant repolarization abnormality. In cardiac tamponade, the ECG may show electrical alternans associated with cardiac motion as the heart "floats" in relation to the recording leads. Electrical alternans is alternate-beat variation in the direction, amplitude, and duration of any component of the ECG waveform (i.e., P, PR, QRS, R-R, ST, T, and U). Chronic constrictive pericarditis presents with low voltage of the QRS complex and diffuse flattening or inversion of the T waves. Atrial fibrillation occurs in one third of patients with pericardial disease. The ECG changes that are unique to pericarditis are listed in Table 30-2.

THERAPY AND PREVENTION

Supportive care is indicated in patients with **viral pericarditis.** Nonsteroidal anti-inflammatory drugs (NSAIDs) can be used to reduce chest pain; however, these drugs should be avoided if the patient also has myocarditis. In patients with **purulent pericarditis** pericardiocentesis and systemic antibiotics are important in helping to resolve the infection. The antibiotic prescribed depends on the organism that is causing the purulent pericarditis. Until the cause is identified, antibiotics used to treat this infection include a penicillinase-resistant β-lactam antibiotic and a third-generation cephalosporin (Table 30-3). To treat chronic pericarditis due to *M tuberculosis*, a four-drug regimen is recommended that includes isoniazid, ethambutol, rifampin, and pyrazinamide. Since constrictive pericarditis is more common in patients with chronic pericarditis, prednisone is also prescribed to prevent constriction.

TABLE 30-3. Antibiotic Therapy (and Microbial Coverage) for Treatment of Acute Purulent Pericarditis*

Penicillinase-resistant β-Lactam Antibiotic	Microbial Coverage	Third-generation Cephalosporins	Microbial Coverage
Oxacillin	Good gram-positive coverage; effective against penicillinase producing staphylococci; poor gram-negative coverage	Cefotaxime	Good gram-negative coverage poor gram-positive coverage
Methicillin	Good gram-positive coverage; effective against penicillinase producing staphylococci; poor gram-negative coverage	Ceftriaxone	Good gram-negative coverage poor gram-positive coverage
Nafcillin	Good gram-positive coverage; effective against penicillinase producing staphylococci; better gram-negative coverage than oxacillin and methicillin		

*Empiric therapy usually includes the use of one penicillinase beta-lactam antibiotic and a third-generation cephalosporin.

MYOCARDITIS

Myocarditis is an infection of the myocardium or the myocytes of the heart. Viruses are the most common cause of myocarditis, and are ingested in fecally contaminated water or food. The viruses then enter the bloodstream and infect the heart myocytes.

ETIOLOGY

Similar to pericarditis, viruses are the most important infectious agents that cause myocarditis. Of these agents, the *Enteroviruses are the single most important group, with coxsackievirus B being the most common cause of myocarditis in the United States*.

Other viruses that have been implicated in causing myocarditis include herpes viruses, HIV, and mumps virus. Bacteria (e.g., *Legionella, Chlamydia,* and *Borrelia burgdorferi*), fungi (e.g., *Aspergillus fumigatus, Candida albicans,* and *Cryptococcus neoformans*), and parasites (e.g., *Trypanosoma cruzi* and *Trichinella spiralis*) can also cause myocarditis, but these are rare causes in the United States and will not be discussed further in this chapter.

MANIFESTATIONS

Most persons with myocarditis are asymptomatic. If symptoms are present, the pace of the illness and the symptoms vary greatly. Symptoms include flu-like illness with chest pain when the pericardium is involved; arrhythmias; or signs of right-sided (e.g., edema in the legs, feet, or abdomen) and left-sided (e.g., shortness of breath, orthopnea) congestive heart failure. Patients with myocarditis often present with manifestations of acute decompensation of heart failure (i.e., tachycardia, gallop, mitral regurgitation, and edema) and pericardial friction rub in patients with concomitant pericarditis. Left ventricular dilatation can lead to expansion of the mitral valve ring and a mitral regurgitant murmur. An S_3 gallop indicates left-sided congestive heart failure.

EPIDEMIOLOGY

- Strenuous exercise, pregnancy, use of steroids or NSAIDs, use of ethanol, and nutritional deficiencies are factors that predispose a patient with asymptomatic myocarditis to progress to symptomatic myocarditis.

- The incidence of myocarditis is estimated to be 1–10 cases per 100,000 persons.

PATHOGENESIS

Viruses directly invade the myocytes and damage the infected cells of patients with myocarditis. The immune response to infection also damages the myocytes. Immune-cell infiltration of the myocytes includes predominantly T lymphocytes accompanied by macrophages and B lymphocytes. Circulating autoantibodies directed against mitochondria and contractile proteins are frequently detected and may cause further damage. Cytokines and oxygen free radicals have also been implicated in causing damage to the myocytes.

DIAGNOSIS

Diagnosis of myocarditis involves identifying the signs and symptoms of cardiac failure. A complete blood cell count (CBC) usually reveals a leukocytosis. About 50% of patients with myocarditis will have elevated levels of cardiac troponin I, and about 5% of patients will have elevated levels of creatine kinase-MB in the bloodstream. Patients with myocarditis usually have an elevated erythrocyte sedimentation rate (ESR) and increased levels of acute phase proteins in the bloodstream (e.g., C-reactive protein, complement, α_2-macroglobulin).

ECGs can be obtained but are usually nonspecific. An abnormal ECG may demonstrate ST and T wave changes, ventricular or atrial arrhythmias, and conduction defects. Chest radiographs can detect pulmonary edema in congestive heart failure and cardiac dilatation. Echocardiography can be used to assess cardiac contractility, chamber size, valve function, and wall thickness and to exclude other causes of heart failure (e.g., valvular, amyloidosis, congenital). Contrast-enhanced MRI can detect the extent and degree of inflammation and determines parameters that correlate with left ventricular function and clinical status. To obtain a definitive diagnosis, an endomyocardial biopsy is needed; however; this usually is not performed.

THERAPY AND PREVENTION

Most cases of viral myocarditis are self-limited and result in full recovery with no long-term complications. Patients with viral myocarditis usually respond well to bed rest. Cardiac monitoring may be required to alert caregivers to potentially life-threatening arrhythmias. ***Glucosteroids and other immunosuppressive drugs are contraindicated in these patients***.

ENDOCARDITIS

Endocarditis is an inflammation of the endothelium that lines the inside of the heart. Certain areas of the endothelium are more likely to be affected in endocarditis, including the surfaces of the heart valves. Some heart valves are more commonly affected than others, as shown in Figure 30-2.

ETIOLOGY

The etiology of endocarditis depends on the condition of the heart valve, including if the person is an intravenous illicit drug user or if the person has a prosthetic heart valve and the length of time the valve has been in place (Table 30-4).

MANIFESTATIONS

There are two types of infectious endocarditis: subacute and acute. Subacute endocarditis is more common and symptoms develop over a longer period of time. The symptoms often are nonspecific. Acute endocarditis progresses very rapidly and with more severe symptoms. It is more common in intravenous drug users and in staphylococcal infections of the heart.

In **subacute endocarditis,** the interval between the time of bacterial colonization of the endocardium and the onset of symptoms is usually less than 2 weeks. Because the symptoms are usually nonspecific, there usually is a delay of 5 weeks between onset of symptoms and diagnosis. The most common symptom is a low-grade fever (range of 38°C), which is usually accompanied by chills and sometimes by night sweats. Fatigue, anorexia, weakness, myalgias, arthralgias, and malaise are common. Debilitating lower back pain is a prominent complaint in a small percentage of patients.

Acute endocarditis has a rapid onset (e.g., hours to days) and is usually caused by *S aureus* or *Enterococcus.* The patient has a high fever (40°C), rigors, and appears very ill. The likelihood of extravascular complications is high.

Nearly all patients with either subacute or acute endocarditis will have an audible **heart murmur.** Although classically described as a changing murmur, the murmur usually does not change significantly over time unless a valve leaflet is destroyed or a chordae tendineae ruptures. Murmurs are less common in patients with right-sided endocarditis.

Complications that occur in most patients with endocarditis include cardiac complications (e.g., congestive heart failure,

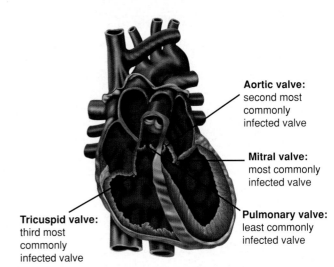

Aortic valve: second most commonly infected valve

Mitral valve: most commonly infected valve

Pulmonary valve: least commonly infected valve

Tricuspid valve: third most commonly infected valve

Figure 30-2. A schematic of the heart showing the most common to the least common valves affected by endocarditis (mitral > aortic > tricuspid > pulmonary).

TABLE 30-4. Causes of Endocarditis by Type of Heart Valve or Patient Condition

Type of Heart Valve or Patient Condition	Common Causes
Native heart valve	*Streptococcus* (viridans streptococci; e.g., *S bovis, S mitis, S anginosus, S mutans, S salivarius*), *Staphylococcus* (usually *S aureus*), *Enterococcus*
Prosthetic valve infections Early (<2 months' post implantation)	*Staphylococcus* (*S aureus* and *S epidermidis*), gram-negative aerobic bacilli
Prosthetic valve infections Late (>2 months' post implantation)	Viridans *Streptococcus, S epidermidis,* and *S aureus*
Intravenous illicit drug users	*S aureus* and gram-negative bacilli (*Pseudomonas aeruginosa* is most the common gram-negative bacilli)

destruction of a heart valve, or perivalvular extension of infection) and complications due to emboli (e.g., mycotic aneurysms, neurologic complications, or renal complications).

Roth spots, petechial hemorrhages, splinter hemorrhages, and Janeway lesions are complications of endocarditis that are relatively rare but can occur when vegetations (i.e., septic emboli) in the heart dislodge from the surface of the heart and lodge in small vessels, causing necrosis and hemorrhage in the tissues served by the blocked blood vessel. **Petechial hemorrhages** can occur in the conjunctiva, buccal mucosa, palate, and extremities. **Splinter hemorrhages** can occur under the nail beds of the hands and feet (Figure 30-3). **Janeway lesions** are painless hemorrhagic plaques on the palms and soles.

Another uncommon extravascular complication, **Osler nodes**, occurs when the host's immune system reacts with bacteria that cause the endocarditis, resulting in a localized inflammation of the blood vessels of the fingers and toes. Osler nodes are small, pea-sized subcutaneous, painful erythematous nodules that occur in the pads of the fingers and toes and the thenar eminence. They are usually present for a brief period of time, lasting only a few hours to a couple of days. **Roth spots**, or flame-shaped hemorrhages with pale centers, can be observed on funduscopic examination of the retina (Figure 30-4).

EPIDEMIOLOGY

- Infective endocarditis is a relatively uncommon infection. The incidence is about 2 cases per 100,000 persons.

- Endocarditis is more common in men than women, and is becoming more a disease of elderly patients.

- Microorganisms growing in the normal flora of the body (e.g., mouth, intestine, skin) cause most cases of infective endocarditis.

- Patients with prior valvular defects or patients with an artificial heart valve are more likely to develop endocarditis. Lip or tongue piercing increases the chances that a patient with a valvular defect or an artificial heart valve will develop endocarditis.

- Patients recovering from endocarditis are at increased risk of having a second episode due to the damage caused by the prior episode of endocarditis.

- Intravenous illicit drug users commonly develop infective endocarditis caused by *S aureus* contracted from contaminated needles.

PATHOGENESIS

Infective endocarditis is usually preceded by the formation of a predisposing cardiac lesion. Endothelial cells that line the inside of the heart and the heart valves can be damaged, leading to the accumulation of platelets and fibrin producing a nonbacterial thrombotic endocarditis. This sterile lesion serves as an ideal site for bacteria to attach to in the bloodstream. Various conditions lead to endothelial cell damage and nonbacterial thrombotic endocarditis and include shear stress, rheumatic heart disease, congenital heart disease (i.e., bicuspid aortic valve, ventricular septal defect, coarctation of the aorta, tetralogy of Fallot), mitral valve prolapse, degenerative heart disease

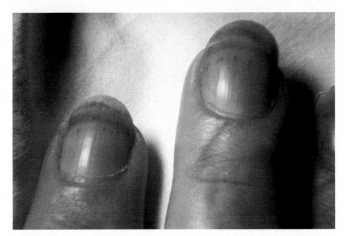

Figure 30-3. A photograph of splinter hemorrhages under finger nails. Image courtesy of the Centers for Disease Control and Prevention.

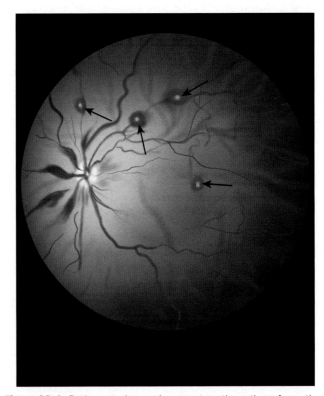

Figure 30-4. Roth spots (*arrows*) present on the retina of a patient with endocarditis.

(e.g., calcific aortic valve disease), prosthetic valve placement, and intravenous illicit drug use. The propensity to develop vegetations occurs in patients who do not have an artificial heart valve in the following order: mitral valve > aortic valve > tricuspid valve > pulmonary valve.

Right-sided endocarditis is uncommon except in intravenous illicit drug users, who are at higher risk of developing endocarditis due to their propensity to inject solutions contaminated with bacteria. Right-sided endocarditis usually occurs on the tricuspid valve.

Microorganisms growing in the normal flora of the body cause most cases of infective endocarditis. The organisms gain access to the blood intermittently as a result of minor trauma to the mucosa of the oropharynx, gastrointestinal tract, or genitourinary tract. Such transient bacteremias usually occur without ill effects, but may lead to endocarditis in patients with an underlying nonbacterial thrombotic endocarditis or artificial heart valve.

Bacteria and platelets tend to accumulate on the downstream or low-pressure side of a patient with valvular nonbacterial thrombotic endocarditis. Bacteria colonize the nonbacterial thrombotic endocarditis and form vegetations (Figure 30-5). Surface adherence factors are essential for the bacteria to colonize the nonbacterial thrombotic endocarditis. Large numbers of bacteria are present in the vegetations. The bulk of the vegetation is an amorphous mass of fibrin and platelets containing colonies of microorganisms. Vegetations vary in size from tiny bodies to masses large enough to occlude valve orifices. These vegetations are soft and friable and loosely attached to the endocardium; they frequently break off to form arterial emboli. The emboli affect perfusion of the tissue causing infarcts in the tissues. Apart from the propensity to generate emboli, there is no correlation between size of vegetation and severity of endocarditis.

The four consequences of valvular vegetations

1. Organisms within the vegetation are protected from elimination by antibodies, complement, and leukocytes and can live for long periods of time in the vegetation (e.g., weeks to months).

2. Organisms within the vegetation are metabolically inactive, replicating at an unusually slow rate. Many antibiotics require the bacteria to rapidly replicate to kill the microorganisms. Because the bacteria in the vegetation replicate very slowly, the bacteria are much less sensitive to killing by antibiotics; therefore, antimicrobial treatment requires a long period (e.g., 4–6 weeks) for successful eradication of the bacteria.

3. Healing is slow because macrophages and fibroblasts must spread through the vegetation, and endothelial cells grow over the surface of the vegetation.

4. Emboli are generated when vegetations break off, and these emboli cause infarcts in other tissues (e.g., brain, kidney, extremities).

Abscesses may develop by direct invasion of the valve rings of the heart near the vegetations, and are common in endocarditis due to pyogenic cocci (e.g., staphylococci and streptococci) but are less likely to develop due to other organisms.

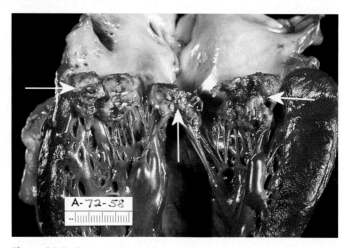

Figure 30-5. Endocarditis of the mitral valve. Notice the large vegetations on the mitral valve (*arrows*). Image courtesy of the Centers for Disease Control and Prevention, Dr Edwin P Ewing Jr.

DIAGNOSIS

Diagnosis of subacute endocarditis can be very difficult and is often misdiagnosed. Acute endocarditis can rapidly cause irreversible damage to the heart valves and must be diagnosed and aggressively treated.

Laboratory values (often nonspecific) associated with endocarditis

- Anemia of chronic disease in patients with subacute endocarditis: normocytic and normochromic erythrocytes, low serum iron, and low iron-binding capacity.
- Peripheral leukocyte count usually is normal except when myocardial abscesses occur, or if an extravascular site of infection exists, or the patient has acute endocarditis.
- ESR and C-reactive protein are elevated in subacute and acute endocarditis.
- About 50% of patients are positive for rheumatoid factor in subacute endocarditis.
- Cryoglobulins, depressed complement levels, and false-positive serology for syphilis can sometimes occur in patients with subacute endocarditis.
- Results of urinalysis are usually abnormal; proteinuria and hematuria are observed in subacute and acute endocarditis.

Laboratory studies that aid in confirming the diagnosis of endocarditis

- **Transesophageal echocardiography is the most sensitive study for detecting valvular vegetations.** It readily detects extravalvular extension of infection and can visualize valve perforations. Chest radiographs may demonstrate distinct round cannonball-like pulmonary emboli in right-sided endocarditis. Pulmonary edema may be present in patients with acute mitral regurgitation or decompensated left-sided heart failure due to aortic valve regurgitation. ECGs should be obtained and closely monitored for conduction defects.
- **Blood cultures are critical in determining the diagnosis of infective endocarditis.** Infective endocarditis is associated with a constant low-level bacteremia. Three blood samples should be obtained over a 24-hour period. The diagnosis is confirmed if good bacterial growth from the blood samples is obtained and if damage to the heart valves is detected by transesophageal echocardiograph.
- The modified Duke criteria can be used if the diagnosis cannot be confirmed (Table 30-5).

THERAPY AND PREVENTION

A combination antibiotic therapy is always used in the treatment of endocarditis and must be given for 4–6 weeks, even if symptoms disappear prior to that time. If no organism has been isolated after repeated attempts, the recommended therapy for subacute bacterial endocarditis is ampicillin and gentamicin. An exception to this treatment schedule is for subacute bacterial endocarditis due to viridans *Streptococcus*, in which case a combination of penicillin G and gentamicin given for 2 weeks

TABLE 30-5. Modified Duke Criteria for Diagnosis of Endocarditis

Diagnosis	Definitions
Definitive	Histologic and/or microbiologic evidence of infection at surgery or autopsy *or* 2 major criteria *or* 1 major criterion and 3 minor criteria *or* 5 minor criteria
Possible	1 major criterion and 1 minor criterion *or* 3 minor criteria

Criteria	Clinical signs and symptoms
Major	**1. Blood cultures positive for infectious endocarditis** Typical microorganism consistent with infectious endocarditis isolated from 2 separate blood cultures, as noted below: • Viridans streptococci, *Streptococcus bovis*, *Staphylococcus aureus*, or HACEK group (*Haemophilus aphrophilus*, *H parainfluenzae*, or *H paraphrophilus*, *Actinobacillus actinomycetemcomitans*, *Cardiobacterium hominis*, *Eikenella corrodens*, *Kingella kingae*) • Community-acquired enterococci in the absence of a primary focus **OR** Microorganisms consistent with infectious endocarditis isolated from persistently positive blood cultures, defined as: • At least 2 positive cultures of blood samples obtained >12 h apart • All of 3 or a majority of ≥4 separate cultures of blood, the first and the last sample obtained >1 h apart
	2. Evidence of endocardial involvement Positive results of echocardiography for infectious endocarditis, defined as: • Oscillating intracardiac mass on the valve or supporting structures in the path of regurgitant jets or on implanted material in the absence of an alternative anatomic explanation • Abscess • New partial dehiscence of a valvular prosthesis **OR** New valvular regurgitation (worsening or changing or preexisting murmur not sufficient)
	3. Single blood culture positive for *Coxiella burnetii* (Q fever) or an antiphase I IgG antibody titer of >1:800 or a single blood culture positive for *C burnetii*.
Minor	1. Predisposing heart disease or intravenous illicit drug use
	2. Temperature of >38°C
	3. Vascular phenomenon: major arterial emboli, septic pulmonary infarcts, mycotic aneurysm, intracranial or conjunctival hemorrhage, Janeway lesions
	4. Immunologic phenomenon: glomerulonephritis, Osler nodes, Roth spots, rheumatoid factor
	5. Microbiologic evidence: positive blood culture that *does not* meet a major criterion (as noted above) or serologic evidence of active infection with an organism consistent with infectious endocarditis

works as well as treatment for 4 weeks. Empiric therapy for acute bacterial endocarditis includes vancomycin, ampicillin, and gentamicin.

If an organism has been isolated, the antibiotic regimen is based on the species of the etiologic agent, the age of the patient, and the extent of the disease. These regimens are complex and beyond the scope of this book. If antibiotic therapy is not successful, surgical removal of infected endocardium may be necessary.

RHEUMATIC FEVER AND RHEUMATIC HEART DISEASE

During the early 1900s, rheumatic fever and the most serious complication associated with rheumatic fever, rheumatic heart disease, were quite common. Rheumatic heart disease is still the leading cause of mitral valve insufficiency and stenosis in the United States.

ETIOLOGY

S pyogenes (group A *Streptococcus*) is the etiologic agent that induces autoimmune reactions that cause rheumatic fever (e.g., fever, arthritis) and rheumatic heart disease (e.g., carditis, valvulitis). Both diseases occur after a pharyngeal infection due to *S pyogenes*. However, **skin infections (e.g., impetigo, cellulitis) caused by this organism do NOT cause rheumatic fever or rheumatic heart disease.**

MANIFESTATIONS

Symptoms of acute rheumatic fever precede acute rheumatic heart disease. Symptoms of acute rheumatic fever can occur within a few days to 5 weeks after *S pyogenes* pharyngeal infection. The patient first presents with fever (38.3–40°C) and migratory polyarthritis, usually in the knees, elbows, or wrists. Other findings can include subcutaneous nodules (Figure 30-6); skin lesions (e.g., erythema marginatum; serpiginous rash) (Figure 30-7); chorea (rapid purposeless movements of the face and upper extremities); and carditis (Figure 30-8).

The most common complication of rheumatic fever is polyarthritis. Rheumatic heart disease can result in a pancarditis, and is the most serious and second most common (50%) complication associated with rheumatic fever (see Figure 30-8). In severe cases of rheumatic heart disease, patients may complain of dyspnea, mild-to-moderate chest discomfort, pleuritic chest pain, edema, cough, or orthopnea. Carditis is most commonly detected when a new heart murmur has been auscultated or when tachycardia out of proportion to the fever is observed. Heart murmurs are usually due to valvular insufficiency. The mitral valve is the most frequently affected valve, followed by the aortic valve, the tricuspid valve, and very rarely, the pulmonary valve (notice the similarity of the order of the valves affected with the order of valves affected in infectious endocarditis). New or changing murmurs are necessary for a diagnosis of rheumatic valvulitis. Patients with chronic rheumatic heart disease can develop valvular stenosis with varying degrees of regurgitation, atrial dilation, arrhythmias, and ventricular dysfunction (Figure 30-9).

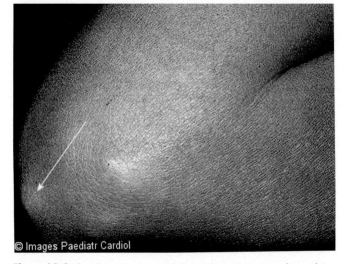

Figure 30-6. A subcutaneous nodule on the extensor surface of the elbow. Image courtesy of MA Binotto et al. Rheumatic Fever. Images Paediatr Cardiol 2002;11:12–25. http://www.impaedcard.com/issue/issue11/1231/1231.htm

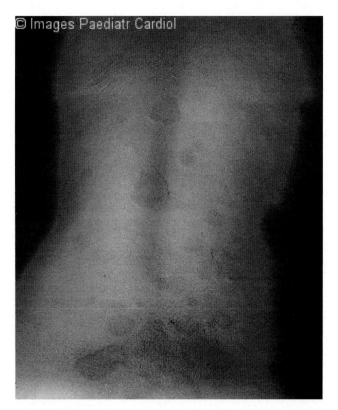

Figure 30-7. The back of a patient with rheumatic fever showing erythema marginatum skin lesions. Image courtesy of MA Binotto et al. Rheumatic Fever. Images Paediatr Cardiol 2002;11:12–25. http://www.impaedcard.com/issue/issue11/1231/1231.htm

Patients may also manifest symptoms of congestive heart failure (e.g., tachypnea, orthopnea, jugular venous distention, rales, hepatomegaly, a gallop rhythm, and peripheral swelling and edema) or pericarditis (e.g., chest pain, fever, dyspnea).

EPIDEMIOLOGY

- Between 0.3% and 3% of cases of untreated streptococcal pharyngitis infection induces the host's immune system to produce antibodies that damage host tissue and elicit the symptoms of acute rheumatic fever.

- Rheumatic fever is principally a disease of childhood, with a median age of 10 years.

- Rheumatic fever affects both males and females equally.

- Prevalence of rheumatic heart disease in the United States is less than 5 cases per 100,000 persons.

- The increased use of antibiotics in treating streptococcal pharyngitis and the change in virulence of the bacterial strains circulating in the population are believed to be the primary reasons for the lower prevalence of rheumatic heart disease and rheumatic fever.

- Valvular insufficiency from acute rheumatic heart disease resolves in 60–80% of patients who adhere to antibiotic prophylaxis.

- Chronic valvular disease can result in progressive valve deformity in adults who have had previous rheumatic heart disease. Rheumatic heart disease remains the leading cause of mitral valve stenosis and valve replacement in adults. Fusion of the valve apparatus results in stenosis or a combination of stenosis or insufficiency and can develop 2–10 years after an episode of acute rheumatic fever.

- Patients tend to have more severe rheumatic heart disease if they have had previous episodes of rheumatic fever, or the length of time between the onset of *S pyogenes* pharyngitis and the start of therapy was more than 9 days, or if the patient is female.

- *S pyogenes* is spread by direct contact with oral or respiratory secretions; crowded living conditions increase person-to-person spread.

- Patients can be colonized by *S pyogenes* weeks after symptomatic resolution of pharyngitis and may serve as a reservoir for infecting others.

PATHOGENESIS

Acute rheumatic fever is an autoimmune response to the *S pyogenes* infection of the pharynx that causes damage to the heart, joints, central nervous system, skin, and subcutaneous tissues. It is characterized by an exudative and proliferative inflammatory lesion of these tissues.

Following pharyngitis caused by *S pyogenes,* the host's immune system produces antibodies that react with bacterial antigens and certain host tissues (i.e., cross-reactive antibodies). Certain rheumatogenic strains of *S pyogenes* are more likely to cause the host to produce the cross-reactive antibodies. The host tissues most likely to be affected are the joints (polyarthritis), heart (pancarditis, valvulitis), skin (erythema marginatum),

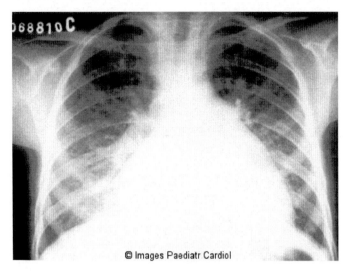

Figure 30-8. A chest radiograph of an 8-year-old patient with acute carditis due to rheumatic fever. Note the severely enlarged silhouette of the heart. Image courtesy of MA Binotto et al. Rheumatic Fever. Images Paediatr Cardiol 2002;11:12–25. http://www.impaedcard.com/ issue/issue11/1231/1231.htm

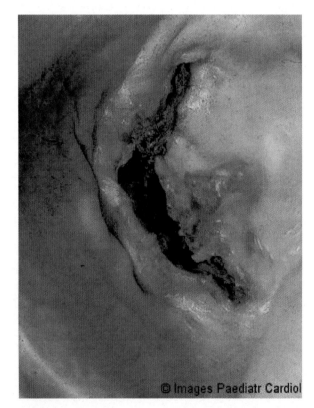

Figure 30-9. A stenotic mitral valve from a patient with rheumatic heart disease. The valve is seen from the left atrium and shows fusion of commissures and thickening and calcification of the cusps. Image courtesy of MA Binotto et al. Rheumatic Fever. Images Paediatr Cardiol 2002;11:12–25. http://www.impaedcard.com/issue/issue11/1231/1231.htm

nerves (chorea), and subcutaneous tissues (subcutaneous nodules). The two bacterial factors that appear to be important in the development of pharyngitis and in acute rheumatic fever and rheumatic heart disease are hyaluronic acid capsule and M protein.

The hyaluronic acid capsule protects the bacteria from phagocytosis; however, it is identical to the hyaluronic acid found in the host's connective tissues. If antibodies are produced to the bacteria's capsule, these antibodies can also cause damage in the host.

S pyogenes is classified by the type of M protein it produces (many serotypes of the M protein have been identified). This protein is important in adherence to host epithelial cells, internalization in host cells, and avoidance of phagocytosis. M proteins are subdivided into class I and class II. Rheumatogenic strains of *S pyogenes* are usually encapsulated strains rich in class I M proteins. These rheumatogenic strains are highly immunogenic and anti–M protein antibodies can cross react with heart tissue. Other streptococcal antigens structurally similar to host tissues include cell-wall polysaccharides (similar to glycoproteins in heart valves) and membrane antigens that share epitopes with the sarcolemma in striated muscle cells and smooth muscle.

DIAGNOSIS

Rheumatic fever is difficult to diagnose, and the Jones Criteria are frequently used to help in determining the diagnosis (Table 30-6). Auscultation of the heart for murmurs, friction rubs, gallops, and irregular rhythms together with the signs and symptoms mentioned above help determine the diagnosis of rheumatic heart disease. Chest radiographs can reveal an

TABLE 30-6. Jones Criteria for Guidance in the Diagnosis of Rheumatic Fever

The presence of 2 major criteria or 1 major criterion and 2 minor criteria indicates a high probability that the patient has acute rheumatic fever, if supported by evidence of preceding group A streptococcal infection.*

Major Manifestations	Minor Manifestations
Carditis	**Clinical**
Polyarthritis	Previous rheumatic fever or rheumatic heart disease
Chorea	Arthralgia
Erythema marginatum	Fever
Subcutaneous nodules	**Laboratory Results**
	Acute phase reactants: increased ESR, increased levels of C-reactive protein in the blood, leukocytosis in CBC
	ECG shows prolonged P-R interval

*Supporting evidence of streptococcal infection: Increased titer of antistreptococcal antibodies (anti-streptolysin O [ASO titers]), positive throat culture, or antigen test for group A *streptococcus* or recent case of scarlet fever.

ESR, erythrocyte sedimentation rate; ECG, electrocardiograph; CBC, complete blood cell count.

enlarged heart (see Figure 30-8), and transesophageal echocardiography can reveal heart valve regurgitation and stenosis. Analysis of synovial fluid may demonstrate an elevated white blood cell count with no crystals or organisms in patients with arthritis.

THERAPY AND PREVENTION

Certain rheumatogenic strains of *S pyogenes* that infect the pharynx are the cause of acute rheumatic fever, and eradication of the organism from the patient's pharynx is the first step in treating these patients. Therapy and prevention of rheumatic fever involves the following:

- Treat *S pyogenes* pharyngitis with antibiotics (e.g., penicillin or erythromycin); treatment within 9 days of the appearance of symptoms prevents development of rheumatic fever.

- Steroids and salicylates are useful in controlling the pain and inflammation associated with the polyarthritis in a patient with rheumatic fever. Naproxen, an NSAID, is effective and may be safer to use than aspirin.

- If the patient has heart failure due to rheumatic heart disease, digitalis may be necessary.

- Patients who have had one episode of acute rheumatic fever are more likely to develop acute rheumatic fever again following an *S pyogenes* infection; therefore, chemoprophylaxis should be given to these patients to prevent recurrences of acute rheumatic fever. Available chemoprophylaxis regimens for patients who have had acute rheumatic fever include monthly intramuscular injections of benzathine penicillin G, oral penicillin V, or oral erythromycin for at least 5 years. Patients who have rheumatic carditis should be given lifelong prophylaxis.

- Haloperidol may help control chorea in a patient with rheumatic fever.

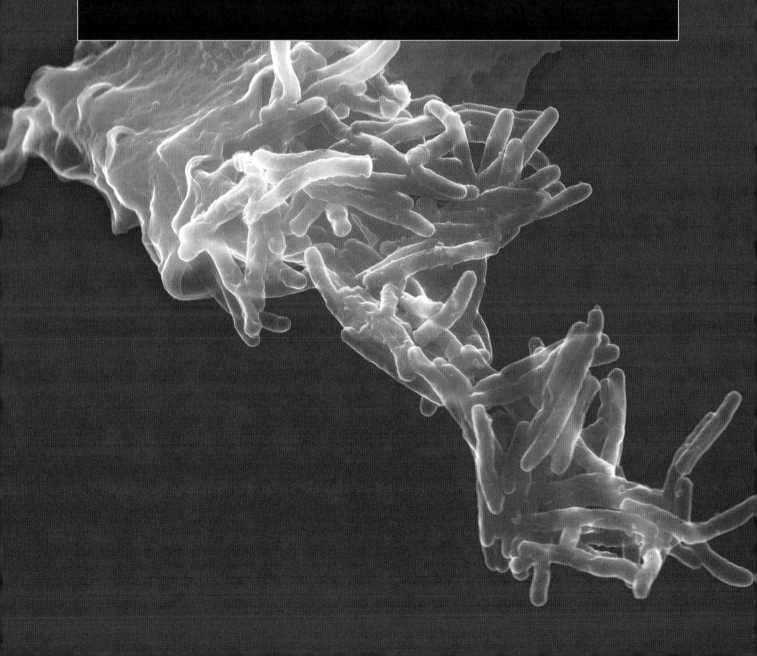

SECTION 9

BONES AND JOINTS

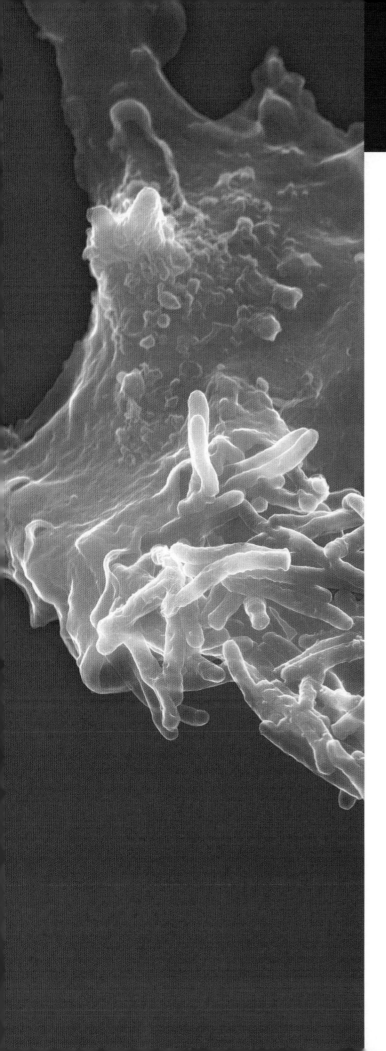

CHAPTER 31

THE BIG PICTURE: INFECTIONS OF THE BONES AND JOINTS

OVERVIEW

The two different infectious diseases that will be discussed in this section are osteomyelitis and septic arthritis. Osteomyelitis is an infection of the bone and includes the periosteum, medullary cavity, and cortical bone. Septic arthritis is an infection of the surface of the cartilage that lines the joint and the synovial fluid that lubricates the joint. **Staphylococcus aureus is the most common cause of infection in both diseases.**

Children and elderly adults are more likely to contract osteomyelitis and septic arthritis. Children usually develop osteomyelitis of the long bones, and elderly persons usually develop osteomyelitis of the vertebral body in the lumbar region of the spine. Osteomyelitis usually requires several weeks to cause extensive damage to the bone (Figure 31-1). Successful treatment of osteomyelitis requires 4–6 weeks of antibiotic therapy. In cases of extensive bone damage, antibiotic therapy plus surgery is required to eliminate the infection.

Two different types of arthritis are associated with microbial infections: reactive arthritis and septic (infectious) arthritis. Reactive arthritis is a sterile inflammatory process in the joint and can occur following a bacterial infection at a distant site in the body. This type of arthritis will not be discussed in Chapter 32, but a short description of the disease is included in this chapter to help to differentiate reactive arthritis from septic arthritis.

Reactive arthritis, or Reiter syndrome, results in urethritis, conjunctivitis, asymmetrical polyarthritis (e.g., ankles, knees, feet, and sacroiliitis), and a rash that occurs weeks after a bacterial infection. The most common cause of this type of arthritis is *Chlamydia trachomatis*. However, *Campylobacter jejuni*, *Yersinia enterocolitica*, *Shigella* or *Salmonella*, and *Streptococcus* can all cause reactive arthritis. It occurs more commonly in patients with human lymphocyte antigen B27 (HLA-B27).

Septic, or infectious, arthritis can be caused by a variety of microorganisms including viruses, fungi, and bacteria; however, bacteria are the most common cause (Figure 31-2). As mentioned above, *S aureus* is the most common cause of septic arthritis, which is more commonly seen in children and in elderly adults. Patients usually present with a triad of fever, joint pain, and impaired range of motion. They do **NOT** have the rash, urethritis, and conjunctivitis that is characteristic of reactive arthritis. Unlike osteomyelitis, septic arthritis can rapidly cause permanent damage to the joint and disability for the patient if not treated quickly and aggressively.

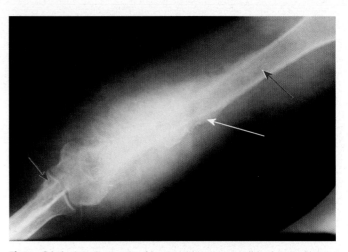

Figure 31-1. A radiograph of bone with osteomyelitis due to *Nocardia asteroides*. Note the moth-eaten appearance of the bone (*red arrows*) and the new bone growth over an area of dead bone (*white arrow*). Image courtesy of the Centers for Disease Control and Prevention, Dr Libero Ajello.

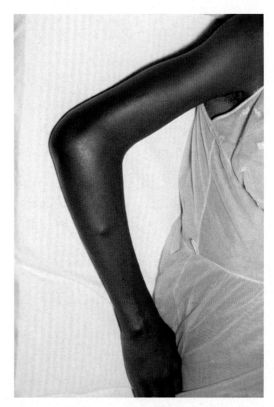

Figure 31-2. A photograph of a patient with gonococcal septic arthritis of the right elbow. Notice the swelling of the patient's arm. Image courtesy of the Centers for Disease Control and Prevention.

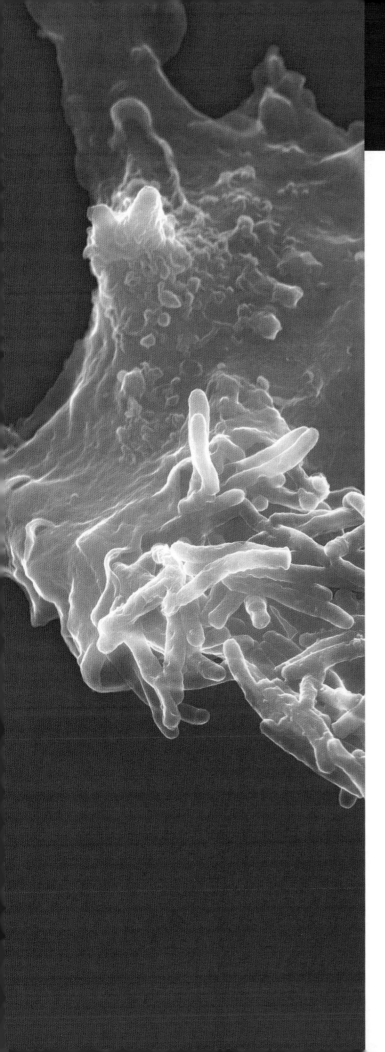

CHAPTER 32

OSTEOMYELITIS AND SEPTIC ARTHRITIS

OVERVIEW

The two infections of the bone that will be discussed in this chapter are osteomyelitis and septic arthritis. Osteomyelitis is a disease of the bone that can develop over a long period of time, and septic arthritis is an infection of the joint that can cause irreversible and debilitating destruction of the joint within 1–2 days. Infections of the bone and joints usually occur in children and older adults.

OSTEOMYELITIS

Osteomyelitis is a progressive infection that can include one or multiple parts of the bone (e.g., periosteum, medullary cavity, and cortical bone). It is usually a subacute to chronic infection that can cause severe disability if not properly treated. If untreated, the disease progresses from inflammatory destruction of bone to necrosis (sequestra), followed by new bone formation (involucrum).

ETIOLOGY

Osteomyelitis is usually a bacterial infection. Table 32-1 lists the various types of osteomyelitis by age group and the common pathogens that cause the infection. **_Overall, Staphylococcus aureus is the most common cause of osteomyelitis._** Other causes of this infection vary depending on the age of the patient. If the vagina of a pregnant woman is colonized with _Streptococcus agalactiae_ (group B _Streptococcus_) or _Escherichia coli,_ the neonate is more likely to aspirate these organisms during labor and delivery. _S agalactiae_ and _E coli_ are frequent causes of meningitis, pneumonia, and sepsis in newborn infants. These two organisms are also more frequent causes of osteomyelitis in newborns when compared with other age groups.

Elderly persons are more frequently infected with _S aureus_ and gram-negative, rod-shaped bacteria (e.g., _E coli, Pseudomonas aeruginosa, Serratia marcescens_), and are more likely to develop gram-negative infections of the bloodstream following diverticulitis, acute prostatitis, and urinary tract infections. These

TABLE 32-1. Osteomyelitis: Type, Patient Profile, and Common Causes

Type of Osteomyelitis/Patient Profile	Common Causes
Hematogenous	Usually only one organism
Infants (<1 year)	*Staphylococcus aureus, Streptococcus agalactiae* (group B *Streptococcus*), *Escherichia coli*
Children (1–16 years)	*S aureus, Streptococcus pyogenes* (group A *Streptococcus*), *Haemophilus influenzae*
Persons >16 years	*S aureus*, coagulase-negative staphylococci (e.g., *Staphylococcus epidermidis*), gram-negative rod-shaped bacteria (e.g., *E coli, Pseudomonas, Serratia*)
Contiguous spread*	More likely to be polymicrobial
Microbiology depends on the primary site of infection	*S aureus, S pyogenes* (group A *Streptococcus*), *Enterococcus* (i.e., group D; *E faecalis* and *E faecium*), coagulase-negative staphylococci (e.g., *Staphylococcus epidermidis*), gram-negative rod-shaped bacteria (e.g., *Escherichia coli, Pseudomonas, Serratia),* anaerobes (e.g., *Prevotella, Bacteroides, Fusobacterium, Peptostreptococcus*)
Diabetic foot	*S aureus, Streptococcus, Enterococcus*, gram-negative rod-shaped bacteria (e.g., *Proteus mirabilis, Pseudomonas),* anaerobes (e.g., *Prevotella, Bacteroides, Fusobacterium, Peptostreptococcus*)

*Contiguous spread is the spread of an infection from a nearby site to the bone. Diabetic foot osteomyelitis is an example of contiguous spread; however, because of the high incidence of this infection, it is mentioned separately.

organisms are also more likely to seed vertebrae in the lumbar region of the spine causing vertebral osteomyelitis.

Some patients are more likely to develop a particular bacterial infection of the bone because of their predisposition to certain factors or behaviors. Intravenous illicit drug users are more likely to acquire *P aeruginosa* infections of the cervical vertebrae. Athletic shoes that are not allowed to dry thoroughly between uses are more likely to harbor increased numbers of *P aeruginosa*. Therefore, puncture wounds to the feet of persons wearing these shoes are more likely to result in infections due to *P aeruginosa* or *S aureus*. The prevalence of osteomyelitis after foot puncture can be as high as 16%, and the prevalence in diabetic patients with peripheral vascular disease can be as high as 30–40%.

Osteomyelitis in patients with sickle cell disease is most likely due to *S aureus* and *Salmonella*. Infections of prosthetic joints are most commonly due to coagulase-negative *Staphylococcus* (e.g., *S epidermidis*); the second most common cause of these infections is *S aureus*.

MANIFESTATIONS

The onset of symptoms of acute osteomyelitis can occur within 1–2 days, or symptoms of chronic osteomyelitis can take weeks to months to develop. Children are more likely to develop acute long bone osteomyelitis, which manifests with symptoms of chills, fever, and malaise. There is usually pain and localized swelling and redness over the site of infection in the bone and guarding of the body part.

Elderly persons are more likely to develop subacute or chronic vertebral osteomyelitis, and usually present with localized lower back pain and tenderness with fever; however, a fever is not always present at the time of presentation. In patients with chronic osteomyelitis, the localized pain may come and go and fever usually is not present.

EPIDEMIOLOGY

- **Acute hematogenous osteomyelitis** occurs most commonly in children and usually results in a single site of infection that involves the metaphysis of the long bones (e.g., tibia, femur, and humerus).

- Osteomyelitis in adults usually involves the vertebral bodies. The lumbar vertebrae are most commonly affected, followed by the thoracic vertebrae, and rarely the cervical vertebrae.

- The overall prevalence of osteomyelitis is 1 per 5000 children, and about 50% of cases occur in preschool-aged children. The prevalence of osteomyelitis in neonates is 1 per 1000.

- The annual incidence of osteomyelitis in patients with sickle cell disease is 0.36%.

- The male to female ratio of osteomyelitis is 2:1.

- Direct trauma and spread to the bone from a contiguous focus are more common among adults and adolescents than in children.

- **Spinal osteomyelitis** is more common in persons older than age 45 than in younger persons.

- Intravenous drug users are more likely to develop vertebral infections in the cervical vertebrae.

PATHOGENESIS

The long bones of children and adolescents increase in length until reaching maturity. At maturity, growth-plate closure occurs at each end of the long bone, and the cartilage in the growth plate is replaced by bone. The nutrient artery supplies the nutrients needed for the growth plate, and connects to the nutrient vein via a venous capillary network. This network of capillaries forms a sharp loop, the site where osteomyelitis usually occurs in children and adolescents (Figure 32-1). The small diameter and the sudden change in the direction of the flow of blood in these blood vessels causes bacteria that may be in the bloodstream to make contact with the endothelium of the blood vessel. After attaching to the surface of the blood vessel, bacteria multiply and then enter the epiphysis of the bone causing osteomyelitis.

After growth-plate closure, the need to supply nutrients to the epiphysis via the bloodstream lessens. Thus, ***adults rarely develop osteomyelitis of the long bones.*** If an adult develops osteomyelitis of the long bone, it is usually due to trauma. The most common site of osteomyelitis by hematogenous spread in adults is the vertebrae, which contain small arteriolar vessels that trap bacteria in the vertebral body. A plexus of veins lacking valves, called Batson plexus, surrounds the vertebrae and drains the bladder and pelvic regions.

As adults age, they are more likely to develop infections of the urinary tract (e.g., cystitis, prostatitis) that are most commonly caused by *E coli,* a gram-negative coliform, although other

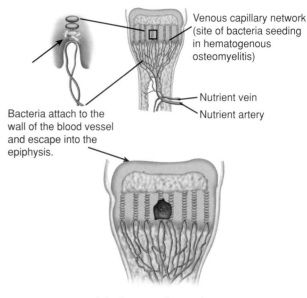

Venous capillary network (site of bacteria seeding in hematogenous osteomyelitis)

Nutrient vein
Nutrient artery

Bacteria attach to the wall of the blood vessel and escape into the epiphysis.

Infection spreads, causing more damage to the bone.

Figure 32-1. A schematic of the epiphysis of the long bone of a child. Note the site of bacterial seeding in the small looping blood vessels that supply nutrients to the epiphysis.

gram-negative coliforms also cause urinary tract infections. These bacteria travel from the urinary tract to the vertebral bodies via Batson plexus and infect the vertebrae. These vertebral arteries usually bifurcate and supply two adjacent vertebral bodies, resulting in osteomyelitis of two adjacent vertebrae and their intervening discs. The vertebrae most commonly infected are the lumbar vertebrae, followed by the thoracic vertebrae, and then the cervical vertebrae. Because urinary tract infections are relatively uncommon in children and adolescents, these age groups rarely develop vertebral osteomyelitis.

DIAGNOSIS

Peripheral white blood cell counts are usually normal in patients with osteomyelitis. In chronic osteomyelitis, patients may have a normochromic normocytic anemia (anemia of chronic disease). In both acute and chronic osteomyelitis, the erythrocyte sedimentation rate (ESR) is usually elevated; however, it is usually higher in patients with acute osteomyelitis. C-reactive protein levels are also elevated in acute and chronic conditions.

Osteomyelitis is usually diagnosed using imaging studies that include plane film radiographs, computed tomography (CT) scans, and magnetic resonance imaging (MRI). Plane radiographs show low sensitivity early in the disease process and require a loss of 50% of the bone calcium before osteomyelitis can be detected, which is usually 2–3 weeks following onset of the disease. In long bone infections, elevation of the periosteum may occur and soft tissue swelling may be detected. Radiographs of a patient with chronic osteomyelitis may show increased calcification (bone sclerosis), sequestra (a portion of dead bone that has become separated during the process of necrosis from normal bone), and involucra (a sheath of new bone that forms around an involucrum) (Figure 32-2).

In **vertebral osteomyelitis,** abnormalities may not be detectable by plane radiographs for 6–8 weeks after infection of the bone. When abnormalities can be detected, the bony plate of the vertebra appears irregular or "moth-eaten," which can also be caused by cancer of the vertebrae. Collapse of the disc space is usually seen as the infection progresses (Figure 32-3) and is best seen on a CT scan. Osteomyelitis almost always involves two adjacent vertebral bodies as well as the disc space, whereas in most cases of vertebral cancer, only one vertebral body is affected and the disc space is usually not affected.

Because MRI is more sensitive than plane films or CT scans, it can be used much earlier in the disease process to detect abnormalities. When bone marrow dies, it creates a unique MRI signal, as shown in Figure 32-4. Bone scans using technetium and gallium are useful; however MRI is now being used as an alternative diagnostic tool.

Once the results of imaging studies are known, the next step in diagnosis is determining which organism is causing the osteomyelitis. Treatment failures are common in patients with osteomyelitis, and the organisms that cause this infection should be isolated from the bone infection to guide antimicrobial treatment. Two or three blood cultures may be useful in determining the cause of the infection. In adults with osteomyelitis, deep tissue samples (e.g., needle biopsies) should be obtained. In spinal osteomyelitis, needle biopsy

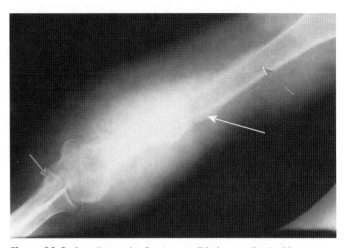

Figure 32-2. A radiograph of osteomyelitis in a patient with a mycetoma due to *Nocardia asteroides*. Note the moth-eaten appearance of the bone (*red arrows*) and the presence of involucrum (*white arrow*). Image courtesy of the Centers for Disease Control and Prevention, Dr Libero Ajello.

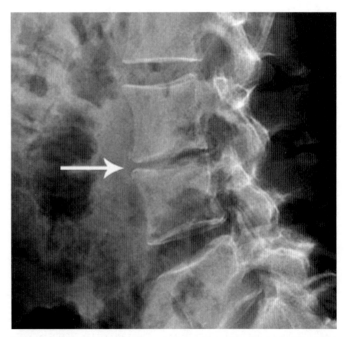

Figure 32-3. A plane film radiograph of spinal discitis and osteomyelitis. The lateral view of the lumbar spine reveals L3–4 disc-space narrowing (*arrow*) and endplate irregularity. Image courtesy of Tara M Lawrimore, MD, et al, 2006. Vertebral Osteomyelitis, vol 4, issue 11, Radiology Rounds. http:www.mghradrounds.org/index.php?src=gendocs&link=nov_dec_2006

using CT guidance is the procedure of choice for obtaining samples, which should be sent for bacteriologic culture and pathologic analysis. Pathology reports can be useful to direct empiric antibiotic therapy for patients with samples that are culture negative. If the patient has a long bone infection, frequently debridement, incision, and drainage of soft-tissue abscesses are required. Samples from this material can be sent for culture.

Deep tissue samples are NOT obtained to diagnose long bone infections in children. The epiphyseal plate can be damaged during the sampling, resulting in impaired bone growth. Instead, blood cultures should be obtained and, if negative, treatment is usually empirical.

TREATMENT AND PREVENTION

There are three important steps to treating osteomyelitis in adults.

1. An adequate sample collected deep in the infected tissue should be obtained for culture and histopathology. (*Note: This technique should not be used to collect samples from children with long bone infections*).

2. A specific antimicrobial regimen should be designed for the patient.

3. Surgery usually is not needed in the treatment of acute hematogenous osteomyelitis; however, antibiotic treatment for 4–6 weeks is required. Patients with chronic osteomyelitis usually require surgery.

A patient with osteomyelitis due to methicillin-sensitive *S aureus* can be treated with nafcillin or oxacillin. However, if the infection is due to methicillin-resistant *S aureus* (MRSA), vancomycin should be given. *Streptococcus* infections can be treated with penicillin G. In gram-negative, rod-shaped bacterial infections, ciprofloxacin should be used to treat the patient. However, if the osteomyelitis is due to *Serratia* or *Pseudomonas,* piperacillin-tazobactam and gentamicin should be used. If anaerobic bacteria are the cause of osteomyelitis, clindamycin or metronidazole should be given.

SEPTIC ARTHRITIS

Viruses, fungi, and bacteria can all cause infectious arthritis. However, bacterial infectious arthritis causes the most injury and is the only cause that will be discussed in this chapter. Bacterial (septic) arthritis is a serious infection, and if not treated quickly, can result in significant permanent damage to the joint and disability.

ETIOLOGY

S aureus is the most common cause of septic arthritis in patients of all ages. There are two major classes of septic arthritis: **gonococcal and nongonococcal arthritis.** *S aureus* is the most common cause of nongonococcal arthritis, and *Neisseria gonorrhoeae* is the most common cause of gonococcal arthritis in sexually active young adults. Gram-negative bacilli are more likely to cause septic arthritis (e.g., *E coli, Proteus,* and *Serratia*) in the elderly. *Streptococcus* (e.g., viridans *Streptococcus,*

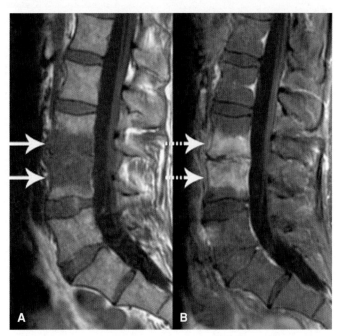

Figure 32-4. A magnetic resonance image (MRI) of lumbar spine discitis and osteomyelitis. **A.** Sagittal T1-weighted image of the lumbar spine of the same patient as shown in Figure 32-3, showing T1-hypointense signal (*solid arrows*) centered around the L3–4 interspace. **B.** Post-gadolinium sagittal fat-suppressed T1-weighted image shows marrow (*dashed arrows*) and disc enhancement with endplate erosions. Image courtesy of Tara M Lawrimore, MD, et al, 2006. Vertebral Osteomyelitis, vol 4, issue 11, Radiology Rounds. http://www.mghradrounds.org/index.php?src=gendocs&link=nov_dec_2006

S pneumoniae, and *S agalactiae*) accounts for 20% of cases of septic arthritis. Infections with anaerobic organisms usually are a consequence of trauma or of abdominal infection.

MANIFESTATIONS

Patients with nongonococcal septic arthritis usually present with the triad of fever, joint pain, and impaired range of motion. Elderly patients may be afebrile. Most patients with nongonococcal septic arthritis present with pain and swelling in a single joint. *S agalactiae* (group B *Streptococcus*) usually infects the sacroiliac and sternoclavicular joints.

Polyarticular arthritis is commonly seen in gonococcal septic arthritis, which is primarily an infection of sexually active young adults and teenagers and may present in one of two ways: either tenosynovitis, dermatitis, and polyarthritis syndrome or monoarticular arthritis.

Patients with **tenosynovitis, dermatitis, and polyarthritis syndrome** (also known as dermatitis-arthritis syndrome) initially present with fever, malaise, and arthralgias following *N gonorrhoeae* infection of the cervix, urethra, or pharynx. Later, inflammation of the tendons (tenosynovitis) in the wrist and fingers can be observed. Tenosynovitis includes tenderness over the tendon sheaths and exacerbation of pain during joint movement. Multiple skin lesions are seen (but seldom more than 12). (*Note: Skin lesions from N meningitidis meningococcemia usually are more numerous.*) Lesions evolve over a few days from papular to pustular or vesicular to necrotic (Figures 32-5 and 32-6), and may recur for several months. *N gonorrhoeae* is usually obtained in cultures of blood and mucosal surfaces but not in cultures of synovial fluid. If untreated, this syndrome can progress to purulent arthritis (*N gonorrhoeae* is present in the synovial fluid of the affected joints).

Monoarticular arthritis has no associated systemic symptoms and usually occurs after untreated tenosynovitis, dermatitis, and polyarthritis syndrome.

EPIDEMIOLOGY

- About 20,000 cases of septic arthritis occur each year in the United States.

- Most cases occur in the very young and the very old and among intravenous drug users. About 45% of cases are persons older than 65 years of age.

- Mortality rates depend on the agent causing the arthritis. In **gonococcal joint infection**, the mortality rate is extremely low. In **septic arthritis** infection due to *S aureus*, the mortality rate can be as high as 50%.

- In adults, the knee is the most commonly infected joint, followed by the hip, shoulder, ankle, and wrists; in children, the hip joint is most commonly affected, followed by the knee.

- Nearly 50% of patients who develop septic arthritis have an underlying chronic joint disease (e.g., rheumatoid arthritis, osteoarthritis).

- Almost all cases of nongonococcal arthritis are monoarticular.

- Gonococcal septic arthritis is more likely to occur following an asymptomatic infection of the pharynx due to *N gonorrhoeae*, and it is more common in females.

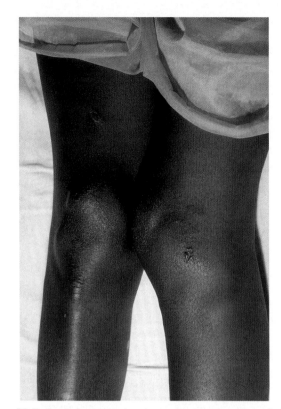

Figure 32-5. A photograph showing gonococcal septic arthritis of the knees. Note the skin lesion on the patient's left knee. Image courtesy of the Centers for Disease Control and Prevention, Dr Thomas F Sellers, Emory University, Atlanta, GA.

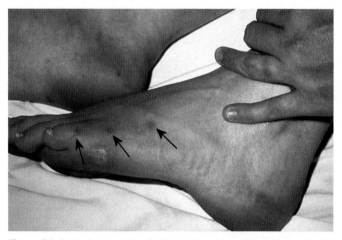

Figure 32-6. A photograph of skin lesions (*arrows*) associated with disseminated gonococcal infections. Image courtesy of the Centers for Disease Control and Prevention, J Pledger, Dr SE Thompson, VDCD.

▓ Polyarticular arthritis usually is observed in patients with gonococcal septic arthritis.

PATHOGENESIS

Organisms can enter the joint by direct inoculation, contiguous spread from infected periarticular tissue, or by bacteremia. However, ***the most common route of infection is following bacteremia.*** Causes of bacteremia leading to septic arthritis include urinary tract infection, intravenous drug use, intravenous catheters, endocarditis, and soft tissue infections.

Some bacteria have surface factors that promote their adherence to the joint. In patients with osteomyelitis, the arteriolar anastomosis between the epiphysis and the synovium allows the organisms to spread into the joint space.

The joint has protective components that can prevent septic arthritis. These components include phagocytic synovial cells and the presence of a phospholipase in the synovial fluid. Synovial cells can phagocytize invaders and produce antibacterial proteins that kill gram-negative organisms. The synovial fluid contains phospholipase A2, which is able to kill many gram-positive organisms (e.g., *S aureus*). Previously damaged joints and especially joints with rheumatoid arthritis are more susceptible to infection. Other underlying conditions that predispose people to the development of septic arthritis include osteoarthritis, systemic lupus erythematosus, minor trauma, and intra-articular injection of corticosteroids.

Damage of joint cartilage is the major debilitating result of septic arthritis. Bacterial growth in the joint causes an acute inflammatory reaction that results in infiltration of polymorphonuclear leukocytes. Injury to joint cartilage is due to the synthesis of cytokines and inflammatory products produced by the polymorphonuclear leukocytes and bacterial production of factors such as chondrocyte proteases of *S aureus,* which cause joint damage.

Most joint injury may be caused by the cytokines and inflammatory products produced by the polymorphonuclear leukocytes. Infection with *N gonorrhoeae* induces a relatively mild influx of polymorphonuclear leukocytes into the joint; thus, minimal joint destruction is usually observed in infections with this organism. In *S aureus* infections, a significant number of polymorphonuclear leukocytes are recruited to the joint resulting in significant damage to the joint cartilage. Cartilage erosion eventually occurs at the lateral margins of the joint and causes significant cartilage damage followed by joint space narrowing. In untreated infections, significant damage to the joint can occur within 3 days.

DIAGNOSIS

A critical laboratory test used to diagnose septic arthritis infections is analysis of the synovial fluid. A white blood cell count, gram stain smear, and culture of the synovial fluid are essential in determining the cause of septic arthritis. The most important use of synovial fluid analysis is to differentiate between noninflammatory, inflammatory, and septic arthritis (Table 32-2).

Blood cultures should also be obtained and are useful in a significant number of cases. In cases of gonococcal septic arthritis, pharyngeal, rectal, cervical, or urethral specimens should be placed on Thayer-Martin plates.

TABLE 32-2. Synovial Fluid Analysis to Differentiate Septic Arthritis from Noninflammatory and Inflammatory Arthritis

Laboratory Test	Normal Synovial Fluid	Septic Arthritis	Noninflammatory Arthritis	Inflammatory Arthritis
Clarity and color	Clear	Opaque, yellow to green	Clear, yellow	Translucent, yellow, or opalescent
Viscosity	High	Variable	High	Low
White blood cells/mm³	<200	>100,000*	200–2000	2000–10,000
Percent polymorphonuclear leukocytes	<25%	>75%	<25%	≥50%
Total protein g/dL	1–2	3–5	1–3	3–5
Glucose concentration (concentration in joint relative to concentration in blood)	Nearly equal	<25%	Nearly equal	50–80%
Culture	Negative	Often positive in nongono-coccal arthritis; usually negative in gonococcal arthritis	Negative	Negative
Disease or condition	Normal	Septic arthritis	Osteoarthritis, trauma to joint	Rheumatoid arthritis Reiter disease Partially treated septic joint Fungal or viral infection Gout or pseudogout Acute rheumatic fever

*Numbers may be lower in partially treated joint infections and in joint infections due to low virulence organisms.

TREATMENT AND PREVENTION

Treatment of **nongonococcal septic arthritis** involves two essential components. First, when possible, *purulent exudate should be completely drained and washed by arthroscopy or surgery.* Allowing the activated polymorphonuclear leukocytes to remain in the joint will allow further release of more inflammatory mediators, causing more joint damage. Then, an *appropriate antibiotic based on gram stain smear, culture results, and clinical presentation should be administered intravenously.* Antibiotic regimens are similar to those mentioned in the information on therapy for osteomyelitis (see above), except antimicrobial treatment for nongonococcal septic arthritis is 3–4 weeks as opposed to 4–6 weeks for osteomyelitis.

Even with appropriate treatment, one third of patients with nongonococcal septic arthritis suffer significant joint damage. Elderly patients, patients with preexisting chronic joint disease, and patients with prosthetic joints are more likely to have adverse outcomes.

Treatment of **gonococcal septic arthritis** requires ***complete drainage and washing of the purulent synovial fluid from the joint and antibiotic therapy with intravenous ceftriaxone*** for 24–48 hours after clinical improvement. Oral cefixime, ciprofloxacin, ofloxacin, or levofloxacin should be used to complete a total of 7–10 days of therapy. Residual joint damage is unusual.

Prevention of nongonococcal arthritis involves avoiding joint trauma and appropriate and timely treatment of infections (e.g., urinary tract infections, soft tissue infections, pneumonia). Prevention of gonococcal arthritis involves avoiding sex partners who have gonorrhea and identifying and treating those with gonorrhea and practicing safe sex.

GENITOURINARY TRACT

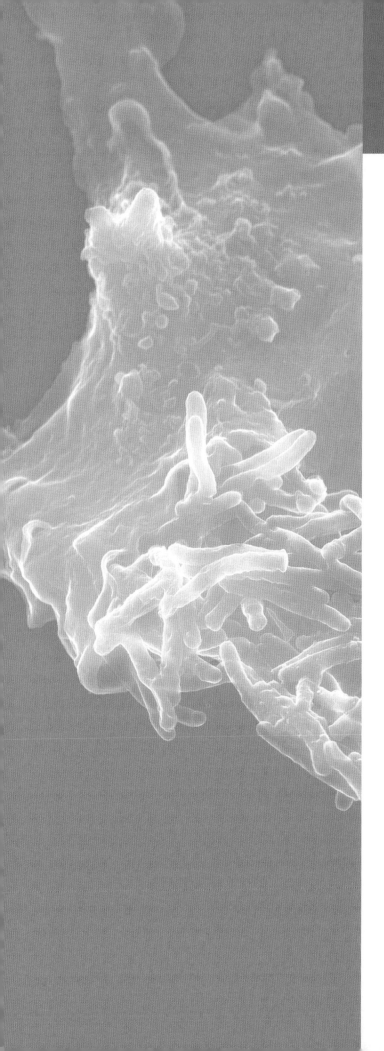

CHAPTER 33

THE BIG PICTURE: INFECTIONS OF THE GENITOURINARY TRACT

OVERVIEW

Infections of the genitourinary tract include infections of the bladder, kidney, and prostate, infections of the vagina, and sexually transmitted infections.

Infections of the urinary tract include urethritis, cystitis, pyelonephritis, and prostatitis and will be discussed in Chapter 34. These infections are very common, and each year result in over 7 million physician office visits and about 1 million hospitalizations. Most urinary tract infections result from contamination of the urethra with organisms found in the colon. ***Escherichia coli is the most common cause of urethritis, cystitis, prostatitis, and pyelonephritis.***

Infections of the vagina will be discussed in Chapter 35 and include bacterial vaginosis, mycotic vulvovaginitis, and trichomoniasis. Vaginal infections are the most common women's health problem, and have been linked to an increasing number of serious health risks such as endometritis, cervicitis, and complications associated with pregnancy.

In the United States, bacterial vaginosis is the most common cause of vaginal infection in females, an infection caused by an overgrowth of organisms that are normal flora in the vaginal mucosa (e.g., *Gardnerella vaginalis*). Mycotic vulvovaginitis is caused by *Candida albicans* and is the second most common cause of vaginitis. Trichomoniasis is caused by a flagellated protozoan, *Trichomonas vaginalis,* and is the least common cause of vaginitis. All three vaginal infections can be sexually transmitted; however, only trichomoniasis is transmitted exclusively by heterosexual interactions.

Sexually transmitted infections will be discussed in Chapter 36. Not all of the sexually transmitted infections discussed in Chapter 36 result in clinical symptoms; therefore these infections will be referred to as sexually transmitted infections (STIs) rather than sexually transmitted diseases (STDs). STIs are among the most common infectious diseases in the United States and affect more than 13 million persons annually. ***Herpes simplex virus type 2 and human papillomavirus are the most common causes of STIs in the United States. Chlamydia trachomatis is the most common bacterial cause of STI.***

TABLE 33-1. Sexually Transmitted Infections (STIs) and the Causative Agent(s)

STI(s)*	Causative Agent
Genital herpes	HSV-1 and HSV-2
Genital warts	HPV
AIDS	HIV
Viral hepatitis	Hepatitis A and hepatitis B viruses
Chlamydial infections	*Chlamydia trachomatis* (serogroups D and K)
Gonorrhea, urethritis, cervicitis	*Neisseria gonorrhoeae*
Pelvic inflammatory disease	*N gonorrhoeae, Chlamydia trachomatis*
Nongonococcal urethritis	*C trachomatis, Ureaplasma urealyticum, Mycoplasma genitalium, Trichomonas vaginalis, Gardnerella vaginalis,* HSV
Bacterial vaginosis	*G vaginalis, Mobiluncus, Mycoplasma hominis, Prevotella*
Syphilis	*Treponema pallidum*
Chancroid	*Haemophilus ducreyi*
Balanitis	*G vaginalis, T vaginalis,* HPV, *Streptococcus agalactiae, Streptococcus pyogenes*
Lymphogranuloma venereum	*C trachomatis* (serogroups L1–L3)
Granuloma inguinale	*Klebsiella granulomatis*
Proctitis, proctocolitis, enteritis	*N gonorrhoeae, T pallidum, C trachomatis,* HSV, *Entamoeba histolytica*
Epididymitis	*C trachomatis, N gonorrhoeae, Escherichia coli*
Trichomoniasis	*T vaginalis*
Pediculosis	*Pediculosis pubis*
Scabies	*Sarcoptes scabiei*

*Sexual transmission includes heterosexual, homosexual, oral-genital, and oral-anal encounters.
HSV, herpes simplex virus; HPV, human papilloma virus; AIDS, acquired immunodeficiency disease; HIV, human immunodeficiency virus.

More than 20 STIs have been identified and are listed in Table 33-1. Some of the diseases listed in this table have been discussed in other chapters of this book and will not be discussed in this section of the book (e.g., viral hepatitis is discussed in Chapter 20 and human immunodeficiency virus is discussed in Chapter 24).

The STIs will be discussed based on their clinical presentation. Infections that cause genital ulcers (i.e., syphilis, genital herpes, and chancroid), cervicitis, and urethritis (i.e., gonorrhea, nongonococcal urethritis, and chlamydial infections) will be discussed in Chapter 36. STIs that do not fit in the classifications above include pelvic inflammatory disease and genital warts and will also be discussed in Chapter 36.

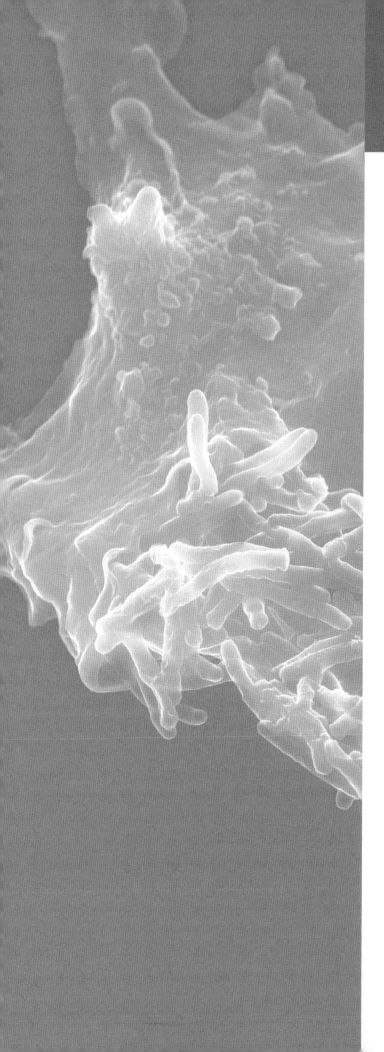

CHAPTER 34

INFECTIONS OF THE URETHRA, BLADDER, KIDNEY, AND PROSTATE

OVERVIEW

The infections discussed in this chapter include the urinary tract infections that affect the urethra, bladder, and kidneys (urethritis, cystitis, and pyelonephritis, respectively), and infections of the prostate such as acute prostatitis. Bacteria are the most common cause of all of these diseases.

URETHRA, BLADDER, AND KIDNEY

A **urinary tract infection** occurs when bacteria and white blood cells are present in the urine of a patient with symptoms of infection of the urethra, urinary bladder, or the kidney. **Bacteriuria** occurs when **bacteria** are present in the urine; **pyuria** occurs when **white blood cells** are present in the urine. The lower urinary tract includes the urethra and urinary bladder. Symptoms of urethritis and cystitis usually occur simultaneously. The upper urinary tract includes the ureters and kidneys. However, infection of the lower urinary tract *does not always* result in infection and symptoms of infection in the upper urinary tract (e.g., pyelonephritis). The bacteria that cause urinary tract infections are usually of fecal origin (e.g., *Escherichia coli*).

ETIOLOGY

The most common cause of urinary tract infections (i.e., urethritis, cystitis, and pyelonephritis) is E coli. *Staphylococcus saprophyticus* is the second most common cause of these infections in sexually active females between the ages of 13 and 40. In complicated cases of urinary tract infections such as those resulting from anatomic obstructions or from catheterization, the most common causes are *E coli*, *Klebsiella pneumoniae*, *Proteus mirabilis*, *Enterococcus*, and *Pseudomonas aeruginosa*. Table 34-1 lists the risk factors for urinary tract infections.

MANIFESTATIONS

Urethritis is an infection of the urethra that causes pain and discomfort during voiding (**dysuria**). **Cystitis** is an infection of the urinary bladder. Signs and symptoms of cystitis include urgency and frequency of urination, voiding small volumes of urine, and suprapubic tenderness just before or immediately after voiding. Patients who have symptoms of cystitis will also have symptoms of urethritis. In most cases of **pyelonephritis,** an infection of the lower urinary tract ascends the ureters to enter the kidneys. As a result, a patient with pyelonephritis will usually experience many of the signs and symptoms of urethritis and cystitis as well as fever, flank pain and tenderness, costovertebral angle tenderness, and nausea and vomiting.

EPIDEMIOLOGY

Urinary tract infections rank second only to respiratory infections in their incidence and cause over 6 million physician office visits per year in the United States.

Most cases of urinary tract infection occur in women (female to male ratio is 30:1). The incidence of urinary tract infections increases with age and with sexual activity.

About 40% of all females have at least one urinary tract infection at some time in their lives.

Postmenopausal women have higher rates of infection because of bladder or uterine prolapse; loss of estrogen, which causes a change in the vaginal flora; loss of lactobacilli in the vaginal flora, which results in periurethral colonization with gram-negative aerobes (e.g., *E coli*); and higher likelihood of concomitant medical illness (e.g., diabetes mellitus).

Males experience a rapid increase in the incidence of urinary tract infections some time in the fifth decade of life due to obstruction of the urethra following development of benign prostatic hypertrophy.

Urinary tract infections are usually endogenous; infection follows contamination of the distal end of the urethra with bacteria from the patient's own fecal organisms.

Urinary tract infections occasionally occur following bacteremia or due to hematogenous spread of a distant infection to the urinary tract.

PATHOGENESIS

The organisms that commonly cause urinary tract infections are found in feces. Contamination of the periurethral region with fecal organisms leads to colonization of the distal end of the urethra. Ascension of the organisms up the urethra to the bladder is the most common means of acquiring a urinary tract infection. Blood-borne infections of the urinary tract can occur but are infrequent and usually lead to renal abscess. Host factors that are important in protection from urinary tract infections include the normal daily flow of urine, the constant sloughing of the uroepithelial cells lining the urinary tract, and the presence of large numbers of *Lactobacillus* in the vaginal mucosa.

Females develop urinary tract infections more frequently than males because of the shorter urethra and the close proximity of the urethra to the anus. Also, sexual intercourse promotes contamination of the urethral opening with fecal organisms and contributes to the increased number of infections in women. Some women have many more urinary tract infections

TABLE 34-1. Risk Factors for Urinary Tract Infections

Female	Male
Sexual intercourse	Enlarged prostate gland
Menopause	Kidney stones
Pregnancy	Diabetes mellitus
Few *Lactobacillus* in vaginal mucosa	Immunosuppression
Immunosuppression	Congenital abnormalities that obstruct or slow urine flow
Diabetes mellitus	Use of Foley catheters
Use of diaphragm and spermicides	
Douching	
Use of Foley catheters	
Bladder or uterine prolapse	
Kidney stones	
Neurogenic bladder or bladder diverticulum	
Congenital abnormalities that obstruct or slow urine flow	

than other sexually active women in their age group. In many cases, women with more frequent urinary tract infections also have more *E coli* receptors on the cells that line the urinary bladder (uroepithelial cells). Uropathogenic *E coli* produce type 1 pili (FimH), which enables the bacteria to attach to uroepithelial cell receptors and avoid being eliminated from the urinary bladder during urination.

Any anatomic obstruction or neurologic disorder leading to incomplete elimination of urine from the bladder can also lead to urinary tract infection. For example, men in their fifth decade and older with prostate gland hypertrophy have difficulty completely emptying the bladder, which predisposes them to developing urinary tract infections (see Table 34-1).

Pyelonephritis, or infection of the kidneys, is due to ascent of bacterial infection from the urinary bladder via the ureters. The kidneys are protected from infection due to the presence of a sphincter at the distal end of each ureter and by movement of urine from the kidneys to the bladder by peristalsis of the ureters rather than by passive flow. Any factor leading to retrograde flow of urine from the urinary bladder to the kidney will predispose the host to pyelonephritis (Table 34-2).

Bacteria that gain access to the kidney can cause damage by production of polysaccharide, hemolysins, and endotoxin. Polysaccharide inhibits phagocytosis, hemolysins can directly cause tissue damage, and endotoxin contributes to inflammation and damage of renal parenchyma. Endotoxin can gain entry into the bloodstream and induce white blood cells into the bloodstream to produce interleukin 1 (IL-1), which causes fever. Fever is seen only in patients who have pyelonephritis and is not seen in patients with only urethritis and cystitis.

Kidney stones can serve as a location in which bacteria can escape antibiotics and cause recurrent urinary tract infections. *Proteus* can cause stones to form when it produces an enzyme called urease, which can catalyze the breakdown of urea to ammonia and carbon dioxide. The ammonia that results from this reaction will increase the pH of urine and cause formation of kidney stones (struvite calculi).

DIAGNOSIS

Signs and symptoms are important in determining a diagnosis in a patient with a urinary tract infection. A patient with dysuria and increased frequency and urgency is likely to have urethritis and cystitis. Treatment differs if a patient has pyelonephritis in addition to urethritis and cystitis. Therefore, symptoms unique to pyelonephritis (i.e., fever, flank pain and tenderness, and costovertebral angle tenderness) indicate that the patient also has a kidney infection.

Urinalysis should be performed in patients symptomatic for urethritis and cystitis without kidney involvement to determine the urine pH and if there is pyuria (white blood cells in urine) and bacteriuria (bacteria in urine). The pH of the urine is usually determined using a dipstick test. If the pH is >7.9 and the urine contains bacteria and white blood cells, the patient usually has a urinary tract infection due to urease-producing *Proteus* species. The pH is not elevated when there are other bacterial causes of urinary tract infection. Pyuria can be determined using traditional urinalysis (i.e., microscopic wet mount examination of spun urine), a cell-counting chamber technique

TABLE 34-2. Predisposing Factors that Cause Pyelonephritis

Colonization with *E coli,* which produce mannose-resistant pili that bind to the P blood group receptor found on uroepithelial cells and erythrocytes
Reflux of urine to the kidney due to incomplete development of the sphincter at the distal end of each ureter
Physiologic malfunctions leading to incomplete emptying of the bladder (e.g., pregnancy)
Urethral catheters
Stones in the urinary tract

(i.e., positive if >8 white blood cells/mm^3), or a dipstick test for leukocyte esterase.

Bacteriuria can be determined using a dipstick test to check for the presence of nitrites in the urine. Many uropathogens convert nitrates to nitrites when growing in urine. The nitrite detection part of the dipstick test demonstrates the presence of the most common uropathogen, *E coli*, and most of the gram-negative, rod-shaped bacteria that can cause a urinary tract infection (e.g., *Proteus*). Unfortunately, not all uropathogens have the ability to reduce nitrates to nitrite. *Enterococcus* and *S saprophyticus* do not produce nitrites in human urine and yield false-negative results. If patients have a **nitrite-negative cystitis,** urine should be obtained using a midstream catch procedure (known as a clean-catch urine specimen), and the specimen should be plated on growth media, incubated, and the resulting colonies counted. If more than 10,000 colony-forming units per mL are obtained, the patient has **bacteriuria.** If there are clinical manifestations such as fever, flank pain, and costovertebral tenderness, the patient may have **pyelonephritis** as well as **cystitis.** The following tests can be performed to confirm the diagnosis of pyelonephritis.

An **antibody-coated bacterial urine test** is based upon the principle that bacteria originating from the urinary bladder are not coated with human antibody; however, if the infection enters the kidney, an antibody response occurs and the antibodies produced by the patient will then coat the bacterial cells in the kidney. The antibody-coated bacteria enter the urinary bladder and can be obtained in the urine specimen. These antibody-coated bacteria are detected by addition of fluorescein-labeled antibody that binds to human antibody and can be seen with a fluorescent microscope.

Microscopic wet mount of spun urine to check for the presence of white blood cell casts. **Blood cultures** positive for bacterial growth. About 20% of patients with pyelonephritis have bacteremia.

Patients submit urine specimens following routine physician examinations (e.g., obstetric examination, annual physical examination). In some patients, urinalysis reveals pyuria and bacteriuria, which is referred to as an **asymptomatic bacteriuria.** Three groups of patients with asymptomatic bacteriuria have been shown to benefit from treatment: (1) pregnant women who are more likely to develop pyelonephritis or preterm delivery following an asymptomatic bacteriuria; (2) patients who have undergone renal transplantation and may reject the transplanted kidney if it becomes infected; and (3) patients who are about to undergo genitourinary tract surgical procedures. To confirm the results of urinalysis, a quantitative bacterial cell count should be performed. If the count is more than 100,000 CFU/mL, the diagnosis is asymptomatic bacteriuria and the patient should be treated with an antimicrobial agent.

THERAPY AND PREVENTION

Treatment depends on the extent of the infection. Patients with only urethritis and cystitis can be treated with an antibiotic on an outpatient basis. However, patients with pyelonephritis may also need antibiotic treatment in the hospital setting.

Patients with **acute symptomatic urethritis and cystitis** should be treated with trimethoprim-sulfamethoxazole, norfloxacin, or ciprofloxacin for 3 days. A 7-day course should be considered for pregnant women, women with diabetes mellitus, and women who have had symptoms for more than 1 week and are at higher risk for pyelonephritis because of the delay in treatment.

A patient who also has **pyelonephritis** and is only moderately ill can often be treated with trimethoprim-sulfamethoxazole, norfloxacin, or ciprofloxacin for 14 days. Patients who have severe pyelonephritis (e.g., high fever, toxic, unable to care for themselves) or who cannot comply with the 14-day outpatient treatment should be treated in a hospital setting with intravenous antibiotics (i.e., ceftriaxone or a fluoroquinolone) until 24 hours after the fever breaks; they should then be given an oral antibiotic for a total treatment time of 14 days. Long-term low-dose antibiotic treatment may be necessary for women with frequent reinfections to prevent future urinary tract infections.

To help prevent future **urinary tract infections,** patients should be encouraged to have a high fluid intake to ensure good urine output (at least 1–2 quarts of fluid within a 24-hour period) and to drink cranberry juice. Tannins in cranberry juice prevent binding of the bacteria to the uroepithelial cell surface receptors. Patients should also be encouraged to empty the bladder as soon as they feel the urge to urinate and to avoid foods that may irritate the bladder such as spicy foods, alcohol, or beverages containing caffeine.

Many pregnant women develop asymptomatic bacteriuria, which may have a role in causing preterm deliveries. Up to 30% of pregnant women with asymptomatic bacteriuria will develop acute pyelonephritis if the bacteruria is not treated with antibiotics. Treatment substantially decreases the risk of pyelonephritis. Urine samples should be obtained periodically from pregnant women to determine if they have bacteriuria.

Sexually active women with recurrent urinary tract infections can prevent recurrences by avoiding the use of spermicide-containing contraceptives and by taking an antimicrobial agent just before having intercourse. Postmenopausal women with recurrent urinary tract infections can prevent recurrences by taking oral or vaginal estrogen, which will shift the vaginal flora from predominantly uropathogens to *Lactobacillus*. The lactobacilli lower the vaginal pH, which reduces colonization of the vagina by uropathogens and protects from urinary tract infections.

PROSTATE

Prostatitis is an inflammation of the prostate gland. The term **prostatitis** describes a wide spectrum of disorders ranging from acute bacterial infection to chronic pain syndromes. Only acute bacterial prostatitis will be discussed in this chapter.

ETIOLOGY

The most common cause of acute bacterial prostatitis is *E coli*. Other pathogens that can cause acute bacterial prostatitis include *K pneumoniae, P aeruginosa, Enterobacter, Serratia, Proteus*, and *Enterococcus*.

MANIFESTATIONS

Because **acute bacterial prostatitis** is usually associated with infection in other parts of the urinary tract, patients may also have symptoms consistent with urethritis, cystitis, or pyelonephritis (Table 34-3). Physical examination usually reveals a warm, tender, diffusely enlarged, irregular, and indurated prostate. Patients with asymptomatic prostatitis detected by the presence of elevated PSA levels in the blood appear to also have an infection in the prostate.

EPIDEMIOLOGY

- Acute bacterial prostatitis occurs in less than 1 in 1000 adult men per year.
- Patients with a previous episode of acute bacterial prostatitis are more likely to experience future episodes of prostatitis.
- Acute bacterial prostatitis is the most common malady of the prostate in patients younger than the age of 35.
- It is more common in sexually active males.
- The organisms that cause prostatitis are usually acquired following ascension of fecal organisms that have colonized the distal end of the urethra.

PATHOGENESIS

The *E coli* strains that cause pyelonephritis appear to use the same virulence factors to cause prostatitis. Two main mechanisms associated with acute bacterial prostatitis include reflux of infected urine into the glandular prostatic tissue via the ejaculatory and prostatic ducts and ascension of a urethral infection from the meatus during sexual intercourse. Numerous polymorphonuclear leukocytes are seen in and around the acini and are associated with intraductal desquamation and cellular debris and tissue invasion by lymphocytes, plasma cells, and macrophages.

DIAGNOSIS

Acute bacterial prostatitis is usually identified based on clinical manifestations. A rectal examination will reveal a prostate that is swollen (boggy), warm, and tender to the touch. ***A vigorous digital examination of the prostate should be avoided because it can induce bacteremia.*** A urine specimen should be obtained using the midstream catch procedure, and the specimen should be quantitatively analyzed for the number of bacterial cells in the urine. The specimen of patients with acute bacterial prostatitis will have more than 100,000 CPU/mL as well as more than 10–20 white blood cells per high-powered field when examined under a microscope. Patients with asymptomatic prostatitis are usually identified following routine PSA testing and have elevated levels of PSA in the bloodstream.

THERAPY AND PREVENTION

Patients with acute bacterial prostatitis usually respond well to treatment with trimethoprim-sulfamethoxazole, ciprofloxacin, levofloxacin, or ofloxacin for 3–4 weeks. Asymptomatic prostatitis can be treated similarly for 14 days with similar antibiotics. Some infections of the prostate can be prevented by using a condom during sexual interactions.

TABLE 34-3. Signs and Symptoms of Acute Bacterial Prostatitis

Fever
Shaking chills
Perineal pain
Lower back pain
Decreased libido or impotence
Painful ejaculation
Varying degrees of bladder outflow obstruction
Symptoms of urethritis and cystitis that frequently occur coincidentally with acute bacterial prostatitis include dysuria and urinary frequency and urgency

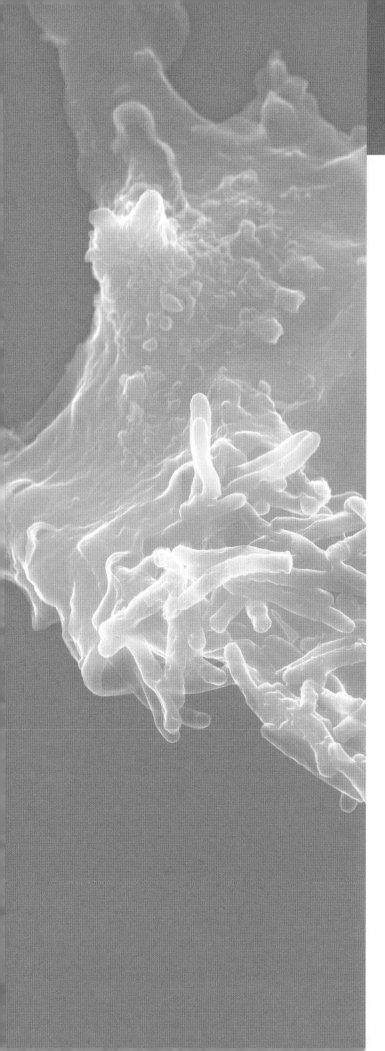

CHAPTER 35

VAGINAL INFECTIONS

OVERVIEW

Daily vaginal discharge is the body's means of maintaining a healthy vaginal mucosa. A normal vaginal discharge is usually clear or milky with no malodor; however, a change in the amount, color, or smell, and irritation, itching, or burning of the vaginal region may be due to an imbalance of the normal bacterial flora and can lead to vaginitis. Vaginitis is the most common women's health problem and is the most common complaint of women seeking health care, resulting in more than 10 million office visits annually in the United States.

This chapter will include discussions of bacterial vaginosis, mycotic vulvovaginitis, and trichomoniasis.

BACTERIAL VAGINOSIS

Bacterial vaginosis (previously called nonspecific vaginitis or *Gardnerella*-associated vaginitis) **is the most common cause of vaginal infection.** Bacterial vaginosis and vaginal discharge occur when there is overgrowth of organisms in the normal flora of the vaginal mucosa. This overgrowth can occur when there are fewer normal floras such as *Lactobacillus* that can no longer restrict growth of the organisms that cause bacterial vaginosis. Bacterial vaginosis can also be transmitted through sexual activity.

ETIOLOGY

Bacterial vaginosis is caused by a facultatively anaerobic gram-positive rod, *Gardnerella vaginalis*, and various anaerobic bacteria (e.g., *Mobiluncus* and *Prevotella*) that are present in the vaginal mucosa.

MANIFESTATIONS

Bacterial vaginosis manifests as an unpleasant vaginal odor and a white or gray vaginal discharge with a milk-like consistency. The odor can become particularly pungent after sexual intercourse because semen combined with vaginal secretions reduce the acidity level of the secretion, causing a strong odor. Odor may also be more noticeable about the time of menses. Vaginal itching or burning may also be present in a patient with bacterial vaginosis. Up to 40% of women with bacterial vaginosis may experience no outward symptoms.

TABLE 35-1. Characteristics of Vaginal Discharge Used in the Diagnose of Vaginitis

Diagnostic Criteria	Normal Vaginal Discharge	Bacterial Vaginosis	Trichomoniasis	Mycotic Vulvovaginitis
Vaginal pH	3.8–4.2	>4.5	4.5	<4.5
Discharge consistency	Thin white, flocculent	Thin white (milky), gray	Yellow-green, frothy (see Figure 35-5)	White, cottage cheese-like (see Figure 35-2)
Amine odor "whiff" test	Absent	Fishy	Fishy	Absent
Microscopic	Lactobacilli, epithelial cells	Clue cells (see Figure 35-1), no WBCs in discharge	Trichomonads, >10 WBCs per high-powered field (see Figure 35-8)	Budding yeast, hyphae or pseudohyphae (see Figure 35-3)

WBC, white blood cells.

Bacterial vaginosis is associated with **pelvic inflammatory disease** (PID), which can result in infertility as well as increased risk of endometritis, cervicitis, pregnancy complications, and postoperative infections. Pregnant women with bacterial vaginosis in gestations weeks 23–26 are also more likely to deliver a low birth weight infant (<2.5 kg).

EPIDEMIOLOGY

Bacterial vaginosis has been diagnosed in 10–26% of patients in primary care settings and in out-patient visits to an obstetrician. It is more common in patients who seek treatment for sexually transmitted infections (STIs) (32–64% of women) in clinics.

It is the most common cause of symptoms of vaginitis among women and causes 40–50% of cases of vaginitis.

Bacterial vaginosis can be caused by vaginal douching, an increased number of sexual partners, and use of intrauterine devices.

PATHOGENESIS

The normal balance of the organisms in the vaginal mucosa of patients with bacterial vaginosis is disrupted so the bacteria that cause this infection overgrow at the expense of protective bacteria known as lactobacilli. Lactobacilli produce hydrogen peroxide to maintain a healthy and normal balance of microorganisms in the vagina. Patients who have been diagnosed with bacterial vaginosis have up to 1000 times more anaerobic bacteria in their vaginal discharge compared with patients who do not have the disease.

DIAGNOSIS

Clinical signs and symptoms are helpful in determining the diagnosis of bacterial vaginosis (Table 35-1). A sample of vaginal discharge should be obtained and tested for pH, consistency, odor following addition of 10% potassium hydroxide, and for the presence of clue cells (Figure 35-1). Three of four criteria listed in Table 35-2 should be positive to obtain a diagnosis of

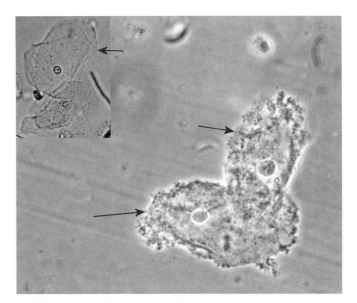

Figure 35-1. A photomicrograph of a specimen of vaginal discharge collected from a patient with bacterial vaginosis. Notice that the clue cells in the lower right-hand corner have a rough cytoplasmic membrane due to attachment of bacteria to the surface of the cells. The cells in the upper left-hand corner are from a patient who does not have bacterial vaginosis. These cells do not have bacteria attached to their surface and, as a result, their cytoplasmic membrane is sharp and clearly defines the edge of the cell. Image courtesy of the Centers for Disease Control and Prevention, M Rein and Dr Stuart Brown.

TABLE 35-2. Criteria for Diagnosis of Bacterial Vaginosis*

1. Thin, homogeneous vaginal discharge
2. pH of vaginal discharge >4.5
3. Clue cells in saline wet mount or Gram stain of vaginal discharge
4. Mixture of vaginal discharge and 10% potassium hydroxide liberates an amine-like or fishy odor

*If 3 of 4 criteria are positive, the diagnosis is bacterial vaginosis.

bacterial vaginosis. The patient should avoid douching or using a feminine hygiene spray for a few days before the sample is obtained because these products can worsen the condition or conceal important clues that may help in the diagnosis of bacterial vaginosis.

TREATMENT AND PREVENTION

Bacterial vaginosis can be treated with metronidazole or clindamycin. Vaginal douches or deodorant sprays that mask vaginal odor should not be used to treat the infection. Although these products may temporarily eliminate odor, they will not cure the condition. Bacterial vaginosis can be prevented by avoiding vaginal douching and limiting the number of sexual partners. Patients who have sexual interactions with several partners should encourage the use of condoms to avoid future infections.

MYCOTIC VULVOVAGINITIS

Mycotic vulvovaginitis (also known as vulvovaginal candidiasis or vaginal yeast infection) is caused by *Candida albicans*. Mycotic vulvovaginitis is the second most common cause of vaginitis.

ETIOLOGY

The causative agent of mycotic vulvovaginitis is a yeast called *C albicans*.

MANIFESTATIONS

The vaginal discharge frequently appears as a thick, curd-like discharge containing epithelial cells and masses of pseudohypha (Figures 35-2 and 35-3). The patient usually has intense pruritus of the vulva and erythematous vagina and labia.

EPIDEMIOLOGY

C albicans causes 20–25% of cases of vaginitis.

Most cases of mycotic vulvovaginitis result from overgrowth of *C albicans,* which is already present in the vaginal mucosa.

Factors that can upset the balance of the normal flora include pregnancy, obesity, diabetes mellitus, oral contraceptives, corticosteroids, antibiotic therapy, prolonged exposure to moisture, and poor feminine hygiene.

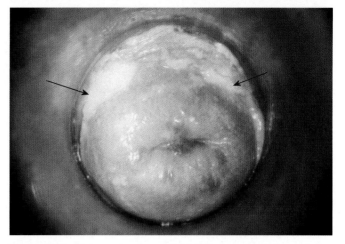

Figure 35-2. The cervix of a patient with mycotic vulvovaginitis. Notice the curd-like substance on the cervix (*arrows*). Image courtesy of the Centers for Disease Control and Prevention.

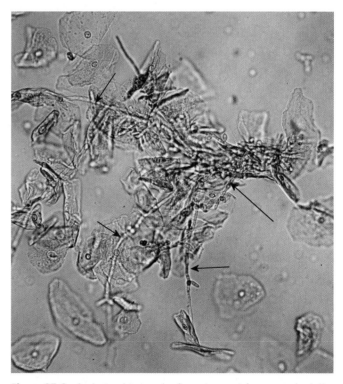

Figure 35-3. A photomicrograph of a wet mount from a vaginal discharge containing a mass of *Candida albicans* pseudohyphae (*arrows*). Image courtesy of the Centers for Disease Control and Prevention, Dr Stuart Brown.

PATHOGENESIS

When the delicate balance of organisms in the vaginal mucosa is upset, *C albicans* can overgrow and cause vaginitis. For example, when a patient is taking an antibiotic to treat a bacterial infection, the antibiotic may also kill the lactobacilli that produce hydrogen peroxide to protect against *C albicans* overgrowth.

DIAGNOSIS

Diagnosis of mycotic vulvovaginitis is frequently determined based on the curd-like nature of the vaginal discharge and on manifestations (e.g., pruritic erythematous labia) (see Figure 35-2 and Table 35-1). A Gram stain or wet mount of the discharge can be performed to determine if yeast cells and pseudohyphae are present (Figure 35-4; see Figure 35-3).

TREATMENT AND PREVENTION

Intravaginal agents such as butoconazole, clotrimazole, nystatin, or terconazole are available for treatment as over-the-counter drugs. Fluconazole, an oral antifungal agent, can also be prescribed to treat mycotic vulvovaginitis. Mycotic vulvovaginitis can be prevented by practicing good feminine hygiene, maintaining a healthy diet and weight, and whenever possible avoiding the use of antibiotics and corticosteroids that cause overgrowth of *C albicans* in the vaginal mucosa.

TRICHOMONIASIS

Trichomonas vaginalis is a very fragile microorganism that can only survive for 20–30 minutes outside the host. It is transmitted primarily by intimate heterosexual contact.

ETIOLOGY

The etiologic agent of trichomoniasis is a flagellated protozoan *T vaginalis*. It is a pear-shaped organism that exhibits a characteristic motility described as a wobbling and rotating motion. Recognition of this motility on wet mounts is helpful in diagnosis of the infection.

MANIFESTATIONS

Proliferation of *T vaginalis* is associated with a low-grade inflammation manifested by itching and burning, painful urination, and a frothy green, creamy vaginal discharge, which is described as being leukorrheic and malodorous (Figure 35-5). Because of the anatomic ease of spread to the urethra, urethritis often results in dysuria and increased frequency and urgency. Many females with this infection may be asymptomatic. In males, symptoms include dysuria and increased frequency and urgency and can be associated with

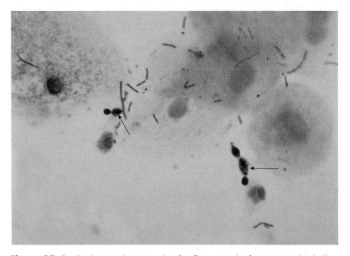

Figure 35-4. A photomicrograph of a Gram stain from a vaginal discharge due to *Candida albicans*. Notice the yeast cells in the Gram-stained image (*arrows*). Image courtesy of the Centers for Disease Control and Prevention, Dr Stuart Brown.

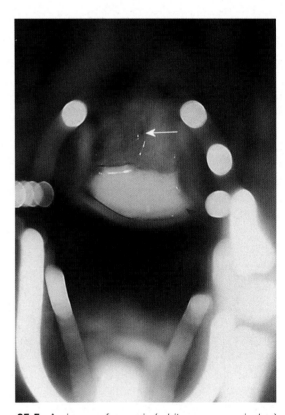

Figure 35-5. An image of a cervix (*white arrow; cervical os*) and a large amount of leukorrheic vaginal discharge due to infection with *Trichomonas vaginalis* (*blue arrow*). Image courtesy of the Centers for Disease Control and Prevention.

urethritis and prostatovesiculitis. Males are usually asymptomatic, however.

EPIDEMIOLOGY

T vaginalis is a common parasite of both males and females, and the incidence is in part related to hygiene. Humans are the only natural host of *T vaginalis*.

T vaginalis causes 10–20% of cases of vaginitis in the United States.

Pregnant women who acquire trichomoniasis are more likely to have low birth weight infants, premature rupture of membranes, or preterm delivery.

Sexual intercourse is the usual method of transmission, especially via asymptomatic males. In rare instances, trichomoniasis may be transmitted by wet towels, washcloths, and bathing suits.

PATHOGENESIS

Low-grade inflammation is associated with the presence of an abundance of trichomonads. *T vaginalis* binds to the cells that line the surface of the vagina and produces proteases and cytotoxic toxins that cause host cells to round up and detach. This damage to the host cells causes an immunologic response. Numerous polymorphonuclear leukocytes are present in the vaginal discharge. Immunity to the infection does occur, but it is only partially protective against subsequent *T vaginalis* infections.

DIAGNOSIS

Clinical diagnosis of trichomoniasis depends upon recognition of the symptoms of dysuria—frothy, creamy, malodorous discharges associated with punctate hemorrhagic lesions and hyperemia of the vagina (Figure 35-6; see Figure 35-5 and Table 35-1). Microscopic examination of the vaginal discharge for motile trichomonads will yield a definitive diagnosis of trichomoniasis (Figure 35-7). The vaginal discharge of a patient with trichomoniasis contains numerous polymorphonuclear leukocytes, which usually are not present in the other causes of vaginitis (Figure 35-8).

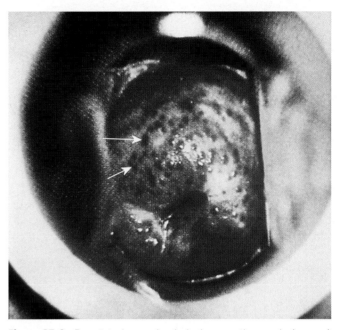

Figure 35-6. Punctate hemorrhagic lesions on the cervix (*arrows*) of a patient with trichomoniasis. Image courtesy of the Centers for Disease Control and Prevention.

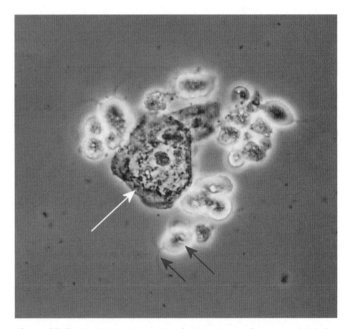

Figure 35-7. A photomicrograph of a wet mount from a vaginal discharge from a patient with trichomoniasis. Note the vaginal epithelial cell (*white arrow*), the trichomonad (*blue arrow*), and the fine flagella of the trichomonad (*red arrow*). Image courtesy of the Centers for Disease Control and Prevention.

TREATMENT AND PREVENTION

Metronidazole is effective in the treatment of trichomoniasis. The infection often persists because the parasite rarely causes symptoms in males, so that reinfection of females by untreated males is common. Some females can be infected for months to years as the infection is passed back and forth between the female and her sexual partner; therefore, both sexual partners must be treated simultaneously, even if they are in a monogamous relationship. The use of male condoms or treatment of the male partner with metronidazole can reduce the chances of transmission from an infected male to the female sexual partner.

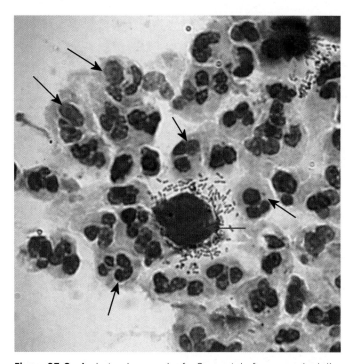

Figure 35-8. A photomicrograph of a Gram stain from a vaginal discharge due to *Trichomonas vaginalis*. Notice the abundance of polymorphonuclear leukocytes (*black arrows*) and the trichomonad (*blue arrow*) surrounded by gram-negative, rod-shaped bacteria. Image courtesy of the Centers for Disease Control and Prevention.

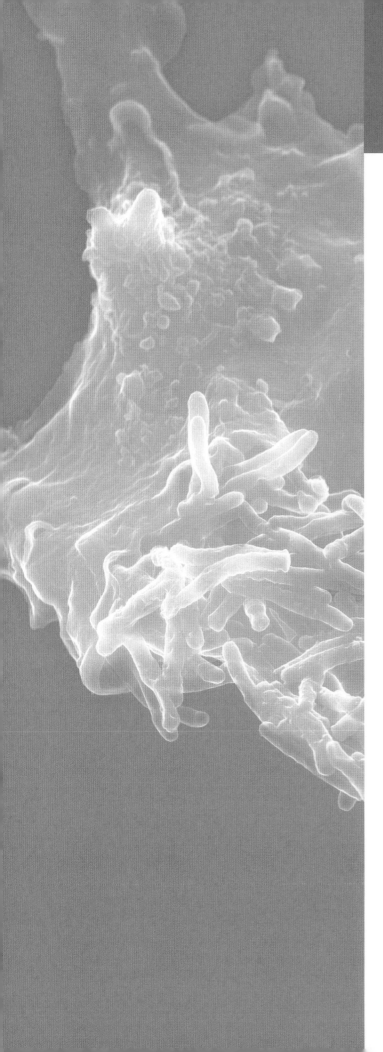

CHAPTER 36

SEXUALLY TRANSMITTED INFECTIONS

OVERVIEW

Sexually transmitted infections (STIs) are among the most common infectious diseases in the United States and infect more than 13 million men and women each year. The term sexually transmitted infections (STI) is replacing the term sexually transmitted diseases (STD), which has been used previously, because many sexually transmitted infections do NOT result in disease and are asymptomatic.

Over 900,000 *Chlamydia trachomatis* infections are sexually transmitted in the United States each year. This infection is asymptomatic in many women; however, eventually women who have been infected may want to become pregnant and find that they are infertile due to scarring of the fallopian tubes as a result of the infection.

The STIs discussed in this chapter are divided into groups based on their clinical presentation: genital ulcers (genital herpes, syphilis, and chancroid), urethritis and cervicitis (gonorrhea, chlamydial infections, and nongonococcal urethritis), and other STIs (pelvic inflammatory disease [PID] and human papillomavirus infections [HPV]).

DISEASES CHARACTERIZED BY GENITAL ULCERS

Most young, sexually active patients who have genital ulcers have genital herpes, syphilis, or chancroid. The frequency of each disease differs by geographic area and patient population; however, ***genital herpes is the most common of these diseases.*** Genital herpes, syphilis, and chancroid have all been associated with an increased risk for acquiring human immunodeficiency virus (HIV) from an HIV-infected sexual partner. The characteristics associated with these infections may aid in determining a correct diagnosis (Table 36-1).

GENITAL HERPES

Genital herpes is a recurrent lifelong inflammatory viral disease of the male and female genital tracts.

TABLE 36-1. Characteristics that Differentiate Genital Ulcerative Diseases

Disease	Occurrence in the United States	Number and Location	Tenderness	Ulcer Appearance	Adenopathy
Herpes simplex virus (HSV)	Most common	Clusters of ulcers on labia and penis	Tender	Uniform size clean base erythematous border	Tender inguinal nodes
Syphilis	Second most common (after HSV)	One or two lesions on vagina and penis	Little to no tenderness	Clean base indurated border	Rubbery, mildly tender
Chancroid	Least common	One or two lesions on labia and penis; may coalesce	Painful	Can be large, ragged, and necrotic base, undermined edge	Very tender, fluctuant inguinal nodes

ETIOLOGY

Genital herpes is caused by herpes simplex virus type 1 (HSV-1) and HSV-2.

MANIFESTATIONS

Primary genital herpes is acquired by sexual contact with an infected partner and has an incubation period of 2–7 days. Initial manifestations include local pain, tenderness, pruritus, and dysuria. A profuse, watery vaginal discharge may occur in females. Initial lesions are papules on a red erythematous base that rapidly develop into vesicles (Figure 36-1). The vesicles break down and develop into ulcers covered with a grayish exudate (Figure 36-2). In females, the vesicles develop on the labia majora and minora, the vaginal mucosa, the cervix, and the perineal region (Figure 36-3). In males, the lesions typically appear on the glans penis, the prepuce, and the shaft of the penis. About 75% of patients present with a painful nonsuppurative inguinal, pelvic, or femoral lymphadenopathy. Constitutional symptoms include headache, malaise, and myalgias. These lesions are self-limiting and heal in about 3 weeks. HSV-1 primary genital infections are less severe than HSV-2 infections.

The manifestations of **recurrent genital herpes** are similar but less severe and resolve more rapidly. Recurrences, which may be hormonally triggered during menses, are usually about 4 months after the first episode and then at intervals of approximately 6–8 weeks. Recurrences of genital herpes in HSV-2 patients are more frequent and more severe than in HSV-1 infected patients.

Newborns who acquire the virus during passage through the birth canal of a symptomatic mother usually develop disseminated disease, which includes disseminated vesicular lesions (Figure 36-4), pneumonitis, hepatitis, and infections of the central nervous system (i.e., meningitis or encephalitis). The virus can also cross the placenta and cause stillbirth or extreme teratogenic effects.

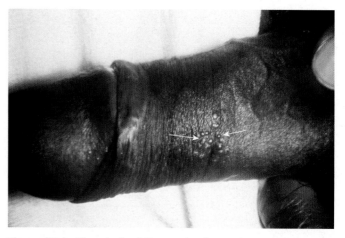

Figure 36-1. The shaft of the penis of a patient with vesicular lesions due to genital herpes. Image courtesy of the Centers for Disease Control and Prevention, Susan Lindsley.

EPIDEMIOLOGY

Genital herpes in adults

About 10% of the adult population in the United States experiences symptomatic genital herpes. At least 50 million people are infected with HSV.

About 80% of patients with genital herpes are infected with HSV-2 and the remaining 20% are infected with HSV-1.

The herpetic vesicles are filled with infectious virus, so contact can spread the infection on the patient to uninfected sexual partners. Risk of infection is approximately 75% following contact with a symptomatic person.

Acquisition of HSV is by sexual contact with an infected person or by transfer to a fetus or newborn from an infected mother.

Most persons infected with genital herpes have not been diagnosed. Many persons have mild or unrecognized infections but shed virus intermittently in the genital tract.

Most people acquire genital herpes by sexual contact with an asymptomatic person infected with HSV.

Genital herpes during pregnancy and in the neonate

Newborns who acquire the virus during passage through the birth canal of a symptomatic mother usually develop disseminated infection and have a 60–70% mortality rate.

About 1 in 20,000 deliveries results in HSV infection of the neonate. There is a 50% chance of infection.

Most mothers of infants who acquire neonatal herpes lack histories of clinically evident genital herpes.

The risk for transmission to the neonate from an infected mother is high among women who have a primary genital herpes infection near the time of delivery (30–50%), and is low among women with a history of recurrent herpes at term or who acquire genital herpes during the first half of pregnancy (<1%).

Recurrent genital herpes is much more common than primary HSV infection during pregnancy; therefore, the proportion of neonatal HSV infections acquired from mothers with recurrent herpes remains high.

PATHOGENESIS

HSV gains access to the genital mucosa by sexual contact with an HSV-infected partner. Symptomatic and asymptomatic HSV infected sexual partners can transmit the infection to an uninfected partner. Viral replication induces an erythematous papule that develops into a fluid-filled vesicle. The vesicular fluid contains many infectious virus particles and degenerating cells containing eosinophilic intranuclear inclusion bodies and multinucleated giant cells. The vesicles eventually rupture, and the remaining small ulcers are covered with a grayish exudate. The lesions heal in about 3 weeks. During primary infection, the patient will have a viremia and regional lymphadenopathy. Interferon alpha, HSV-specific antibody, and cell-mediated immunity will eventually curtail viral replication.

During the primary infection, HSV invades local nerve endings, ascends the axons, and establishes latency in the sacral

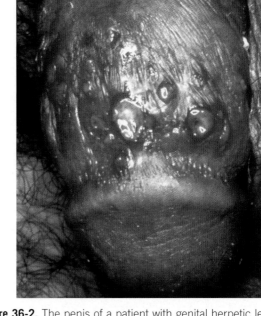

Figure 36-2. The penis of a patient with genital herpetic lesions in which the vesicles have broken, resulting in herpetic ulcers. Image courtesy of the Centers for Disease Control and Prevention, Dr NJ Fiumara and Dr Gavin Hart.

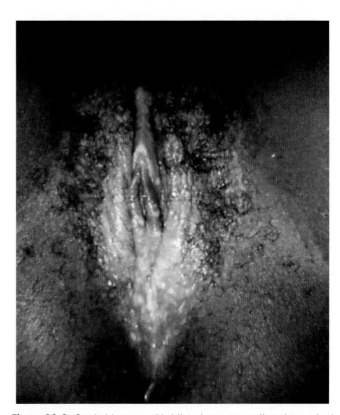

Figure 36-3. Genital herpes with blistering surrounding the vaginal introitus. Image courtesy of the Centers for Disease Control and Prevention, Susan Lindsley.

ganglia. Following an immunosuppressive event such as menses or stress, viral replication occurs in the sacral ganglia, and HSV travels down the axon and causes a recurrence of lesions in the epidermis. In most patients, recurrent lesions heal within a shorter period of time than lesions that occur during a primary infection.

DIAGNOSIS

A clinical diagnosis is based upon presence of vesicular lesions in the genital area and a sexual history suggestive of genital herpes. Laboratory approaches for determining the diagnosis of genital herpes include culturing for the virus, detection of multinucleated giant cells in the herpetic lesions by a positive Tzanck test (Figure 36-5), immunofluorescent staining of cells from the herpetic lesions, and type-specific serologic testing for antibody to G1 glycoprotein produced by HSV-1 and G2 glycoprotein produced by HSV-2.

THERAPY AND PREVENTION

Patients experiencing the initial episode of genital herpes should be advised that episodic antiviral therapy during recurrent episodes may shorten the duration of lesions and that suppressive antiviral therapy can ameliorate or prevent recurrent outbreaks. ***Treatment does NOT cure, however, and even if given early in the primary HSV infection, it will not prevent the establishment of viral latency.*** Treatment for primary infections, for recurrences, and for daily suppressive therapy includes acyclovir, famciclovir, or valacyclovir.

Intravenous acyclovir therapy should be provided to patients who have severe disease or complications necessitating hospitalization such as disseminated infection, pneumonitis, hepatitis, or infections of the central nervous system (i.e., meningitis and encephalitis).

To prevent further spread of the infection, patients should be advised to abstain from sexual activity when lesions or prodromal symptoms are present and are encouraged to inform their sexual partners that they have genital herpes. Sexual transmission of HSV can occur during asymptomatic periods; however, asymptomatic viral shedding occurs more frequently in patients who have genital HSV-2 infection than in patients with HSV-1 infection and in patients who have had genital herpes for less than 12 months. The use of condoms during all sexual exposures with new or uninfected sex partners should be encouraged.

Prevention of neonatal herpes depends both on preventing acquisition of genital herpes during the third trimester of pregnancy and avoiding exposure of the infant to herpetic lesions during delivery. Pregnant women who are negative for HSV-2 infection should be counseled to avoid intercourse during the third trimester with partners known or suspected of having genital herpes. In addition, pregnant women without known orolabial herpes should be advised to avoid cunnilingus during the third trimester with partners known or suspected of having orolabial herpes.

At the onset of labor, all pregnant women with genital herpes should be questioned carefully about symptoms of genital herpes, including prodrome, and all women should be examined carefully for herpetic lesions. Women without symptoms or

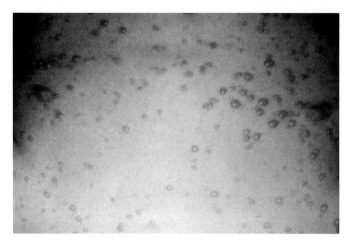

Figure 36-4. Disseminated herpes simplex vesiculopapular rash over the trunk of a patient. Image courtesy of the Centers for Disease Control and Prevention, Dr KL Hermann.

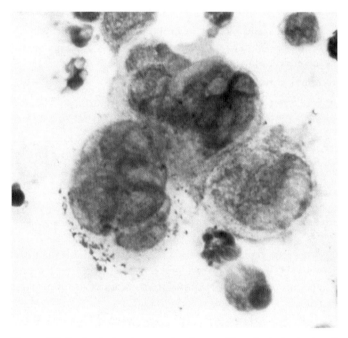

Figure 36-5. A photomicrograph of a multinucleated giant cell scraped from a herpetic lesion. Image courtesy of the Centers for Disease Control and Prevention, Dr KL Hermann.

signs of genital herpes or its prodrome can have vaginal delivery. Women with recurrent genital herpetic lesions at the onset of labor should have cesarean section.

SYPHILIS

Syphilis is caused by the stealth pathogen *Treponema pallidum*. The outer surface of *T pallidum* contains no antigenic molecules that can be easily recognized by the host's immune system. As a result, this bacterial pathogen can evade detection for decades much like the United States stealth B2 bomber airplane can evade detection by radar.

ETIOLOGY

T pallidum has a number of characteristics that are important for diagnosis. The spiral-shaped morphology and characteristic corkscrew motility pattern of these bacteria are important for diagnosis via darkfield microscopy.

MANIFESTATIONS

The manifestations of syphilis depend on the stage of disease the patient is experiencing. There are four stages of syphilis in adults: primary, secondary, latent, and tertiary syphilis. Manifestations of **primary syphilis** include a highly infectious hard painless chancre and regional lymphadenitis. The hard chancre develops after an incubation period of approximately 3 weeks (Figure 36-6) and will usually heal within 3–6 weeks. Regional lymphadenopathy with swollen and firm, nonsuppurative lymph nodes may also develop during primary syphilis. Lymphadenopathy may persist for months, despite healing of the chancre.

The manifestations of **secondary syphilis** usually begin 6–8 weeks after the appearance of the initial chancre and may overlap the time when the primary chancre is present. The principal manifestations of secondary syphilis are skin and mucous membrane lesions as well as manifestations of systemic disease. Systemic manifestations include malaise, anorexia, headache, sore throat, arthralgia, low-grade fever, and generalized lymphadenopathy. The skin and mucous membrane lesions occur over the entire body and are usually macular, but can be papular or nodular (Figure 36-7). These lesions are also found on the palms and soles (Figure 36-8). Other lesions include condyloma lata (Figure 36-9), which are moist flat, raised lesions usually seen around the anus and on mucous patches in the mouth and on the tongue (Figure 36-10). The first stage of secondary syphilis lasts 2–6 weeks, and the patient then enters the latent phase.

Latent syphilis is by definition the stage in which the results of a serologic test are positive for syphilis in the absence of any clinical symptoms. The duration of the infection is highly variable. Approximately one fourth of patients experience a relapse of secondary syphilis during this latent period, and only about one third of patients who progress to latent syphilis have signs and symptoms of tertiary syphilis.

Tertiary, or late, syphilis is a noncontagious but highly destructive phase of syphilis that develops over many years. Tertiary

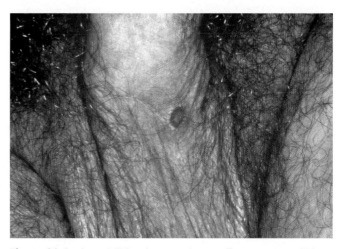

Figure 36-6. A syphilitic chancre due to *Treponema pallidum.* Image courtesy of the Centers for Disease Control and Prevention, Dr NJ Fiumara and Dr Gavin Hart.

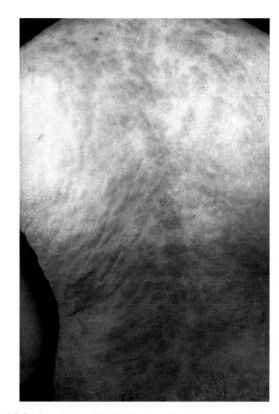

Figure 36-7. A patient with skin lesions due to secondary syphilis. Image courtesy of the Centers for Disease Control and Prevention, Dr Gavin Hart.

syphilis presents in three basic forms: gummatous syphilis (granulomatous lesions that coalesce in the skin, bone, and mucous membranes), cardiovascular syphilis, and neurosyphilis. Tertiary syphilis is extremely rare and will not be discussed in detail in this book.

Congenital syphilis results when maternal syphilis is transmitted in utero to the fetus after 16 weeks' gestation. If the mother is highly infective, the infant will be stillborn or present with early congenital syphilis manifested during the first 2 years of life by rhinitis (snuffles). Rhinitis is followed by skin and mucocutaneous lesions similar to those of an adult with secondary syphilis and by osteochondritis, hepatosplenomegaly and lymphadenopathy, immune complex-induced glomerulonephritis, or death.

Late congenital syphilis occurs in children after age 2. Manifestations include Clutton joints (painless symmetrical hydrarthrosis of the knee joint), deafness, Hutchinson teeth (notched and narrow edged permanent incisors) and mulberry-shaped molars, and bone abnormalities that include saddle nose, saber shins, and rhagades (fissures, cracks, or fine linear scars in the skin especially around the mouth).

EPIDEMIOLOGY

The highest incidence of syphilis occurs in young, sexually active persons aged 20–29 years of age.

There are approximately 30,000–40,000 new cases of primary and secondary syphilis diagnosed each year in the United States. The highest incidence occurs in southern states, with minority populations disproportionately affected.

About 300–400 cases of congenital syphilis are reported each year in the United States.

Humans are the only known host of *T pallidum,* and transmission is by sexual contact.

PATHOGENESIS

T pallidum enters the body via minute abrasions of epithelial cell linings, via penetration of mucous membranes, or via hair follicles. The organisms slowly multiply at the site of the infection, and eventually some organisms will enter the bloodstream and the lymphatics and infect the skin, endothelial cells, cartilage, joints, bones, neurons, and mucous membranes.

The organisms that multiply at the initial site of infection will cause the hard chancre seen in primary syphilis. The bacteria that are carried by the lymphatics and bloodstream to the lymph nodes will cause regional lymphadenopathy that occurs in patients with primary syphilis and the generalized lymphadenopathy that is seen in patients in the later stages of the disease. The organisms carried through the bloodstream to the skin and mucous membranes cause the lesions seen in secondary and tertiary syphilis. The organisms carried to the neurons and brain can cause the neurologic symptoms seen in tertiary syphilis. Bacteria carried to the endothelial cells weaken the wall of the blood vessel and cause the aneurysms that occur in cardiovascular syphilis.

In untreated cases of syphilis, one fourth of patients experience one or more relapses of secondary syphilis and develop

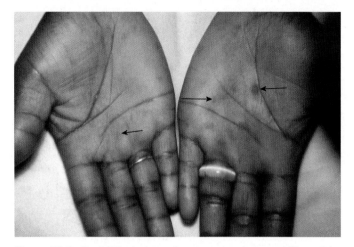

Figure 36-8. Syphilitic lesions due to secondary syphilis on the palms of the hands. Image courtesy of the Centers for Disease Control and Prevention.

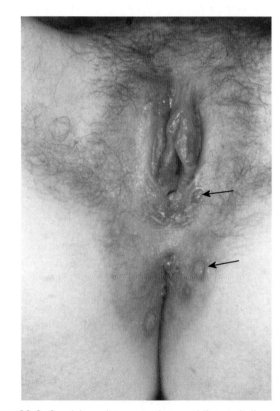

Figure 36-9. Condyloma lata on and around the genitalia and anus (*arrows*) of a patient with secondary syphilis. Image courtesy of the Centers for Disease Control and Prevention.

mucocutaneous lesions during the first 4 years. Antibiotic treatment in primary and secondary syphilis aborts the process; however, the changes associated with tertiary syphilis, except for gumma formation, are irreversible.

Congenital syphilis occurs following infection of the placenta. *T pallidum* is then spread through the bloodstream of the fetus to the skin, endothelial cells, cartilage, joints, bones, neurons, and mucous membranes. Because infection from the onset is systemic rather than localized, symptoms in the neonate with early onset disease are similar to symptoms of secondary syphilis in adults. Late onset symptoms in the infant are similar to those of tertiary syphilis in adults except that because the bones in an infant are still developing, there is more damage to the teeth, long bones, and joints in the infant.

DIAGNOSIS

Diagnosis of syphilis involves evaluation of presenting signs and symptoms. An examination of exudative material in syphilitic lesions using a dark field microscope (Figure 36-11) or a fluorescence microscope using fluorescein labeled anti-*T pallidum* antibodies will confirm diagnosis of a patient in early primary syphilis before serologic test results are positive.

Serologic tests are frequently used and are positive within 1 week after the appearance of the chancre in primary syphilis. The two different types of serologic tests used are the treponemal and the nontreponemal tests. Nontreponemal, or reagin tests, are used for screening and to determine treatment efficacy. Treponemal tests are used to confirm a positive nontreponemal test. Reagin tests measure antibodies that develop to cardiolipin lecithin following damage of host cells by *T pallidum*. Unfortunately, several other conditions, including viral hepatitis, infectious mononucleosis, malaria, pregnancy, and patients with connective tissue disease, can cause the body to produce anticardiolipin antibody and require the use of a treponemal serologic test to confirm a diagnosis of syphilis.

THERAPY AND PREVENTION

Penicillin is the drug of choice for treatment of syphilis. Reagin serologic tests for syphilis will become negative if the treatment has helped to eliminate the infection. Treatment of the pregnant mother before gestation week 16 will prevent congenital syphilis. Treatment after the 16th week also helps the fetus but may not alleviate all of the manifestations of congenital syphilis. Treatment of the neonate with penicillin is required if maternal treatment is inadequate or unknown, treatment has been with drugs other than penicillin, or if follow-up cannot be ensured.

Posttreatment follow-up is important because some patients may experience the Jarisch-Herxheimer reaction to therapy. This reaction is an intensification of existing syphilitic lesions or exacerbation of previous (old) syphilitic lesions following administration of penicillin. The Jarisch-Herxheimer reaction usually subsides within 24 hours. Spread of syphilis can be prevented by treating infected persons and identifying and treating their infected sexual partners.

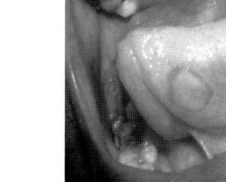

Figure 36-10. A mucous patch on the tongue of a patient with secondary syphilis. Image courtesy of the Centers for Disease Control and Prevention, Susan Lindsley.

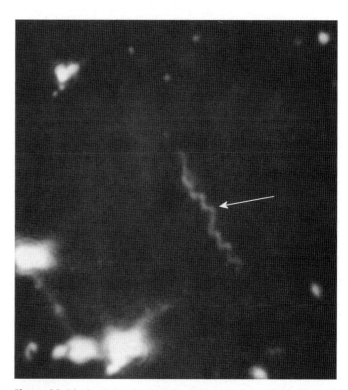

Figure 36-11. A photomicrograph of *Treponema pallidum* (*arrow*) using darkfield microscopy. Image courtesy of the Centers for Disease Control and Prevention, VDRL Department.

CHANCROID

Chancroid or soft chancre is a rare disease caused by *Haemophilus ducreyi*, and is usually present in urban areas with a high incidence of prostitution.

ETIOLOGY

Chancroid is an acute sexually transmitted infection that is caused by the gram-negative coccobacillus *H ducreyi*, which is similar to *H influenzae* in that neither can grow on blood agar but can only grow on chocolate agar plates or on plates supplemented with hemin and nicotinamide adenine dinucleotide (NAD).

MANIFESTATIONS

There is an incubation period of 1–14 days after exposure to *H ducreyi*. The soft chancre begins as a small inflammatory papule and eventually develops into a chancre (Figure 36-12). In contrast to the chancre seen in primary syphilis, chancroid chancres are painful and lack induration. Initially, the lesion is a solitary chancre, but multiple lesions can develop when uninfected skin comes in contact with the chancre. The chancre is accompanied by an acute, painful inflammatory inguinal lymphadenopathy that develops in over half of patients (Figure 36-13).

EPIDEMIOLOGY

About 20 cases of chancroid are reported each year in the United States.

Transmission of *H ducreyi* is by sexual contact. Prostitution is a major cause of the increase in cases of chancroid.

PATHOGENESIS

The organism, *H ducreyi*, enters the body through skin abrasions and produces a papule or vesicle that ulcerates to form the soft chancre. There is a dense inflammatory exudate with polymorphonuclear leukocytes. The soft chancres may heal quickly and spontaneously or they may persist and induce deep scars. Severe inguinal lymphadenopathy can be caused by bacteria that are transported by the lymphatics from the site of initial infection.

DIAGNOSIS

Diagnosis includes evaluation of the lesions for pain upon touch and induration. Specific diagnosis requires culture of *H ducreyi* on chocolate agar plates.

THERAPY AND PREVENTION

Chancroid can be treated with azithromycin, ceftriaxone, ciprofloxacin, or erythromycin. If treatment is successful, chancres usually improve within 7 days after therapy. Clinical resolution of regional lymphadenopathy is slower than that of chancres and may require needle aspiration or incision and drainage. Finding and treating the patient's infected sexual partners will prevent further spread of the disease.

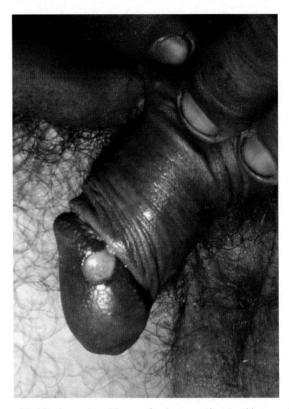

Figure 36-12. A penis with a soft chancre due to *Haemophilus ducreyi*. Image courtesy of the Centers for Disease Control and Prevention, Joe Miller.

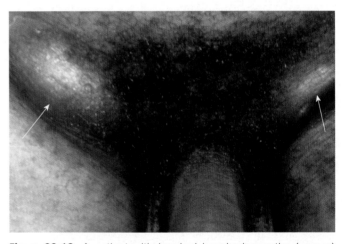

Figure 36-13. A patient with inguinal lymphadenopathy (*arrows*) due to chancroid. Image courtesy of the Centers for Disease Control and Prevention, Susan Lindsley.

DISEASES CHARACTERIZED BY URETHRITIS OR CERVICITIS

OVERVIEW

Urethritis is an infection characterized by urethral discharge of mucopurulent or purulent material and by dysuria or urethral pruritus. The most common causes of urethritis in men are *Neisseria gonorrhoeae* and *Chlamydia trachomatis*. Two diseases cause urethritis in men and will be discussed in this section—gonorrhea and nongonococcal urethritis. All of these diseases facilitate transmission of the human immunodeficiency virus (HIV).

Mucopurulent cervicitis is a purulent or mucopurulent endocervical exudate visible in the endocervical canal or in an endocervical swab specimen. It is frequently asymptomatic; however, if symptomatic, patients will have an abnormal vaginal discharge and vaginal bleeding. The most common causes of infectious mucopurulent cervicitis are *C trachomatis* and *N gonorrhoeae*. Mucopurulent cervicitis can be observed in gonorrhea and chlamydial infections.

GONORRHEA

Gonorrhea is a sexually transmitted disease involving infection by *N gonorrhoeae* of the epithelial cells that line the mucosa of the cervix and urethra.

ETIOLOGY

N gonorrhoeae is a small gram-negative diplococcus that has flattened surfaces between the adjacent individual cocci (shaped similar to a kidney bean or a coffee bean). Thayer-Martin medium (chocolate agar containing vancomycin, colistin, and nystatin) must be used to grow *N gonorrhoeae* from clinical samples. *N gonorrhoeae* will not grow on blood plates.

EPIDEMIOLOGY

- About 300,000–500,000 cases of gonorrhea are reported annually in the United States.
- Gonorrhea is more common in inner cities and in homosexual populations.
- The risk of contracting gonorrhea from an infected partner by heterosexual intercourse is 50% for women and 20% for men following a single exposure.
- Humans are the only known host of *N gonorrhoeae*, and infection is by sexual contact.

MANIFESTATIONS

Gonococcal infection in heterosexual men usually involves only the urethra. Patients present with inflammation and erythema around the opening of the urethra, a profuse purulent urethral discharge, and dysuria (Figure 36-14). Some men with gonorrhea are asymptomatic and are more likely to develop complications that include inguinal lymphadenitis, urethral stricture, epididymitis, prostatitis, septic arthritis, or disseminated gonococcemia with skin lesions (Figure 36-15).

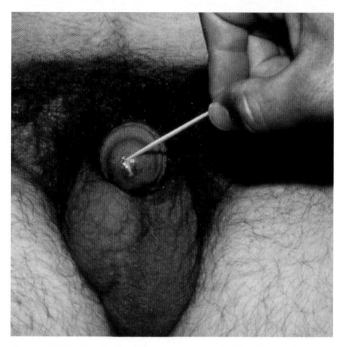

Figure 36-14. A patient with gonococcal urethritis. The urethra was stripped with a thin sterile urethral swab. The swab was inserted into the urethra, rotated, and pulled toward the orifice of the urethra to express purulent material. Image courtesy of the Centers for Disease Control and Prevention, Renelle Woodall.

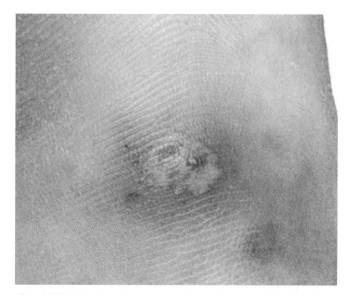

Figure 36-15. A skin lesion on a patient with a disseminated gonococcal infection. Image courtesy of the Centers for Disease Control and Prevention, Dr Wiesner.

Infection in homosexual men involves the urethra, the anal canal, and the pharynx. Anorectal infection is manifested by rectal pain and mucopurulent rectal discharge. Patients with pharyngeal gonorrhea are more likely to develop disseminated gonorrhea.

Women with gonorrhea are asymptomatic approximately one third of the time. In many cases, patients present with only vague, nonspecific symptoms and thus often do not seek medical treatment. The usual site of infection is the cervix, manifested upon examination by a purulent vaginal discharge or an inflamed and purulent cervix (Figure 36-16). Infection of the cervix frequently results in contiguous spread along mucous membranes to the urethra and rectum resulting in anorectal infection manifested by pain, purulent discharges, and rectal bleeding. Urethral infection includes signs and symptoms of purulent exudates, dysuria, increased urinary frequency, and bartholinitis. About 10–20% of cervical infections result in PID due to upward spread of the bacteria resulting in endometritis, salpingitis, tuboovarian abscesses, and pelvic peritonitis. The Fitz-Hugh-Curtis syndrome is associated with PID and is a form of perihepatitis resulting from direct inoculation of gonococci on the surface of the liver, which causes adhesions that form between the surface of the liver and the peritoneum lining the peritoneal space of the lower abdomen.

Disseminated gonococcal infections occur in about 1–3% cases of gonorrhea. Most patients are initially asymptomatic. Manifestations include low-grade fever, migratory polyarthralgia, septic arthritis with increased pain and swelling of the joints, purulent synovial fluids, and tenosynovitis, and petechial skin lesions (see Chapter 32).

If a pregnant woman is infected with gonococci, the organisms can infect the neonate during childbirth. These neonatal infections can include conjunctivitis and pharyngitis of the respiratory and gastrointestinal tracts of the neonate. Conjunctival infections (e.g., ophthalmia neonatorum) can rapidly cause blindness (Figure 36-17). The most severe manifestations of *N gonorrhoeae* infection in newborns are ophthalmia neonatorum, sepsis, arthritis, and meningitis.

PATHOGENESIS

The pathogenesis of gonorrhea is related to the ability of gonococci to attach to mucosal cells via their pili and then penetrate to submucosal areas to induce a strong influx of polymorphonuclear leukocytes. Many cases of gonorrhea will resolve without treatment; however complications are more likely to occur if gonorrhea is not treated with antibiotics.

DIAGNOSIS

Diagnosis of gonorrhea involves a threefold approach.

1. Evaluation of the patient's presenting signs and symptoms and sexual history.

2. Gram stain of a smear of the patient's purulent exudate (Figure 36-18). The smear is positive for gonorrhea if gram-negative diplococci are seen within polymorphonuclear leukocytes.

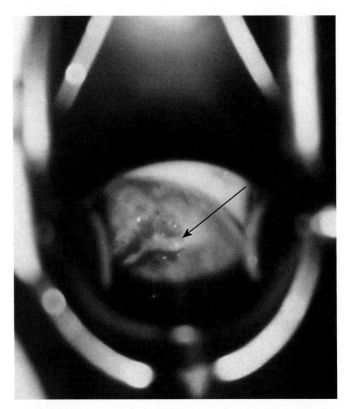

Figure 36-16. A photograph of a patient with cervicitis due to *Neisseria gonorrhoeae*. Note the purulent exudate on the cervix (*arrow*). Image courtesy of the Centers for Disease Control and Prevention.

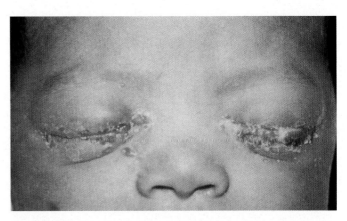

Figure 36-17. A newborn with ophthalmia neonatorum, an infection of the eyes due to *Neisseria gonorrhoeae*. Image courtesy of the Centers for Disease Control and Prevention, J Pledger.

3. Culture exudates for *N gonorrhoeae* using Thayer-Martin medium or testing the exudates for *N gonorrhoeae* infection by nucleic acid amplification techniques.

TREATMENT AND PREVENTION

Because many strains of *N gonorrhoeae* are resistant to penicillin (e.g., penicillinase-producing *N gonorrhoeae*), cephalosporins and quinolone antibiotics are now commonly used to treat these infections. The drugs of choice for uncomplicated cases of cervicitis, pharyngitis, urethritis, and proctitis are ceftriaxone or ciprofloxacin. If chlamydial infection cannot be ruled out, pharyngeal infections can be treated with ceftriaxone or ciprofloxacin plus azithromycin or doxycycline. Disseminated infections require a parenteral antibiotic treatment with ceftriaxone until 24–48 hours after improvement begins. Then oral treatment with ciprofloxacin should be given for at least 1 week.

Ophthalmia neonatorum can be treated with ceftriaxone. Routine treatment with silver nitrate ($AgNO_4$), erythromycin, or tetracycline applied directly to the eye following birth prevents ophthalmia neonatorum.

Preventing transmittal requires improved education of sexually active individuals, proper reporting, follow-up of patients and their contacts, use of condoms, and chemoprophylaxis to prevent ophthalmia neonatorum. Culturing pregnant women for gonorrheal infection before delivery and treating those who are infected can prevent gonorrheal infections of the newborn.

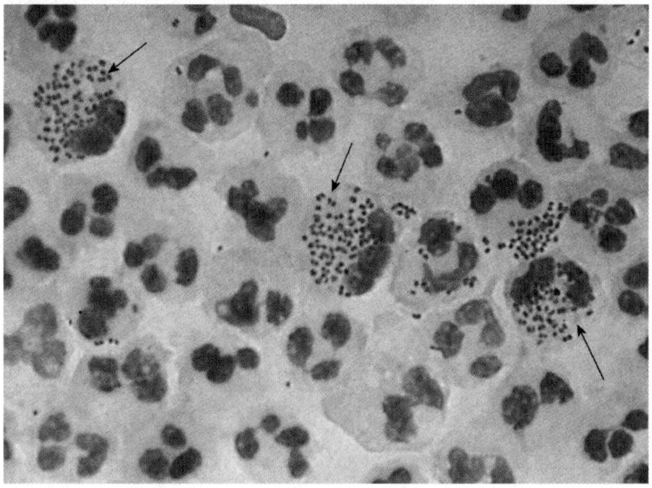

NONGONOCOCCAL URETHRITIS

Nongonococcal urethritis (NGU) is the most frequent cause of urethritis in heterosexual men. Nearly one half of patients with gonococcal urethritis also have nongonococcal urethritis.

ETIOLOGY

Chlamydia trachomatis is the most frequent cause of NGU, but there are a number of other organisms that can cause the infection including *Ureaplasma urealyticum, Mycoplasma genitalium, Trichomonas vaginalis, Gardnerella vaginalis,* and HSV.

MANIFESTATIONS

The patient usually has a history of urethral discharge and may have pain on urination and pruritus in the meatal region of the urethra. *The urethral discharge of a patient with NGU can be differentiated from a patient with gonococcal urethritis in that the patient with gonorrhea has a purulent discharge, whereas the patient with NGU will have a serous and clear discharge.* Complications of NGU among patients infected with *C trachomatis* include epididymitis and Reiter syndrome (arthritis, urethritis, and conjunctivitis).

EPIDEMIOLOGY

The prevalence of NGU differs by age group, with patients between the ages of 15 and 30 with multiple sex partners at highest risk.

Figure 36-18. A photomicrograph of a Gram stain of urethral discharge due to *Neisseria gonorrhoeae*. Notice the large number of polymorphonuclear leukocytes and the intracellular gram-negative diplococci in some cells (*arrows*). Image courtesy of the Centers for Disease Control and Prevention, Joe Miller.

- In the United States, over of 50% of cases of urethritis are nongonococcal.

- The incidence of NGU is more common in heterosexual populations such as college students and in suburban or rural populations.

- NGU is unusual in monogamous relationships. Most cases occur if the man or his partner has had one or more new partners in the preceding months.

- NGU is transmitted almost exclusively through sexual contact involving penis-to-vagina or penis-to-rectum contact.

DIAGNOSIS

Diagnosis of NGU requires demonstration of a polymorphonuclear leukocyte response in the urethral discharge or urine and exclusion of *N gonorrhoeae* urethritis. Urethral inflammation may be diagnosed by the presence of one of the following: a visible abnormal clear serous urethral discharge and a positive leukocyte esterase test in the urine from a man younger than age 60 or microscopic evidence of urethritis (i.e., ≥5 white blood cells per high-power field) on a Gram stain of a urethral smear. No evidence of *N gonorrhoeae* urethritis as demonstrated by culture, Gram stain of a smear of the urethral discharge, or nucleic acid detection should be detected.

TREATMENT AND PREVENTION

Patients with NGU can be treated with azithromycin or doxycycline. All sexual partners should be examined for STIs and promptly treated to prevent recurrences of NGU. If the patient with NGU has been treated and continues to complain of dysuria, less common causes of NGU should be sought. For instance, NGU due to *Trichomonas vaginalis* should be treated with metronidazole plus azithromycin.

CHLAMYDIAL INFECTIONS

Chlamydial genital infections are the most frequently reported infectious disease in the United States. Most persons infected with this bacterial pathogen have no symptoms of infection, although serious and life-threatening complications occur in thousands of women after untreated infection with *Chlamydia trachomatis*.

ETIOLOGY

C trachomatis serovars D and K cause these infections.

MANIFESTATIONS

Asymptomatic infection is common among both males and females. Symptomatic chlamydial infection is rare in females; however, if symptomatic, it is usually mucopurulent cervicitis (Figure 36-19). If not treated, several important sequelae can result from symptomatic and asymptomatic *C trachomatis* infection in females, with the most serious including PID, ectopic pregnancy, and infertility. Symptomatic males usually have urethritis, as described in the above discussion of NGU.

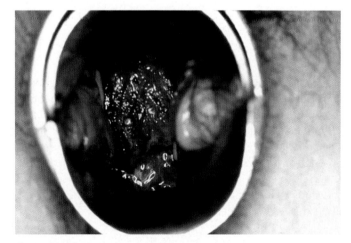

Figure 36-19. A photograph of the cervix of a patient with cervicitis due to *Chlamydia trachomatis*. Note the erosion and erythema on the cervix. Image courtesy of the Centers for Disease Control and Prevention, Dr Lourdes Fraw and Jim Pledger.

EPIDEMIOLOGY

The prevalence of chlamydial infections is highest in sexually active persons younger than 25 years of age.

Over 900,000 chlamydial infections were reported in the United States in 2005. The reported rate of infection was 496.5 cases per 100,000 persons.

C trachomatis is a sexually transmitted bacterial infection.

DIAGNOSIS

Sensitive and specific methods used to diagnose chlamydial infections include both tissue culture used to grow the organism and nonculture tests that detect the presence of *C trachomatis* or its DNA from clinical samples. *C trachomatis* urogenital infections can be diagnosed in females by testing urine or swab specimens collected from the endocervix. Urethral infection in males can be diagnosed by testing a urethral swab specimen or urine specimen. Rectal infections can be diagnosed by testing a rectal swab specimen. Culture, direct immunofluorescence, enzyme immunoadsorbent assay, nucleic acid hybridization tests, and nucleic acid amplification tests are available for the detection of *C trachomatis* on endocervical and urethral swab specimens. Chlamydial culture is rarely used to confirm a diagnosis of *C trachomatis* infection.

TREATMENT AND PREVENTION

Patients with chlamydial infections can be treated with azithromycin or doxycycline. Treatment of this bacterial infection in pregnant women prevents transmission of *C trachomatis* to infants during birth. Treatment of sexual partners helps to prevent reinfection of the treated patient and infection of other partners.

Screening and treatment of cervical infection can reduce the number of patients who develop PID due to chlamydial infection. Sexually active females from 13 to 25 years of age and older women with risk factors that predispose them to chlamydial infection (e.g., new or multiple sexual partners) should be screened annually and treated if positive for *C trachomatis* infection.

OTHER SEXUALLY TRANSMITTED INFECTIONS

OVERVIEW

The remaining diseases discussed in this chapter cause diseases that cannot be placed in the categories discussed previously. PID manifests in any number of ways, including fever, adnexal masses, pain on cervical motion, vaginal bleeding, and abdominal pain. The human papillomaviruses (HPV) can cause warty lesions or infect the cervix and penis without producing any detectable signs and symptoms. However, it is the undetected HPV infections that can in time lead to invasive cervical carcinoma and in rare cases penile carcinoma. This section of the chapter will include a discussion of PID and HPV.

PELVIC INFLAMMATORY DISEASE

PID is a disease of females and is defined as the clinical syndrome resulting from the ascending spread of microorganisms from the vagina and endocervix to the endometrium, the fallopian tubes, and other contiguous structures. It can include any combination of endometritis, salpingitis, tubo-ovarian abscess, and pelvic peritonitis.

ETIOLOGY

N gonorrhoeae and *C trachomatis* serovars D and K are the most common causes of PID. Other causes include anaerobic bacteria (e.g., *Bacteroides, Prevotella, Peptostreptococcus,* and *Peptococcus*), *Streptococcus*, facultative gram-negative and gram-positive rods (e.g., *Gardnerella vaginalis, Escherichia coli,* and *Haemophilus influenzae*), *Mycoplasma hominis*, and *Actinomyces israelii*.

MANIFESTATIONS

The signs and symptoms of PID vary depending on the location and extent of the infection (Figure 36-20). Many women with PID have minimal symptoms, and some may be asymptomatic ("silent PID"). Symptoms that may occur in a patient with PID include moderate fever (>38.3°C), bilateral lower abdominal pain that is maximal in the region of the fallopian tubes, increased vaginal discharge, irregular bleeding, tenderness on cervical motion, dyspareunia, tender adnexal mass, purulent endocervical discharge, and nausea and vomiting. Only about 20% of females with PID manifest all these signs. If the infection is limited to the cervix and endometrium, the patient usually has vaginal discharge and irregular bleeding. If the infection has ascended up into the fallopian tubes and gained access to the peritoneum, the patient usually has fever, irregular bleeding, bilateral lower abdominal pain, tenderness on cervical motion, tender adnexal masses, nausea and vomiting, and abdominal rebound tenderness. Dissemination to the liver can result in a perihepatitis called Fitz-Hugh-Curtis syndrome in which adhesions appear similar to "violin strings" and are found between the abdominal wall and the liver capsule. Other complications include unilateral or bilateral ovarian abscesses, tubal occlusion and scarring, adhesions, chronic abdominal pain, and death.

EPIDEMIOLOGY

PID is the most common cause of involuntary infertility in women. Approximately 12% of women are infertile after a single episode of PID, almost 25% after two episodes, and over 50% after three or more episodes.

Over 1 million women have at least one episode of PID per year. Complications associated with PID require more than 212,000 hospital admissions and 115,000 surgical procedures annually.

Over 100,000 women become infertile each year due to PID, and more than 150 women die due to the infection.

Sexually active teenagers are three times more likely than sexually active 25- to 29-year-old women to develop PID following an untreated *C trachomatis* or *N gonorrhoeae* infection.

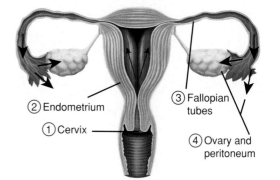

**PID
Ascension of Infection**

② Endometrium
① Cervix
③ Fallopian tubes
④ Ovary and peritoneum

Figure 36-20. A schematic showing the female genital tract with symptoms that may be present when infection enters a particular area of the genital tract. **1,** The bacteria infect the cells lining the cervix and vagina, causing vaginal discharge and cervicitis. **2,** The infection ascends into the endometrium, causing irregular vaginal bleeding and pain associated with endometritis. **3,** The infection spreads to the fallopian tubes, causing abdominal pain, adnexal masses, and pain on cervical motion associated with salpingitis or abscess in the fallopian tubes. **4,** The infection leaves the fallopian tubes, causing abdominal pain, nausea, vomiting, adnexal masses, pain on cervical motion, and rebound abdominal tenderness associated with tubo-ovarian abscess, peritonitis, or Fitz-Hugh-Curtis syndrome.

- After one episode of PID, a woman's risk of ectopic pregnancy increases sevenfold, compared with the risk for women who have no history of PID.
- PID develops following an untreated sexually transmitted infection.

PATHOGENESIS

PID occurs in a woman when an infection of the vagina and cervix ascends to the upper genital tract. Prior asymptomatic infections of the fallopian tubes due to *N gonorrhoeae* or *C trachomatis* result in damage to the ciliary cells lining the fallopian tubes. If another infection occurs, the organisms are then able to ascend the fallopian tubes and cause infections in contiguous structures. Sexually active women in their childbearing years are most at risk; women younger than age 25 as opposed to women older than age 25 are more likely to develop PID. The cervix of teenage girls and young women is not fully matured, and as a result, these patients are more likely to develop STIs that result in PID. Hormonal changes that occur during menses lead to cervical alterations that may result in loss of a mechanical barrier preventing ascent of the infection. The bacteriostatic effect of cervical mucus is lowest at the onset of menses. Uterine instrumentation (e.g., insertion of an intrauterine device) also facilitates upward spread of vaginal and cervical bacteria.

DIAGNOSIS

Clinical diagnosis of PID is difficult because of the wide variation in signs and symptoms among patients with this condition. Most patients with PID have either mucopurulent cervical discharge or evidence of inflammation when white blood cells are observed on a microscopic evaluation of a saline preparation of vaginal fluid. A diagnosis of PID is unlikely if the cervical discharge appears normal and there are no white blood cells on the vaginal fluid saline preparation,

Definitive diagnosis requires endometrial biopsy with histopathologic evidence of endometritis—transvaginal sonography or magnetic resonance imaging techniques showing thickened, fluid-filled tubes; direct visualization of inflamed fallopian tubes seen on laparoscopy or laparotomy; or biopsy evidence of salpingitis. Only a confirmed culture of a biopsy of the fallopian tube positively identifies the etiology of salpingitis. Unfortunately, these means of confirming the diagnosis are often not readily available for acute cases nor easily justified when symptoms and signs are mild or vague. Therefore, the diagnosis of PID is often based on clinical findings supplemented with results of cultures or nonculture tests of specimens obtained from the endocervix (e.g., enzyme immunoadsorbent assay, nucleic acid hybridization tests, and nucleic acid amplification tests).

Empiric treatment for PID should be given to sexually active adolescents and young women or other women at risk for PID (Table 36-2) when no other cause for illness can be identified (e.g., negative pregnancy test; no acute appendicitis) and if the following minimum criteria are met: uterine or adnexal tenderness and cervical motion tenderness. Requiring both of these criteria may result in low sensitivity in some patients who are at high risk for infection. A more elaborate diagnostic evaluation

TABLE 36-2. Risk Factors or Behaviors that Predispose a Person to Development of PID

- Multiple sex partners or new sex partner
- History of previous PID
- Menstruation
- IUD (for contraception) (more likely the first few months after insertion of the device)
- Single, divorced, and separated women are at higher risk
- Use of vaginal douching
- Asymptomatic gonococcal or chlamydial infection in either sexual partner

PID, pelvic inflammatory disease; IUD, intrauterine device.

may be necessary, since an incorrect diagnosis and inappropriate management can cause unwanted patient morbidity. Additional criteria that can be used to enhance the sensitivity of the minimum criteria are listed in Table 36-3.

TREATMENT AND PREVENTION

Treatment of PID is often empiric and should cover the wide variety of possible etiologies. To prevent the long-term sequelae that result from PID, antibiotic therapy should be administered as soon as a presumptive diagnosis has been made. PID can be treated on an outpatient basis but only if the patient's temperature is lower than 38°C, the white blood cell count in the peripheral blood sample is <11,000/mm³, there is minimal evidence of peritonitis and there are active bowel sounds, and the patient is able to tolerate oral nourishment and treatment. However, if the conditions identified in Table 36-4 are present, the patient should be hospitalized for treatment.

Due to the many different pathogens capable of causing PID, broad-spectrum antibiotic treatment should be employed. Inpatient therapy includes intravenous administration of cefotetan or cefoxitin and oral doxycycline or intravenous clindamycin and gentamicin. Parenteral therapy is usually given until 24–48 hours after the patient shows clinical improvement, and then oral therapy is initiated.

Oral therapy can be utilized to initiate therapy in many patients; however, if there is no response to this therapy within 72 hours, the patient should be reevaluated to confirm the diagnosis and should then be given parenteral therapy. Oral therapy includes ofloxacin or levofloxacin with or without metronidazole or ceftriaxone or cefoxitin plus doxycycline with or without metronidazole. Follow-up of the patient after therapy is essential due to the higher failure rates of therapeutic regimens.

To prevent future episodes of PID, the patient's sexual partners should be tested for STIs. If the patient has an intrauterine device to prevent pregnancy, the device should be removed during therapy. Annual or biannual chlamydial screening of sexually active adolescent girls can reduce the incidence of the chlamydial infections that cause scarring and put patients at risk of acquiring PID.

HUMAN PAPILLOMAVIRUS INFECTIONS

There are over 100 different types of HPV and about 30 of these types can infect the genitalia. Some types will produce the raised rough verrucae (cauliflower-like) genital warts called condyloma acuminata. Other types do not initially produce any observable lesion; however, they do infect the epithelial cells of the cervix and penis and can in time cause carcinoma of these organs.

ETIOLOGY

HPV types 6 and 11 are the most common types that cause genital warts. HPV-16 and HPV-18 are the most common causes of cervical and penile carcinoma.

TABLE 36-3. Additional Criteria that Support a Diagnosis of PID

- Oral temperature >38.3°C
- Abnormal cervical or vaginal mucopurulent discharge
- Presence of white blood cells on saline microscopy of vaginal secretions
- Elevated ESR
- Elevated C-reactive protein
- Laboratory documentation of cervical infection with *Neisseria gonorrhoeae* or *Chlamydia trachomatis*

PID, pelvic inflammatory disease; ESR, erythrocyte sedimentation rate.

TABLE 36-4. Conditions that Require Hospitalization in the Treatment of the Patient with PID

- Pregnant patient
- Patient does not respond clinically to oral antimicrobial therapy
- Patient is unable to follow or tolerate an outpatient oral regimen
- Patient has severe illness, nausea and vomiting, or high fever
- Patient has a tubo-ovarian abscess
- There is a surgical emergency (e.g., appendicitis)

PID, pelvic inflammatory disease.

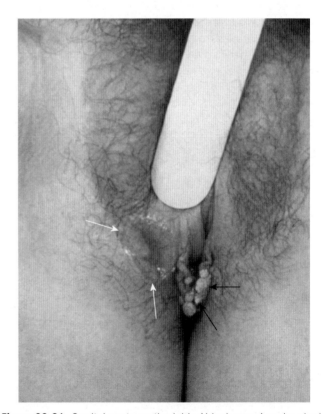

Figure 36-21. Genital warts on the labia (*black arrow*) and a single chancre due to *Treponema pallidum* (*white arrow*). Image courtesy of the Centers for Disease Control and Prevention, Susan Lindsley.

MANIFESTATIONS

Condyloma acuminata are usually soft, fleshy, cauliflower-like lesions (exophytic) that may be present on skin, external genitalia, perineum, perianal, and intra-anal regions (Figure 36-21). The genital warts may also be painful, friable, and pruritic.

In many cases, HPV-16 and HPV-18 infections of the cervix and penis do not produce any recognizable lesions. These HPV types have been associated with vaginal, anal, and cervical intraepithelial dysplasia and squamous cell carcinoma.

EPIDEMIOLOGY

- **Genital warts** caused by HPV-6 and HPV-11 are the most common viral STIs in the United States. Over 1 million cases of genital warts are reported annually.

- HPV-6 and HPV-11 cause external genital warts and are only rarely associated with invasive squamous cell carcinoma.

- Recurrence of genital warts within the first several months after treatment is common and usually indicates recurrence rather than reinfection.

- Infection with HPV-6 and HPV-11 is almost always by sexual contact.

- HPV-16 or HPV-18 viral DNA has been found in over 85% of cases of cervical carcinomas and is believed to be the major cause of invasive cervical carcinoma.

- **Cervical carcinoma** is the third most common gynecologic malignancy and the eighth most common malignancy among women in the United States.

- The average age of developing cervical cancer is about 50 years.

- HPV-16 and HPV-18 viral DNA has been found in between 60 and 90% of cases of **penile carcinoma.**

- Risk of cervical cancer is inversely related to age at first intercourse and directly related to the lifetime number of sexual partners. Risk of cervical cancer is also increased for sexual partners of men whose previous partners had cervical cancer.

- Cervical carcinoma due to HPV is a sexually transmitted infection.

PATHOGENESIS

HPV infects and replicates in the squamous epithelial cells (keratinocytes) that are present in the skin and mucous membranes. The incubation period for genital wart formation is from 3 to 4 months. HPV types 6 and 11, which cause genital warts, induce the keratinocytes to proliferate. HPV-induced keratinocyte proliferation thickens the stratum granulosum as well as the basal and prickle cell layers in the stratum spinosum, resulting in the verrucae that are seen in patients with genital warts. The virus causes keratinocytes to become koilocytes, described as enlarged keratinocytes with a halo around a smaller than normal nucleus. Genital warts remain localized and usually recede spontaneously. Recurrences of genital warts are more common in immunosuppressed patients.

The neoplastic HPV types 16 and 18 also infect the keratinocytes and then integrate into the host chromosome. The

E6 and E7 genes of these HPV viruses are expressed and their protein products bind to and inactivate host cell proteins that suppress cell growth and multiplication (i.e., p53 and p105). Cell-growth suppressors p53 and p105 are essential in limiting keratinocyte multiplication, and without active suppressor proteins p53 and p105, the keratinocytes grow rapidly and are more susceptible to mutation, chromosomal aberrations, or action of some other cofactor (e.g., toxins from tobacco smoke) and develop into neoplastic cells.

DIAGNOSIS

Diagnosis of the cauliflower-like lesions of HPV is usually clinically determined; however, these lesions should be differentiated from condyloma lata (e.g., condyloma lata are soft, unlike the rough genital wart) and molluscum contagiosum (molluscum contagiosum has an umbilicated lesion). Diagnosis of genital warts can be confirmed by biopsy.

Placing a solution of 3–5% acetic acid on the cervix or penis can reveal the acetowhite epithelium of patients with HPV-16 and HPV-18. A Papanicolaou test, or "PAP" smear as it is often called, should be performed to determine if there is koilocytosis in the cells obtained from the cervix. A definitive diagnosis of HPV infection is based on detection of viral nucleic acid (DNA or RNA) or capsid protein in samples taken from the cervix or penis.

TREATMENT AND PREVENTION

The goal of treating genital warts is removal of the lesions. If left untreated, genital warts can resolve, remain unchanged, or increase in size and number. Currently available therapies for genital warts reduce infectivity but do not eradicate infectivity. The various treatments that exist to remove genital warts include cryotherapy, surgical excision, laser vaporization, or chemical cautery with podophyllin, podophyllotoxin, or trichloroacetic acid.

If there are no genital warts or cervical squamous intraepithelial lesions present in women, treatment is not recommended whether diagnosed by colposcopy, biopsy, acetic acid application, or by detection of HPV with laboratory tests. Genital HPV infection often resolves spontaneously, and no therapy has been identified that can eradicate infection. Annual PAP smears should be performed to stage HPV infections and to treat the patient based on the stage of the disease. Treatment may include cryotherapy, laser vaporization, loop excision, cone biopsy, or hysterectomy.

To avoid transmission, avoid contact with lesions. The use of latex condoms has been associated with a lower rate of cervical cancer. A quadrivalent vaccine against HPV types 6, 11, 16, 18 is available and licensed for females aged 9–26 years.

SECTION 11

QUESTIONS AND DISCUSSIONS

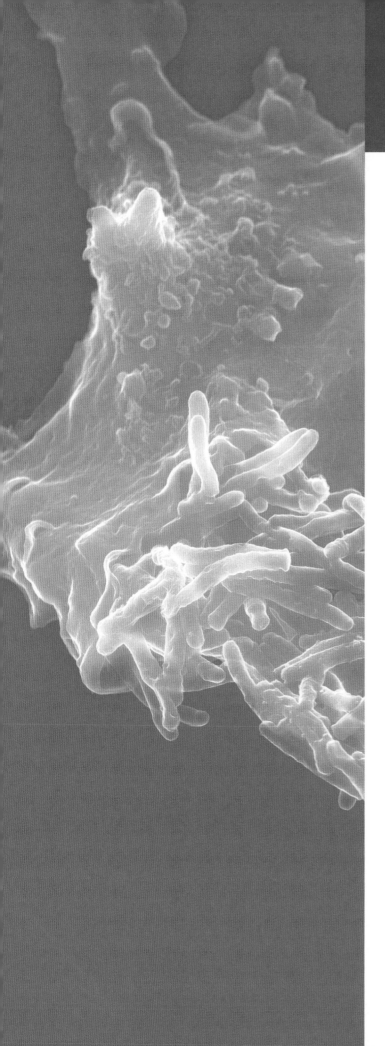

CHAPTER 37

PRACTICE EXAMINATION

DIRECTIONS

Each numbered item is followed by options. Select the best answer to each question. Some options may be partially correct, but there is only *ONE BEST* answer.

Questions 1 and 2

A 6-year-old girl is taken to the pediatrician because of a swollen and painful upper eyelid, similar to that shown in the figure below. The eyelid began bothering her about 2 days ago. Her vital signs are normal.

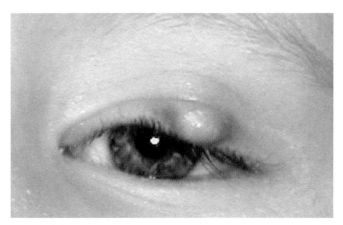

1. Which of the following is the most likely diagnosis of this patient's condition?
   A. Hordeolum
   B. Blepharitis
   C. Periorbital cellulitis
   D. Orbital cellulitis
   E. Conjunctivitis

2. Culture of the purulent material from the lesion is grown aerobically on blood agar plates. Only one colony type grew on the plate, and those colonies are beta hemolytic and produce a gold pigment. The colonies are gram-positive cocci in clumps and are catalase positive and coagulase positive. Which of the following organisms is the mostly likely cause of this patient's infection?

   A. *Streptococcus pyogenes*

   B. *Streptococcus pneumoniae*

   C. *Staphylococcus aureus*

   D. *Staphylococcus epidermidis*

   E. *Propionibacterium acne*

Questions 3 and 4

A 5-year-old boy is brought into the clinic with a rash that started on his trunk and now has spread to his face and extremities. Other than the rash, he appears healthy. His vital signs are temperature of 37.8°C, pulse 100/min, blood pressure 110/80 mm Hg, and respirations 21/min. He started kindergarten 3 weeks ago and mentions that some of his classmates have had a similar rash and had to miss school. A physical examination reveals a rash that is primarily on the boy's abdomen; there are a few lesions on his face and extremities, similar to those shown in the figure below. This child has no history of immunizations.

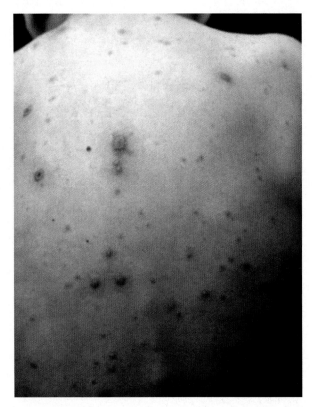

Image courtesy of the Centers for Disease Control and Prevention.

3. Which of the following is the most likely disease affecting this patient?

   A. Chickenpox

   B. Rubella

   C. Rubeola

   D. Shingles

   E. Systemic herpes

4. Which virus is the most likely cause of this patient's infection?

   A. Rubella virus

   B. Measles virus

   C. Herpes simplex virus

   D. Cytomegalovirus

   E. Varicella-zoster virus

5. A 35-year-old man complains that his left hip is painful after being punctured by a tool when he was at work 4 days ago. After cleaning the wound quickly, he went on about his work. The wound now has pus in it, and it is erythematous and swollen. Physical examination reveals a purulent and relatively deep skin lesion with an erythematous swollen region around the puncture that extends up to 2 cm from the wound, similar to that shown in the figure below. A sample of the purulent material obtained from the lesion is cultured on a blood agar plate and Gram stained. The resulting colonies are gram-positive cocci in clusters that are beta hemolytic, catalase positive, and coagulase positive. Which of the following organisms is the most likely cause of this patient's infection?

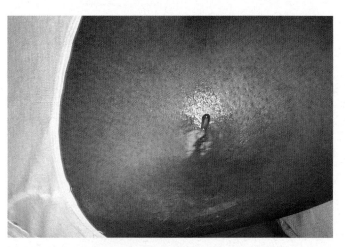

Image courtesy of the Centers for Disease Control and Prevention, Bruno Coignard, MD, and Jeff Hageman, MHS.

   A. *Streptococcus pyogenes*

   B. *Staphylococcus epidermidis*

   C. *Staphylococcus aureus*

   D. *Corynebacterium* sp.

   E. *Clostridium perfringens*

6. A 24-year-old woman comes to the clinic with complaints of a runny nose and congestion. Physical examination reveals erythematous nasal passages with clear mucus draining from the patient's nose. No pain on palpation of the sinuses is noted. Her vital signs are temperature 37°C, pulse 73/min, blood pressure 120/85 mm Hg, and respirations 18/min. Which of the following is the most common cause of this patient's condition?

A. Respiratory syncytial virus

B. Rhinovirus

C. Coxsackie virus

D. Echovirus

E. *Mycoplasma pneumoniae*

7. A 60-year-old woman sees her physician because of complaints of difficulty walking up stairs and being out of breath. She has a productive cough. Her vital signs are temperature 38.9°C, pulse 120/min, blood pressure 130/90 mm Hg, and respirations 24/min. Auscultation of the patient's lungs reveals rales and dullness to percussion in the left lower lobe. Chest radiograph reveals consolidations in the left lower lobe. An image of the Gram stain of a smear of the patient's sputum is shown in the photomicrograph below. Which of the following organisms is the most likely cause of this patient's infection?

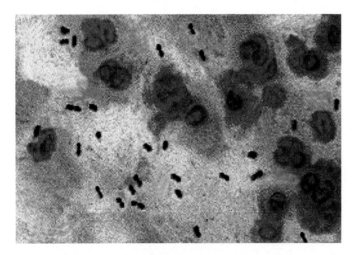

A. *Staphylococcus aureus*

B. *Streptococcus agalactiae*

C. *Streptococcus pneumoniae*

D. *Mycoplasma pneumoniae*

E. *Enterococcus faecalis*

Questions 8 and 9

A 72-year-old man with diabetes mellitus sees his physician because of complaints of intense pain and swelling in the right ear. The patient mentions that he has participated in a water aerobics class three times a week for the past 2 weeks. His vital signs are temperature 38.9°C, pulse 110/min, blood pressure 140/90 mm Hg, and respirations 21/min. Lymphadenopathy is noted just anterior to the tragus, and there is significant swelling and purulent material in the ear canal.

8. Which of the following is the most likely diagnosis of this patient's current infection?

A. Otitis media

B. Otitis externa

C. Mastoiditis

D. Sinusitis with extension to the ear

E. Subdural empyema

9. Culture of a sample of the purulent material in the ear canal contained many lactose-negative, oxidase-positive colonies on MacConkey agar. A Gram stain of one of the colonies contained many gram-negative, rod-shaped bacteria. Which of the following organisms is the most likely cause of this patient's current infection?

A. *Escherichia coli*

B. *Proteus mirabilis*

C. *Pseudomonas aeruginosa*

D. *Staphylococcus aureus*

E. *Streptococcus pneumoniae*

10. A 65-year-old woman goes to the clinic because she has a cough and says that she feels like she has a fever. She mentions that she had a headache and a runny nose a few hours before the cough began. The cough initially was nonproductive, but the woman now mentions that she is coughing up something that looks like pus. Her vital signs are temperature 37.8°C, pulse 90/min, blood pressure 110/80 mm Hg, and respirations 17/min. Auscultation reveals moist crackles in both lungs. After receiving a breathing treatment with albuterol, the crackles are not auscultated. Chest radiographs are negative for infiltrates and consolidations. Which of the following best describes this patient's condition?

A. Common cold

B. Pharyngitis

C. Bronchiolitis

D. Bronchitis

E. Pneumonia

11. A 2-year-old girl is brought to the emergency department because of a paroxysmal cough and fever. She has had a runny nose and a mild, occasional cough for the past week. She is sneezing. Her temperature is 37.8°C. The mother says the cough is now much worse, with the coughing episodes lasting up to 1 minute. She says that the child sometimes turns "blue" when coughing and yesterday fainted following a particularly severe episode. A physical examination reveals a very ill and distressed child. A coughing episode began in the emergency department and lasted for about 30 seconds. The coughing was short and rapid and ended with a high pitched sound associated with inhalation. Significant inspiratory stridor was noted, but no other abnormal breath sounds were auscultated. No dullness to lung percussion was noted. The patient's vital signs are temperature 38.9°C, pulse 130/min, blood pressure 130/90 mm Hg, and respirations 27/min. The child has no history of immunization. A complete blood count reveals a significant lymphocytosis. Which of the following is the most likely diagnosis for this patient's condition?

A. Viral croup

B. Pertussis

C. Bronchitis

D. Bronchiolitis

E. Pneumonia

Questions 12 and 13

12. A 5-year-old boy is brought to the pediatrician with lesions just under his nostrils (refer to the figure top right). His vital signs are temperature 37°C, pulse 80/min, blood pressure 110/80 mm Hg, and respirations 20/min. Which of the following is the most likely diagnosis of this patient's condition?

A. Cellulitis

B. Oral herpes

C. Carbuncle

D. Impetigo

E. Furuncle

13. If a culture of the patient's lesion contains many gram-positive, catalase-negative, beta-hemolytic, and bacitracin-sensitive cocci, which of the following is the most likely cause of this patient's infection?

A. *Staphylococcus aureus*

B. *Streptococcus pyogenes*

C. *Streptococcus pneumoniae*

D. *Enterococcus faecalis*

E. *Neisseria meningitidis*

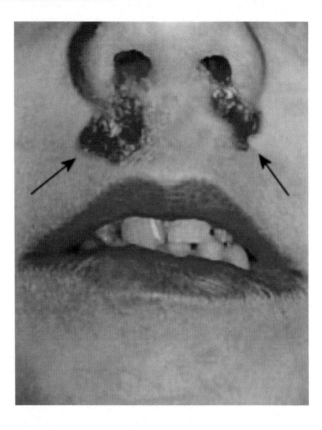

Questions 14–16

A 15-year-old boy sees his physician because of complaints of sore throat and pain when he moves his jaw. The boy mentions feeling tired and having a fever for the past 3 days. The jaw pain has increased over the past 24 hours. His vital signs are temperature 38.3°C, pulse 90/min, blood pressure 110/80 mm Hg, and respirations 18/min. Physical examination reveals a nonexudative erythematous pharynx with petechia on the hard palate. There is significant bilateral anterior cervical lymphadenopathy. A complete blood cell count is significant for a lymphocytosis with large numbers of atypical lymphocytes. Results of a heterophile antibody test are negative.

14. Which of the following Epstein-Barr virus (EBV) titers would indicate that this patient has acute infectious mononucleosis?

A. No antibodies to viral capsid antigen (VCA) and Epstein-Barr nuclear antigen (EBNA)

B. Immunoglobulin M (IgM) to EBNA and no antibodies to VCA

C. IgM to VCA and no antibodies to EBNA

D. IgG to both VCA and EBNA

E. IgM to both VCA and EBNA

15. Which of the following could also cause an increase in atypical lymphocytes and result in similar clinical symptoms manifested by this 15-year-old patient?

 A. Coxsackievirus

 B. Herpes simplex virus

 C. Varicella-zoster virus

 D. Cytomegalovirus

 E. Hepatitis B virus

16. If this patient has an Epstein-Barr virus infection, in which of the following cell types would this virus cause cell multiplication?

 A. Erythrocytes

 B. Neutrophils

 C. Macrophages

 D. T lymphocytes

 E. B lymphocytes

17. A 55-year-old man came to the clinic with complaints of pain on the right lower portion of his rib cage. Physical examination elicits pain to the touch along the intercostal dermatome. Vesicular skin lesions similar to those shown in the figure below are also observed. Which of the following is the most likely cause of this patient's condition?

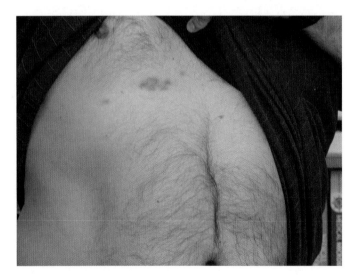

 A. Herpes simplex virus 1

 B. Herpes simplex virus 2

 C. Cytomegalovirus

 D. Epstein-Barr virus

 E. Varicella-zoster virus

Questions 18–21

A 28-year-old pregnant woman arrives at the clinic in need of prenatal care. She is in week 6 of gestation. After reading the patient's history, you notice that she has refused all vaccinations.

18. Which of the following could cause a congenital infection in her fetus if she has not been infected by this microorganism prior to the pregnancy?

 A. *Toxoplasma gondii*

 B. Cytomegalovirus

 C. Herpes simplex viruses

 D. Rubella virus

 E. *Treponema pallidum*

19. Which of the following organisms should be swabbed from the vagina and rectum of a patient when she is at gestation week 35 to see if she is colonized with this common cause of neonatal disease?

 A. *Escherichia coli*

 B. *Streptococcus agalactiae*

 C. Herpes simplex virus 2

 D. *Treponema pallidum*

 E. *Neisseria gonorrhoeae*

20. During the patient interview, the patient discloses that about 1 year ago she used intravenous drugs and that she had used methamphetamine about 12 months ago for a period of 3 months. She says that she successfully completed a drug rehabilitation program and has not used intravenous drugs for the past 9 months. If two different blood samples are collected from this patient and ELISA results are positive for human immunodeficiency virus (HIV), which of the following must be conducted to confirm a diagnosis of HIV infection?

 A. Western blot

 B. Southern blot

 C. Northern blot

 D. Culture

 E. A second ELISA

21. If this pregnant patient is positive for human immunodeficiency infection (HIV), which of the following drugs most significantly reduces the rate of transmission from mother to child?

 A. Zidovudine and nevirapine

 B. Zidovudine alone

 C. Nevirapine alone

 D. Abacavir

 E. Efavirenz

22. A 25-year-old man who is an intravenous drug user is about to enter a drug rehabilitation program and must have a blood test to determine his hepatitis B virus (HBV) serologic status. The results of his serologic tests are HBs-Ag negative, anti-HBs positive, and positive anti-HBc. What is this patient's current HBV status?

   A. The patient was previously vaccinated for HBV

   B. He has an acute HBV infection

   C. He is in the "window period" of HBV infection

   D. He has chronic HBV infection

   E. He had a previous HBV infection

23. A 25-year-old man presents with a lesion on his right forearm. Physical examination reveals a lesion similar to that seen in the figure below. Pain can be elicited when the center of the lesion is pricked with a pin. A KOH wet mount confirms what you thought was causing this lesion. Which of the following is the most likely diagnosis of this patient's condition?

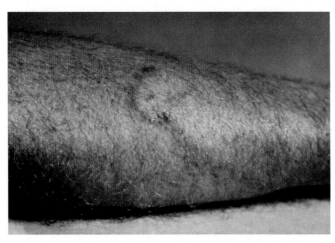

Image courtesy of the Centers for Disease Control and Prevention.

   A. Leprosy

   B. Anthrax

   C. Tinea capitis

   D. Tinea corporis

   E. Tinea versicolor

Questions 24 and 25

A 21-year-old woman at 16 weeks' gestation presents with several vesicular lesions on her labia majora. When asked if the lesions have appeared previously, she mentions that she has had them at other times. Results of a Tzanck test are positive.

24. Which of the following organisms is the most common cause of this patient's infection?

   A. Herpes simplex virus 1

   B. Herpes simplex virus 2

   C. Cytomegalovirus

   D. *Treponema pallidum*

   E. *Microsporum gypseum*

25. Knowing that this patient is pregnant and has a recurring infection and to prevent infection of her child, the physician should advise the patient about which of the following?

   A. Deliver the infant vaginally even if these lesions are present during labor and delivery

   B. Deliver the infant by caesarian section if the lesions are present during labor and delivery

   C. Deliver the infant vaginally while treating the mother with acyclovir

   D. Avoid sexual relations with partners who have lesions similar to these

   E. Have the pregnancy terminated because the lesions are a sign that the fetus has been infected in utero and is highly likely to be adversely affected or die

26. A 32-year-old man presents with a vesicular lesion on his lower lip (refer to the figure below). He mentions getting this type of lesion about five or six times a year. Which of the following organisms is the most common cause of this patient's current infection?

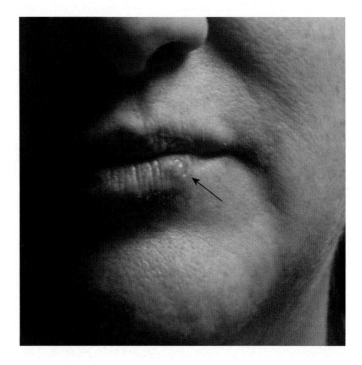

   A. Herpes simplex virus 1

   B. Herpes simplex virus 2

   C. Cytomegalovirus

   D. *Candida albicans*

   E. *Microsporum gypseum*

27. A 65-year-old man sees his physician because he is having perineal pain and difficulty urinating. Rectal examination of the prostate gland reveals a prostate that is enlarged, tender, and warm to the touch. He mentions only having had the problem for the past 2 days. Which of the following organisms is the most common cause of this patient's condition?

    A. *Staphylococcus saprophyticus*

    B. *Staphylococcus aureus*

    C. *Proteus mirabilis*

    D. *Pseudomonas aeruginosa*

    E. *Escherichia coli*

28. A 24-year-old woman sees her physician because of pruritus and erythema of her genitalia. Physical examination reveals erythematous labia majora and minora. A gynecologic examination is performed. The patient's cervix appears similar to that shown in the figure on the right. A sample of the white material collected from the cervix is smeared on a slide and Gram stained, similar to that shown in the figure on the right. Which of the following organisms is the most likely cause of this patient's infection?

    A. *Candida albicans*

    B. *Gardnerella vaginalis*

    C. *Trichomonas vaginalis*

    D. Herpes simplex virus 2

    E. *Lactobacillus acidophilus*

29. A 42-year-old man presents to a clinic with acute onset of low-grade fever (37.8°C), watery nonbloody diarrhea, abdominal cramping, and nausea and vomiting. No fecal leukocytes are observed in his stool sample. He mentions just returning from a cruise ship tour of islands in the Bahamas. Which of the following organisms is the most common cause of this patient's condition?

    A. Rotavirus

    B. Adenovirus

    C. Norovirus

    D. *Entamoeba histolytica*

    E. *Shigella sonnei*

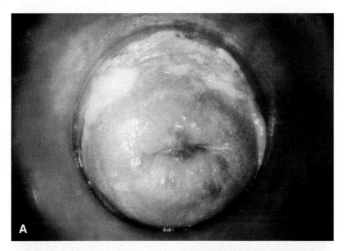

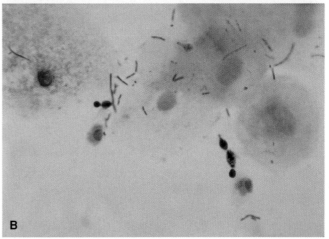

Image A courtesy of the Centers for Disease Control and Prevention. Image B courtesy of the Centers for Disease Control and Prevention, Dr Stuart Brown.

30. A 29-year-old woman presents with areas of hyperpigmentation on her chest (refer to the figure A below). The erythematous lesions are neither pruritic nor edematous. A skin scraping is smeared on a slide and H&E stained (the results are shown in the figure B below). Which of the following organisms is the most likely cause of this patient's infection?

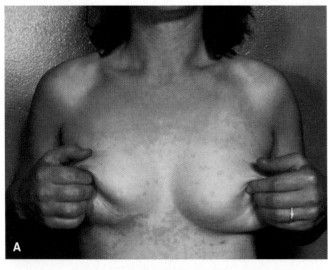

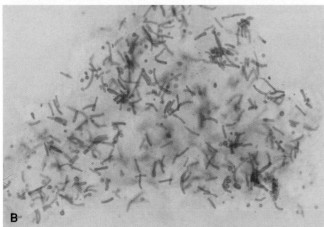

Images courtesy of the Centers for Disease Control and Prevention, Dr Lucille K Georg.

A. *Candida albicans*

B. *Streptococcus pyogenes*

C. *Staphylococcus aureus*

D. *Malassezia furfur*

E. *Blastomyces dermatitides*

31. A 45-year-old woman goes to a clinic because she has many pus-filled lesions on the inner aspects of both thighs, similar to those shown in the figure below. She has just returned from a 5-day cruise. When asked what activities she participated in while on the cruise, she states that she did a lot of shopping on the islands, sunbathing on the ship, and at night she spent several evenings in the ship's hot tub. Some of the pustules were opened, and the purulent material was collected and sent to the laboratory for culture. Many gram-negative, rod-shaped, nonlactose fermenting colonies were obtained. Which of the following organisms is the most likely cause of this patient's condition?

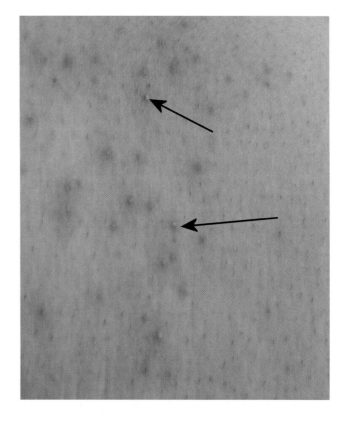

A. *Staphylococcus aureus*

B. *Streptococcus pyogenes*

C. *Moraxella catarrhalis*

D. *Escherichia coli*

E. *Pseudomonas aeruginosa*

Questions 32 and 33

A 20-year-old woman at 12 weeks' gestation arrived in the clinic for a routine prenatal care visit. She mentioned having no major problems other than morning sickness. A urine sample is obtained. A dipstick test reveals pyuria and the presence of nitrites. A quantitative assay for bacteria in the urine reveals 500,000 CFU/mL in the sample. A Gram stain of the lactose-fermenting bacteria contained many gram-negative rods.

32. Which of the following organisms is the most common cause of her asymptomatic bacteriuria?

A. *Staphylococcus saprophyticus*

B. *Escherichia coli*

C. *Proteus mirabilis*

D. *Klebsiella pneumoniae*

E. *Pseudomonas aeruginosa*

33. Which of the following complications is most likely to occur in a pregnant woman who has asymptomatic bacteriuria?

A. Pneumonia

B. Stillbirth of the fetus

C. Peritonitis

D. Pyelonephritis

E. Spinal osteomyelitis

34. A 5-year-old boy was taken to the pediatrician because of fever and runny nose. His parents mentioned that he had a cold about 2 weeks ago. Other than the runny nose, he seemed to be fine until about 2 days ago when he developed a fever and complained of pain just below his right eye. His vital signs are temperature 38.9°C, pulse 110/min, blood pressure 110/80 mm Hg, and respirations 21/min. Physical examination reveals pain when pressure is applied over the right maxillary sinus. The nasal passages are both inflamed. The right nasal passage contains purulent material that is draining from a partially blocked nasal ostium. Which of the following organisms is the most likely cause of this patient's current condition?

A. *Streptococcus pneumoniae*

B. *Staphylococcus aureus*

C. *Streptococcus pyogenes*

D. *Escherichia coli*

E. *Aspergillus niger*

Questions 35 and 36

A 72-year-old man presented to his physician with complaints of severe generalized headache, stiff neck, and fever. He says that the headache and fever began about 2 hours before he came to the clinic. His vital signs are temperature 40°C, pulse 130/min, blood pressure 160/95 mm Hg, and respirations 21/min. Kernig and Brudzinski signs are both positive. No papilledema or skin lesions are noted. A lumbar puncture is performed, and the opening pressure is noted as 200 mm H_2O. The cerebrospinal fluid (CSF) appears turbid. An analysis of the CSF reveals an increase in protein, a decrease in glucose concentration, and 1500 white blood cells/mm^3. Most of the leukocytes are polymorphonuclear leukocytes.

35. Based on this patient's signs and symptoms and the findings of the cerebrospinal fluid analysis, which of the following is the most likely diagnosis of this patient's infection?

A. Acute bacterial meningitis

B. Aseptic meningitis

C. Chronic meningitis

D. Viral encephalitis

E. Rabies

36. A Gram stain of some of the cerebrospinal fluid is performed, and appears similar to that shown in the figure below. Which of the following organisms is the most likely cause of this patient's infection?

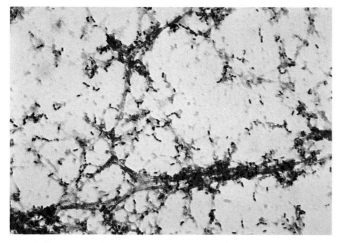

Image courtesy of the Centers for Disease Control and Prevention, Dr Mike Miller.

    A. *Neisseria meningitidis*

    B. *Streptococcus pneumoniae*

    C. *Streptococcus pyogenes*

    D. *Staphylococcus aureus*

    E. *Enterococcus faecalis*

Questions 37 and 38

A 55-year-old woman saw her physician because of complaints of bloody diarrhea and malaise. She states that she has had severe abdominal cramps and watery diarrhea for the past 2 days. When she had a bowel movement this morning, she said that she noticed blood in her stool. When asked about what she may have eaten or drunk recently, she remembered drinking unpasteurized apple juice about 4 days ago. Her vital signs are temperature 37°C, pulse 100/min, blood pressure 120/85 mm Hg, and respirations 19/min. Fecal specimens grown on sorbitol containing MacConkey agar isolated several lactose fermenting gram-negative, rod-shaped organisms.

37. Which of the following organisms is the most likely cause of this patient's condition?

    A. *Campylobacter duodenale*

    B. *Shigella sonnei*

    C. *Escherichia coli* (an enterohemorrhagic strain)

    D. *Escherichia coli* (an enterotoxigenic strain)

    E. *Escherichia coli* (an enteropathogenic strain)

38. If this patient is treated with an antibiotic, more toxin is released from the bacteria and can result in renal failure. Which toxin causes this syndrome?

    A. Endotoxin

    B. Shiga toxin

    C. Toxin A

    D. Labile toxin

    E. Exotoxin B

Questions 39 and 40

A 43-year-old woman went to a clinic because of conjunctivitis in her left eye, similar to that shown in the figure below. She also has pharyngitis. She mentions to the physician that it feels like something is in her eye and it feels itchy. Upon examination, no exudate is seen in the eye. When asked, she does not mention any exudate being present when she awakened that morning. Physical examination reveals a nonexudative erythematous pharynx. Preauricular lymphadenopathy is noted on the left side. On closer inspection, follicles are seen in the palpebral conjunctiva of the left eye. Her vital signs are temperature 37°C, pulse 85/min, blood pressure 120/85 mm Hg, and respirations 18/min.

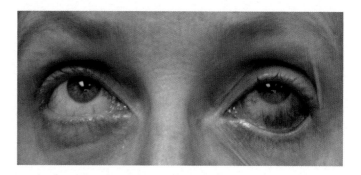

39. Which of the following is the most likely diagnosis of this patient's condition, as shown in the above figure?

    A. Hordeolum

    B. Anterior blepharitis

    C. Posterior blepharitis

    D. Dacryocystitis

    E. Conjunctivitis

40. Which of the following organisms is the most likely infectious cause of this patient's condition?

    A. Adenovirus

    B. *Staphylococcus aureus*

    C. *Haemophilus influenzae*

    D. *Chlamydia trachomatis*

    E. Herpes simplex virus

Questions 41–46

A 32-year-old woman saw her physician because of complaints of soreness in her mouth that started about 1 month ago. She does not complain about any other problems except that she has been bothered from time to time with fatigue and she notices that her lymph nodes are frequently swollen in several areas on her body. Physical examination reveals lymphadenopathy of the cervical, axillary, and inguinal lymph nodes. Her pharynx appears similar to that shown in the figure below.

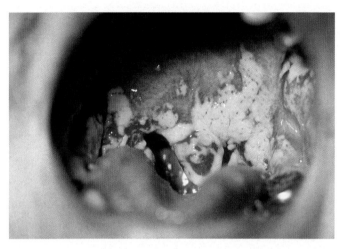

Image courtesy of the Centers for Disease Control and Prevention.

41. Which of the following is the most likely diagnosis of this patient's condition?

    A. Perlèche

    B. Thrush

    C. Gingivostomatitis (viral)

    D. Diphtheria

    E. Streptococcal pharyngitis

42. A sample of the material obtained from the patient's pharynx was sent to the laboratory for culture and Gram stain. The material grew as creamy white colonies on blood agar and Sabouraud dextrose agar with chloramphenicol. A Gram stain of one of the colonies contains large oval gram-positive budding organisms. Which of the following organisms is the most likely cause of this patient's current pharyngeal problems?

    A. Herpes simplex virus

    B. *Corynebacterium diphtheria*

    C. *Streptococcus pyogenes*

    D. *Candida albicans*

    E. *Neisseria gonorrhoeae*

43. The patient first mentioned that the exudate in her mouth has been there for about 4 weeks. However, about 2 days ago, she stated that it has become difficult and painful for her to swallow. She mentions having epigastric pain and has experienced nausea and vomiting. Which of the following is the most likely diagnosis of a patient with these signs and symptoms?

    A. Esophagitis

    B. Gastric ulcer

    C. Duodenal ulcer

    D. Gastroenteritis

    E. Gastroesophageal reflux disease

44. Upon further questioning, you discover that the patient is a recovering intravenous drug user. She mentions earning money as a prostitute to buy drugs. She states that she has not taken any illegal drugs for the past 8 months. If this patient's serologic test results are positive for human immunodeficiency virus ((HIV) using both ELISA and Western blot assays, which of the following would best describe her current condition?

    A. Primary HIV infection

    B. Asymptomatic HIV infection (clinical category A)

    C. Symptomatic HIV but not clinical category A or C (clinical category B)

    D. Acquired immunodeficiency syndrome (AIDS) (clinical category C)

    E. Indeterminate HIV infection

45. When examining the patient for the presence of skin lesions, you notice several dark purple lesions on her back. Which of the following is the most likely cause of these skin lesions?

    A. Human immunodeficiency virus (HIV)

    B. Human herpes virus 2 (HHV-2)

    C. HHV-3

    D. HHV-4

    E. HHV-5

    F. HHV-6

    G. HHV-7

    H. HHV-8

46. Which of the following would be appropriate provided the patient is willing to comply with treatment of her HIV infection?

    A. Wait and see because she is not far enough along in the disease process

    B. Single anti-HIV drug therapy

    C. Dual anti-HIV drug therapy

    D. Triple anti-HIV drug therapy

47. A 35-year-old man goes to a clinic because he is nauseated and has been vomiting for the past 2 hours. He states that about an hour after eating at a Chinese restaurant, he began feeling nauseated and vomited. While being examined, he experiences an episode of projectile vomiting. He states that his noon meal at the restaurant consisted of fried rice and chicken. His vital signs are temperature 37°C, pulse 90/min, blood pressure 130/90 mm Hg, and respirations 18/min. Cultures of the chicken contained no significant contamination; however, gram-positive, rod shaped bacterial colonies were obtained from the fried rice. Which of the following organisms is the most likely cause of this patient's condition?

A. *Staphylococcus aureus*

B. *Bacillus cereus*

C. *Clostridium perfringens*

D. *Campylobacter jejuni*

E. *Clostridium botulinum*

48. Which of the following is the most common cause of food poisoning in the United States?

A. *Staphylococcus aureus*

B. *Bacillus cereus*

C. *Clostridium perfringens*

D. *Campylobacter jejuni*

E. *Clostridium botulinum*

Questions 49 and 50
A 2-year-old boy is brought to the pediatrician by his parents because he has a temperature of 38.3°C. He is limping and complains of pain in the left knee. The parents state that the child has been limping for the past day and now refuses to walk. When the physician asks the child to walk, the child has a noticeable limp but does not complain of pain when at rest. No history of trauma is reported. There is no history of joint stiffness or chronic fatigue. No other joints are involved. Upon examination of the left knee, there is no limitation in flexion or extension. There is mild diffuse tenderness that is poorly localized over the medial femoral condyle. No soft tissue swelling or joint effusion is noted. No pain is elicited with range of motion testing of the left knee. The remaining extremities do not have any tenderness or swelling. His vital signs are temperature 38.3°C, pulse 110/min, blood pressure 100/80 mm Hg, and respirations 22/min. A complete blood count reveals a white blood cell count of 13,400 μL and a differential of 75% polymorphonuclear leukocytes, 5% lymphocytes, and 1% bands. The erythrocyte sedimentation rate is 45 mm/h. The boy is taken to the hospital for a bone scan, which shows significant inflammation in the epiphysis of the lower left femur.

49. Which of the following organisms is the most common cause of this patient's condition?

A. *Neisseria gonorrhoeae*

B. *Streptococcus pyogenes*

C. *Streptococcus agalactiae*

D. *Escherichia coli*

E. *Staphylococcus aureus*

50. Which of the following would be the most appropriate duration of antibiotic therapy for this patient's condition?

A. No antibiotic treatment is necessary

B. 5 days

C. 10 days

D. 2 weeks

E. 4–6 weeks

Questions 51 and 52
A 36-year-old man sees his physician because he is experiencing pain upon urination. Physical examination reveals a purulent urethral discharge from the penis, shown in figure A below. Further questioning reveals that the patient has had several sexual partners while he was recently estranged from his wife. Physical examination of the patient's penis shows a discharge, which is collected and sent to the laboratory. The patient denies having had sexual relations with his wife for the past 2 months. His vital signs are all within normal range. A smear and Gram stain of the urethral discharge is similar to that shown in figure B below.

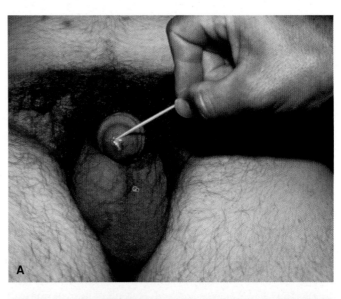

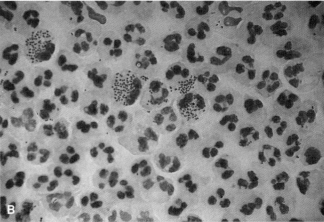

Images courtesy of the Centers for Disease Control and Prevention, Renelle Woodall.

51. Which of the following is the most likely diagnosis of this patient's infection?

A. Syphilis

B. Chlamydia

C. Gonorrhea

D. Genital herpes

E. Genital warts

52. A 31-year-old woman, the wife of the patient in Question 51, goes to the clinic because of fever and joint pain. She states that over the past 2 weeks her ankles have been swollen and painful, and she is now experiencing similar pain and swelling in her knees. She mentions that just before the fever and joint pain began that she had a sore throat. Further questioning reveals that she has not had sexual relations with anyone for the past 5 months; however, she states that she did perform oral sex on her husband recently. Her vital signs are temperature 37.8°C, pulse 90/min, blood pressure 110/80 mm Hg, and respirations 18/min. Physical examination reveals several lesions on her feet and ankles and both knees are swollen and red, similar to that shown in the figure below. Passive range of motion testing is painful for the patient. Synovial fluid is removed from both knees, Gram stained, and cultured. Which of the following media would be most helpful in isolating the causative agent from the synovial fluid?

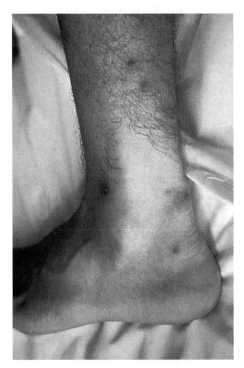

Image courtesy of the Centers for Disease Control and Prevention, Dr SE Thompson, VCCD, and J Pledger

A. Blood agar plates

B. Campy medium

C. MacConkey agar plates

D. Thayer-Martin plates

E. Bordet-Gengou agar plates

Questions 53 and 54

A 40-year-old man has spent the past week hiking various trails in Connecticut, Rhode Island, and Massachusetts. Toward the end of the trip, he states that he began to experience fever, malaise, and myalgia. While taking a shower this morning, he said that he noticed a rash on his upper right arm, similar to that shown in the figure below. After further questioning, the patient remembers removing a tick from his arm 2 days ago.

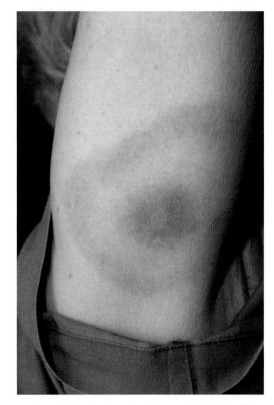

Image courtesy of the Centers for Disease Control and Prevention, James Gathany.

53. Which of the following organisms is the most likely cause of this patient's condition?

A. *Rickettsia rickettsii*

B. Varicella-zoster virus

C. *Borrelia burgdorferi*

D. *Borrelia hermsii*

E. *Francisella tularensis*

54. Which of the following is the most appropriate treatment for this patient's condition?

A. Doxycycline

B. Penicillin

C. Tobramycin

D. Erythromycin

E. Vancomycin

Questions 55–57

About 5 days after returning from a camping trip to Arkansas in June, a 25-year-old man sees his physician because of fever, severe headache, myalgia, nausea and vomiting, and anorexia. His vital signs are temperature 40°C, pulse 120/min, blood pressure 130/90 mm Hg, and respirations 21/min. Physical examination reveals several petechial lesions on his wrists and ankles. You also notice the lesions are present on the soles of his feet and palms of his hands. A complete blood count indicates that the platelet count is 75,000/mL and the hematocrit is 35%, but other values are within normal range.

55. Which of the following is the most common means of transmitting the causative agent of this patient's condition?

  A. Fleas

  B. Rabbits

  C. Flies

  D. Ticks

  E. Kissing beetles

56. Which of the following is the most likely cause of this patient's current condition?

  A. *Francisella tularensis*

  B. *Babesia microti*

  C. *Rickettsia rickettsii*

  D. *Bartonella henselae*

  E. *Ehrlichia chaffeensis*

57. Which of the following would be the most appropriate treatment for this patient's condition?

  A. Penicillin

  B. Ceftriaxone

  C. Kanamycin

  D. Streptomycin

  E. Doxycycline

Questions 58–60

A 10-year-old boy is taken to a clinic because of fever and pharyngitis. His vital signs are temperature 38.9°C, pulse 120/min, blood pressure 120/85 mm Hg, and respirations 21/min. His parents state that he vomited several times last night and that he seems to feel much worse today than he did yesterday. Physical examination reveals tender cervical lymphadenopathy and an erythematous pharynx, similar to that shown in figure A above. He has no cough, conjunctivitis, or runny nose. A throat swab is plated on blood agar plates and a bacitracin disk is placed on the plate, as shown in the following figure B above and on the right. Gram stain of the etiologic agent contains gram-positive cocci in chains.

58. Which of the following is the most likely causative organism of this patient's current condition?

  A. Adenovirus

  B. Epstein-Barr virus

  C. *Arcanobacterium haemolyticum*

  D. *Streptococcus pyogenes*

  E. *Corynebacterium diphtheriae*

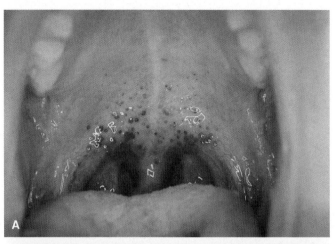

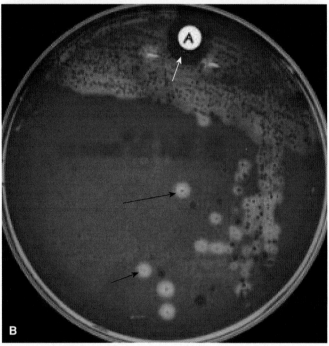

Image on the left courtesy of the Centers for Disease Control and Prevention, Dr Heinz F Eichenwald

59. Treatment of this patient with antibiotics will reduce the chances that he will develop which of the following conditions?

  A. Glomerulonephritis

  B. Rheumatic fever

  C. Scarlet fever

  D. Hemolytic uremic syndrome

  E. Erythema chronicum migrans

60. Which of the following agents would be used to treat this patient's condition?

  A. Penicillin

  B. Ciprofloxacin

  C. Gentamicin

  D. Vancomycin

  E. Rifampin

Questions 61–63

An 8-year-old girl with no history of childhood immunizations presents with pharyngitis and a low-grade fever (38°C). Physical examination reveals a severely swollen and edematous neck region. Her cervical lymph nodes can be palpated and are also swollen. Her pharynx is erythematous, and it is painful for her to swallow. The gray material at the back of her throat caused some bleeding when removed for cultures. The patient also mentioned not being able to feel the roof of her mouth. Her breath has an unpleasant odor, and she has a dry cough. An inspiratory stridor is noted upon auscultation of the lungs.

61. Which of the following is the most likely diagnosis of this patient's condition?

- A. Diphtheria
- B. Pertussis
- C. Streptococcal pharyngitis
- D. Thrush
- E. Hand, foot, and mouth disease

62. Which of the following vaccines would have prevented the disease in this patient?

- A. *Haemophilus influenzae* type b (Hib)
- B. Hepatitis B (Hep B)
- C. Diphtheria, tetanus toxoids, and acellular pertussis (DTaP)
- D. Pneumovac
- E. Poliomyelitis vaccine

63. Treatment of this patient first involves the administration of

- A. antitoxin
- B. antibiotics
- C. diphtheria, tetanus toxoids, and acellular pertussis vaccine (DTaP)
- D. corticosteroids
- E. antiepileptics

Questions 64 and 65

A 33-year-old man sees his physician because he says that he has a "high fever." He states that he felt fine 2 days ago but that by yesterday afternoon he started feeling sick. His vital signs are temperature 40°C, pulse 130/min, blood pressure 130/90 mm Hg, and respirations 22/min. Physical examination reveals some needle track marks on his arms. When the patient is asked about the marks, he admits to having used intravenous drugs several times over the past week. Auscultation of his heart reveals a high pitched holosystolic murmur that is louder during inspiration and softer during exhalation.

64. Which of the following is the most likely diagnosis of this patient's condition?

- A. Pericarditis
- B. Myocarditis
- C. Subacute endocarditis
- D. Acute endocarditis
- E. Rheumatic heart disease

65. Which of the following is the most likely cause of this patient's current condition?

- A. Coxsackievirus
- B. Human immunodeficiency virus (HIV)
- C. *Streptococcus mitis*
- D. *Enterococcus faecalis*
- E. *Staphylococcus aureus*

Questions 66 and 67

A 41-year-old man presented to his physician with crampy bilateral lower quadrant pain that decreased after bowel movements. He has a low-grade fever of 37.8°C. He states that his bowel movements are watery but there is no blood in them, and that he has had about 15 bowel movements in the past 24 hours. About 1 week before he began having diarrhea, the patient finished a 3-week course of antibiotic to treat acute bacterial prostatitis. A complete blood count reveals a leukocytosis of 20,000 white blood cells/µL. A colonoscope shows numerous elevated yellow-white plaques with the intervening mucosa being hyperemic and edematous.

66. Which of the following is the most likely causative organism of this patient's condition?

- A. *Staphylococcus aureus*
- B. *Shigella sonnei*
- C. *Vibrio cholera*
- D. *Clostridium difficile*
- E. *Campylobacter jejuni*

67. If detected by ELISA in a stool sample, which of the following toxins would confirm your diagnosis?

- A. Cholera toxin
- B. Exotoxin A
- C. Toxin A and B
- D. Shiga toxin
- E. Staphylococcal enterotoxin

68. A 27-year-old woman presented to her physician with dysuria and increased frequency of urination. A dipstick test of the patient's urine specimen is positive for leukocyte esterase and nitrites. The pH of her urine sample is 8.1. Which of the following organisms is the most likely cause of this patient's condition?

- A. *Staphylococcus saprophyticus*
- B. *Escherichia coli*
- C. *Klebsiella pneumoniae*
- D. *Proteus mirabilis*
- E. *Candida albicans*

69. A 12-year-old boy from New York presented with shaking chills, fatigue, arthralgia, anorexia, nausea and vomiting, cough, and dyspnea. He has no history of foreign travel. A urine sample collected from the patient is a dark color. His vital signs are temperature 38.9°C, pulse 120/min, blood pressure 120/85 mm Hg, and respirations 22/min. Physical examination reveals hepatosplenomegaly and yellow sclera and yellowing of his skin. A complete blood cell count indicates that the patient had a normochromic normocytic anemia, thrombocytopenia, and a leukopenia with a large number of atypical lymphocytes present. The photomicrograph below shows a smear of a blood sample taken from the patient. Which of the following is the most likely cause of this patient's condition?

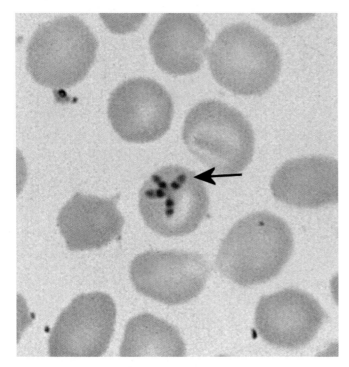

Image courtesy of the Centers for Disease Control and Prevention, Steven Glenn, Laboratory & Consultation Division.

    A. *Plasmodium*

    B. *Babesia*

    C. *Listeria*

    D. *Yersinia*

    E. *Bartonella*

Questions 70–73

A 75-year-old woman was brought to a clinic because she was experiencing chills and confusion. The patient's medical record indicates that she had been diagnosed with cystitis 2 weeks ago. When the patient's daughter was asked if her mother took the medication prescribed, the daughter stated that her mother could not afford the medicine and said that she would "ride out the pain." The patient's vital signs are temperature 35°C, pulse 130/min, blood pressure 95/75 mm Hg, and respirations 25/min. Physical examination of the patient reveals costovertebral angle tenderness. Blood cultures and a complete blood count (CBC) are obtained. The CBC contains a leukocyte count of 25,000/mm^3 and 11% bands.

70. Which of the following is the best description of this patient's condition?

    A. Systemic inflammatory response syndrome (SIRS)

    B. Sepsis

    C. Severe sepsis

    D. Septic shock

    E. Multiorgan dysfunction syndrome (MODS)

71. The patient is admitted to the hospital and antibiotic treatment is begun immediately. Which of the following would be the most appropriate antimicrobial treatment for this patient?

    A. Ceftriaxone and gentamicin

    B. Cefepime and gentamicin

    C. Piperacillin-tazobactam and gentamicin

    D. Ciprofloxacin and gentamicin

    E. Vancomycin and cefepime

72. Which of the following tests would be the most specific in determining if this patient has developed disseminated intravascular coagulation (DIC)?

    A. Complete blood cell count

    B. Serum electrolytes

    C. D-dimers

    D. Partial thromboplastin time

    E. Lactic acid levels

73. The patient's blood culture contained many lactose fermenting colonies that were shown by Gram stain to be gram-negative rods. Which of the following is the most likely cause of this patient's current condition?

    A. *Escherichia coli*

    B. *Proteus mirabilis*

    C. *Klebsiella pneumoniae*

    D. *Staphylococcus saprophyticus*

    E. *Streptococcus pneumoniae*

74. A 70-year-old man presents to his physician with dyspnea, confusion, a nonproductive cough, and chest pain. About 1 week ago, the weather became very hot so the man took a window air conditioner that had been stored in the basement and put it in the living room window so he could get some relief from the heat. A family member mentions that the patient complained of abdominal pain and diarrhea and vomiting yesterday and that today they noticed that his urine was pink. His vital signs are temperature 40°C, pulse 60/min, blood pressure 110/90 mm Hg, and respirations 27/min. Auscultation of his lungs reveals bilateral rales in the upper lobes of both lungs. A chest radiograph shows patchy infiltrates bilaterally in the upper lobes of both lungs. A Gram stain of a sputum sample contains many polymorphonuclear leukocytes but few bacteria. A Dieterle silver stain of the same sample can be seen in figure below. A urine antigen test of this etiologic agent is positive. Which of the following is the most likely causative agent of this patient's condition?

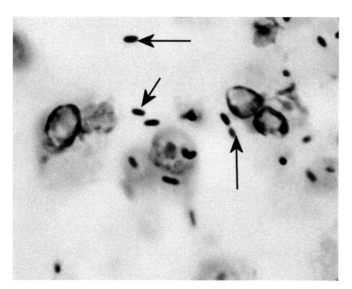

Image courtesy of the Centers for Disease Control and Prevention.

- A. *Streptococcus pneumoniae*
- B. *Mycoplasma pneumoniae*
- C. *Legionella pneumophila*
- D. *Chlamydia psittaci*
- E. *Coxiella burnetii*

Questions 75 and 76

A 35-year-old man who is a cross-country truck driver presents with a painful lesion on the shaft of his penis. The patient admits having had sexual intercourse with several prostitutes at a truck stop in the past 2 weeks. Physical examination reveals a bilateral inguinal lymphadenopathy. Palpation of the lesion, similar to that shown in the figure below, elicits pain from the patient. The lesion was neither indurated nor hard to the touch.

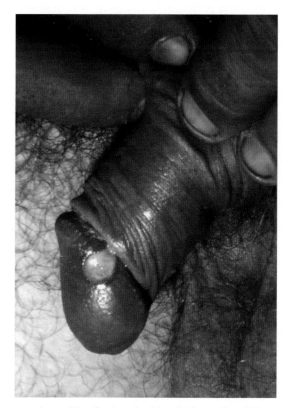

Image courtesy of the Centers for Disease Control and Prevention, Joe Miller.

75. Which of the following is the most likely diagnosis of this patient's condition?
- A. Syphilis
- B. Genital herpes
- C. Chancroid
- D. Granuloma inguinale
- E. Lymphogranuloma venereum

76. A Gram-stain smear of a sample from the lesion on the man's penis contained many pleomorphic gram-negative, rod-shaped organisms. Which of the following organisms is the most likely cause of this patient's condition?
- A. *Treponema pallidum*
- B. Herpes simplex virus 2
- C. *Haemophilus ducreyi*
- D. *Klebsiella granulomatis*
- E. *Chlamydia trachomatis*

Questions 77 and 78

A 7-year-old boy arrives in your office with complaints of chest pain and a rash that looks similar to that shown in the figure below. The rash is limited to his trunk. No skin lesions are observed in his mouth or on the palms of his hands or soles of his feet. No history of tick bite is noted. His vital signs are temperature 38.3°C, pulse 100/min, blood pressure 110/80 mm Hg, and respirations 20/min. When questioned about his chest pain, the patient indicates that when he does not breathe deeply, the pain is not as intense. He also states that if he leans forward while seated, it hurts less. When asked to lie down, the patient mentions that the sharp substernal left-sided chest pain is much worse. A friction rub is noted upon auscultation of the patient's heart. An electrocardiogram reveals a diffuse elevated ST segment and depression of the PR segment.

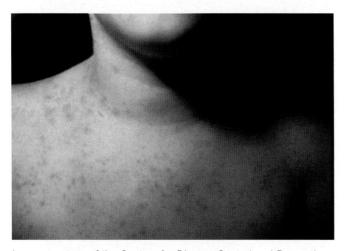

Image courtesy of the Centers for Disease Control and Prevention.

77. Which of the following is the most likely diagnosis of this patient's condition?

   A. Myocarditis

   B. Pericarditis

   C. Endocarditis

   D. Rheumatic heart disease

   E. Pneumonia

78. Which of the following is the most likely causative organism of this patient's condition?

   A. Echovirus

   B. *Staphylococcus aureus*

   C. *Streptococcus pneumoniae*

   D. *Mycobacterium tuberculosis*

   E. *Candida albicans*

Questions 79 and 80

A 34-year-old woman presents to her physician with complaints of a malodorous vaginal discharge that began about 3 days ago. Gynecologic examination reveals a frothy vaginal discharge. A sample was obtained and a wet mount was made of the discharge, shown in the figure below.

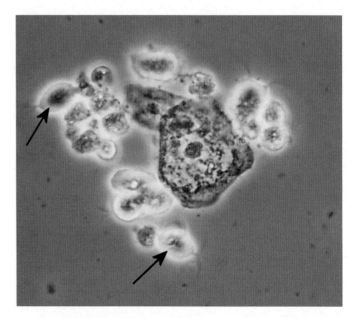

Image courtesy of the Centers for Disease Control and Prevention.

79. Which of the following organisms is the mostly likely cause of this patient's infection?

   A. *Candida albicans*

   B. *Trichomonas vaginalis*

   C. *Gardnerella vaginalis*

   D. *Neisseria gonorrhoeae*

   E. *Chlamydia trachomatis*

80. Which of the following would be the most appropriate treatment if the diagnosis of this patient is determined to be protozoan vaginitis?

   A. Doxycycline

   B. Metronidazole

   C. Penicillin

   D. Ceftriaxone

   E. Azithromycin

81. A 35-year-old woman who is infected with the human immunodeficiency virus (HIV) presents at a clinic with a large red nodule near the Achilles tendon near her left ankle. She says that the only thing different about her life in the past month has been getting used to a stray kitten she adopted. She mentions that the cat has a strange need to grab hold of her feet and ankles whenever she walks around the house barefoot. You note several scratches on her feet and ankles. The results of a biopsy of a fine needle aspirate indicate that there is significant proliferation of blood vessels lined with plump endothelial cells. The interstitial space is occupied by neutrophilic infiltrate, leukocytoclastic debris, and clumps of amphophilic, granular material. A Warthin-Starry stain demonstrates clusters of bacilli. Which of the following is the most likely diagnosis of this patient's foot lesion?

A. Kaposi sarcoma

B. Bacillary angiomatosis

C. Hepatica peliosis

D. Angioma

E. Port wine stain

82. A 55-year-old man arrives in the clinic complaining of toenail discoloration. He says that for the past year he has been using various over-the-counter agents to try to eliminate the problem himself. He asks you to determine why his toenails are so abnormal (refer to figure A on the *right*). You scrape some of his toenail on a slide, treat the scraping with 10% KOH, and stain with lactophenol cotton blue (refer to figure B on the *right*). Which of the following organisms is the mostly likely cause of this patient's condition?

A. *Candida albicans*

B. *Malassezia furfur*

C. *Epidermophyton floccosum*

D. *Sporothrix schenckii*

E. *Blastomyces dermatitidis*

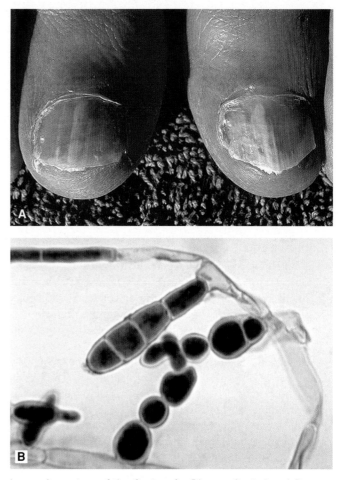

Image A courtesy of the Centers for Disease Control and Prevention, Dr Edwin P Ewing, Jr. Image B courtesy of the Centers for Disease Control and Prevention, Dr Libero Ajello.

Questions 83–86

A 29-year-old pregnant woman at 35 weeks' gestation arrives for a routine prenatal visit. The physician examines the patient to see if she is colonized by microbes that could cause her or her child significant problems. Samples of the vaginal and cervical mucosa are placed on blood agar plates and incubated at 37°C. Many gram-positive, aerobic catalase-negative bacterial colonies are observed on the plates. Results of the CAMP (Christie, Atkinson, Munch, Peterson) test are positive.

83. Which of the following organisms is currently colonizing the patient's vaginal mucosa?

A. *Staphylococcus aureus*

B. *Streptococcus pyogenes*

C. *Enterococcus faecalis*

D. *Streptococcus agalactiae*

E. *Candida albicans*

84. Which of the following would be the most appropriate treatment for the bacterial colonization of this patient?

    A. Immediately give her penicillin to eliminate the organism colonizing her vaginal mucosa

    B. Encourage her to have a caesarian section when she goes into labor

    C. Give her penicillin immediately and during labor and delivery

    D. Give her penicillin only during labor and delivery

    E. Do nothing since colonization with this microorganism is harmless to the mother and her infant

85. The pregnant patient at 38 weeks' gestation called your office this morning stating that her membranes had ruptured. You encouraged her to come to the hospital immediately where you said that you would meet her. The patient informs you that she would rather have her infant delivered at home and has already contacted a midwife. You express your concerns and inform her of the potential problems that she and her infant could have based on previous tests. Two days after the infant was delivered vaginally at home, the mother arrives in the emergency department with her newborn male infant. The infant, who weighs 3.2 kg, has a temperature of 40°C and is unwilling to eat. The mother received no medications during labor and delivery. Examination reveals a bulging fontanelle; however, before the examination can be completed, the infant begins to convulse. Once the convulsions are stopped, a head CT scan is performed. No intracerebral masses are noted. A lumbar puncture is performed, and the opening pressure is 200 mm H_2O. The cerebrospinal fluid is turbid and contains 140 mg/dL of protein, 30 mg/dL of glucose, and a white blood cell count of 1100/mm^3. Which of the following is the most likely diagnosis of this infant?

    A. Aseptic meningitis

    B. Chronic bacterial meningitis

    C. Chronic fungal meningitis

    D. Acute bacterial meningitis

    E. Viral encephalitis

86. If the Gram stain of the infant's cerebrospinal fluid contains many polymorphonuclear leukocytes and gram-negative rods, which of the following organisms is most likely causing the infant's current condition?

    A. *Streptococcus pneumoniae*

    B. *Streptococcus agalactiae*

    C. *Neisseria meningitidis*

    D. *Listeria monocytogenes*

    E. *Escherichia coli*

Questions 87 and 88

A 2-year-old girl is brought to the clinic by her parents who state that for the past 2 days the child has had a temperature of 38.9°C, a hacking cough, conjunctivitis, a runny nose, and a rash. The child's fever began 2 days before the rash appeared. The rash began on her face and has now spread all over her trunk. The child has no history of immunizations.

87. Which of the following is the most likely diagnosis of this child's condition?

    A. Rubella

    B. Rubeola

    C. Scarlet fever

    D. Erythema infectiosum

    E. Exanthem subitum

88. The 2-year-old girl has a brother who is 4 days old. The mother is concerned that her newborn may also contract the rash. The mother's medical history indicates that she had a similar rash 10 years ago. What advice would you give the mother concerning her newborn and his risk of being infected by the microbe that is causing her 2-year-old daughter's current infection?

    A. The newborn is at significant risk of contracting the rash and should be given gamma globulin immediately

    B. The newborn is at significant risk of contracting the rash and should be given the mumps-measles-rubella (MMR) vaccine immediately

    C. The newborn is at significant risk of contracting the rash and the 2-year-old sister should be kept apart from the infant until she shows no signs of illness

    D. The newborn is not at significant risk of contracting the rash because IgM to the microbe that causes this illness was passively acquired from the mother via the placenta and will protect the newborn

    E. The newborn is not at significant risk of contracting the rash because IgG to the microbe that causes this illness was passively acquired from the mother via the placenta and will protect the newborn

89. If acquired by a pregnant woman during her first trimester, which of the following organisms could cause significant fetal damage?

    A. Rubella virus

    B. Measles virus

    C. *Streptococcus pyogenes*

    D. Erythrovirus B19

    E. Human herpes virus 6

Questions 90–92

A 50-year-old man visits a clinic because he has an ulcerous lesion on the shaft of his penis. The lesion is painless and hard to the touch (refer to figure A below). A dark-field microscope visualized the etiologic agent in a sample taken from the lesion (refer to figure B below).

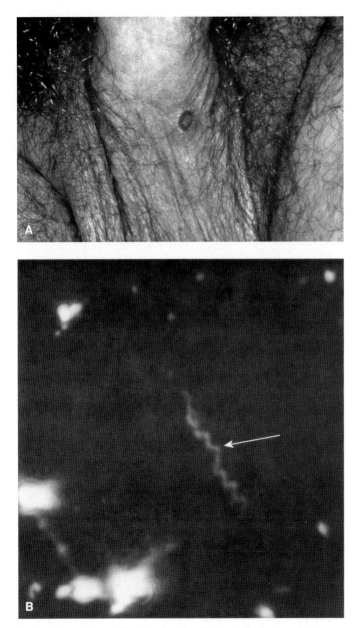

Image A courtesy of the Centers for Disease Control and Prevention, Dr NJ Fiumara, Dr Gavin Hart. Image B courtesy of the Centers for Disease Control and Prevention, VDRL Department.

90. Which of the following is the most likely causative organism of this patient's condition?

A. *Chlamydia trachomatis*

B. *Neisseria gonorrhoeae*

C. Herpes simples virus 2

D. *Treponema pallidum*

E. *Haemophilus ducreyi*

91. Which of the following serologic tests would be a good screening test to use for this patient's condition?

A. Western blot

B. ELISA

C. Reagin test

D. Treponemal test

E. Radial immunodiffusion test

92. After treatment, which of following tests could be used to determine if the treatment of this patient was effective?

A. Western blot

B. ELISA

C. Reagin test

D. Treponemal test

E. Radial immunodiffusion test

93. Treatment of a neonate's eyes with an antibiotic ointment at birth will prevent which of the following conditions?

A. Ophthalmia neonatorium due to *Neisseria gonorrhoeae*

B. Meningitis due to *Streptococcus agalactiae*

C. Sepsis due to *Streptococcus agalactiae*

D. Sepsis due to *Escherichia coli*

E. Pneumonia due to *Escherichia coli*

Questions 94 and 95

A 2-month-old girl is brought to the pediatrician by her parents because she is lethargic and does not want to eat. She also has a sharp staccato-like cough. Her vital signs are temperature 37°C, pulse 160/min, blood pressure 80/50 mm Hg, and respirations 75/min. Physical examination reveals dyspnea. Auscultation of her lungs reveals bilateral rales and wheezing. After obtaining an AP chest radiograph (similar to that shown in the figure on page 394), the child is admitted to the hospital. A Gram stain smear of a bronchoscopy specimen from the child contains many polymorphonuclear leukocytes but no stainable bacteria.

94. Which of the following is the most likely causative organism of this child's condition?

A. *Streptococcus agalactiae*

B. *Chlamydia trachomatis*

C. *Escherichia coli*

D. *Streptococcus pneumoniae*

E. *Staphylococcus aureus*

95. Which of the following agents would be the most appropriate treatment for this child's condition?

A. Ceftriaxone

B. Doxycycline

C. Erythromycin

D. Penicillin

E. Tobramycin

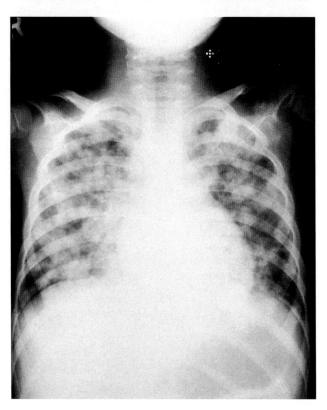

Image courtesy of the Centers for Disease Control and Prevention, Dr Joel D Myers.

96. A 2-month-old boy is brought to the clinic by his parents because he has a weak pulse, sunken fontanelle, and lethargy. When he cries, he produces no tears. The infant has a low-grade fever. For the past 6 days, he has been vomiting and has had diarrhea. Which organism is the most likely cause of this child's condition?

A. Adenovirus

B. Astrovirus

C. Norovirus

D. Norwalk virus

E. Rotavirus

97. A 21-year-old woman came to a clinic because she has had dyspnea, a nonproductive paroxysmal cough, and chills. Her temperature is 37.8°C. She states that she has been sick for the past 5 days but has been going to work. A chest radiograph shows infiltrates in both lungs. Which organism is the most common cause of this patient's condition?

A. *Haemophilus influenzae*

B. *Legionella pneumophila*

C. *Mycoplasma pneumoniae*

D. Parainfluenza virus

E. *Streptococcus pneumoniae*

98. A 29-year-old woman presented to her physician with complaints of malaise and upper right quadrant pain. Physical examination reveals a jaundiced female with icterus and hepatomegaly. Serologic tests are performed, with the results shown in the table below.

Hepatitis B Test	Result
HBs antigen	Positive
Antibody to HBs	Negative
IgM to HBc	Positive
IgG to HBc	Negative

Which of the following is the most appropriate diagnosis of this patient's condition?

A. Chronic hepatitis B virus (HBV)

B. A patient vaccinated with the hepatitis B vaccine (HepB)

C. Convalescent HBV

D. Early acute HBV

E. "Window" period HBV

99. A 56-year-old farmer from Iowa traveled to southern California for a 1-week vacation. He began feeling ill on his return trip. About 2 weeks later, he went to see his physician because of a cough, chest pain, and night sweats. He states that he has no appetite and has had a 9.1-kg weight loss over a 2-week period, without dieting. His temperature is 38.3°C. A chest radiograph shows consolidations in the apical region of the upper right lung. A sputum sample contains several spherules. Which organism is the most likely cause of this patient's condition?

A. *Actinomyces israelii*

B. *Blastomyces dermatitidis*

C. *Coccidioides immitis*

D. *Histoplasma capsulatum*

E. *Mycobacterium tuberculosis*

100. Which of the following organisms is most often related to fatalities in children younger than 1 year of age that are associated with ingestion of honey?

A. *Bacillus cereus*

B. *Clostridium botulinum*

C. *Clostridium perfringens*

D. *Clostridium tetani*

E. *Staphylococcus aureus*

PRACTICE EXAMINATION ANSWERS

Question 1

Answer A: The infection is localized to the eyelid, which is characteristic of a hordeolum (stye). The infection has not affected the eyelashes (e.g., blepharitis), the orbit around the eye (i.e., periorbital or orbital cellulitis), or the conjunctiva (i.e., conjunctivitis).

Question 2

Answer C: The most common cause of a hordeolum is *Staphylococcus aureus*. *S aureus* produces a golden pigment and is beta hemolytic. The coccal morphology and the colonies grew aerobically, which eliminates *Propionibacterium acne*, an anaerobe that is a gram-positive rod. Only the *Staphylococcus* genera are catalase positive, eliminating the *Streptococcus* genera. *S aureus* is coagulase positive, whereas *Staphylococcus epidermidis* is coagulase negative.

Question 3

Answer A: The patient has vesicular lesions that are in different stages of development. The lesions began on the trunk and moved to the face and extremities. This presentation is what is commonly seen in a patient with chickenpox (varicella). This child is beyond the age of a person who would normally have systemic herpes; the lesions shown in the figure are not indicative of herpetic lesions. Rubella and rubeola do not form vesicles but rather form an erythematous rash in the skin.

Question 4

Answer E: The cause of chickenpox is the varicella-zoster virus.

Question 5

Answer C: The cause of this patient's cellulitis is *Staphylococcus aureus*. *Corynebacterium* and *Clostridium* are gram-positive rods. *Streptococcus pyogenes* is catalase negative, and *Staphylococcus epidermidis* is coagulase negative.

Question 6

Answer B: Rhinitis with clear mucosal secretions and congestion with no fever or a low-grade fever indicate that the patient has the common cold. The most common cause of the common cold is rhinovirus.

Question 7

Answer C: The patient has typical pneumonia caused by a gram-positive diplococcus. After considering the results of the chest radiograph and the Gram stain, the most likely cause of pneumonia in this patient is *Streptococcus pneumoniae*.

Question 8

Answer B: The signs and symptoms of this patient are indicative of otitis externa, an infection of the ear canal.

Question 9

Answer C: The most common cause of otitis externa is *Pseudomonas aeruginosa*. The Gram stain reveals that the organism in the ear canal was a gram-negative rod, thus eliminating choices D and E (*Staphylococcus aureus* and *Streptococcus pneumoniae*, respectively). *Escherichia coli* is a lactose fermenting gram-negative rod. *Proteus mirabilis* is not oxidase positive.

Question 10

Answer D: The patient's signs and symptoms indicate that she has an inflammation that extends down into the lungs. Answers A and B (common cold and pharyngitis, respectively) can be eliminated because the common cold and pharyngitis cause only upper respiratory tract symptoms. The patient is beyond an age group that would be diagnosed as having significant problems associated with bronchiolitis. Bronchiolitis is usually most problematic in infants younger than 1 year of age. The signs and symptoms in this patient indicate she could have either bronchitis or pneumonia. Since no infiltrates or consolidations are observed on chest radiographs, the patient would not be diagnosed as having pneumonia. Thus, choice E (pneumonia) has been eliminated, leaving only choice D (bronchitis) as the correct answer.

Question 11

Answer B: The paroxysmal cough with inspiratory stridor and high pitched sound produced at the end of the coughing spell are indicative of pertussis (whooping cough). The child's cough was neither harsh nor "barky" sounding, which are indicative of viral croup. She did not have any signs of lower respiratory tract infection in that no crackles or wheezing were noted, nor did she have any dullness to percussion. These manifestations would eliminate bronchitis, bronchiolitis, and pneumonia, leaving only pertussis (choice B) as the correct answer.

Question 12

Answer D: The lesions are superficial and a honey brown color, which is indicative of impetigo. There is no significant edema or erythema around the lesions, which will exclude cellulitis and carbuncles. The lesions are neither vesicular nor are they ulcerous in nature, thus excluding oral herpetic lesions. There is no purulent center to the lesions and furuncles, which excludes those choices.

Question 13

Answer B: The most common causes of impetigo are *Staphylococcus aureus* and *Streptococcus pyogenes*. Choices C, D, and E (*Streptococcus pneumoniae*, *Enterococcus faecalis*, and *Neisseria meningitidis*, respectively) do not cause impetigo. The laboratory results indicate that *S aureus* can be excluded since it is catalase negative.

Question 14

Answer C: A patient with an acute infection due to Epstein-Barr virus (EBV) would have IgM antibodies to VCA, but no antibodies to EBNA. Anti-EBNA antibodies are not detectable until most patients have recovered from the infection. Therefore, the presence of anti-EBNA would indicate a past infection with EBV.

Question 15

Answer D: Cytomegalovirus (CMV) and hepatitis B virus infections both induce production of atypical lymphocytes. Coxsackievirus, herpes simplex virus, and varicella-zoster virus do not induce production of atypical lymphocytes, which eliminates these choices. The triad of pharyngitis, fever, and cervical lymphadenopathy is common in patients with infectious mononucleosis. Primary CMV infections can appear very similar to Epstein-Barr virus infections and have often been called heterophile-negative mononucleosis. Hepatitis B virus infections usually do not manifest this triad of symptoms

Question 16

Answer E: Epstein-Barr virus (EBV) is a B-lymphocyte mitogen. EBV can cause multiplication and activation of B lymphocytes without binding to the B lymphocyte's antibody receptor. It is this ability to cause the multiplication of many different B lymphocytes that results in the heterophile antibody response.

Question 17

Answer E: The patient's lesions are vesicular and are located along an intercostal dermatome. He also mentions pain along that dermatome. This is indicative of a patient with varicella-zoster virus. Cytomegalovirus and Epstein-Barr virus do not produce such localized skin lesions. Herpes simplex virus type 1 and type 2 produce vesicular lesions, but they tend to produce lesions around the mouth and genitalia.

Question 18

Answer D: The most common cause of viral congenital defects prior to universal vaccination with the mumps-measles-rubella (MMR) vaccine was rubella. Currently, there are no vaccines for any of these other causes of congenital infection.

Question 19

Answer B: Group B *Streptococcus agalactiae* is a common infection of neonates that causes pneumonia, sepsis, and meningitis. Laboratory examination of samples from a pregnant patient to determine if she is colonized can alert the physician to institute treatment during labor and delivery. Antibiotic treatment with penicillin has been shown to significantly reduce the rate of intrapartum transmission.

Question 20

Answer A: After two different blood samples have tested positive for human immunodeficiency test (HIV) by ELISA, the confirmatory test for determining the diagnosis of HIV infection is a Western blot.

Question 21

Answer A: The recommended treatment that results in the lowest rate of transmission of human immunodeficiency infection (HIV) to the fetus during labor and delivery and following delivery is zidovudine and nevirapine. When used alone, zidovudine and nevirapine significantly reduce the rate of transmission; however, the drugs used in combination most significantly reduce the rate of transmission.

Question 22

Answer E: The patient's serum contained antibodies to HBs and HBc. A patient immunized with the hepatitis B (HBV) vaccine would only have antibodies to HBs, since that is the only antigen in the recombinant vaccine. No HBs antigen could be detected in this patient's serum, thus eliminating choices B (he has an acute HBV infection) and D (he has chronic HBV infection). During acute and chronic HBV infections, the patient's serum will contain detectable levels of HBs antigen. Choice C (he is in the "window period" of HBV infection) can be eliminated because the patient's serum would not contain any detectable levels of anti-HBs but would contain anti-HBc.

Question 23

Answer D: The lesion shown in the figure is a fungal infection known as tinea corporis, or ringworm. It can be differentiated from leprosy in that the nerves that sense pain are still viable in a tinea infection but have been destroyed in a patient with leprosy. Anthrax lesions are raised and have a black center, called a black eschar. Tinea capitis is found on the head, not the arm. Tinea versicolor is either a hypopigmented or hyperpigmented region of the skin and does not have the scaly center seen in tinea corporis or tinea capitis.

Question 24

Answer B: The most common cause of genital herpes is herpes simplex virus (HSV) type 2. HSV-1 can also cause genital herpes; however, it is the cause of only about 20% cases of genital herpes.

Question 25

Answer B: To prevent transmission of the virus to the neonate, vaginal delivery should not be attempted if the patient is in the prodromal period of a recurrence or has genital lesions present during labor. Therefore, the physician should advise the woman to have a caesarian section.

Question 26

Answer A: The most common cause of oral vesicular lesions is herpes simplex virus (HSV) type 1. HSV-2 is a more common cause of genital herpes. Cytomegalovirus does not cause recurrent perioral lesions. *Candida albicans* produces lesions inside the mouth or at the corners of the mouth. *Microsporum gypseum* produces scaly lesions on the skin that are not recurrent.

Question 27

Answer E: The most common cause of acute bacterial prostatitis is *Escherichia coli*.

Question 28

Answer A: The curd-like appearance of the vaginal secretions and the results of the Gram stain of the yeast-shaped cells are indicative of a vaginitis due to *Candida albicans*. The vaginal discharges caused by *Gardnerella vaginalis* and *Trichomonas vaginalis* are less curd-like in appearance. Herpes simplex type 2 would also produce vesicular or ulcerous lesions and the discharge, if any, would be clear, but it is not purulent and curd-like. *Lactobacillus acidophilus* is normal flora that maintains a healthy vaginal mucosa and does not cause vaginitis.

Question 29

Answer C: The most common cause of noninflammatory diarrhea and nausea and vomiting in adults is norovirus. Rotaviruses are the most common cause of these symptoms in infants. Adenovirus can also cause these symptoms, but it is not as common as norovirus. *Entamoeba histolytica* and *Shigella sonnei* cause an inflammatory bloody diarrhea that usually contains fecal leukocytes.

Question 30

Answer D: The hypo- or hyperpigmented areas on this patient's chest are indicative of tinea versicolor, which is caused by *Malassezia furfur. Staphylococcus aureus* and *Streptococcus pyogenes* produce skin lesions that involve erythema and edema of the tissues. In many cases, the lesions are filled with a purulent material. Skin lesions due to *Candida albicans* are similar but are usually found in the moist regions of the body and not on the regions of the chest, as described in this case. The stained smear of the skin scraping shows the classic "spaghetti and meatball" appearance of *M furfur. C albicans* does not have this appearance. *Blastomyces dermatitides* causes rough verrucae that appear very different from these lesions; a skin scraping would reveal broad-based budding yeast.

Question 31

Answer E: This patient has "hot tub folliculitis." She had been on a cruise and had frequented a hot tub. The pus obtained from her folliculitis lesions contained gram-negative bacterial cells. *Escherichia coli* does not cause hot tub folliculitis; it is a lactose fermenter. *Pseudomonas aeruginosa* is a nonlactose fermenting, gram-negative rod that is frequently obtained from aqueous environments.

Question 32

Answer B: The most common cause of asymptomatic bacteriuria is *Escherichia coli. E coli* is also the most common cause of symptomatic urinary tract infection. *Proteus mirabilis* would have raised the pH of the patient's urine. This was not the case in this patient, thus eliminating this organism. *Staphylococcus saprophyticus* does not produce nitrites in the urine; the urine sample contained nitrites, thus eliminating that choice. *Klebsiella pneumoniae* and *Pseudomonas aeruginosa* rarely, if ever, cause urinary tract infections.

Question 33

Answer D: The most common complication that occurs in pregnant women with asymptomatic bacteruria is pyelonephritis. During pregnancy, the ureters tend to dilate and peristalsis of the ureters is less effective in preventing ascension of an infection of the urinary bladder to the kidneys.

Question 34

Answer A: The common causes of acute bacterial rhinosinusitis are *Streptococcus pneumoniae* and *Haemophilus influenzae*. None of the other organisms listed commonly cause acute bacterial rhinosinusitis.

Question 35

Answer A: Because the onset of meningeal irritation was rapid, chronic meningitis would be eliminated as a choice. The cerebrospinal fluid findings as turbid with a decrease in glucose concentration would also eliminate viral encephalitis, rabies, and aseptic meningitis. Only acute bacterial meningitis would have such a rapid onset that would result in high opening pressures on lumbar tap, low glucose concentration, high numbers of polymorphonuclear leukocytes, and a turbid appearance.

Question 36

Answer B: The Gram stain obtained from this patient reveals the presence of a gram-positive diplococcus in the cerebrospinal fluid. The most common cause of bacterial meningitis in adults is *Streptococcus pneumoniae*, and it is a gram-positive diplococcus.

Question 37

Answer C: Based on the hemorrhagic nature of this patient's stool specimen, the most likely causes of this patient's current condition could be enterohemorrhagic *Escherichia coli, Campylobacter duodenale*, or *Shigella sonnei*. The other *E coli* strains usually do not cause a bloody diarrhea. The patient in this case did not have a fever, which is common for a patient with enterohemorrhagic *E coli*. This patient also mentions consuming an unpasteurized apple juice, which makes it more likely that the patient is infected with enterohemorrhagic *E coli. C duodenale* requires special growth media, temperature, and aeration, and does not grow at standard conditions (i.e., room air at 37°C) on MacConkey agar. *S sonnei* will grow on this medium but is not a lactose fermenter.

Question 38

Answer B: All gram-negative bacteria produce endotoxin; however, this is not the reason antibiotics are not suggested for treating these patients. Toxins A and B are produced by *Clostridium difficile* and are not produced by *Escherichia coli*. Labile toxin produced by *E coli* has not been associated with renal failure. Only shiga toxin has been shown to be associated with renal failure in patients with enterohemorrhagic *E coli* infections.

Question 39

Answer E: The capillaries are dilated in the conjunctiva, indicating that the patient has conjunctivitis. No pathology can be seen in the eyelids or the eyelashes, thus eliminating hordeolum and anterior and posterior blepharitis. Dacryocystis is a blockage of the lacrimal duct and would show swelling between the bridge of the nose and the affected eye. No swelling is noted, thus eliminating dacryocystitis as a likely diagnosis.

Question 40

Answer A: Bacterial causes of conjunctivitis would result in a significant amount of purulent exudate draining from the eye. This would eliminate *Staphylococcus aureus* and *Haemophilus influenzae* as potential causes of this patient's conjunctivitis. Herpes simplex virus is not as common as adenovirus, and the pharyngitis in this patient makes it even more likely that she has an adenovirus infection. The preauricular lymphadenopathy makes it more likely that she has conjunctivitis due to adenovirus and not to *Chlamydia trachomatis*.

Question 41

Answer B: The curd-like material in the patient's throat is commonly seen in a patient with thrush. A patient with gingivostomatitis would present with vesicular lesions or ulcers with an erythematous base. Diphtheria would produce a gray pseudomembrane. Streptococcal pharyngitis could produce an exudate, but it would usually be restricted to the tonsils.

Question 42

Answer D: Of the choices (herpes simplex virus, *Corynebacterium diphtheria*, *Streptococcus pyogenes*, *Candida albicans*, and *Neisseria gonorrhoea*), only *Candida albicans* will grow on Sabouraud dextrose agar and produce colonies with large oval gram-positive organisms.

Question 43

Answer A: Of the choices listed (esophagitis, gastric ulcer, duodenal ulcer, gastroenteritis, and gastroesophageal reflux disease), the only disease that that causes dysphagia and odynophagia is esophagitis.

Question 44

Answer D: A patient whose serologic test results are positive using ELISA and Western blot assays is infected with human immunodeficiency virus (HIV), which eliminates a diagnosis of indeterminate HIV infection (choice E). A patient infected with HIV who has symptoms of infectious esophagitis has a category C condition (choice D, acquired immunodeficiency syndrome, or AIDS). Without even knowing the patient's CD4$^+$ cell count, category C conditions are enough to define the patient's current condition as AIDS.

Question 45

Answer H: The patient has Kaposi sarcoma. The causative agent of these cancerous lesions is human herpes virus 8.

Question 46

Answer D: If this patient with acquired immunodeficiency syndrome (AIDS) is able to tolerate the complex treatment regimen, she should be treated with triple anti-HIV drug therapy. Mono- and dual drug therapies have not been shown to be as effective in lowering viremia, preventing opportunistic infections, and prolonging the life of the patient.

Question 47

Answer B: The rapidity of onset of this patient's symptoms indicates that he has food poisoning caused by *Bacillus cereus*. *Campylobacter jejuni* infection is associated with consumption of chicken; however, it is an infectious process and would take 24–48 hours for symptoms to appear, rather than 1 hour as was seen in this patient. *Clostridium botulinum* would not cause nausea and vomiting but rather a flaccid paralysis. *Clostridium perfringens* can cause food poisoning, but the onset of symptoms is usually longer than 1 hour. *Staphylococcus aureus* and *Bacillus cereus* could have caused this patient's problem. However the results of the culture of the fried rice show that *B cereus*, a gram-positive, rod-shaped bacteria, is the cause of this patient's current condition.

Question 48

Answer A: *Staphylococcus aureus* is the most common cause of food poisoning in the United States.

Question 49

Answer E: The most common cause of osteomyelitis of the long bone is *Staphylococcus aureus*. *Neisseria gonorrhoeae* is a common cause of septic arthritis in sexually active individuals but not a common cause of osteomyelitis. *Streptococcus agalactiae* and *Escherichia coli* would be more likely in a patient younger than 1 year of age; however, this patient is 2 years old, making these causes of osteomyelitis less likely than *S aureus*. *Streptococcus pyogenes* is a rare cause of osteomyelitis.

Question 50

Answer E: The most effective therapy for osteomyelitis requires 4–6 weeks of treatment with antibiotics.

Question 51

Answer C: The presence of a purulent urethral discharge and intracellular gram-negative diplococci is indicative of a patient with urethritis due to *Neisseria gonorrhoeae*.

Question 52

Answer D: The only media that allows for growth of *Neisseria gonorrhoeae* is Thayer-Martin agar plates.

Question 53

Answer C: The target-like erythematous lesion seen on this patient's upper right arm and the history of a tick bite are classic examples of a patient with Lyme disease. *Rickettsia rickettsii* causes small petechial lesions starting at the ankles and wrists. Varicella-zoster virus produces vesicular skin lesions that form all over the body or occur over a dermatome. *Borrelia hermsii* causes relapsing fever and does not cause any skin rash. *Francisella tularensis* produces an ulcer in the skin.

Question 54

Answer B: Penicillin is the recommended treatment for Lyme disease.

Question 55

Answer D: The vector that caused this patient's current condition is a tick.

Question 56

Answer C: The petechial skin lesions starting at the wrists and ankles that are also present on the soles and palms is a classic example of a patient with Rocky Mountain spotted fever due to *Rickettsia rickettsii*. *Francisella tularensis* produces ulcers, not petechial lesions. *Babesia microti* does not cause skin lesions. *Ehrlichia chaffeensis* causes the same signs and symptoms as *R rickettsii*; however, a leukopenia is usually seen in a complete blood cell count and the rash is less common.

Question 57

Answer E: The recommended treatment for Rocky Mountain spotted fever is doxycycline.

Question 58

Answer D: The presence of gram-positive group A *Streptococcus* (*S pyogenes*) confirms a diagnosis of streptococcal pharyngitis.

Question 59

Answer B: Treatment of patients with streptococcal pharyngitis will reduce their chances of developing rheumatic fever. Treatment does not affect the occurrence of glomerulonephritis. Scarlet fever is caused by *Streptococcus pyogenes* and would likely be present at the time the patient presented with the streptococcal pharyngitis. Hemolytic uremic syndrome is caused by shiga toxin-producing strains of *Escherichia coli*. Erythema chronicum migrans although similar in name to the rash seen in rheumatic fever, erythema marginatum, it is not caused by *S pyogenes* but rather by *Borrelia burgdorferi*.

Question 60

Answer A: The recommended treatment for streptococcal pharyngitis is penicillin.

Question 61

Answer A: The presence of palatine palsy and the pseudomembrane in the pharyngeal region that causes some bleeding when removed is indicative of diphtheria. Pertussis and streptococcal pharyngitis do not produce a pseudomembrane. Thrush can produce a pseudomembrane, but it does not cause bleeding when removed.

Question 62

Answer C: The DTaP (diphtheria, tetanus toxoids, and acellular pertussis) vaccine contains the diphtheria toxoid that would have protected the patient from developing diphtheria.

Question 63

Answer A: Treatment of a patient with diphtheria first requires administration of antitoxin, followed by antibiotics, and then the vaccine. Antibiotic treatment will kill the organisms in the patient's pharynx, releasing more toxins and potentially creating a worsening situation. The diphtheria, tetanus toxoids, and acellular pertussis vaccine (DTaP) is given, since the infection has not been allowed to run its course and provide adequate protection against future infections with *Corynebacterium diphtheriae*.

Question 64

Answer D: The presence of the new murmur and high fever in an intravenous drug user with an acute onset is acute endocarditis, the most likely diagnosis for this patient's signs and symptoms. Pericarditis would have resulted in a friction rub rather than a heart murmur. If there were signs of heart failure, then myocarditis would have been a more likely diagnosis. Rheumatic fever can be excluded in that this patient has no history of prior streptococcal pharyngitis.

Question 65

Answer E: The most common cause of acute endocarditis in an intravenous drug user is *Staphylococcus aureus*. Coxsackievirus is the most common cause of myocarditis. Human immunodeficiency virus (HIV) does not cause an acute endocarditis. The other bacteria listed as choices (i.e., *Streptococcus mitis* and *Enterococcus faecalis*) are more common causes of subacute endocarditis, not acute endocarditis.

Question 66

Answer D: The most likely cause of diarrhea after antibiotic therapy is *Clostridium difficile*.

Question 67

Answer C: Toxin A and B are produced by *Clostridium difficile*. The other toxins are produced by other bacteria; cholera toxin by *Vibrio cholerae*; exotoxin A by *Pseudomonas aeruginosa*; shiga toxin by *Shigella* and *Escherichia*; and staphylococcal enterotoxin by *Staphylococcus aureus*.

Question 68

Answer D: The most likely cause of urinary tract infection is *Escherichia coli*. However, in this case, the pH of the urine reveals a different cause of the patient's current condition. *Proteus mirabilis* produces urease. Urease catalyses the breakdown of urea to ammonia and carbon dioxide. Ammonia causes the pH of the urine to increase and is indicative of a urinary tract infection due to *Proteus* species that produce urease.

Question 69

Answer B: The presence of protozoan parasites in the blood indicates that the patient could have malaria or babesiosis. This patient has no history of foreign travel, making the diagnosis of malaria unlikely. The characteristic Maltese-cross configuration seen in the blood smear image of the merozoites in the erythrocytes of this patient is pathognomonic for babesiosis.

Question 70

Answer C: This patient meets the definition for diagnosis of severe sepsis in that she has two or more signs of systemic inflammatory response syndrome (SIRS). Her temperature is lower than 36°C and she has tachycardia; she has a documented site of infection (a previously untreated cystitis that appears to now be in the kidneys), and organ dysfunction (confusion indicating hypoperfusion of the brain). She would not be diagnosed with septic shock because her blood pressure is not low enough at this point.

Question 71

Answer D: The recommended treatment for a patient with severe sepsis due to a urinary tract infection is ciprofloxacin and an aminoglycoside (e.g., gentamicin).

Question 72

Answer C: D-dimers are the most specific test of the choices given for determining if a patient has disseminated intravascular coagulation (DIC).

Question 73

Answer A: Only *Escherichia coli, Proteus mirabilis,* and *Klebsiella pneumoniae* are gram-negative rods. Of those, only *P mirabilis* and *E coli* are lactose fermenters. The remaining two choices, *Staphylococcus saprophyticus* and *Streptococcus pneumoniae,* are gram-positive cocci and can be eliminated as correct choices. *E coli* is the most common cause of cystitis and pyelonephritis making choice A the best answer to this question.

Question 74

Answer C: This patient is diagnosed with pneumonia, which he exhibited with a few rather unique signs and symptoms: bradycardia, hematuria, and vomiting and diarrhea. The history of the recent use of a window air conditioner hints that *Legionella* is the cause of the pneumonia. Many rod-shaped bacteria were seen by Dieterle silver stain. This is significant in a patient with interstitial pneumonia for a diagnosis of Legionnaire disease or pneumonia due to *Legionella pneumophila.*

Question 75

Answer C: The ulcer seen on the shaft of this patient's penis is painful but not indurated, which is a common presentation of chancroid. Syphilis can also result in an ulcerous lesion; however, the lesions of syphilis are indurated and painless. Once the vesicles are broken, genital herpes can become ulcers; however, there are usually many lesions that coalesce to form irregularly shaped painful ulcers that are bordered by an erythematous inflammation of the tissues surrounding the ulcers. Granuloma inguinale and lymphogranuloma venereum do not result in ulcerous lesions of the genitalia.

Question 76

Answer C: Many pleomorphic gram-negative, rod-shaped bacteria were observed in a Gram stained sample of the lesion. The ability of this organism to produce cells of different lengths (pleomorphic) is common in the genera *Haemophilus* and confirms that this patient's current condition is due to *H ducreyi.*

Question 77

Answer B: The patient's signs and symptoms of sharp substernal pain that is made worse by lying supine and the auscultation of a friction rub is indicative of pericarditis. Endocarditis and rheumatic heart disease usually result in heart murmurs rather than a friction rub. Myocarditis does not produce a friction rub but rather produces signs and symptoms of heart failure. Pneumonia produces certain adventitious sounds, but they are lung sounds similar to rales and wheezes.

Question 78

Answer A: Viruses are the most common cause of pericarditis. Among the viral causes of pericarditis, the enteroviruses, coxsackievirus and echovirus, are the most common cause of pericarditis. The child's skin rash also makes it more likely that the child has an echoviral rash rather than a coxsackie viral rash. Coxsackievirus tends to cause stomatitis and a vesicular skin rash rather than the maculopapular rash seen in this patient.

Question 79

Answer B: The malodorous frothy vaginal discharge is indicative of trichomoniasis. The wet mount of the vaginal discharge contains many of the protozoan parasites that surround the vaginal epithelial cells. No clue cells were present in the wet mount, thus eliminating *Gardnerella vaginalis. Candida albicans* vaginitis produces a curd-like discharge that contains budding yeasts and yeasts with pseudohyphae on wet mount. *Neisseria gonorrhoeae* and *Chlamydia trachomatis* can be excluded based on the results of the wet mount.

Question 80

Answer B: Metronidazole is the drug of choice for treating *Trichomonas vaginalis* vaginitis.

Question 81

Answer B: The most likely cause of this patient's current condition is bacillary angiomatosis. The history of human immunodeficiency virus (HIV) infection and being the owner of a cat indicates that she could have been infected with *Bartonella henselae.* The bacilli seen after Warthin-Starry stain is diagnostic of bacillary angiomatosis.

Question 82

Answer C: This patient has tinea unguium, a fungal infection, and the most common cause of this infection is *Epidermophyton floccosum.* The wet mount and stain of the macroconidia is diagnostic for *Epidermophyton.*

Question 83

Answer D: A CAMP (Christie, Atkinson, Munch, Peterson) test is used to determine if the woman is colonized by group B streptococci, also known as *Streptococcus agalactiae.* An arrow-head shape will appear in the agar when group B streptococci are streaked in a direction perpendicular to a streak of beta hemolytic *Staphylococcus aureus.*

Question 84

Answer D: *Streptococcus agalactiae* is a common cause of sepsis, pneumonia, and meningitis in neonates who acquire the organism from their mother's vaginal mucosa during delivery. Doing nothing is not an appropriate option. Performing a caesarian section is more likely to result in more serious complications than simply giving the patient penicillin during labor and delivery. Giving penicillin at 35 weeks' gestation will eliminate the organism from the vaginal mucosa but only for a short period of time, because many women are recolonized by the time they deliver the infant. Giving the mother an antibiotic at 35 weeks' gestation and during labor and delivery does not provide any more protection to the infant and would be an excessive use of antibiotics in this case. Therefore, the appropriate treatment is to give the woman penicillin during labor and delivery.

Question 85

Answer D: The infant has acute onset bacterial meningitis. The cerebrospinal fluid was turbid and had a high protein concentration and a low glucose concentration. This is indicative of a bacterial meningitis rather than chronic fungal meningitis, aseptic meningitis, or viral encephalitis. Chronic bacterial meningitis would take longer than 2 days for the patient to manifest signs and symptoms.

Question 86

Answer E: The most common cause of acute bacterial meningitis that is gram-negative and rod-shaped, as seen on Gram stain, is *Escherichia coli*. Although the neonate's mother was colonized by *Streptococcus agalactiae*, this finding does not require that the resulting meningitis will always be due to this organism. Also, not every woman who is colonized by *S agalactiae* will infect her newborn. *Neisseria meningitidis* is a gram-negative coccus, and *Listeria monocytogenes* is a gram-positive rod; therefore, both of these choices can be eliminated. *Streptococcus pneumoniae* is alpha hemolytic and is negative by CAMP (Christie, Atkinson, Munch, Peterson) testing.

Question 87

Answer B: The child's symptoms began with cough, coryza (runny nose), and conjunctivitis, known as the three Cs of rubeola. The child then developed a rash that has coalesced and appears morbilliform in nature, which is indicative of rubeola or measles. Rubella rashes are less noticeable and are not preceded by the three Cs. Scarlet fever is a sandpaper-like rash that appears uniformly over most of the body with circumoral pallor and Pastia sign under the arms and behind the knees. In exanthem subitum, the rash appears after the fever recedes. A child with erythema infectiosum will have a slapped-cheek appearance and a rash on the extremities rather than on the trunk.

Question 88

Answer E: The mother contracted the rash when she was younger (10 years ago), and IgG to this illness can cross the placenta and will provide protection to the newborn. If present, IgM does not cross the placenta and is unable to provide protection to the newborn.

Question 89

Answer A: Rubella virus causes significant damage when acquired early in a pregnancy.

Question 90

Answer D: The lesion is painless and indurated. This lesion is classic in a patient who has primary syphilis. It can be differentiated from herpes simplex virus and *Haemophilus ducreyi* infections because lesions caused by these pathogens are painful. *Neisseria gonorrhoeae* and *Chlamydia trachomatis* do not cause ulcerous lesions of the genitalia.

Question 91

Answer C: Reagin tests are used to screen patients to see if they have syphilis. The radial immunodiffusion test is used to quantify the amount of an antigen in a sample using an agar plate containing antibodies reactive with the antigen. This test is not used to identify a patient with syphilis. Western blot and ELISA assays are not used to screen for syphilis. The treponemal tests are too expensive to be used to screen for syphilis but are used to confirm a case of syphilis if the result of the reagin screening test is positive.

Question 92

Answer C: The results of treponemal tests are positive for the lifetime of the patient, even after effective treatment. Levels of antibody to reagin do decrease with successful treatment, and this is the only test that can demonstrate if the treatment was effective. The other tests are not used to measure the effectiveness of treatment of syphilis.

Question 93

Answer A: A topical ointment containing erythromycin will prevent the development of ophthalmia neonatorium due to *Neisseria gonorrhoeae* in the eyes of a neonate delivered to a woman infected with *Neisseria gonorrhoeae*. Application of this ointment will not prevent any of the other diseases listed (meningitis due to *Streptococcus agalactiae*, sepsis due to *S agalactiae* or to *Escherichia coli*, or pneumonia due to *E coli*).

Question 94

Answer B: An afebrile pneumonia that causes a staccato-like cough is due to *Chlamydia trachomatis*. Other causes of pneumonia would result in a fever and there would be stainable bacterial cells in the sputum.

Question 95

Answer B: The most effective antibiotic to treat afebrile pneumonia due to *Chlamydia trachomatis* is doxycycline.

Question 96

Answer E: The most common cause of diarrhea in children younger than 1 year of age is rotavirus. Norovirus, astrovirus, and Norwalk virus are more common in adults as a cause of diarrhea. Compared to rotavirus infection, adenovirus is not very common in children and usually also causes a conjunctivitis which this patient does not have.

Question 97

Answer C: The woman is diagnosed as having interstitial pneumonia. The most common cause of interstitial pneumonia is *Mycoplasma pneumoniae*. *Haemophilus influenzae* and *Streptococcus pneumoniae* cause a lobar pneumonia with a productive cough. *Legionella pneumophila* also causes vomiting and diarrhea. Parainfluenza virus can cause interstitial pneumonia, but is not the most common cause of this type of pneumonia.

Question 98

Answer D: The presence of HBs antigen and IgM to HBc indicates that this patient is in the early acute phase of hepatitis B virus (HBV). A patient with chronic HBV would have HBs antigen in their bloodstream for at least 6 months and by that time would have no signs or symptoms of hepatitis. A patient who had been vaccinated with the HBV vaccine would have antibody to HBs but no antibody to HBc. Convalescent HBV patients have positive antibody to HBs and are negative for HBs antigen. Patients in the "window" period of HBV will be positive for antibody to HBc but negative for antibody to HBs and for the HBs antigen.

Question 99

Answer C: Recent travel to the southwestern United States and the presence of spherules in the sputum in a patient with chronic onset of pneumonia is indicative of *Coccidioides immitis* infection. *Actinomyces israelii* and *Mycobacterium tuberculosis* would be acid-fast positive in a sputum sample. *Actinomyces israelii* would produce filamentous rod-shaped bacterial cells, and *Mycobacterium tuberculosis* would produce slender rod-shaped bacterial cells in the sputum. *Blastomyces dermatitidis* would produce broad-based budding yeasts in the sputum; it is found in the southeastern and midwestern areas of the United States. *Histoplasma capsulatum* would produce yeast cells in the sputum and is found in the midwestern areas of the United States.

Question 100

Answer B: Honey contains high concentrations of carbohydrate and does not allow the growth of bacteria. *Clostridium botulinum* spores can survive in the honey and will begin growing in a young child's small intestine after ingestion. These spores are not killed during passage through the child's stomach because a young child produces less acid. While growing in the intestine, *Clostridium botulinum* produces the neurotoxin that causes flaccid paralysis and can result in the death of the child.

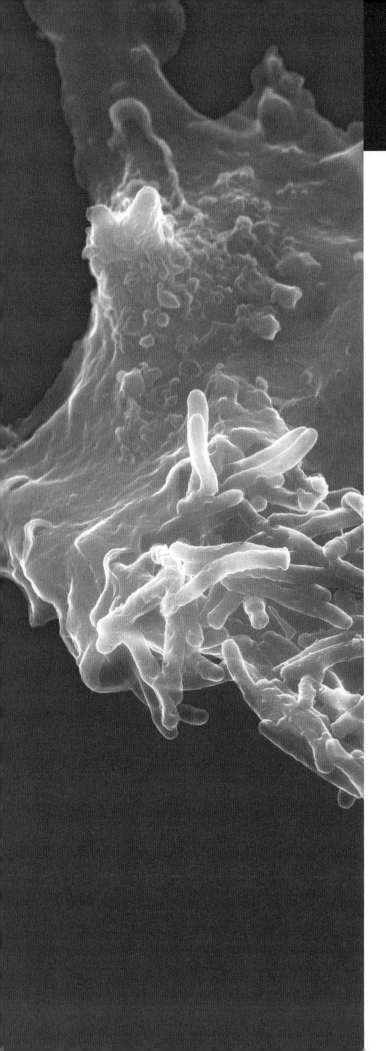

IMPORTANT MEDICAL MICROBIOLOGY LABORATORY TESTS

The Appendix contains a variety of tables and brief discussions that will help you prepare for the United States Medical Licensing Examination (USMLE) and the Comprehensive Osteopathic Medical Licensing Examination (COMLEX) and may also be helpful in studying for course examinations during medical school. Many case-based microbiology examination questions require you to think through several steps to correctly respond to the question. Frequently, you will be given the patient's history, signs and symptoms, and physical examination and laboratory findings, all of which provide information needed to determine a clinical diagnosis. For example, information about a patient who presents with dyspnea, productive cough, and rales and has a chest radiograph that shows consolidations will help you to establish that the patient has pneumonia. The cough, dyspnea, and rales are manifestations that help to determine that the respiratory tract is infected and that it is likely from hearing rales that the lower respiratory tract is infected. In this case, the chest radiograph confirms that the patient has pneumonia.

Once you have determined a diagnosis, it is important for you to know the microbial causes that result in that diagnosis. With many diagnoses, there are several different organisms that can cause the patient's condition. In the patient with pneumonia, the most common group of microorganisms that cause pneumonia is bacteria. Several different bacteria, including *Streptococcus pneumoniae*, *Haemophilus influenzae*, *Mycoplasma pneumoniae*, and *Klebsiella pneumoniae*, can cause pneumonia and, based on the patient's history, you can frequently narrow the possible correct answer to two or three of the possible choices. To arrive at the one best answer, usually the final one or two sentences in the case will describe certain characteristics of the specific microbe that is causing the patient's condition. For the patient with pneumonia who has a productive cough, the findings of a Gram stain of sputum are usually used to direct you to the one best answer. In the above example of the patient with pneumonia, a Gram stain of the sputum would contain many gram-positive diplococci—this information should then point you to the one best answer, *Streptococcus pneumoniae*.

Table A-1 and the section on unique bacterial characteristics contain diagnostic, clinical, and microbiologic findings that are usually helpful in identifying the correct answer from the other one or two distractors. The rules of thumb section on Gram staining and acid-fast staining and Table A-2 should help refresh your memory about these very important microbiologic characteristics.

In some examination questions, there may be two organisms that may be the likely cause of the patient's condition. For example, impetigo can be caused by *Streptococcus pyogenes* and *Staphylococcus aureus*. Both of these organisms are gram-positive cocci. Knowing that *Staphylococcus aureus* is catalase positive and that *Streptococcus pyogenes* is catalase negative can help you determine the best answer. The sections of the Appendix that include Tables A-3 through A-8 and the flow charts that identify common gram-positive and gram-

negative bacterial pathogens contain some important microbiology laboratory tests. Tables A-9 and A-10 include information on organisms that are transmitted by arthropod vectors and by raw milk.

Tables A-11 through A-19 list the common causes of various diseases by organ system. The causes have been identified previously in chapters throughout the book, and these tables may seem somewhat redundant to include here in the Appendix. However, placing summary tables of the diseases of an organ system in one place can help you see trends regarding the common causes of various diseases. For example, in Table A-17, you will quickly realize that *Staphylococcus aureus* is the most common cause of all the infectious bone and joint infections discussed in this book.

IMPORTANT DIAGNOSTIC FINDING OR LABORATORY TEST

TABLE A-1. Diagnostic Test or Clinical Finding Highly Suggestive of a Particular Disease

Disease	Finding and/or Test	Organism
Atypical pneumonia	Cold hemagglutinins; bullous myringitis	*Mycoplasma pneumoniae*
Typical pneumonia	Currant jelly sputum; alcohol abuse	*Klebsiella pneumoniae*
Typical pneumonia	Green sputum; cystic fibrosis	*Pseudomonas aeruginosa*
Aspiration pneumonia	Consolidations in dependent lung segments; foul-smelling sputum	Anaerobic bacteria
Pertussis (whooping cough)	Inspiratory stridor that results in a whooping sound; lymphocytosis	*Bordetella pertussis*
Tuberculosis	Coin lesions on chest radiograph or Ghon complexes (cheese-like necrosis); acid-fast rods in sputum; positive Mantoux or PPD test	*Mycobacterium tuberculosis*
Bacterial vaginosis	Clue cells	*Gardnerella vaginalis*
Granuloma inguinale	Donovan bodies: safety-pin appearance of bacteria in an intracellular vacuole in a leukocyte	*Klebsiella granulomatis* (formerly *Calymmatobacterium granulomatis*)
Plague	Safety pin-appearance of bacteria in leukocytes from aspirate of a bubo	*Yersinia pestis*
Gonorrhea	Gram-negative diplococci in polymorphonuclear leukocytes	*Neisseria gonorrhoeae*
Cholera	Rice water stools	*Vibrio cholerae*
Herpes virus infection	Tzanck test	Herpes simplex virus 1 and 2
Cytomegalovirus infection	Owl's eye cell	Cytomegalovirus
Rabies encephalitis	Negri bodies	Rabies virus

Disease	Finding and/or Test	Organism
Amebiasis (parasitic dysentery)	Flask-shaped ulcers in colon; amoeba with intracellular erythrocytes; anchovy paste-like or chocolate milk-like substance from liver abscess aspirate	*Entamoeba histolytica*
Cryptosporidiosis: chronic diarrhea in AIDS patients	Acid–fast-positive round oocytes in stools	*Cryptosporidium parvum*
Blastomycosis: fungal pneumonia and skin lesions	Broad-based budding yeast cells	*Blastomyces dermatitides*
Histoplasmosis: fungal pneumonia	Tuberculate macroconidia in vitro	*Histoplasma capsulatum*
Coccidioidomycosis: fungal pneumonia	Spherule in tissue; arthroconidia in vitro	*Coccidioides immitis*
Fungal meningitis	India ink test; only encapsulated pathogenic yeast	*Cryptococcus neoformans*
Candidiasis	Germ tube formation when grown in serum in vitro; produces pseudohyphae in human tissue	*Candida albicans*

UNIQUE CHARACTERISTICS OF BACTERIA

SOME UNIQUE FEATURES OF THE PATHOGENIC BACTERIA

1. Two medically important bacterial genera produce spores: *Bacillus* and *Clostridium*.

2. *Mycoplasma* and *Ureaplasma* do NOT produce a cell wall.

3. *Chlamydia, Chlamydophila, Ehrlichia, Anaplasma, Orientia, Coxiella,* and *Rickettsia* are obligate intracellular bacteria.

4. *Chlamydia* and *Chlamydophila* produce elementary and reticulate bodies. Elementary bodies are infectious.

5. *Listeria monocytogenes* can grow at 4°C and has a tumbling motility. The ability to grow at low temperatures helps it to grow in food at refrigerator temperatures.

6. *Campylobacter* is a seagull-shaped rod that grows best at 42°C and requires an atmosphere that has reduced levels of oxygen and increased levels of hydrogen and carbon dioxide.

7. *Haemophilus influenzae* does NOT grow on blood agar plates because the medium lacks hemin and nicotinamide adenine dinucleotide (NAD). This genus grows best on chocolate agar plates.

8. *Bordetella pertussis* requires Bordet Gengou agar media to grow.

9. *Mycobacterium tuberculosis* is often grown on Lowenstein-Jenson-Gruft medium.

10. *Neisseria gonorrhoeae* does NOT grow on blood agar but will best grow on chocolate agar, called Thayer-Martin agar plates, which have antibiotic added to suppress the normal flora.

11. *Legionella* grow best on charcoal yeast extract agar plates.

12. *Corynebacterium diphtheriae* is grown on Loffler medium, tellurite plates, or blood agar plates.

13. Pathogenic *Vibrio* species are comma-shaped (curved) rods that grow best on thiosulfate-citrate-bile salts-sucrose agar (TCBS agar). *Vibrio cholerae* turns medium yellow color; other *Vibrio* species do not.

14. *Treponema pallidum* and *Mycobacterium leprae* cannot be grown in vitro.

15. *Escherichia coli* O157:H7 requires sorbitol in the media to grow.

16. Only a few pathogenic bacteria are oxidase positive and include *Neisseria, Pseudomonas, Campylobacter, Helicobacter,* and *Vibrio*.

17. Three bacteria produce pigments that can be helpful in identification of these pathogens. *Staphylococcus aureus* produces a golden colored water-insoluble pigment. *Pseudomonas aeruginosa* produces a green water-soluble pigment. *Serratia marcescens* produces a red water-insoluble pigment.

RULES OF THUMB FOR GRAM STAINING

1. **Gram-positive organisms are purple. Gram-negative organisms are red.** Hint: *Keep your "P's" together; purple is positive.* Gram stains are never pink; if they are, it destroys the "P" rule.

2. **Only a few pathogenic bacteria cannot be Gram stained or are visible if they are stainable.**

   Organisms that are NOT Gram stainable or are NOT routinely Gram stained are the spirochetes (*Borrelia, Treponema, Leptospira*), the obligate intracellular parasites (*Chlamydia, Chlamydophila, Ehrlichia, Anaplasma, Orientia, Coxiella,* and *Rickettsia*), and *Bartonella, Mycobacterium, Legionella, Mycoplasma,* and *Ureaplasma*.

3. **Most pathogenic bacteria are rod-shaped, so know which organisms are cocci.**

   ▪ *Streptococcus, Staphylococcus, Enterococcus, Peptostreptococcus, Neisseria,* and *Moraxella.*

   ▪ *NOTE.* Only 2 of the common pathogenic cocci are gram negative: *Neisseria* and *Moraxella.* All others are gram positive.

4. **There are many gram-negative rods but only a few gram-positive rods, so know the gram-positive, rod-shaped bacteria.**

   ▪ The gram-positive rods: *Clostridium, Bacillus, Corynebacterium, Listeria, Lactobacillus, Nocardia, Actinomyces, Propionibacterium, Gardnerella,* and *Erysipelothrix.*

5. **All others are gram-negative rods.**

TABLE A-2. Grouping Common Bacterial Pathogens by Gram-stain Reaction

Gram-positive Bacteria	Gram-negative Bacteria	Bacteria Usually *not* Gram-stained
Aerobic gram-positive rods *Bacillus* *Corynebacterium* *Listeria*	**Gram-negative cocci** *Neisseria* *Moraxella*	**Elementary body/reticulate body** *Chlamydia* *Chlamydophila*
Anaerobic spore-forming gram-positive rods *Clostridium*	**Enteric gram-negative rods** *Escherichia* *Proteus* *Campylobacter* *Yersinia enterocolitica* *Salmonella* *Shigella* *Helicobacter* *Vibrio* *Bacteroides*	**Spirochetes** *Borrelia* *Treponema* **No cell wall** *Mycoplasma* *Ureaplasma* **Unique cell wall** *Mycobacterium*
Gram-positive cocci *Staphylococcus* *Streptococcus* *Enterococcus*	**Nonenteric gram-negative rods** *Haemophilus* *Legionella* *Francisella* *Pasteurella* *Brucella* *Pseudomonas* *Klebsiella* *Yersinia pestis*	

RULES FOR ACID-FAST STAINING

1. Acid-fast or acid–fast-positive organisms are red. Non–acid-fast or acid–fast-negative organisms are blue.

2. Almost all human pathogens are non–acid-fast.

3. The acid-fast organisms, when using the Ziehl-Neelsen method, are *Mycobacteria* and *Nocardia.* Both these genera produce rod-shaped organisms.

LABORATORY TESTS USED TO DIFFERENTIATE THE GRAM-POSITIVE COCCI

There are three genera of gram-positive cocci that are of clinical significance: **Staphylococcus**, **Streptococcus**, and **Enterococcus**. Staphylococci are **catalase positive** and appear as large clusters. They are categorized by their ability to produce coagulase and whether they are resistant to novobiocin. There are three clinically significant species in this genus: **S aureus, S epidermidis,** and **S saprophyticus.**

TABLE A-3. Laboratory Tests Used to Differentiate the Pathogenic Staphylococcal Species

Organism	Hemolysis on Blood Agar Plates	Catalase Production	Coagulase Production/Mannitol Fermentation	Novobiocin Sensitivity
Staphylococcus aureus	Beta or gamma	Positive	Positive/ positive	Sensitive
Staphylococcus epidermidis	Gamma	Positive	Negative/negative	Sensitive
Staphylococcus saprophyticus	Gamma	Positive	Negative/negative	Resistant

Streptococci are **catalase negative** and grow in chains. They are categorized by their group-specific carbohydrates (Lancefield groupings: group A to W) and by their hemolysis patterns on blood agar plates (alpha, beta, or gamma hemolysis). There are three common clinically significant species in this genus: *S pyogenes* (group A, beta hemolytic), *S agalactiae* (group B, beta hemolytic), and *S pneumoniae* (viridans group or non-groupable with Lancefield groupings, alpha hemolytic).

Enterococci are closely related to the streptococci. They are **catalase negative,** in the Lancefield group D, and gamma hemolytic. There are two common clinically significant species in this genus: *E faecalis* and *E faecium*. **Note the importance of the catalase test in determining whether a particular gram-positive coccus is a *Staphylococcus*, a *Streptococcus*, or an *Enterococcus*.**

TABLE A-4. Laboratory Tests Used to Differentiate the Pathogenic Streptococcal Species

Organism	Lancefield Grouping	Hemolysis* on Blood Agar Plates	Biochemical Tests
S pyogenes	A	Beta	Sensitive to bacitracin (A disc)
S agalactiae	B	Beta usually; gamma sometimes	Positive CAMP-test; hippurate hydrolysis
S pneumoniae	Nongroupable; Viridans group	Alpha	Soluble in bile; sensitive to Optochin (P disc)

CAMP, Christie, Atkinson, Munch, Peterson.
*There are three different types of hemolysis. **Alpha hemolysis** is not really hemolysis of the erythrocytes in the blood agar plates but rather a conversion of hemoglobin to a form of hemoglobin that appears green in the agar around the bacterial colony. **Beta hemolysis** is true hemolysis with actual lysis of the erythrocytes in the blood agar around the bacterial colony. **Gamma hemolysis** is not really a hemolytic event either. The organism is gamma hemolytic when no lysis of the erythrocytes or color change occurs in the media around the colony. In other words, these organisms are nonhemolytic.

LABORATORY TESTS USED TO DIFFERENTIATE GRAM-NEGATIVE COCCI

TABLE A-5. Laboratory Tests Used to Differentiate the Pathogenic Gram-negative Cocci

Organism	Shape	Oxidase Reaction	Acid Via Oxidation of Carbohydrate	Media Requirements
Neisseria gonorrhoeae	Diplococcus (coffee bean)	+	Glucose positive and maltose negative	Chocolate and Thayer-Martin agar
Neisseria meningitidis	Diplococcus (kidney bean)	+	Glucose and maltose positive	Blood or chocolate agar
Moraxella catarrhalis	Diplococcus (kidney bean)	+	Glucose and maltose negative	Blood or chocolate agar

LABORATORY TESTS USED TO DIFFERENTIATE GRAM-POSITIVE RODS

TABLE A-6. Physical Properties of Aerobic Gram-Positive Rods

Organism	Morphology	Spore Production	Motility	Unique Properties
Bacillus anthracis	Large: end-to-end chains	Yes	No	Poly-D-glutamic acid capsule; spores
Bacillus cereus	Large	Yes	Yes; 50% of strains	Spores
Corynebacterium diphtheriae	Small, narrow	No	No	Pleomorphic; Chinese characters (snapping fission)
Listeria monocytogenes	Small	No	Yes; tumbling motility	Grows at 4°C; grows intracellularly

LABORATORY TESTS USED TO DIFFERENTIATE GRAM-NEGATIVE RODS

ENTERIC GRAM-NEGATIVE RODS

This group of gram-negative organisms is found either as normal flora that can cause disease in the gastrointestinal tract or can cause disease in the gastrointestinal tract following inges-tion. Some of the enteric gram-negative rods belong to the Enterobacteriaceae: *Escherichia, Klebsiella, Salmonella, Shigella,* and *Yersinia*. The Enterobacteriaceae are a group of gram-negative, rod-shaped bacteria that for the most part have simple nutritional requirements. They all ferment glucose, reduce nitrates to nitrites, and are oxidase negative. Four genera, *Vibrio, Campylobacter, Helicobacter,* and *Bacteroides,* are NOT members of the Enterobacteriaceae.

TABLE A-7. Physical Properties of Enteric Gram-Negative Rods

Genera	Pathogenic Species	Shape	Motile	Glucose Fermentation	Oxidase	Lactose Fermentation	H_2S Gas	Special
Escherichia	E coli	Rod	Yes	Yes	No	Yes	No	
Salmonella	S enterica, S typhi	Rod	Yes	Yes	No	No	Yes	
Shigella	S flexneri, S dysenteriae, S boydii, S sonnei	Rod	No	Yes	No	No	No	
Yersinia	Y enterocolitica,	Rod	No	Yes	No	No	No	
Campylobacter	C jejuni, C coli, C fetus	Comma-shaped rod, or S-shaped rod, or corkscrew	Yes	No	Yes	No	No	Grows best at 42°C, microaerophile
Helicobacter	H pylori	Spiral-shaped rod	Yes	No	Yes	No	No	Urease producer
Vibrio	V parahaemolyticus, V vulnificus, V cholerae	Comma-shaped rod	Yes	Yes	Yes	No, Yes, No	No	Grows best in high salt
Bacteroides	B fragilis	Rod	No	Not applicable	No	Not applicable	No	Obligate anaerobe

TABLE A-8. Important Groups of *Escherichia Coli*

Organism	Major Clinical Disease
Enterotoxigenic ETEC	Watery diarrhea
Enterohemorrhagic EHEC (O157:H7 and non-O157:H7 strains)	Hemorrhagic colitis Hemolytic uremic syndrome
Enteroinvasive EIEC	Begins with diarrhea, which then develops into dysentery
Enteropathogenic EPEC	Infant watery diarrhea
Enteroaggregative EAEC	Infant watery diarrhea

Organism	Major Clinical Disease
Uropathogenic UPEC	Urinary tract infections
E coli K1	Neonatal meningitis
Host flora *E coli*	Sepsis

IDENTIFICATION OF COMMON GRAM-POSITIVE BACTERIAL PATHOGENS (FIGURE A-1)

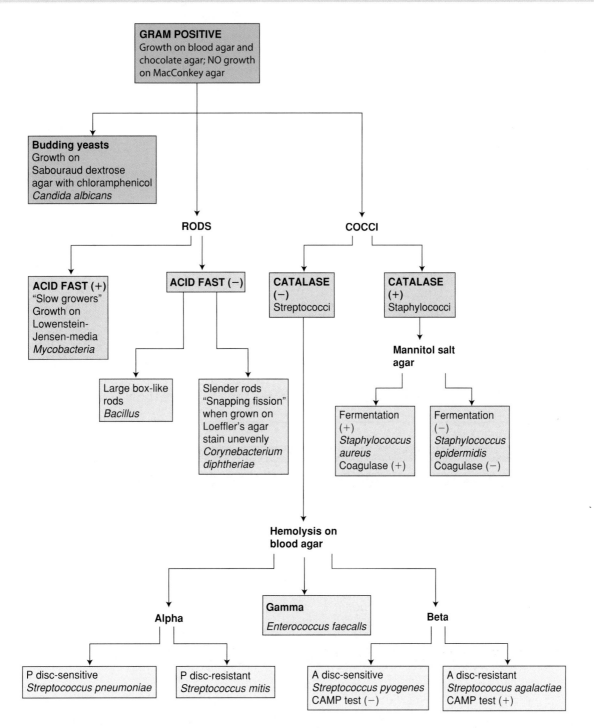

IDENTIFICATION OF COMMON GRAM-NEGATIVE BACTERIAL PATHOGENS (FIGURE A-2)

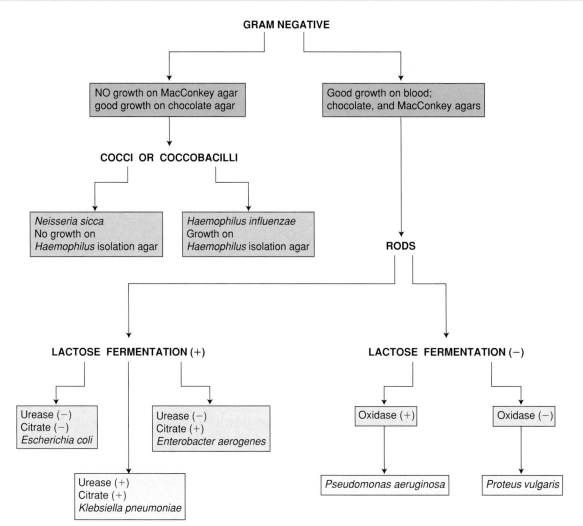

ORGANISMS TRANSMITTED BY ARTHROPOD VECTORS

TABLE A-9. Arthropod-Borne Diseases

Arthropod Vector	Disease	Disease Agent	Method of Human Exposure
Arachnida			
Tick: *Dermacentor*	Tularemia	*Francisella tularensis* (Gram-negative bacteria)	Bite of tick
Tick: *Dermacentor* and other Ixodid ticks	Rocky Mountain spotted fever	*Rickettsia rickettsii* (bacteria)	Bite of tick
Tick: *Ornithodoros*	Endemic relapsing fever	*Borrelia sp.* (bacteria, spiral shaped)	Bite of tick
Arachnida			
Tick: *Ixodes*	Babesiosis	*Babesia microti* (parasite, protozoan)	Bite of tick

Arthropod Vector	Disease	Disease Agent	Method of Human Exposure
Tick: *Ixodes*	Lyme disease	*Borrelia burgdorferi* (bacteria, spiral shape)	Bite of tick
Tick: *Ornithodoros* various species	Tick-borne relapsing fever or endemic relapsing fever	*Borrelia* various species	Bite of tick
Tick: *Dermacentor variabilis, Amblyomma americanum*	Ehrlichiosis, anaplasmosis	*Ehrlichia canis, E chaffeensis, Anaplasma phagocytophilum* (bacteria, intracellular)	Bite of tick
Tick: *Dermacentor*	Colorado tick fever	Colorado tick fever virus, Eyach virus, or strain S6-14-03 (Reoviridae)	Bite of tick
Tick	Powassan Encephalitis	Powassan virus	Bite of tick
Crustacea			
Copepod: *Cyclops*	Diphyllobothriasis, fish tapeworm	*Diphyllobothrium latum* (parasite, cestode, tapeworm)	Arthropod is first intermediate host, then human swallows infected fish
Copepod: *Cyclops*	Sparganosis	*Diphyllobothrium spirometra* (parasite, cestode, tapeworm)	Human swallows infected *Cyclops*
Copepod: *Cyclops*	Dracunculosis	*Dracunculus medinensis* (parasite, nematode)	Human swallows infected *Cyclops*
Crabs, crayfish: various freshwater species	Paragonimiasis	*Paragonimus westermani* (parasite, trematode, lung fluke)	Human eats infected crustacean
Insecta			
Lice: *Pediculus humanus*	Trench fever, bacillary angiomatosis, bacillary peliosis	*Bartonella quintana* (Gram-negative bacteria)	"Bite," contaminated by louse feces or crushing louse on skin
Lice: *Pediculus humanus*	Louse-borne relapsing fever or epidemic relapsing fever	*Borrelia recurrentis* (bacteria; spiral shape)	"Bite," contaminated by louse feces or crushing louse on skin
Flea: *Xenopsylla cheopis*, and various other rodent fleas	Plague	*Yersinia pestis* (Gram-negative, rod-shaped bacteria)	"Bite" and feces of flea
Flea: *Xenopsylla cheopis*, and various other rodent fleas	Rat tapeworm infection	*Hymenolepsis diminuta* (parasite, cestode, tapeworm)	Swallowing infected flea
Flea: various species	Dog tapeworm infection, Dipylidiasis	*Dipylidium caninum* (parasite, cestode, tapeworm)	Swallowing infected flea

(*continued*)

TABLE A-9. Arthropod-Borne Diseases (*cont.*)

Arthropod Vector	Disease	Disease Agent	Method of Human Exposure
Insecta			
Beetles: flour beetle	Hymenolepsis	*Hymenolepsis nana* (parasite; tapeworm; cestode)	Swallowing infected beetle
Deer fly: *Chrysops*	Tularemia	*Francisella tularensis* (Gram-negative, rod-shaped bacteria)	Bite of infected fly
Mosquito: *Anopheles*	Malaria	*Plasmodium falciparum, P malariae, P vivax, P ovale* (parasite; protozoan)	Bite of infected mosquito
Mosquito: *Culiseta melanura, Coquillettidia pertubans, Aedes vexans*	Eastern equine encephalitis	Eastern equine encephalitis virus (Togaviridae)	Bite of infected mosquito
Mosquito: *Aedes triseriatus*	La Crosse encephalitis	La Crosse encephalitis virus (Bunyaviridae)	Bite of infected mosquito
Mosquito: *Culex*	St. Louis encephalitis	St. Louis encephalitis virus (Flaviviridae)	Bite of infected mosquito
Mosquito: *Culex*	Western equine encephalitis	Western equine encephalitis virus (Togaviridae)	Bite of infected mosquito

ORGANISMS TRANSMITTED BY RAW MILK

TABLE A-10. Diseases Contracted from Consumption of Raw Milk

Disease	Organism	Symptoms and Complications
Campylobacteriosis	*Campylobacter*	Bloody diarrhea
Salmonellosis	*Salmonella*	Bloody diarrhea
Hemolytic uremic syndrome	*Escherichia coli* O157:H7	Diarrhea; kidney failure; death
Yersiniosis	*Yersinia enterocolitica*	Diarrhea
Listeriosis	*Listeria monocytogenes*	Meningitis; blood infections
Tuberculosis	*Mycobacterium tuberculosis*	Tuberculosis; pneumonia
Brucellosis	*Brucella*	Blood infections; heart infections
Cryptosporidiosis	*Cryptosporidium parvum*	Diarrhea
Staphylococcal enterotoxin poisoning	*Staphylococcus aureus*	Vomiting
Q fever	*Coxiella brunetti*	High fever, severe headache, muscle aches; can infect the liver and/or heart

COMMON CAUSES OF INFECTIOUS DISEASES BY ORGAN SYSTEM

TABLE A-11. Common Causes of Infectious Diseases of the Central Nervous System*

Disease	Age of Patient	Common Cause(s) and/or Comments
Bacterial meningitis	Neonates (< 1 month)	*Streptococcus agalactiae* (Group B *streptococcus*) *Escherichia coli*
	Children and adults	*Streptococcus pneumoniae* *Neisseria meningitidis*
	Elderly (> 60 years)	*Streptococcus pneumoniae* Gram-negative bacilli
Viral (aseptic) meningitis and encephalitis	90% of cases in patients < 30 years	Enteroviruses; 70%; occurs in late summer and early fall Arboviral meningoencephalitis are the **most common cause of episodic encephalitis in the United States** Herpes simplex virus (sporadic)
Chronic meningitis		*Mycobacterium tuberculosis* *Cryptococcus neoformans*
Spinal cord		*Clostridium tetanus* Polio virus

*Note that this is not an exhaustive list and does not include all possible etiologies for a particular disease.

TABLE A-12. Common Causes of Infectious Diseases of Skin or Integument*

Microorganism	Common Cause(s)	Disease(s)
Bacteria	*Staphylococcus aureus*	Impetigo, bullous impetigo, scalded-skin syndrome, folliculitis, furuncles, carbuncles, cellulitis, myositis, and toxic shock syndrome
	Streptococcus pyogenes	Impetigo, scarlet fever, erysipelas, necrotizing fasciitis, and streptococcal toxic shock syndrome
	Propionibacterium acne	Acne
Viruses	Herpes simplex 1 and 2 viruses	Oral and genital herpes
	Human papillomaviruses	Warts, genital warts, cervical dysplasia, and cervical carcinoma
Fungi	*Malassezia furfur*	Tinea versicolor
	The dermatophytes: *Microsporum, Trichophyton* and *Epidermophyton*	Tinea pedis, tinea corporis, tinea capitis, tinea manus, tinea unguium, and tinea cruris
	Candida albicans	Intertrigo, thrush, perlèche, folliculitis, paronychia, and onychomycosis

*Note this is not an exhaustive list and does not include all possible etiologies for a particular disease.

TABLE A-13. Childhood Exanthems*

Disease (Number)	Alternative Name(s) for the Disease	Etiology(ies)
First disease	Rubeola, measles, hard measles, 14-day measles, Morbilli	Measles virus
Second disease	Scarlet fever, scarlatina	*Streptococcus pyogenes*
Third disease	Rubella, German measles, 3-day measles	Rubella virus
Fourth disease	Filatov-Dukes disease, staphylococcal scalded-skin syndrome, Ritter disease	Some authorities say the disease does not exist; others believe it is due to *Staphylococcus aureus* strains that produce epidermolytic (exfoliative) toxin
Fifth disease	Erythema infectiosum	Erythrovirus (parvovirus) B19
Sixth disease	Exanthem subitum, roseola infantum, "sudden rash," rose rash of infants, 3-day fever	Human herpes virus 6B or human herpes virus 7

*The terminology for all but fifth disease is not used anymore. However, if ever caught in a medical trivia battle, this information could come in handy!

TABLE A-14. Common Causes of Infectious Diseases of Ears and Eyes*

Disease and Location	Common Cause(s)
Ear: otitis media	*Streptococcus pneumoniae* *Moraxella catarrhalis* *Haemophilus influenzae*
Ear: otitis externa	*Pseudomonas aeruginosa* *Staphylococcus aureus*
Eye: anterior blepharitis	*Staphylococcus aureus* *Staphylococcus epidermidis*
Eye: hordeola (stye)	*Staphylococcus aureus*
Eye: periorbital (preseptal) cellulitis	*Streptococcus pneumoniae* in young children *Staphylococcus aureus* or *Streptococcus pyogenes* posttraumatic
Eye: orbital (postseptal) cellulitis	*Staphylococcus aureus, Streptococcus pyogenes, Streptococcus pneumoniae, Haemophilus influenzae,* and *Enterobacteriaceae*
Eye: dacryocystitis	*Streptococcus pneumoniae, Staphylococcus aureus, Haemophilus influenzae, Streptococcus pyogenes,* and *Pseudomonas aeruginosa*
Eye: conjunctivitis	**Viral:** adenoviruses, herpes simplex viruses types 1 and 2 **Bacterial (pinkeye):** *Staphylococcus aureus, Streptococcus pneumoniae, Haemophilus influenzae, Moraxella catarrhalis, Pseudomonas aeruginosa, Neisseria gonorrhoeae,* and *Neisseria meningitidis* **Chlamydial:** *Chlamydia trachomatis*

Disease and Location	Common Cause(s)
Eye: keratitis	**Bacteria:** most common of all causes • Gram-positive bacteria *Staphylococcus aureus* • Gram-positive bacilli that cause keratitis include *Corynebacterium diphtheriae, Bacillus,* and *Clostridium* • Gram-negative bacilli: *Pseudomonas aeruginosa* is one of the most destructive of the bacterial causes of keratitis • Gram-negative cocci: *Neisseria gonorrhoeae, Neisseria meningitidis, Moraxella, Pasteurella multocida,* and *Acinetobacter* • Ophthalmia neonatorum: *Neisseria gonorrhoeae* and *Chlamydia trachomatis* **Viruses** • Herpes simplex 1 and 2, most common of viruses

*Note this is not an exhaustive list and does not include all possible etiologies for a particular disease.

TABLE A-15. Common Causes of Infectious Diseases of the Respiratory Tract*

Disease	Common Cause(s)
Common cold (rhinitis)	Rhinoviruses
Acute rhinosinusitis	Rhinoviruses, adenoviruses, parainfluenza viruses, influenza viruses, respiratory syncytial virus, coronaviruses
Acute bacterial rhinosinusitis	*Streptococcus pneumoniae* *Haemophilus influenzae*
Pharyngitis	Adenovirus Herpes simplex virus Epstein-Barr virus Coxsackie viruses *Streptococcus pyogenes* (group A *Streptococcus* is important because of the complications that can result (e.g., rheumatic fever, infections of contiguous tissues)
Viral croup	Parainfluenza virus Influenza virus Respiratory syncytial virus
Bacterial tracheitis	*Staphylococcus aureus*
Epiglottitis (bacterial croup)	*Haemophilus influenzae* type b
Bronchitis	Influenza viruses, parainfluenza viruses, adenovirus, respiratory syncytial virus, herpes simplex virus, rhinovirus, coxsackieviruses, and echovirus *Mycoplasma pneumoniae* *Chlamydophila pneumoniae* *Streptococcus pyogenes*
Bronchiolitis	Respiratory syncytial virus
Pneumonia	**Neonatal (0–1 month):** *Escherichia coli* and *Streptococcus agalactiae* **Infants (1–6 months):** *Chlamydia trachomatis* and respiratory syncytial virus **Children (6 months–5 years):** Respiratory syncytial virus and parainfluenza virus **Children (5–15 years):** *Mycoplasma pneumoniae* and influenza A virus **Young adults (16–30 years):** *Mycoplasma pneumoniae* **Older adults (> 30 years):** *Streptococcus pneumoniae*

*Note that this is not an exhaustive list and does not include all possible etiologies for a particular disease.

TABLE A-16. Common Causes of Infectious Diseases of the Gastrointestinal Tract*

Disease	Common Cause(s)
Teeth: dental caries	*Streptococcus mutans*
Gums: gingivitis and periodontal disease	Polymicrobial infection involving may anaerobic bacteria found in the oropharynx
Sublingual and submaxillary space: Ludwig angina	*Streptococcus, Bacteroides, Fusobacterium* and/or *Staphylococcus aureus*
Mouth and tongue: gingivostomatitis or oral herpes	Herpes simplex virus
Mouth: stomatitis or oral candidiasis (thrush)	*Candida albicans*
Salivary glands: parotitis	Mumps virus: benign viral parotitis *Staphylococcus aureus:* acute bacterial parotitis
Esophagus: esophagitis	*Candida albicans*
Stomach and upper duodenum: gastritis and peptic ulcer disease	*Helicobacter pylori*
Intestine: food poisoning	*Staphylococcus aureus* *Bacillus cereus* *Clostridium perfringens*
Intestine: viral gastroenteritis	Rotavirus (winter infant diarrhea) Noroviruses (winter vomiting disease) Norwalk virus (summer diarrhea)
Intestine: noninflammatory bacterial infections	*Escherichia coli* (EPEC), *E coli* (ETEC), and *E coli* (EAEC) *Vibrio cholerae* *Clostridium difficile*
Intestine: inflammatory bacterial infections	*Campylobacter jejuni* *Escherichia coli* (EIEC) and *E coli* (EHEC) *Salmonella typhimurium* *Shigella dysenteriae, S sonnei,* and *S flexneri* *Yersinia enterocolitica* *Clostridium difficile*
Intestine: parasitic infections	*Giardia lamblia* *Entamoeba histolytica* *Cryptosporidium parvum* *Enterobius vermicularis* *Ascaris lumbricoides*
Liver: viral hepatitis	Hepatitis A, B, and C virus

*Note that this is not an exhaustive list and does not include all possible etiologies for a particular disease.

TABLE A-17. Common Causes of Infectious Diseases of Bone and Joints*

Disease	Common Cause(s)
Osteomyelitis	*Staphylococcus aureus*
Septic arthritis	*Staphylococcus aureus* *Neisseria gonorrhoeae* (most common in sexually active young adults)

*Note that this is not an exhaustive list and does not include all possible etiologies for a particular disease.

TABLE A-18. Common Causes of Infectious Diseases of the Heart*

Disease	Common Cause(s)
Pericarditis: viral	Enteroviruses: coxsackieviruses A and B and echovirus type 8
Pericarditis: purulent	*Staphylococcus aureus, Streptococcus pneumoniae*
Pericarditis: chronic	*Mycobacterium tuberculosis*
Myocarditis	Coxsackievirus B
Endocarditis: native valve	*Streptococcus viridans, Enterococcus,* and *Staphylococcus aureus*
Endocarditis: prosthetic valve < 2 months post surgery	*Staphylococcus* and gram-negative aerobic bacilli
Endocarditis: prosthetic valve > 2 months post surgery	Viridans *Streptococcus, Staphylococcus epidermidis,* and *Staphylococcus aureus*
Endocarditis: intravenous drug users	*Staphylococcus aureus* and gram-negative bacilli
Rheumatic heart disease	*Streptococcus pyogenes*

*Note that this is not an exhaustive list and does not include all possible etiologies for a particular disease.

TABLE A-19. Common Causes of Infectious Diseases of the Genitourinary Tract*

Disease	Common Cause(s)
Cystitis and pyelonephritis	*Escherichia coli*
Acute bacterial prostatitis	*Escherichia coli*
Vaginitis	Bacterial vaginosis: *Gardnerella vaginalis, Mycoplasma hominis, Mobiluncus,* and *Prevotella* *Candida albicans* *Trichomonas vaginalis*
Sexually transmitted infections of the genitourinary tract	
Genital ulcerative diseases: genital herpes	Herpes simplex virus 2
Genital ulcerative diseases: syphilis	*Treponema pallidum*
Genital ulcerative diseases: chancroid	*Haemophilus ducreyi*

Disease	Common Cause(s)
Sexually transmitted infections of the genitourinary tract	
Urethritis	*Chlamydia trachomatis* *Neisseria gonorrhoeae*
Cervicitis	*Chlamydia trachomatis* *Neisseria gonorrhoeae*
Pelvic inflammatory disease	*Chlamydia trachomatis* *Neisseria gonorrhoeae*
Genital warts	Human papillomavirus types 6, 11, 16, and 18
Epididymitis	Sexually active men < 35 years: *Chlamydia trachomatis* or *Neisseria gonorrhoeae* Men > 35 years: gram-negative enteric bacteria
Scabies	*Sarcoptes scabiei*
Pediculosis	*Pthirus pubis* (pubic louse)

*Note this is not an exhaustive list and does not include all possible etiologies for a particular disease.

INDEX

Page numbers followed by *f* indicate figures; page numbers followed by *t* indicate tables.